AF326901

AANN's NEUROSCIENCE NURSING:
Human Responses to Neurologic Dysfunction

AANN's NEUROSCIENCE NURSING:
Human Responses to Neurologic Dysfunction

SECOND EDITION

Chris Stewart-Amidei, RN, MSN, CNRN, CCRN
Clinical Nurse Specialist
Department of Neurosurgery
University of Chicago
Chicago, Illinois

Joyce A. Kunkel, RN, MS
Clinical Nurse Specialist
Miami Valley Neurosurgery, Inc.
Dayton, Ohio

W.B. SAUNDERS COMPANY
A Harcourt Health Sciences Company
Philadelphia   London   New York   St. Louis   Sydney   Toronto

W.B. SAUNDERS COMPANY
A Harcourt Health Sciences Company

The Curtis Center
Independence Square West
Philadelphia, Pennsylvania 19106

Library of Congress Cataloging-in-Publication Data

AANN's neuroscience nursing : human responses to neurologic dysfunction / American
Association of Neuroscience Nursing; editor, Chris Stewart-Amidei.—2nd ed.

   p.   cm.

Includes bibliographical references and index.

ISBN 0–7216–2288–7

   1. Neurological nursing. I. Title: Neuroscience nursing. II. Stewart-Amidei, Christina.
III. American Association of Neuroscience Nurses.
   [DNLM: 1. Nervous System Diseases—nursing. 2. Nursing Assessment. 3. Nursing
Diagnosis. WY 160.5 A112 2001]

RC350.5 .A22 2001

610.73′68—dc21   99–057047

Acquisitions Editor: Robin Carter
Editorial Assistant: Ross Landy
Manuscript Editor: Jennifer Ehlers
Production Manager: Frank Polizzano
Illustration Specialist: Robert F. Quinn
Book Designer: Kevin O'Malley

AANN'S NEUROSCIENCE NURSING:
HUMAN RESPONSES TO NEUROLOGIC DYSFUNCTION   0–7216–2288–7

Printed in the United States of America

Last digit is the print number: 9   8   7   6   5   4   3   2   1

Contributors

CONTRIBUTORS

Gerald A. Banet, MSN(R)
Clinical Instructor, School of Medicine, Washington University, St. Louis, MO;
Clinical Instructor, School of Nursing, St. Louis University, St. Louis, MO
Integrated Regulation and Altered Integrated Regulation

A. Susan Bidwell, EdD, MSN, RN, CS
Professor of Nursing, Marymount University, Arlington, VA; Therapist,
Cascades Counseling/Cascades Mediation, Sterling, VA
Affiliative Relationships: An Overview

Barbara J. Boss, BSN, MSN, PhD
Professor of Nursing, School of Nursing, University of Mississippi Medical
Center, Jackson, MS; Family Nurse Practitioner, UNACARE Health Center,
Jackson, MS
Cognition: An Overview

Kathryn S. Bronstein, PhD
Medical Scientific Associate, Novartis Pharmaceuticals, East Hanover, NJ
Human Mobility: An Overview

Margaret Auld Bruya, DNSc, MN, BSN
Professor, Graduate Program Faculty; Comanager, The Children's Transition
Clinic Project, Intercollegiate Center for Nursing Education, Washington State
University College of Nursing, Spokane, WA
Self-Care: An Overview

Margarethe Cammermeyer, PhD, RN
Former Clinical Faculty, University of Washington, Seattle, WA; University of
California–San Francisco, CA; Pacific Lutheran University, Tacoma, WA
Assessment of Cognition

Wen Yun Cheng, MS, RN
Doctoral Candidate, University of Minnesota School of Nursing,
Minneapolis, MN
Nursing Therapeutics: An Overview

Catherine Ecock Connelly, DNSc, MSN, BSN
Dean and Professor, School of Health Professions, Marymount University,
Arlington, VA
Affiliative Relationships: An Overview and *Alterations in Affiliative Relationships*

Cheryl S. Deeley, MS, RNc, CNRN
Clinical Associate, University of Rochester, Rochester, NY; Nurse Practitioner, Movement and Inherited Neurologic Disorders, University of Rochester, Rochester, NY
Chronic Alterations in Mobility

Andrew K. Gruen
Director of Restorative Services, Mediplex-Milford Meadows, Milford, MA
Communication Disorders: An Overview, Alterations and Management of Cognitive-Language Disorders, and *Alterations and Management of Neurologic Swallowing Disorders*

Barbara Habermann, PhD, RN
Postdoctoral Scholar, University of Washington, Seattle, WA
Human Responses: Phenomena of Neuroscience Nursing

Jeanette C. Hartshorn, PhD, RN, FAAN
Associate Dean for Academic Administration, Graduate Program Director, Professor, University of Texas Medical Branch, School of Nursing, Galveston, TX
Abrupt Alterations in Mobility

Ann D. Hollerbach, PhD
Associate Professor of Nursing, Medical University of South Carolina, College of Nursing, Charleston, SC
Assessment of Human Mobility

Donald D. Kautz, PhD, RN
Assistant Professor, Department of Nursing, Winston-Salem State University, Winston-Salem, NC
Human Sexuality: An Overview and *Alterations in Human Sexuality*

Catherine A. Kernich, MSN
Clinical Faculty, Frances Payne Bolton School of Nursing, Case Western Reserve University, Cleveland, OH; Director, Ambulatory Practice, Department of Medicine, University Hospitals Health System, Cleveland, OH
Chronic Alterations in Mobility

Hillary Lipe, BSN, MN
Clinical Faculty, University of Washington School of Nursing, Seattle, WA; Clinical Nurse Specialist—Neuroscience, VA Puget Sound Health Care System, Seattle, WA
Common Neurologic Health Problems: Phenomena of Neuroscience Medicine

Norma D. McNair, MSN, RN
Assistant Clinical Professor, University of California–Los Angeles School of Nursing, Los Angeles, CA; Clinical Nurse III, Liver Transplant/Surgical Subspecialties Intensive Care Unit, University of California–Los Angeles Medical Center, Los Angeles, CA
Pain: Acute and Chronic

Michaelene Pheifer Mirr, PhD, RN, CS
Professor, University of Wisconsin, Eau Claire, WI; Gerontological Nurse
Practitioner, South Side Medical Clinic, Eau Claire, WI
Abnormally Increased Behavioral Arousal

Pamela H. Mitchell, PhD, RN, CNRN, FAAN
Professor of Biobehavioral Nursing and Health Systems, University of
Washington, Seattle, WA; Professor of Clinical Education, Harborview
Medical Center, Seattle, WA
Consciousness: An Overview and *Decreased Behavioral Arousal*

Ruth A. Mulnard, RN, DNSc
Associate Director, Institute for Brain Aging and Dementia, University of
California Irvine, Irvine, CA
Sensation: An Overview and *Alterations in the Special Senses*

Christina Mumma, PhD, RN, CRRN
Associate Professor, School of Nursing, University of Alaska–Anchorage,
Anchorage, AK
Alterations in Self-Care

Judy Ozuna, BSN, MN
Clinical Assistant Professor, Department of Biobehavioral Nursing and
Health Systems, University of Washington School of Nursing, Seattle, WA;
Clinical Nurse Specialist—Neurology, Veterans Affairs Medical Center,
Seattle, WA
Intermittent Loss of Arousal

Marlene Reimer, PhD, RN, CNN(C)
Associate Professor, Faculty of Nursing, University of Calgary, Calgary,
Alberta, Canada
On Being Human: Alterations in the Sense of Being

Ann E. Rogers, PhD, RN
Associate Professor, University of Pennsylvania School of Nursing,
Philadelphia, PA
Rhythmic Alterations in Consciousness: Sleep

Sr. Callista Roy, PhD, RN, FAAN
Professor and Nurse Theorist, Boston College, Chestnut Hill, MA
Alterations in Cognitive Processing

Rose Rossi Schwartz, MSN, RN
Lecturer, University of Pennsylvania, School of Nursing, Philadelphia, PA;
Ambulatory Quality Improvement Coordinator, University of Pennsylvania
Health Systems, Philadelphia, PA
Elimination: An Overview, Alterations in Bladder Elimination, and *Alterations in
Bowel Elimination*

Roberta Schwartz-Cowley
Maryland State Department of Health, Baltimore, MD
Communication Disorders: An Overview, Alterations and Management of Cognitive-Language Disorders, and *Alterations and Management of Neurologic Swallowing Disorders*

Rebecca A. Sisson, PhD, RN
Associate Professor, College of Nursing, University of South Florida, Tampa, FL
Alterations in Memory

Mariah Snyder, PhD, RN, FAAN
Professor and Division Head for Adult, Gerontological, and Psychiatric/Mental Health Nursing, University of Minnesota, Minneapolis, MN
Nursing Therapeutics: An Overview

Chris Stewart-Amidei, RN, MSN, CNRN, CCRN
Clinical Nurse Specialist, Department of Neurosurgery, University of Chicago, Chicago, IL
Integrated Regulation and Altered Integrated Regulation

Yueh-hsia Tseng, MS, RN
Doctoral Candidate, University of Minnesota School of Nursing, Minneapolis, MN
Nursing Therapeutics: An Overview

Deborah Webb, MSN
Neuroscience Clinical Nurse Specialist, Harborview Medical Center, Seattle, WA
Scope of Neuroscience Nursing

Preface

Neuroscience nursing was formally recognized as a specialty in 1968 through the formation of the American Association of Neurosurgical Nurses. To reflect its evolving nature, the name was later changed to the American Association of Neuroscience Nurses (AANN). The AANN has been a leader in advancing the specialty of neuroscience nursing, not only in nursing and in the health care profession, but in the public realm as well.

Specialization in nursing is a concentrated focus on one aspect of the entire field of nursing. Characteristics of a specialty include a unique body of knowledge, specialized training and skills, certification, and a focused body of literature. There are many texts devoted to the specialized field of neuroscience nursing, with a focus on the fundamental aspects of care, and they are usually written from a disease or medical model focus. Some time ago, the AANN recognized the need to have an advanced text that approached the specialty from a conceptual basis. This culminated in the first edition of *AANN's Neuroscience Nursing,* published in 1988, which integrated the phenomena unique to neuroscience nursing and described human responses to these phenomena within a conceptual framework. This text successfully linked organized knowledge necessary for clinical care around the patient's medical diagnosis within the context of human responses to health problems specifically affecting the nervous system.

This, the second edition, has built on the framework of the first text, not only with updated material, but with new approaches as well. The second edition is again formatted around core phenomena: consciousness and mentation, communication, affiliative relationships, mobility, sensation, elimination, sexuality, and self-care. An additional phenomenon has been added to reflect the regulatory nature of the nervous system: integrated regulation. A final chapter has been added to tie together the phenomena from the perspective of "human being and being human."

Chapters are organized around the phenomena, addressing the nature of the phenomena (definition, anatomy, and physiology) and the characteristics of the phenomena (assessment). Further chapters address alterations in the phenomena and resulting diagnoses, as well as management of human responses. Case studies are incorporated to illustrate specific situations. Management is addressed from patient, family, and societal perspectives.

Beyond updates in this second edition, the chapters have been expanded to include how the nurse assists the patient in adapting to responses. Many of the interventions have been reformatted into tables for easy reference. The nursing diagnoses, using North American Nursing Diagnosis Association (NANDA) nomenclature, are further developed, with defining characteristics, related factors, outcome criteria, interventions (including teaching), and evaluations. Additionally, the text more fully explores the phenomena through the full continuum from prevention through acute care to rehabilitation, home and community reintegration, and long-term or chronic care. The effects of health care reform in the last decade have affected where and how the care is delivered as well as the availability of care; these developments are reflected in discussions on the effects of the phenomena on the individual, family, and community. The material now addresses the full life trajectory from birth through late adulthood.

This text has been several years in the making, with contributions from previous and new authors. It has been comforting to learn that even with the necessary updates, the conceptual framework has remained, supporting the importance of the integrated phenomena to neuroscience nursing. We would like to thank the editors and authors of the first edition who pioneered the text and envisioned the whole of neuroscience nursing, developing this text as a conceptual approach to practice: Pamela Holsclaw Mitchell, RN, MS, CNRN, FAAN; Linda C. Hodges, RN, EdD; Marylou Muwaswes, RN, MS, CNRN; and Connie A. Walleck, RN, MS, CNRN. We would also like to thank all the contributors to this text, especially Kathryn Bronstein for her substantial contributions as an editor to revisions of this text.

Chris Stewart-Amidei
Joyce A. Kunkel

Contents

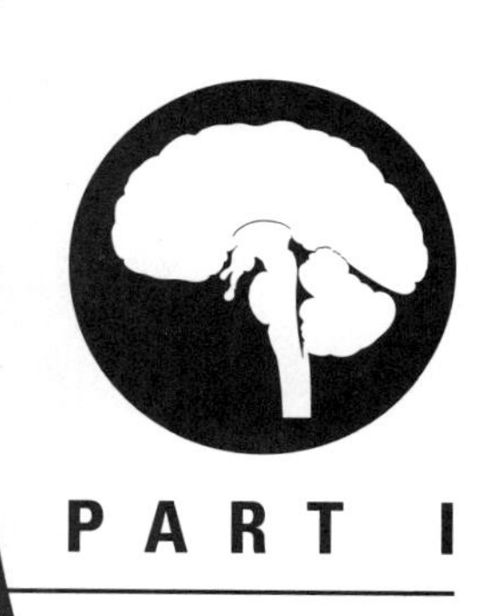

PART I

Neuroscience Nursing in Modern Health Care

Scope of Neuroscience Nursing

DEBORAH WEBB

NEUROSCIENCE NURSING PRACTICE IN RELATION TO THE PROFESSION

Nursing has been striving to be recognized as a profession since its beginnings. Questions such as "What is nursing?" "What do nurses do?" and "What is nursing practice?" are being asked today as they were a century ago. Nursing is at last beginning to explore and answer these and other questions. In 1980, the American Nurses Association (ANA) published a document titled *Nursing: A Social Policy Statement,* in which the nature and scope of nursing practice and the characteristics of specialization in nursing were delineated. This document was intended as a fundamental and undergirding delineation, providing a foundation that promotes unity in nursing by setting forth a basic and common approach to practice. It provided enabling definitions and descriptions, seeking to clarify the direction in which nursing had evolved and to provide a means for distinguishing between desirable and undesirable directions for future development. The ANA revised the social policy statement in 1995, with particular attention to input from specialty nursing organizations (ANA, 1995).

Historically, the focus of nursing has been on the individual's optimal functioning in the environment. Florence Nightingale's *Notes on Nursing: What It Is and What It Is Not,* published in 1859, defined nursing as having "charge of the personal health of somebody and what nursing has to do is to put the patient in the best condition for nature to act upon him" (Nightingale, 1859). More than 100 years later, Virginia Henderson (1961) defined nursing as an action

> *to assist the individual, sick or well, in the performance of those activities contributing to health or its recovery (or a peaceful death) that he would perform unaided if he had the necessary strength, will or knowledge. And to do this in such a way as to help him gain independence as rapidly as possible*

The ANA definition of nursing, contained in the social policy statement, maintains this historical orientation of Nightingale and Henderson and at the same time reflects the evolution of nursing over time (ANA, 1995). This definition identifies four "essential features" of nursing practice:

- "attention to the full range of human experiences and responses to health and illness without restriction to a problem-focused orientation
- integration of objective data with knowledge gained from an understanding of the patient's or group's subjective experience
- application of scientific knowledge to the processes of diagnosis and treatment, and
- provision of a caring relationship that facilitates health and healing" (ANA, 1995, p. 6).

The ANA definition of nursing and the characteristics derived from the definition continue to describe the current practice of nursing. The approach to this practice is reflected in the use of the nursing process, which serves as an organizing framework for practice. Nursing process encompasses all significant steps taken in providing care to individuals and to the families and communities in which they function: systematic assessment, diagnosis, planning to achieve specific outcomes, implementation of the plan, and continual evaluation of progress toward achieving outcomes. This process is used by all of nursing and reflects both independent and interdependent care provided for the patient. Care within this scope may be of a restorative, supportive, or promotive type (ANA, 1995).

Since the late 1960s, nursing has moved from the realm of rote behavior to the era of nursing diagnosis, application of theory, and establishment of evidence-based practice. Nursing practice demands professional intention and commitment. Although all nurses are responsible for practice in accordance with the *Standards of Clinical Nursing Practice* first published by the ANA in 1973 (and revised in 1991), the level and sophistication of application vary with the education and skills of the individual nurse. Nursing is practiced by nurses in basic and advanced practice with flexible boundaries. Nurses who practice basic nursing are graduates of approved nursing education programs and have successfully tested for registered nurse licensure. Basic level nursing practice may be applied in any patient care setting. Advanced practice nurses have acquired the knowledge and experience that affords specialization, expansion, and advancement in practice. Advanced practice roles incorporate all three components and have a specific clinical focus (ANA, 1995). Advanced practice nursing, regardless of the setting, is characterized by autonomy.

Specialization

Just as the field of medicine developed to allow for quality delivery of care to all types of people, so nursing had a need for specialization. Specialization arises in five main ways:

1. The amount and complexity of knowledge and technology create a demand for some professionals to give special attention to applications in delineated practice areas.

2. A few professional pioneers seek to obtain greater depth of understanding of phenomena related to a segment of nursing and to test new practices intended to correct or ameliorate recognized conditions.

3. Public attention and available funds become focused on an area of practice in which there has been a lack of interest, knowledge, and skilled practitioners.

4. The complexity of services exceeds the prevailing knowledge and skills of general practitioners, and this problem is approached by intense personal studies or post–basic study by a few interested professionals.

5. A part of a professional field expands, and, simultaneously, some of its members seek ways for increased use of their intellectual and other capacities (ANA, 1980).

Specialists in nursing are experts in providing care focused on specific clusters of phenomena drawn from the area of general practice. The phenomena of concerns selected by specialists in a nursing practice may relate either to a specialized field or to the "interprofessional intersections across which collegial, collaborative practice occurs" (ANA, 1980; ANA, 1995, p. 12). Specialization in nursing marks its growth as a profession. The specialty practice of neuroscience nursing can be traced back to the latter part of the 19th century in England and France (Hartshorn, 1986). From that time until the 1960s, nurses learned the special knowledge and skills needed to care for the neurologic patient through informal courses taught by physicians and nurses and through on-the-job training. As the subspecialties of neurosurgery and neurology continued to grow, formal courses to educate nurses caring for these patients were developed, and in 1967 the University of California at San Francisco initiated a master's degree program in neurologic and neurosurgical nursing (Hartshorn, 1986). Since that time, more opportunities have appeared for those with training in neuroscience nursing at both the basic and the advanced practice levels as new practice settings (e.g., neuroscience patient care units in acute settings, specialty clinics) have proliferated. This in turn has supported more graduate programs and increasing numbers of continuing education programs targeting the specialty.

To recognize the common needs of nurses caring for neurologic patients and to provide a forum for these nurses to share concerns, the American Association of Neurosurgical Nurses (AANN) was founded in 1968 in affiliation with the American Association of Neurologic Surgeons. The AANN was renamed the American Association of Neuroscience Nurses in 1983. The mission of the AANN is to work for the highest standard of care for neuroscience patients by advancing the science and practice of neuroscience nurses. The association accomplishes its mission through continuing education, information dissemination, standard setting, and advocacy on behalf of neuroscience patients, families, and nurses. Since its establishment, the AANN has developed a number of documents to assist the nurse caring for the neuroscience patient.

DEFINING NEUROSCIENCE NURSING PRACTICE

The first document, published in 1977 by the AANN in conjunction with the ANA, was *Standards of Neurological and Neurosurgical Nursing Practice*. These standards reflected generic standards established by the ANA in 1973 as they were applied to the neurologic patient. With the publication of the ANA's revised *Standards of Clinical Nursing Practice* in 1991, the AANN retired its 1977 standards. Since that time, emphasis has been on developing practice guidelines on a variety of topics such as intracranial pressure monitoring and seizure assessment.

Conceptual Framework

To further clarify the domains of the specialty's practice, a conceptual framework for neuroscience nursing was developed. The conceptual framework identifies and links the concepts inherent in the art and science of neuroscience nursing practice. The six essential components of the conceptual framework are (1) recipients of care, (2) settings for practice, (3) definition of nursing, (4) human responses, (5) responsibilities of nurses, and (6) characteristics of nurses (AANN, 1984).

The framework identifies the recipients of neuroscience nursing care as the individual with nervous system dysfunction, the individual's family or significant others, and the community and society in which the individual lives. When these three groups of recipients are identified, the framework can be applied to the various settings in which the neuroscience nurse practices, including primary care, secondary care, and tertiary care facilities.

The AANN has adopted the evolving ANA definition of nursing found in *Nursing: A Social Policy Statement* (ANA, 1980 & 1995). This broad definition allows for the specialty organization to specify the health problems, human responses, nursing diagnoses, and interventions unique to the neurologic patient as well as to the other recipients of neuroscience nursing care.

The framework helped clarify the focus of nursing intervention as the human response rather than the health problem. The phenomena of concern to neuroscience nurses include communication, consciousness and cognition, mobility, protective reflexes, rest and sleep, sensation, sexuality, and integrated regulation. From these phenomena, the neuroscience nurse derives the specific human responses to the identified problem, determines the appropriate nursing diagnoses, and states the nursing interventions that are needed to achieve the desired outcome. The nursing focus is on the biopsychosocial response of the recipient of care rather than on the medical diagnosis. The following is the heart of the conceptual framework:

The essence of neuroscience nursing practice is its theory developed on sound principles of nursing science and research as well as those derived from the fields of neuroanatomy, neurophysiology, pharmacology, nutrition, rehabilitation, biologic science, behavioral and social sciences, and learning theories. Nursing is an applied science, so neuroscience nurses apply knowledge and theory from other fields to care for their clients in various roles and settings. Their practice may encompass clinical teaching, administrative, consultative, and research roles. Nursing responsibilities, in any of the roles identified, may include the following: to care for, to support, and to teach.

Advocacy and accountability are characteristics inherent in professional behavior and, therefore, are salient characteristics of neuroscience nurses. Advocacy is demonstrated by collaborating with, or acting for, the recipient of neuroscience nursing care to (1) establish goals, (2) identify options and resources, (3) choose treatments, (4) make decisions and implement plans, and (5) formulate opinions and evaluations. Accountability requires that each neuroscience nurse ensure the quality of his or her own practice by identifying and applying requisite knowledge and using evaluation criteria. Individual responsibility and commitment are essential to the development of advocacy and accountability and are demonstrated by involvement in continuing education activities, academic education, certification, professional nursing organizations, development of standards and quality improvement guidelines, or nursing research.

The nursing process is the vehicle used to operationalize neuroscience nursing practice. Initial and ongoing assessment includes physical assessment, especially of the nervous system aspects; assessment of emotional and behavioral responses to illness; and assessment of sociocultural parameters. The nursing diagnoses, with their associated etiologies and defining characteristics, are based on such assessment data and reflect current nursing knowledge. Goals are established that demonstrate patient and family involvement as well as a projected time frame for attainment. The intervention process and patient outcome criteria are developed mutually with and reflect the participation of the patient and the family. Outcome criteria, which describe a measurable change in either the biologic or the psychosocial state of the recipient of nursing care, are used by the professional nurse in evaluating the quality of his or her nursing care. The following statements are identified as essential to neuroscience nursing practice and serve as the basis for the AANN conceptual framework:

1. Neuroscience nurses diagnose and treat responses to actual or potential health problems.

2. The phenomena of concern to neuroscience nurses include consciousness and cognition, mobility, protective reflexes, rest and sleep, sensation, and sexuality.

3. The potential recipients of neuroscience nursing care include the individual with nervous system dysfunction, the individual's family or significant others, and society.

4. Responsibilities of neuroscience nurses are to care for, to support, and to teach.

5. The settings for neuroscience nursing practice include those for primary, secondary, and tertiary care.

6. Advocacy and accountability are characteristics inherent in professional behavior and are salient characteristics of neuroscience nurses.

7. Professional responsibility is demonstrated by involvement in continuing education activities, academic education, certification, professional nursing organizations, development of standards and quality improvement guidelines, or nursing research.

8. The nursing process is the framework under which nursing care is provided.

9. Standards of practice, which incorporate patient outcomes and the nursing process, direct and guide neuroscience nursing care.

Scope of Neuroscience Nursing Practice

The development of the conceptual framework for neuroscience nursing practice was a landmark activity for a specialty nursing organization. The framework moved neuroscience nursing practice into the realm of scientific care delivery based on a conceptual approach to the care provided. From this conceptual framework, the AANN, through the Nursing Practice Committee, developed the Scope of Practice Statement in 1985 and then revised it in 1993. Copies of the Scope of Practice Statement may be obtained by writing to the AANN at 4700 West Lake Avenue, Glenview, Illinois 60025-1485 or by calling (847) 375-4733.

NEUROSCIENCE NURSING SCOPE OF PRACTICE

Neuroscience nursing is a unique area within the nursing discipline that specializes in the care of individuals who have biopsychosocial alterations as a result of nervous system dysfunction. This encompasses all levels of human existence, from basic bodily functions to advanced processes of the human mind. Neuroscience nurses diagnose and treat human responses to actual or potential health problems concerned with phenomena affected by nervous system dysfunction, such as consciousness and cognition, communication, mobility, protective mechanisms, rest and sleep, sensation, and sexuality. Potential recipients of neuroscience nursing care are individuals with nervous system dysfunction, their families and significant others, and the society in which they live.

The nature of patient or client dysfunction mandates that the neuroscience nurse be a registered professional nurse, have requisite knowledge and clinical competency in the discipline's standards of practice, and use the nursing process to implement these standards. The neuroscience nurse gains such knowledge and competency by formal and informal continuing education endeavors, by implementation and utilization of research, and by participation in the specialty's professional organization. Professionalism is demonstrated by the assumption of accountability for maintaining excellence in practice through self-motivated ventures such as participation in the specialty's certification process as well as through collaborative efforts with other nursing colleagues, organizations, and intraprofessional associates.

The parameters of nursing practice for the neuroscience nurse depend on basic academic preparation, advanced formal or informal educational pursuits, and clinical experiences entered into and mastered while rendering care to the patient and family. These parameters encompass using the nursing process to include neurologic assessment in all care delivery and planning and implementing nursing interventions specific to the patient's neurologic dysfunction. Also included are interventions to support bodily functions and to promote healing and recovery of the acutely ill, to enhance adaptation to persistent neurologic deficits, to facilitate patient and family coping, and to teach patients and families about disease processes, adaptation techniques, and therapies. The neuroscience nurse evaluates the quality of nursing care on an ongoing basis.

The neuroscience nurse may practice in a variety of settings and roles, such as teacher, administrator, researcher, consultant, and clinical practitioner. Advanced practice in these roles requires additional formal education as well as knowledge of nursing theory and the applied, social, and behavioral sciences. Each advanced nursing role is also based on increased clinical expertise through experience and additional education in assessment, pathology, and nursing therapies. All this, plus continual review and application of all related clinical research, results in the promotion of creative therapeutic nursing interventions and improved patient outcomes.

In clinical practice, nurses with basic educational preparation may deliver care in outpatient, rehabilitation, or acute care settings, working either with a broad range of patients with neurologic dysfunction or with a specific population. With experience, the nurse may have responsibility for teaching staff or community members as well as patients and families. Role titles may include staff nurse and nurse clinician. With advanced formal educational preparation and training as described above, nurses may assume clinical nurse specialist or nurse practitioner roles.

In all the identified roles, settings, and levels of practice, the primary intent of the settings is to care for, support, teach, and serve as an advocate for the patient. The goal of all interventions in neuroscience nursing practice is consistent with and flows from the goal of the entire nursing profession: to provide the highest quality of care to patients and to achieve a state of wellness consistent with the quality of life desired by the patient, which may be a peaceful death.

The Scope of Practice Statement reflects current neuroscience nursing. The future may hold new, greater roles for the neuroscience nurse. The fields of neurosurgery and neurology are expanding and changing. New diagnostic methodologies, new treatment techniques, and the rapidly growing research base in the neurosciences have already had an impact on the role of the nurse.

The move from the era of needing only to provide good physical, hygienic care to the patient with severe neurologic dysfunction to the era of explicit incorporation of rehabilitation techniques in the intensive care unit is one mark of the change in the nurse's role. Advances in neurogenetics are also rapidly changing the face of neuroscience nursing practice; alternative medicine may have similar options. Another difference is the number of patients surviving the devastating effects of many neurologic diseases. Survivors will possibly create new phenomena of concern for the neuroscience nurses of the future. A recent theorized understanding of the complex interactions between the brain and other organ systems has led to a proposed addition to the conceptual framework—integrated regulation.

Another major impact on the scope of practice in neuroscience nursing is the changing health care delivery system. Societal, economic, and political pressures are forcing the development of more cost-effective means to meet the health care needs of the public. One strategy for containing costs is to use specialists to deliver care. Theoretically, nurse specialists, with their expanded knowledge base and expertise in areas of specialty, can provide high-quality care to patients in a more cost-effective manner. Specialists can also function as consultants to nurse generalists caring for the neurologic patient and to other health care team members involved in providing the care needed. Collaboration, along with effective use of resources, cost containment, increased participation by recipients of care, timely achievement of goals, and continuity of care, is a concept critical to nursing as well as to current health care systems (Hegyvary, 1990; Jones, 1991). Neuroscience nurses will be key players in the collaborative effort to determine appropriate care for those with neurologic dysfunction.

The changing health care market will also have an impact on the practice of the neuroscience nurse. As the population of the United States ages, chronic illness has become predominant, and a paradigm shift from an acuity model to a chronicity model is critical (Detmer, 1986). The focus of health care providers is becoming prevention and management of health and health problems across the entire life spectrum of an individual, as opposed to episodic care. Neuroscience nurses will provide care in a variety of settings and may carry caseloads across settings. Indeed, a major shift from inpatient to outpatient care has occurred. More expanded roles in community-based neuroscience nursing practice will be developed (Hickey, 1993). In all these roles, the major responsibility of the neuroscience nurse remains the realm of human responses to actual or potential health problems.

Nursing has defined its practice, and the AANN has defined the practice of neuroscience nursing using a conceptual framework to link the concepts inherent in the art and science of neuroscience nursing. The boundaries of practice are changing and expanding in response to the needs and demands of the times.

References

American Association of Neuroscience Nurses. (1984). The AANN conceptual framework. *Journal of Neuroscience Nursing, 16*(2), 117–120.

American Association of Neuroscience Nurses. (1994). Scope of practice statement. *Journal of Neuroscience Nursing, 26*(1), 47.

American Nurses Association. (1980). *Nursing: A social policy statement.* Washington, DC: Author.

American Nurses Association. (1995). *Nursing: A social policy statement.* Washington, DC: Author.

Detmer, S. S. (1986). The future of health care delivery systems and settings. *Journal of Professional Nursing, 2*(1), 20–27.

Hartshorn, J. C. (1986). Aspects of the historical development of neuroscience nursing. *Journal of Neuroscience Nursing, 18*(1), 45–48.

Hegyvary, S. T. (1990). Education. Redefining community. *Journal of Professional Nursing, 6*(1), 7.

Henderson, V. (1961). *Basic principles of nursing care.* London, England: International Council of Nurses.

Hickey, J. V. (1993). The changing health care system: Neuroscience nursing practice in the 1990's. *Journal of Neuroscience Nursing, 25*(2), 73–77.

Jones, K. R. (1991). Maintaining quality in a changing environment. *Nursing Economist, 9*(3), 159–164.

Nightingale, F. (1859). *Notes on nursing: What it is and what it is not.* London: Harrison and Sons.

2 Human Responses: Phenomena of Relevance to Neuroscience Nursing

BARBARA HABERMANN

Nursing has been defined as "the diagnosis and treatment of human responses to potential or actual health problems" (American Nurses Association, 1980). Neuroscience nursing is concerned with those responses that are experienced by clients with nervous system dysfunction or potential dysfunction. Because nervous system functioning is essential to human beings, the phenomena of relevance to neuroscience nursing are those most essential to life. But because of the integrative nature of the nervous system, the phenomena may also be the most complex.

This chapter lays the foundation for understanding those human responses or phenomena of relevance to neuroscience nursing. This book uses a phenomenon approach for several reasons. First, the approach helps nurses focus on health problems or states and responses to these across various disease categories. Rather than emphasizing the specific diseases or disorders of the nervous system, as in the practice of medicine, the clinical problem or phenomenon (such as mobility) is presented. The phenomena of concern often present in several different disorders. Although neuroscience nurses need to have knowledge of the various disorders, the focus of nursing practice is not the disorder but the human response experienced. Likewise, the approach helps nurses relate phenomena across different populations, including individuals and families, and across the life span from birth to old age. In addition, this approach delineates the central concepts within neuroscience nursing as part of a larger discipline. There has been a plea for a greater focus on knowledge development in nursing (Hinshaw, 1989; Meleis, 1987; Woods, 1987). Many nursing authors suggest that this focus must be specialty based, concentrating on the phenomena and concepts that are of substance to practicing nurses (Hinshaw, 1989; Stevenson, 1988). Lastly, the phenomenon approach demonstrates how knowledge relevant to neuroscience nursing can be developed. The phenomena presented in this book are human responses, which neuroscience nurses are responsible for assessing, diagnosing, monitoring, intervening for, and evaluating. They are the central problems that neuroscience nurses focus on in their daily practice.

And, likewise, they should be areas of priority for neuroscience nursing research. This will ultimately lead to the development of a specialty knowledge base that is germane to nursing practice and has relevance for the discipline as a whole.

IDENTIFICATION OF PHENOMENA: HISTORICAL PERSPECTIVE

The American Nurses Association (ANA) has identified two types of human responses that are of concern to nursing: (1) health-restoring responses and (2) health-supporting responses (ANA, 1980). Health-restoring responses are reactions of individuals and groups to actual health care problems, whereas health-supporting responses are concerns of individuals and groups about potential health problems.

The ANA social policy statement includes an illustrative list of human response phenomena that are the focus of nursing. Although not attempting to be comprehensive in the identification of phenomena, the policy statement is seminal from a historical viewpoint. The phenomena identified include self-care limitations; impaired functioning in areas such as rest, sleep, ventilation, circulation, activity, nutrition, elimination, skin integrity, and sexuality; pain and discomfort; emotional problems related to illness and treatment; distortion of symbolic functions; deficiencies in ability to make personal choices; self-image changes required by health status; dysfunctional perceptual orientations to health; strains related to life processes; and problematic affiliative relationships. The phenomena are suggested as the focus for nursing intervention in all substantive and practice areas.

Building on the framework that the ANA provided, the American Association of Neuroscience Nurses (AANN), in collaboration with the ANA, identified phenomena that are frequently encountered in neuroscience nursing practice. An initial list of 17 phenomena was narrowed to a core list of 6 phenomena that were judged to be the most essential by a joint committee. These six phenomena were consciousness and cognition, communication, mobility, sensation, rest and sleep, and sexuality. In 1985, a joint publication of the AANN and the ANA used these phenomena as a model for developing process and outcome criteria (ANA Council on Medical-Surgical Nursing Practice & AANN, 1985). This effort was followed by another publication, *AANN's Neuroscience Nursing: Phenomena and Practice*, which was aimed at meeting an identified need for a comprehensive text (Mitchell, Hodges, Muwaswes, & Walleck, 1988). Because most texts of the time were organized around diseases or categories of disease, the editors identified the need to structure this publication according to the phenomena of nursing (i.e., human responses). The human response categories discussed were consciousness and cognition, communication, affiliative relationships, mobility, sensation, elimination, sexuality, and self-care.

Research has led to increased knowledge related to the human response categories most relevant to neuroscience nursing. In 1993, a role delineation study was jointly undertaken by the AANN and the American Board of Neuroscience Nursing (ABNN), the corporation that administers the certification program for neuroscience nurses. The purpose of the study was to gather and organize knowledge about what neuroscience nurses are doing in practice to (1) develop a certification examination and (2) describe the specialty as it evolves within the profession. Study participants were asked to indicate the importance and frequency of selected human response categories and selected health problem categories in their practice areas. Seven human response categories were included in the matrix: consciousness and cognition, communication, nutrition, mobility, sensation, elimination, and social role. Preliminary results indicate that although all human response categories are of relevance to practice, cognition and consciousness, communication, and mobility are the primary areas of focus for neuroscience nursing practice.

This second edition of *AANN's Neuroscience Nursing* includes chapters on the phenomena discussed in the earlier edition. Two additional sections—integrated regulation and the human experience of neurologic illness—are included because nursing research has increased in these areas. In addition, the complex interactions between the nervous system and other body systems continue to be explored.

This book has several goals: It aims to gather the most current knowledge about the phenomena of concern to neuroscience nurses. It provides a discussion of the general phenomena (e.g., consciousness), the specific manifestations of the phenomena (e.g., intermittent loss of arousal), and the relevant interventions. Each chapter summarizes nursing research and related interdisciplinary research. In doing so, the book aims to challenge practitioners and researchers to be informed of what knowledge exists in the specialty of neuroscience nursing and to participate in systematic knowledge development for the 21st century.

NURSING KNOWLEDGE DEVELOPMENT

Nursing scholars have suggested that nursing is entering a new era of knowledge development (Hinshaw, 1989; Stevenson, 1988). For the purpose of understanding the progress and the challenges involved, some underlying definitions and relationships must be stated.

Knowledge generation results from the interface between nursing science and research. Nursing science as a body of knowledge has been defined in several ways. It has been characterized as "defined concepts/constructs describing various human responses to health and illness as well as therapeutic nursing actions in systematically specified relationships" (Hinshaw, 1989). Nursing science can also be defined as the body of knowledge generated and tested to provide relevant, accurate, and reliable information to guide nursing practice (Hinshaw, 1989). Research or systematic inquiry shapes nursing science by investigating the questions and phenomena of interest to nursing (DeGroot, 1988).

In discussing nursing knowledge development, several scholars have noted a shift or revision (Meleis, 1987; Mitchell, Gallucci, & Fought, 1991). Early debates in the literature focused on the nature of nursing knowledge, the congruent methodologies for nursing research, and the philosophical underpinnings of methodologies for building nursing science. Meleis (1987) proposed that the passion for methodology, science, and philosophy be revised to a passion for substance and content. Another way of stating this is that the focus needs to switch from how we develop knowledge to the identification of the substance and the major phenomena of nursing, that is, the knowledge itself.

Simultaneous to the theoretical, philosophical, and methodological debates in the literature, activity and energy were focused on the development and training of nurse scholars and the creation of resources, such as research centers and laboratories, to support scholarship. Stevenson (1988), while acknowledging the importance and timeliness of these efforts, noted that little progress had been made in contributing to nursing's knowledge base. Instead, she saw these early efforts as laying the foundation that, along with the establishment of the National Center for Nursing Research of the National Institutes of Health (NIH) in 1986, served as a turning point in shifting the priority to developing the substantive content of the knowledge base through systematic inquiry.

Human Responses: Substance for Developing a Science of Nursing

Since the ANA first categorized health-restoring and health-supporting human responses, various authors have suggested that these categories need expanding. Several authors have suggested that some physiologic responses are neither health restoring nor health supporting but are nonetheless human responses (Carrieri-Kohlman, Lindsey, & West, 1993).

Perhaps the most complete categorization of human responses is one that involves multiple perspectives. Mitchell et al. (1991) suggested that human responses be viewed from behavioral, experiential, pathophysiologic, and physiologic perspectives. These authors believed that research pertaining to each of these four perspectives is appropriate for nursing and can lead to knowledge that will guide the practice of nursing. The authors suggested that the science of individual human responses is part of the science of nursing, and they recommended the study of human responses as a way to build a substantive knowledge base. They clearly explicated four aims of studying and developing a science of human responses. The first aim is to understand from four perspectives (physiologic, pathophysiologic, experiential, and behavioral) the spectrum of responses to illness and to maintaining health. The second aim is to understand how social, cultural, and environmental contexts influence human responses. The third aim involves predicting changes in health status as a result of nursing interventions with specific human responses. The final aim is to measure the effectiveness of specific nursing interventions in promoting healthy responses and in altering or changing health-damaging responses (Mitchell et al., 1991).

Ways of Knowing in Practice

In 1978, Carper identified four patterns or ways of knowing in nursing. These patterns were *empirics,* or the science of nursing; *esthetics,* or the art of nursing; *personal knowledge;* and *moral knowledge* (Carper, 1978). Her work has been extensively cited, discussed, and debated. It has laid the foundation for nursing scholars to examine ways of knowing in nursing practice. Chinn (1994), in an editorial, noted that Carper's work has stood the test of time and debate and that the true value of her work is its opening the door for knowledge development beyond the boundaries of empirical inquiry.

Although Carper's work identified additional ways of knowing beyond empirics, much of nursing literature has continued to be dominated by a discussion of the nature of nursing science. More recently, several nursing authors have demonstrated the limits of nursing science in explaining or answering the concerns of nursing as a practice discipline (Johnson, 1994; Tanner, Benner, Chesla, & Gordon, 1993). These authors did not discredit the significance of empirics or science but rather reiterated the need to examine multiple ways of knowing in nursing practice. Nursing, first and foremost, is a practice discipline. Questions, concerns, or problems arise from practice, and for this reason nursing problems will never be answered solely by the application of scientific findings.

Role of Experience and Expertise

Throughout the 1990s, the role of experience and the development of expertise in nursing emerged as recurring themes in nursing clinical knowledge (Benner, Tanner, & Chesla, 1992; Jenny & Logan, 1992; Tanner et al., 1993). It has been suggested that both experience and expertise are aspects of nursing art and personal knowledge (Gadow, 1990; Johnson, 1994; Moch, 1990).

In nursing, the importance of experience in clinical knowledge development is evident. Although formal knowledge gained through education is critical, nurses with limited clinical experience generally do not demonstrate skills and judgment comparable to those of nurses who have gained expertise in a clinical arena. Studies of nurses have explicated the significance of clinical knowledge gained from experience (Benner, 1984; Benner & Wrubel, 1989).

Some suggest that experiential knowledge is personal and subjective in nature (Carper, 1978; Schultz & Meleis, 1988). Although acknowledging experiential knowledge as a way of knowing, this viewpoint does not allow experiential knowing as equally legitimate to scientific inquiry, which leads to theory generation and propositional relationships. Gadow (1990) has stated that personal or experiential knowing practiced in nursing tends to be regarded as a "fallback" position, that is, as a secondary form of knowing rather than as a mode of inquiry valid in its own right.

A contrasting viewpoint claims that experience (and the knowledge that results from it) is not idiosyncratic or purely subjective; rather, the clinical world has shared languages, practices, and meanings (Benner, 1984; Benner et al., 1992; Tanner et al., 1993). Thus, experiential knowledge is not private or inaccessible to inquiry. Experiential knowledge goes both before and after science (Benner et al., 1992). The clinical world is always more complex than what can be captured in a controlled, experimental setting. Acknowledging and valuing experiential and personal knowledge as an area ripe for inquiry in nursing may ultimately lead to a better understanding of the substance of neuroscience nursing.

In nursing literature, an area receiving focus involves knowing the patient as an essential component of clinical knowledge and skilled clinical judgment (Liaschenko & Fisher, 1999; Tanner et al., 1993). Knowing the patient involves having an understanding of the individual's patterns of response and an understanding of the individual as a person (Tanner et al., 1993). Knowing the patient, including how this particular patient responds in a particular circumstance or outcome, is an important dimension of expertise in nursing practice. By studying phenomena such as knowing the patient in specific practice contexts, much can be learned about patient populations and human responses experienced by such populations. Research of this nature will articulate the practical and experiential knowledge that exists in expert nursing practice.

Expanding areas of inquiry to include experiential knowledge along with other ways of knowing can contribute significantly to the development of nursing science. An example illustrates this best. One area of inquiry in neuroscience nursing research has been the effects of various interventions and stimuli on intracranial pressure. Studies have examined how routine nursing activities such as turning, suctioning, and talking influence intracranial pressure (Mitchell, 1986). The results from the growing number of studies in this area are contributing to a beginning knowledge base relative to the physiologic variables involved. Additional research that explores expert neuroscience nurses' knowledge of how particular patients will respond to certain nursing activities would complement and expand knowledge relative to this clinical problem. Combining observational studies, experimental designs, and descriptive research that explores the knowledge embedded in expert neuroscience nursing practice would advance understanding of a phenomenon of substance to the specialty practice.

Current Status of Nursing Knowledge

The emphasis in nursing research on the substance and the phenomena of concern to practicing nurses has been a relatively recent development. Therefore, the depth and breadth of knowledge that can direct practice are limited. Certain phenomena have been studied more extensively than others. Pain, for example, has been an area of inquiry in nursing research for more than 20 years. Other phenomena have not been studied as extensively. Efforts such as those of the National Center for Nursing Research at the NIH to identify priority areas for nursing research will ultimately lead to the development of knowledge in those identified areas.

Neuroscience nursing research, much like nursing research in general, has lacked organized programs of research (DiIorio, 1990). Although the number of neuroscience nursing studies has increased significantly, the studies have been of a noncumulative nature. The need for long-term research programs and supporting clusters of studies relative to specific phenomena of concern has been identified (Hinshaw, 1990). Developing conferences around specific phenomena such as pain or mobility and designing curricula, especially at the graduate level, around human responses are two additional strategies for adapting knowledge to direct practice.

SUMMARY

Understanding human responses to potential or actual nervous system dysfunction is the essence of neuroscience nursing practice and is central to the development of science within the specialty and the larger discipline. In the 1990s, a shift occurred within the profession to a greater focus on knowledge development regarding the phenomena of nursing. Neuroscience nurses are best suited to ask questions that seek to describe, explain, and predict human responses to neurologic illness and to maintain health. Only with a deep understanding of the spectrum of responses experienced by neuroscience patients can clinicians and researchers begin to evaluate the effectiveness of specific nursing therapeutics. These are the challenges that await neuroscience nurses in the 21st century.

References

American Nurses Association. (1980). *A social policy statement* (ANA Publication No. NP-63). Washington, DC: Author.

American Nurses Association Council on Medical-Surgical Nursing Practice & American Association of Neuroscience Nurses (1985). *Neuroscience nursing practice: Process and outcome for selected diagnosis.* Washington, DC: American Nurses Association.

Benner, P. (1984). *From novice to expert: Power and excellence in clinical nursing practice.* Don Mills, Canada: Addison Wesley Longman.

Benner, P., Tanner, C., & Chesla, C. (1992). From beginner to expert: Gaining a differentiated clinical world in critical care nursing. *Advances in Nursing Science, 14*(3), 13–28.

Benner, P., & Wrubel, J. (1989). *The primacy of caring: Stress and coping in health and illness.* Don Mills, Canada: Addison Wesley Longman.

Carper, B. (1978). Fundamental patterns of knowing in nursing. *Advances in Nursing Science, 1*(1), 13–23.

Carrieri-Kohlman, V., Lindsey, A. M., & West, C. M. (1993). *Pathophysiological phenomena in nursing.* Philadelphia: W. B. Saunders.

Chinn, P. L. (1994). Art and esthetics in nursing. *Advances in Nursing Science, 17*(1), viii.

DeGroot, H. A. (1988). Scientific inquiry in nursing: A model for a new age. *Advances in Nursing Science, 10*(3), 1–21.

DiIorio, C. (1990). An analysis of trends in neuroscience nursing research: 1960–1988. *Journal of Neuroscience Nursing, 22*(3), 139–146.

Gadow, S. (1990). Response to "Personal knowing: Evolving research and practice." *Scholarly Inquiry for Nursing Practice, 4,* 167–170.

Hinshaw, A. S. (1989). Nursing science: The challenge to develop knowledge. *Nursing Science Quarterly, 2,* 162–171.

Hinshaw, A. S. (1990). Exciting challenges ahead: Neuroscience nursing research. *Journal of Neuroscience Nursing, 22*(3), 137–138.

Jenny, J., & Logan, J. (1992). Knowing the patient: One aspect of clinical knowledge. *Image, 24*(4), 254–258.

Johnson, J. L. (1994). A dialectical examination of nursing art. *Advances in Nursing Science, 17*(1), 1–14.

Liaschenko J., & Fisher, A. (1999). Theorizing the knowledge that nurses use in the conduct of their work. *Scholarly Inquiry for Nursing Practice, 13*(1), 29–41.

Meleis, A. I. (1987). Revisions in knowledge development: A passion for substance. *Scholarly Inquiry for Nursing Practice, 1,* 5–19.

Mitchell, P. H. (1986). Intracranial hypertension: Influence of nursing care activities. *Nursing Clinics of North America, 21,* 563–574.

Mitchell, P. H., Gallucci, B., & Fought, S. G. (1991). Perspectives on human responses to health and illness. *Nursing Outlook, 39*(4), 154–157.

Mitchell, P. H., Hodges, L. C., Muwaswes, M., & Walleck, C. A. (1988). *AANN's neuroscience nursing: Phenomena and practice.* Stamford, CT: Appleton & Lange.

Moch, S. D. (1990). Personal knowing: Evolving research and practice. *Scholarly Inquiry for Nursing Practice, 4,* 155–165.

Schultz, P., & Meleis, A. (1988). Nursing epistemology: Traditions, insights and questions. *Image, 20*(4), 217–221.

Stevenson, J. S. (1988). Nursing knowledge development: Into era II. *Journal of Professional Nursing, 4,* 152–162.

Tanner, C., Benner, P., Chesla, C., & Gordon, D. (1993). The phenomenology of knowing the patient. *Image, 25*(4), 273–280.

Woods, N. F. (1987). Response: Early morning musing on the passion for substance. *Scholarly Inquiry for Nursing Practice, 1,* 25–28.

Common Neurologic Health Problems: Phenomena of Relevance to Neuroscience Medicine

HILLARY LIPE

Most nursing practice requires considerable knowledge of both health problems and human responses to those problems. Neuroscience nurses care for people with disorders of the nervous system. Diagnosis and treatment of neurologic disease are directed by a physician specialist—neurologist, neuroradiologist, or neurosurgeon—or, in some cases, by a physician generalist—internist, family practitioner, or general surgeon. Diagnosis and treatment of human responses to actual or potential neurologic disease are directed by nurses who specialize in neuroscience nursing or, in many cases, by nurse generalists who sometimes encounter patients with neurologic disorders.

The purpose of this chapter is to present an overview of common neurologic and neurosurgical health problems and medical treatments, with reference to the categories of human responses (nursing diagnoses) often associated with those health problems. The remainder of this book concentrates on the phenomena of human functioning in which those nursing diagnoses cluster. Textbooks of neurology and neurosurgery should be consulted for details on the pathophysiology and the medical diagnostics and therapeutics of specific medical diagnoses.

This chapter is organized according to classifications of neurologic disorders, with reference to the parts of the neuraxis affected. The term *neuraxis* refers to the following subsets of the nervous system:

Axis I: Cerebral hemispheres and diencephalon

Axis II: Brain stem and cerebellum

Axis III: Spinal cord

Axis IV: Peripheral nerves and junctions with innervated organs

Because the human functions served differ with each of the segments of the neuraxis, the nursing diagnoses tend to cluster with respect to the part of the neuraxis affected rather than by the disease classification. The purpose of including both disease and neuraxis classifications is to assist nurses in correlating medical and nursing diagnoses.

CEREBROVASCULAR DISORDERS

Any abnormality of the brain resulting from a lesion in the vessel wall, an occlusion of the vessel lumen, a rupture of the vessel, or a change in the quality of the blood is considered cerebrovascular disease. More than any other organ, the brain depends on an adequate supply of oxygenated blood. Brain tissue deprived of blood undergoes ischemia or infarction. Failure of the circulation, for whatever reason, can produce focal and diffuse ischemic changes. In cerebral hemorrhage, blood leaks from the vessel directly into the brain, a ventricle, or the subarachnoid space. After the leakage, the blood slowly disintegrates and is absorbed over time. The mass effect causes physical disruption of the tissue and increased intracranial pressure. Cerebrovascular disease affects both sexes. Various types of cerebrovascular disease are characteristic at different stages of life. Stroke and vascular headache are the primary categories of cerebrovascular disorders resulting in human responses of concern to neuroscience nurses.

Stroke

Stroke is the third most common cause of death in the United States (American Heart Association, 1993). In 1990, 145,000 Americans died from stroke of all types. Stroke is a major cause of disability, accounting for one half of all patients hospitalized for acute neurologic disease.

Stroke is defined as a sudden, nonconvulsive focal neurologic deficit (Adams & Victor, 1993). Known risk factors include hypertension, heart disease, diabetes mellitus, hyperlipidemia, and cigarette smoking for many years. The three main types of stroke are thrombotic stroke, embolic stroke, and rupture of a vessel. Thrombotic and embolic strokes are the most common, although the highest mortality occurs with vessel rupture.

Cerebral thrombosis usually occurs in cerebral vessels damaged by atherosclerosis. Onset is usually at night or early in the morning, when systemic blood pressure is low. Thrombotic strokes often are preceded by transient ischemic attacks (focal neurologic deficits that resolve within minutes to hours) and occur in people at high risk for other forms of vascular disease (e.g., myocardial infarction, peripheral vascular insufficiency). Cerebral embolism accounts for 5% to 14% of all strokes, with cardiac valvular emboli and atrial fibrillation being the most common sources of the embolus.

Subarachnoid and cerebral hemorrhage account for 7% and 10%, respectively, of all strokes. Spontaneous subarachnoid hemorrhage is associated with ruptured cerebral aneurysm or arteriovenous malformation in younger people and with systemic hypertension in older people. Intracerebral hemorrhage may result from rupture of aneurysms, less commonly from arteriovenous malformations, and from hypertension. Head injury is also a common source of traumatic subarachnoid and intracerebral hemorrhage.

The amount and location of the hemorrhage determine the severity of symptoms in vessel rupture. In subarachnoid hemorrhage, vasospasm of cerebral vessels 4 to 7 days after hemorrhage can worsen symptoms by producing cerebral ischemia.

ALTERED HUMAN RESPONSES WITH STROKE IN AXIS I

Strokes of all types that affect axis I produce symptoms referable to the portions of the cerebral hemispheres and diencephalon supplied by the vascular distribution of the affected extracerebral or intracerebral vessels. The majority of strokes are in the distribution of the anterior circulation to the brain, supplied by the common and internal carotid arteries: the middle cerebral, anterior cerebral, and penetrating arteries. These arteries and their branches supply circulation to the frontal and parietal lobes, lateral temporal lobe, basal ganglia, and internal capsule. The posterior circulation, supplied from the vertebral arteries, provides blood to the caudal portion of the brain—occipital lobes, thalamus, and inferior temporal lobes—as well as to axis II.

The internal carotid artery supplies the ophthalmic artery and the vessels of the ipsilateral hemisphere. Sudden occlusion of the artery thus produces severe contralateral hemiplegia and hemianesthesia, profound aphasia if occlusion occurs in the dominant hemisphere, and often unilateral blindness. Nurses should expect, therefore, to see alterations in communication, mobility, sensation, vision, and perhaps cognition (see Chapters 13, 15, 20, and 24).

The middle cerebral artery is the major branch of the internal carotid artery and supplies most of the lateral cortex of the brain: the lateral frontal and parietal lobes, the temporal pole and insula of the temporal lobe, and the caudate nucleus and putamen via penetrating branches. These structures serve the majority of higher cerebral processes of communication; interpretation of language; perception and interpretation of space, form, and sensation; and voluntary movement. Depending on the hemisphere involved, one can expect stroke of the middle cerebral artery distribution to alter communication, cognition, mobility, and sensation.

The anterior cerebral artery supplies the medial surfaces and the upper convexities of the frontal and parietal lobes and the cingulate gyrus (medial surface of the hemisphere), which includes the motor and somesthetic cortex serving the legs. Stroke in this distribution affects mobility and sensation of the lower extremities more than in the upper extremities, may produce urinary incontinence secondary to loss of inhibition of the micturition reflex, and may produce emotional lability and confusion. Altered human responses will thus be possible in the categories of cognition, mobility, and elimination.

The posterior cerebral artery supplies the medial and inferior temporal lobe and the medial occipital lobe, including the visual receptive area, the thalamus, and the posterior portion of the hypothalamus. Occlusion of portions of or all of this artery can result in hemianesthesia (resulting from involvement of the sensory portions of the thalamus); hemiplegia (as fibers pass through the cerebral peduncle); homonymous hemianopsia (visual radiations as they pass through the temporal lobe); receptive aphasia, particularly with written language; and cortical blindness (inability to interpret visual events). Thus, altered responses may occur in the areas of mobility, sensation, and language.

ALTERED HUMAN RESPONSES WITH STROKE IN AXIS II

The posterior circulation derives from the vertebral arteries, which give rise to the basilar artery, supplying axis II, and the posterior cerebral artery (described under axis I). The posterior and anterior circulations are joined by the posterior communicating arteries to form the circle of Willis at the base of the brain. Disruption of circulation to the brain stem has the potential to alter all primary human functions except cognition. The nerve fibers carrying motor and autonomic information to and sensory information from the periphery must all pass through the compact tracts of the brain stem. In addition, the nuclei and peripheral branches of all the cranial nerves except I and II are in the brain stem.

A variety of vascular syndromes of the brain stem are possible, depending on the particular vascular distribution involved. Partial occlusion of the vertebral or basilar arteries can produce transient ischemic attacks characterized by unilateral or bilateral weakness of limbs or even total loss of tone, diplopia, nausea, vertigo, tinnitus, dysphagia, or dysarthria and sometimes confusion or drowsiness. These symptoms all reflect transient ischemia to corticospinal tracts in the brain stem or the brain stem consciousness system and cranial nerve dysfunction.

Basilar artery occlusion or hemorrhage affects all functions of the brain stem and, if complete, results in coma, miotic pupils, decerebrate rigidity, respiratory and circulatory abnormalities, and, ultimately, death. Partial basilar artery thrombosis can produce the *locked-in syndrome*, in which anterior portions of the pons are affected, thus precluding all movement except that of the eyelids. Sensation and consciousness are preserved.

A number of medullary syndromes are produced by vascular disorders of the cerebellar arteries, which are branches of the vertebral artery. The most common syndrome is the lateral medullary syndrome, or Wallenberg's syndrome, produced by thrombosis of the posterior inferior cerebellar artery. Circulation to the lateral and posterior portion of the medulla is disrupted, resulting in dysfunction of the ambiguous nucleus; the fibers and tracts of cranial nerves V, IX, and X; the descending sympathetic pathways; the afferent spinocerebellar tracts; and the lateral spinothalamic tract. The person thus exhibits dysphagia and dysphonia related to ipsilateral paralysis of the soft palate, larynx, and pharynx; ipsilateral anesthesia of the face and cornea for pain and temperature but not touch; ipsilateral Horner's syndrome (miosis, ptosis, and anhidrosis); ipsilateral cerebellar dyssynergy (decomposition of movement); and contralateral loss of pain and temperature sensations in the trunk and limbs. The primary alterations in human response are in communication, swallowing (see Chapters 14, 15, and 22), and unilateral lack of coordination, with potential safety problems related to the loss of pain and temperature sensations. Cognition and most aspects of mobility are intact.

Hemorrhage into or ischemia of the cerebellum can occur from thrombosis or aneurysms of the posterior inferior, anterior inferior, or superior cerebellar arteries, all of which are branches of the vertebral arteries. Problems in motor coordination, synergy, tone, station, and gait can occur with cerebellar vascular lesions. These may be manifested in difficulties in articulation (resulting from dyssynergies of speech), swallowing, eye movement (nystagmus), or gross motor movements of the limbs.

ALTERED HUMAN RESPONSES WITH STROKE IN AXIS III

Spinal cord (axis III) circulation is supplied by the anterior and posterior spinal arteries. The anterior spinal artery branches from the vertebral arteries and travels the length of the anterior spinal cord, reinforced by branches of the lateral spinal arteries. The anterior spinal cord controls voluntary and reflex movement via the anterior horn motor neurons and carries descending motor sensations and ascending touch, pain, and temperature sensations. Thrombosis of the anterior spinal artery results in a transverse myelitis with flaccid paralysis at the level of the lesion; spastic paralysis below the lesion; and loss of pain, touch, and temperature sensations but sparing of proprioception (posterior columns). Dissecting aortic aneurysm, complications of arteriography, and disseminated atherosclerosis are the most common causes. Human responses are altered in a pattern similar to that in acute spinal cord injury (see Chapter 20), but with preservation of proprioceptive sensation.

The posterior spinal arteries are really a series of plexiform channels, rather than single vessels, and arise from the vertebral arteries. Isolated ischemia or thrombosis of posterior vessels in disseminated vascular disease produces sensory loss, particularly of proprioception, vibration, touch, and pressure, with preservation of movement.

Vascular Headache

A vascular etiology for migraine and cluster headaches has come to be accepted. Vasodilation and pulsation of the external carotid artery during an attack have been documented in about one third of patients. Decreased pulsation results in disappearance of the headache. In Olmstead County, Minnesota, overall age-adjusted incidence of migraine headache was 137 per 100,000 person-years for males and 294 per 100,000 person-years for females (Stang, 1992). Cluster headaches (severe vascular headaches that occur in seasonal clusters) occur most commonly in men.

Although numerous symptom constellations are described in the literature, migraine headache is usually characterized by periodic, commonly unilateral, throbbing or pounding head pain. Symptom onset is typically early in life (childhood, adolescence, or early adulthood), with attacks diminishing with advancing age. Often a family history of similar headaches exists. The classic syndrome begins with an alteration in neurologic function (flashing lights, zigzag lights, less commonly speech arrest or unilateral weakness), followed in 15 to 20 minutes by hemicranial pain and often nausea and vomiting. The neurologic symptoms abate with the onset of the headache. Common migraine is typified by the onset of throbbing headache without prodromal neurologic symptoms.

Nonpharmacologic therapy includes biofeedback and progressive muscle relaxation to reduce sympathetic activity. Analysis of diet to identify food implicated in triggering attacks and supportive psychotherapy may also be used. Such approaches may be more effective in reducing the muscle contraction component of the headache than in directly affecting the vascular headache itself.

Drug therapy is directed toward blocking the 5-HT system. Substances administered at the onset of headache to promote constriction of extracranial vessels include ergot derivatives (ergotamine tartrate) and sumatriptan, or related 5-HT receptor agonists. Beta blockers (propranolol HCl), calcium channel blockers (verapamil), methysergide maleate, cyproheptadine HCl, and antidepressants can be taken prophylactically to prevent swings in vascular reactivity thought to cause vascular headaches (Schulman & Silberstein, 1992).

Human responses to vascular headache are all referable to axis I, the cerebral hemispheres and diencephalon, because both the pain and its interpretation are a function of these structures. Responses can be classified into two categories: (1) concerns about the meaning of the pain and (2) behaviors in response to or in anticipation of head pain. Vascular reactivity is the source of chronic but intermittent head pain, often accompanied by transient neurologic dysfunction and gastrointestinal symptoms.

Before definitive medical diagnosis of the cause of the vascular headache, many people fear that it is a sign of a brain tumor or some other fatal brain disease. If the source is indeed an arteriovenous malformation or an aneurysm, definitive neurosurgical intervention may be life saving. In the vast majority of cases, however, the pain is a symptom of a non–life-threatening condition that can be managed reasonably well with either vasoactive drugs or nonpharmacologic techniques. Chronic pain and its nursing management are discussed in Chapter 26.

DEGENERATIVE DISORDERS

Degenerative disorders are those characterized by loss of neurons or neuronal processes after a long period of normal nervous system function. They usually exhibit a gradually progressive loss of both structure and associated human function over many years. Establishing familial occurrence of the disorder may be of great importance. However, familial occurrence of a disease does not prove heredity and may instead indicate exposure to the same infectious or toxic agent by more than one member of a family. Clinical manifestations are generally bilaterally symmetrical. Demyelinating diseases and peripheral neuropathies might be considered special cases of degenerative disorders in that portions of the nerve processes (axons and dendrites) or their coverings (myelin) undergo degenerative changes.

Degenerative Disorders of Axis I

PARKINSON'S DISEASE

Parkinson's disease is a common disorder, affecting about 1% of the population older than 50 years (Adams & Victor, 1993). Onset usually occurs between 40 and 70 years of age, with the peak onset in the sixth decade. The disease affects men and women of all ethnic and socioeconomic groups equally.

A loss of pigmented, dopamine-producing cells in the substantia nigra and other pigmented nuclei in the basal ganglia is believed to be responsible for the clinical symptoms. Some cases are directly attributable to conditions known to destroy the substantia nigra (e.g., carbon monoxide poisoning, manganese poisoning, and use of certain illegal "designer" drugs such as 1-methyl-4-phenyl-1,2,3,6-tetrahydropyridine [MPTP]) or to block the action of dopamine (use of phenothiazine-type antipsychotic agents). An inherited predisposition to environmental or endogenous toxic agents is suspected as the cause (Jenner, Schapira, & Marsden, 1992).

Early symptoms of aching, fatigue, and slowness are often overlooked and attributed to arthritis or other effects of aging. Eventually, stiffness and slowness progress into the classic triad of tremor, rigidity, and bradykinesia. Loss of automatic movement and postural instability are prominent as well. Symptoms are frequently unilateral in the beginning and then progress to bilateral involvement. It is not uncommon for the classic pill-rolling tremor to be absent or very minor. Bradykinesia is the most disabling symptom for most people. Although the course of the disease does not shorten the life span appreciably, as the disorder progresses, all spheres of function mediated by the brain may be affected: mood, cognition, social and work ability, sleep, and sexual function.

Medical treatment is most commonly pharmacologic, with symptomatic therapy using anticholinergic agents (trihexyphenidyl, benztropine mesylate) and amantadine as well as dopamine precursors (levodopa, levodopa-carbidopa combinations), including the controlled-release preparations that induce fewer fluctuations in the plasma concentration of levodopa, resulting in a smoother therapeutic response. There is debate about when to begin levodopa therapy as it loses effectiveness over time and might be neurotoxic. Dopamine agonists (bromocriptine, pramipexole, ropinirole, and pergolide) are useful adjuncts (Lang, 1998). Protective therapy using deprenyl, an inhibitor of monoamine oxidase B, is controversial as a means to prevent or delay neurodegeneration. Occasionally, thalamotomy is used for severe unilateral tremor. Transplantation of fetal catecholamine-producing tissue into the brain is being explored. Therapies do not alter the basic degenerative process but supplement the body's waning ability to produce neurotransmitters that control movement. Function can be maintained for a longer period than was the case before their use, but the disease process continues to progress slowly, resulting in severe disability.

Human responses can occur in all areas directly and indirectly mediated by the cerebral dopamine and acetylcholine neurotransmitter systems: movement, cognition, mood, sleep, and hypothalamically integrated autonomic functions (e.g., blood pressure control, appetite, sexual function), with mobility problems being the most prominent. Chapter 21 illustrates some of these problems.

DEMENTIAS

Collectively, many of the degenerative disorders of axis I compose the dementias or produce generalized cognitive and intellectual deterioration. Clinically, the term *dementia* denotes a syndrome involving intellectual deterioration, changes in personality, and a variety of behavioral abnormalities. Examples of dementing diseases include Alzheimer's disease (AD), multi-infarct dementia, alcoholism, intracranial tumors, normal pressure hydrocephalus, and Huntington's disease (HD). However, it should not be assumed that memory impairment is the same for all diseases. The incidence of the dementias collectively in the United States is estimated to be 17.7 cases/1000 person-years by age 80 (Jorm & Jolley, 1998). This incidence increases with age.

Dementias of the AD type are the most common, with 3.75 million individuals estimated to be afflicted currently. That number is expected to increase to 9 million by the year 2040 (Max, 1993). The overall annual costs associated with all types of dementia patients are approximately $20 billion for direct care and $38 billion for informal care. AD is inherited in 5% to 10% of individuals and is consistent with an autosomal dominant mode of inheritance. Despite the abundance of data from families with AD, most cases of AD are sporadic, and the cause is unknown. Genetic factors might influence the pathogenic process, along with other biochemical factors, such as inflammation, oxidative stress, and estrogen (Farlow, 1998). Several chromosomes are responsible for familial AD, which demonstrates genetic heterogeneity. Early-onset disease has been linked to the amyloid gene on chromosome 21 and to an unidentified gene on chromosome 14. Late-onset disease may be regulated by a gene on chromosome 19 associated with apolipoprotein E. Other familial AD disorders do not map to any of these sites (Martin, 1993).

The U.S. Food and Drug Administration has approved the use of tacrine for AD. Clinical trials suggest an association with modest improvement in cognitive function or a delay in expected progression of the disorder (Schneider, 1993). Additional cholinergic agents, as well as anti-inflammatories, antioxidants, and estrogen, are under investigation.

HD is a disorder of movement, mentation, and behavior. It is inherited in an autosomal dominant pattern. The HD mutation has been found to be an unstable expansion of the DNA known as a trinucleotide repeat (Huntington's Disease Research Collaborative Group, 1993). Coronal cuts using magnetic resonance imaging (MRI) show atrophy of the caudate nucleus in the middle to later stages of HD. HD occurs worldwide, with a prevalence of 5 to 10 per

100,000 population. In the United States, approximately 25,000 people have clinical features of HD, and another 125,000 people are immediately at risk (i.e., have parents with the disorder). Age at onset is approximately 40 years, with a duration of illness ranging from 10 to 25 years. However, juvenile onset may occur, with symptoms of diminishing school performance and rigidity. Progression in these cases is more rapid, leading to death in 5 to 10 years. The father is consistently the affected parent.

Movement abnormalities associated with the disease consist primarily of chorea and, in the later stages, rigidity. Individuals are slow to respond both verbally and with movement. The abnormal movements interfere with safety, speech, swallowing, nutrition, and self-care skills. Psychiatric manifestations may precede the chorea or occur subsequent to the abnormal movements. Poor judgment and dyscontrol syndromes are common.

The clinical course of the dementias is variable and may occur rapidly over a few years or slowly over 15 or more years. The earliest symptoms include gradual development of forgetfulness, lack of initiative, and neglect of routine tasks and are so subtle as to be noticed only in retrospect. As the disorder progresses, the person experiences increased deficits in recent memory, decreased ability to concentrate, and inability to manage personal, work, and financial affairs. It is in this phase that family members often experience the strain of coping with the changing person and seek professional help. Eventually, the person becomes unable to function independently, experiences difficulties in simple activities of daily living (such as dressing), may experience hallucinations or delusions, and exhibits socially problematic behaviors. In the final phases, the person becomes bedridden and incontinent.

The symptoms of the various dementias are related to structural degeneration of neurons in the cerebrum and diencephalon, with the specific structures varying with the particular disease. For example, HD is characterized by degeneration of neurons in the caudate nucleus and has both cognitive and motor symptoms (involuntary choreiform movements). In contrast, AD involves loss of neurons and accumulation of argyophil plaques and neurofibrillary tangles, primarily in the hippocampus (Kwentus, Hart, Lingpon, Taylor, & Silverman, 1986).

Although the dementing diseases have varying pathologic and structural markers that differentiate them at autopsy, the human responses are much the same. They all affect cognition and mood because of their effects on the cerebral hemispheres, diencephalon, and limbic system. Some, such as Parkinson's disease with dementia and HD, also affect movement because of the involvement of the basal ganglia in the pathologic process.

Caregiving issues and the extent of home care support make a difference in the costs of the dementing diseases. Efforts to keep the affected individual at home as long as possible can help contain costs. Attention to the stresses and health of the caregiver has an impact on the well-being of the demented individual and his or her family. Early exploration of end-of-life decisions such as resuscitation, use of antibiotics to treat terminal pneumonia, and nutritional options such as tube-feeding is necessary for total care of the patient and family (Baillie, Norbeck, & Barnes, 1988; Norberg, Asplund, & Waxman, 1987;

Robinson, 1989; Wilson, 1989). Chapters 10 through 13 and Chapter 33 discuss cognitive responses and self-care alterations relevant to this group of disorders.

Degenerative Disorders of Axes II and III

Axes II and III are the brain stem and cerebellum and the spinal cord, respectively. Each performs various roles in the integration of motor and sensory function in the peripheral and central nervous systems.

MULTIPLE SCLEROSIS

Multiple sclerosis (MS) is the most prominent of the diseases that destroy the myelin covering of axons and dendrites in the central nervous system. It is the third most common cause (after trauma and stroke) of severe disability in persons between the ages of 15 and 60 years. Approximately 250,000 to 350,000 persons were estimated to be affected by MS in the United States in 1990 (Anderson et al., 1992). Given the early age at onset (in the second and third decades of life) and the chronicity (approximately 30 years' duration), MS has been estimated to cost greater than $6.8 billion annually in the United States (Rudick, 1999).

The risk of developing MS is related to environment in a complicated manner. Prevalence studies in many countries have demonstrated that there is a high risk of MS above 40 degrees in latitude and the Tropics of Capricorn and Cancer and a low risk of MS between the tropics (McDonald, 1984). Migration studies have shown that moving to a lower prevalence region before age 15 years results in a decreased incidence of the disease. A more recent study of the epidemiology of MS shows that a significant portion of the state-by-state variations in MS risk can be explained by differences in ancestry among state populations, even when geographic latitude is included in the analyses (Page, Kurtzke, Murphy, & Norman, 1993). These results suggest a mixture of genetic susceptibility, cultural, and environmental factors in the etiology of the disease. Another theory of MS causation is late activation of a slow virus or, more likely, an autoimmune response triggered by a virus.

MS is a disease of the white matter (myelinated tissue) associated with multifocal inflammatory demyelinating lesions or diffuse axonal demyelinating lesions that leave the nerve cell process itself intact. It is not strictly a disorder of axes II and III, because there may be lesions in the white matter of the cerebrum as well. Manifestations, however, are most commonly related to formation of plaques (areas of demyelination) in the spinal cord, brain stem, cerebellum, and visual pathways.

The earliest clinical signs are often vague, such as weakness or numbness and tingling in one or more limbs, visual blurring, difficulty walking, or urinary frequency and urgency. The diagnosis has been considerably aided by the use of MRI, which often demonstrates plaques; visual evoked responses; and special techniques of cerebrospinal fluid examination. Diagnostic criteria include visualization of plaques that are consistent with clinical signs, episodes of neurologic deficit that are separated in space and time, and symptoms in more than one neurologic system that cannot be explained on the basis of a single lesion. Clinical syndromes can be classified into the following types: mixed or generalized (50% of cases, with involvement of the optic nerve, brain stem, cerebellum, and spinal cord); spinal (30% to 40% of cases, characterized by spastic ataxia and deep sensory changes); cerebellar or pontobulbar cerebellar (5% of cases, characterized by problems with coordination, equilibrium, speech, and swallowing); and amaurotic (5% of cases, characterized by unilateral visual deficits). Seventy percent of patients experience the typical acute-onset exacerbating and remitting type. Fewer than 10% suffer from the malignant form with early cerebellar signs and rapid progression to severe disability (Smith & Sheinberg, 1985).

A large number of treatments of MS have been attempted, all of which are difficult to evaluate because of the exacerbating and remitting natural course of the disease. Adrenocorticotropic hormone (ACTH) and corticosteroids are often administered to shorten the course of an exacerbation. Immunosuppressive therapy and plasmapheresis have been evaluated on the basis of the theory of autoimmune response. Symptomatic treatment includes antispasmodics (e.g., baclofen), anticholinergics for urinary symptoms, antiepileptics for neuralgia, stimulants to reduce fatigue (e.g., amantadine), antidepressants, and drugs to reduce tremor (e.g., clonazepam) (Smith & Darlington, 1999).

In a multicenter, randomized, double-blind, placebo-controlled trial of interferon beta-1b (IFNB) in patients with relapsing-remitting MS, there was a reduction in exacerbation rates, severity of exacerbations, and MRI abnormalities without serious side effects (IFNB Multiple Sclerosis Study Group, 1993). Further research is planned using this agent, as well as others (alpha interferon, copolymer-1), for the various forms of MS.

As is evident from the large portion of the central nervous system that can be affected by MS, human responses vary widely. There may be alterations in vision, cognition, mobility (related to weakness or coordination), somatic sensation, communication (related to coordination of speaking mechanisms), nutrition (related to swallowing difficulties), elimination, and self-care. Alterations in human responses discussed in Chapters 11, 14, 15, 21, 24, 28, 31, and 33 are relevant to people with MS.

ATAXIAS

Although the term *ataxia* literally means disorder of confusion, there is a complex group of diseases, many genetically determined, that result in the symptom combination of dysarthria, poor coordination, nystagmus, and wide-based gait. Neuropathologic characteristics and changes in the MRI results can show loss of cells in the cerebellum, brain stem, and pontine areas (Harding, 1993). There are both early-onset and late-onset types. Chronic alcohol abuse can cause loss of cells in the cerebellum and therefore ataxia.

Therapies include treatment for alcoholism, genetic counseling, and various supportive interventions to enhance mobility. Generally, cognition is spared. Nursing care focuses on alterations in vision (resulting from nystagmus), mobility (related to incoordination rather than weakness), communication (related to interference with speaking mechanisms), and self-care.

MOTOR NEURON DISEASE

Motor neuron (or motor system) diseases are characterized by progressive degeneration of motor neurons in the anterior horns of the spinal cord and brain stem. Since the 1950s, motor neuron diseases have replaced poliomyelitis as the most frequent cause of anterior horn cell dysfunction. *Amyotrophic lateral sclerosis* (ALS, or Lou Gehrig's disease) is the most common form of adult motor neuron disease in the United States, accounting for 1.5 of the 2 cases per 100,000 of all motor neuron disorders. The prevalence is estimated at 5 of the 6 cases per 100,000 population for all motor neuron disorders (Kurtzke, 1982). The mean duration of survival with ALS is about 3 years, although some patients live as long as 10 to 15 years and some die as soon as 1 year after diagnosis.

About 10% of cases are inherited as an autosomal dominant trait, with clinical similarities to the sporadic form. In 11 of 13 familial ALS kindreds, a missense mutation was found on chromosome 21 in a gene that encodes Cu/Zn-binding superoxide dismutase (Rosen, Siddique, & Patterson, 1993).

Pathologically, motor neurons in the brain stem or spinal cord atrophy and die, with subsequent loss of their peripheral axons. Sensory neurons are not affected. Muscles atrophy as a result of loss of trophic influences from the nerve fiber, and progressive muscular weakness ensues. Symptoms may begin in the periphery (usually the arms), with difficulty performing fine finger movements and wasting of the hands. Cramping and fasciculations of the muscles of the limbs or trunk are evident. Reflexes may be absent in the affected limbs and hyperactive in the more distal limbs. The atrophic weakness progresses to involve the neck, tongue, pharyngeal and laryngeal muscles, trunk, and lower extremities. Ultimately, the patient is unable to move, speak, swallow, and, eventually, breathe. Mentation, sensation, and usually bowel and bladder control are intact throughout the course of the disease. Respiratory insufficiency is frequently the cause of death, although long-term ventilatory support can be offered if the patient wishes. Antiglutamate drugs (e.g., riluzole) offer some benefit in prolonging survival (Miller, 1997).

The *spinal muscular atrophies* are several types of more slowly progressing motor neuron diseases. These are inherited. Symptoms are evident in early infancy, in adolescence, or in adulthood. The childhood form, called Werdnig-Hoffmann disease, and the juvenile spinal muscular atrophy, called Kugelberg-Welander disease, are the result of a duplicate chromosome 5 and are autosomal recessive disorders (Campbell, Potter, Ignatius, Dubowitz, & Davies, 1997). The genetics of adult forms are unclear and require further investigation. Patients have significant deficits in mobility and self-care. Some can have respiratory failure. Chapters 15, 21, and 33 are most relevant to human responses common in persons with motor neuron diseases.

Degenerative Disorders of Axis IV

Neuropathy indicates damage to the peripheral nerves, regardless of cause. Infectious disorders are referred to as neuritis (as in trigeminal neuritis, a sequela of varicella). The neuropathies may be caused by entrapment of the nerve, with subsequent degeneration of either the myelin covering or the axons themselves. Trauma, repetitive use in various occupations or recreational activities, pressure or severing of the nerve, metabolic processes that cause degeneration of myelin or axonal tissue, and genetic factors can be the cause. Other causative factors include exposure to toxins or nutritional deficiency. Diagnostic testing, such as electromyography, is useful in characterizing the nature of the damage (Chalk, 1997). Some neuropathies are reversible.

POLYNEUROPATHIES

Polyneuropathies (involvement of multiple peripheral nerves) have an annual incidence rate of 40 cases per 100,000 population in the United States (Kurtzke, 1982). Most polyneuropathies exhibit a characteristic distribution of weakness, paralysis, and often sensory changes. The pathologic process begins at the most distal parts of the largest and longest nerves and advances headward along the affected fiber to the cell body. Regeneration and functional reconnections are possible unless the cell body itself dies.

Some cases of acquired immunodeficiency syndrome (AIDS) manifest as a distal symmetrical polyneuropathy or mononeuritis multiplex (American Academy of Neurology Task Force, 1989). Human immunodeficiency virus (HIV) testing is included in the battery of blood tests used to evaluate symptoms of polyneuropathy. Treatment includes medications to slow the progression of the disease. The varied neurologic manifestations of AIDS are beyond the scope of this chapter. Alterations in human responses covered in subsequent chapters are relevant to persons with AIDS. Consideration of the symptoms and portions of the neuraxis involved determines nursing approaches.

Guillain-Barré syndrome, also called acute febrile polyneuritis, serves as a prototype for the problems patients face with acute polyneuropathies. The incidence of Guillain-Barré syndrome is approximately 1.7 cases per 100,000 population in the United States (Alter, 1990). It is most common in adults but has been described in adolescents.

The major clinical manifestation is symmetrical weakness that ascends and becomes more severe over 2 to 14 days. Distal muscles of the lower extremities are usually affected first, with progression to the lower proximal muscles and then to the trunk, intercostal, upper extremity, neck, and cranial muscles. Peak severity, which can be complete flaccid paralysis, is reached in 90% of patients within 10 to 14 days. Weakness can progress more rapidly, however, leading to total motor paralysis and respiratory muscle failure within days. The disorder affects primarily motor and autonomic peripheral nerves, leaving sensation intact. Autonomic disturbances (tachycardia, fluctuating blood pressure control, elimination problems) are common.

Most evidence suggests that the disorder results from a cell-mediated immunologic reaction to peripheral nerve myelin. The majority of cases remit spontaneously, with full recovery. Treatment may include plasmapheresis or immune serum globulin and supportive interventions to maintain vital respiratory function, mobility, and self-care activities. The disorder has the potential to alter responses in all areas of human function except consciousness, cognition, and sensation.

MONONEUROPATHIES

Mononeuropathies are disorders of single peripheral nerves secondary to trauma, entrapment, and some metabolic processes, such as diabetes or postinfectious syndromes. The symptoms depend on the specific motor, sensory, or mixed functions of the involved nerve. Most commonly, mononeuropathies occur in the cranial nerves (particularly nerves V and VI) and in the brachial and lumbosacral plexuses. Such disorders produce problems in movement and, in some cases, pain or anesthesia. The incidence of mononeuropathies is estimated at 40 per 100,000 population in the United States (Kurtzke, 1982).

TUMORS

Tumors are abnormal growths of neural or nonneural tissues in the cranial cavity or on the spinal cord or the peripheral nerves. Although many central nervous system tumors are not malignant in the sense that they spread to other parts of the body, the local growth and extension of a tumor may threaten function and life because of compression and destruction of tissues around it by the tumor itself and by the vasogenic brain swelling surrounding the tumor. Tumors from other parts of the body may also metastasize to the central nervous system.

Kurtzke (1982) provided the following general estimates of incidence of tumors in the central nervous system in the United States:

Type	Incidence per 100,000 Population
Metastatic brain tumor	15
Benign brain tumor	10
Malignant brain tumor	5
Metastatic spinal cord tumor	5
Benign spinal cord tumor	1
Malignant spinal cord tumor	0.5

Tumors of the central nervous system occur in great pathologic variety, but their symptoms are based on their size, location, and invasiveness. Common symptoms of tumors in axis I are changes in cognition and motor function, headaches, vomiting, and seizures. Increased intracranial pressure, with papilledema, is often a concomitant sign of slowly growing tumors of the cerebral hemispheres. If tumors continue to grow, they may alter consciousness (see Chapter 6) and ultimately produce brain herniation and death. Central nervous system neoplasms are classified in many ways. This discussion classifies them, first, by type of neural or supporting tissue involved and, second, by area of the nervous system affected. The classification of tumors by type of tissue is helpful to neuroscience physicians in anticipating the relative responsiveness of specific tumors to adjuvant therapies (chemotherapy, radiotherapy). Classification by area of the nervous system involved is useful to neuroscience nurses in anticipating specific alterations in human responses related to location of specific kinds of neoplasms.

Neoplasms Classified by Type of Tissue Involved

Tumors of the nervous system may derive from neuronal tissue, supportive brain tissue, the reticuloendothelial system, brain and spinal cord coverings, residual developmental tissue, glandular structures, or nerve sheaths. In addition, tumors of either the brain or the spinal cord may metastasize from systemic carcinomas.

TUMORS OF NEURONS OR PRIMITIVE NEURONAL ELEMENTS

Medulloblastomas and neuroastrocytomas are tumors derived from primitive neuronal blast cells or from neurons. Medulloblastomas account for about 7% of all central nervous system tumors and occur primarily in children. Generally arising in the fourth ventricle, medulloblastomas thus cause symptoms referable to the posterior fossa: ataxia, nystagmus, and impairment of cerebrospinal fluid flow. These tumors may metastasize throughout the neuraxis and are treated with resection and radiation or chemotherapy. Survival has improved remarkably since the 1930s (Duffner & Cohen, 1992). Consequently, the long-term consequences of neurotoxic treatments, such as dementia, endocrinopathies, and leukoencephalopathy, become considerations when choosing therapies for children. Neuroastrocytomas (or gangliogliomas) are extremely rare and occur primarily in children. They are generally located in the frontal and temporal lobes and the hypothalamus. Excision may or may not be possible, depending on accessibility of the tumor. Radiation may increase length of survival.

TUMORS OF CENTRAL NERVOUS SYSTEM SUPPORTIVE TISSUE

The most frequent central nervous system tumors are those of the supportive tissue: gliomas and tumors of the choroid plexus. Gliomas are tumors of the glial tissues and are subdivided into astrocytomas (grades I and II), glioblastoma multiforme (grades III and IV, or malignant astrocytomas), oligodendrogliomas, and ependymal tumors. Together, the gliomas account for about 46% of all central nervous system tumors. Astrocytomas grades I and II account for 10% to 15% of central nervous system tumors and are found most commonly in children and young adults. Astrocytomas are the most common type of posterior fossa tumor in children (33% of tumors in children). About 1% of astrocytomas are optic gliomas, also found in children. Grades III and IV astrocytomas (glioblastoma multiforme) are seen almost entirely in adults and account for 25% of central nervous system tumors. Although grades I and II astrocytomas are often resectable and sensitive to radiation, glioblastomas are much more invasive and are virtually never eradicated. Excision and subsequent chemotherapy or irradiation are used to prolong life.

Oligodendrogliomas are slowly growing lesions, usually found in the cerebral hemispheres in young adults. About 3% of tumors are of this type. Excision and irradiation are used to prolong life but are rarely curative. Likewise, ependymomas are relatively uncommon (3% of all tumors) and derive from the ependymal cells lining the ventricles. Ventricular obstruction is common, and the tumor can often be completely resected, although metastasis is possible during excision. Irradiation may be used if complete resection is not possible. Colloid cysts and choroid plexus papillomas are rare tumors of supportive tissues that occur in childhood and adolescence. Colloid cysts occur in the third ventricle, and choroid plexus papillomas occur most commonly in the lateral or fourth ventricle. Both are apt to produce hydrocephalus and may be cured if surgical excision is complete.

TUMORS OF THE RETICULOENDOTHELIAL SYSTEM

Systemic diseases, such as leukemia, lymphoma, and myeloma, may involve the nervous system, infiltrating either the brain or the meninges. Such involvement is more likely to occur when there is a generalized immunosuppression, such as with therapeutic immunosuppression or with AIDS. Irradiation, chemotherapy, and shunting to reduce intracranial pressure are all used as adjuvant therapy.

TUMORS OF CENTRAL NERVOUS SYSTEM COVERINGS

Tumors of skull elements, such as osteomas and chondrosarcomas, are relatively rare central nervous system tumors, whereas meningiomas (tumors of the leptomeninges) account for about 15% of central nervous system tumors. Most bony tumors are found in children and young adults, and meningiomas are found only in adults. Meningiomas are rarely malignant, and cure is the rule when excision is complete. Meningiomas of the areas around the brain stem and base of the skull may not be amenable to complete excision, however.

TUMORS OF DEVELOPMENTAL REMNANTS

Congenital tumors include craniopharyngiomas (about 3% of all tumors) and the more rare cholesteatomas (epidermoid cysts), teratomas, and chordomas. All are present from birth but may not be detected until later in life because of their slow growth. Craniopharyngiomas are believed to be remnants of Rathke's pouch and thus develop in the suprasellar region. Pituitary dysfunction, bitemporal visual deficits, and hydrocephalus from obstruction of the third ventricle may all occur. Complete excision is often possible. Cholesteatomas and teratomas derive from remnants of epidermoid cells or germinal cells and are found in the cerebellopontine angle and pineal or suprasellar regions, respectively. Teratomas are usually malignant but are radiosensitive. Cholesteatomas are benign and can often be completely excised.

TUMORS OF GLANDULAR STRUCTURES

Pituitary adenomas account for 5% to 15% of cranial tumors and are found in adults. Pinealomas are rare and are seen in children. Pituitary dysfunction (Cushing's syndrome, acromegaly, amenorrhea) and visual defects are indications for transsphenoidal resection. Hormonal replacement is usually necessary postoperatively.

TUMORS OF NERVE SHEATHS

Tumors of nerve sheaths include acoustic neuromas (vestibular schwannoma) and fifth nerve tumors. Acoustic neuroma is the most common tumor of the cerebellopontine angle in adults and accounts for 5% to 8% of all central nervous system tumors. About 5% of vestibular schwannomas are bilateral and inherited as a dominant genetic disorder called *neurofibromatosis type II*, the result of a mutation on chromosome 22. Acoustic neuroma usually originates on the vestibular portion of cranial nerve VIII within the auditory canal. It grows into the posterior fossa to occupy the cerebellopontine angle and may grow to impinge on cranial nerves V and VII (and occasionally cranial nerves IX and X). If not resected, it will eventually displace the pons and medulla and obstruct cerebrospinal fluid circulation. Unilateral loss of hearing, disturbed balance, ipsilateral loss of coordination, and ipsilateral facial weakness are common symptoms.

Fifth nerve tumors are rare and are usually associated with severe facial pain. Surgical resection is possible but may be limited by access to the junction of the middle and posterior fossa.

METASTATIC TUMORS

Tumors metastasize to the brain most commonly from the lung, followed by breast, skin, kidney, gastrointestinal tract, prostate, and thyroid. Metastatic tumors constitute about 10% of intracranial neoplasms that come to surgery. Single lesions may be excised surgically to extend life or to reduce symptoms. The edema surrounding such lesions is responsive to corticosteroid therapy.

Neoplasms Classified by Neural Structures

AXIS I

Tumors of the cerebral hemispheres may occur in any of the lobes of the brain or in the diencephalon, with the symptoms referable to the particular brain area involved. Gliomas and meningiomas are the most common tumors of the hemispheres. Tumors of the sella or parasella area are the most likely to produce hypothalamic, optic, and pituitary dysfunction. Craniopharyngiomas and pituitary adenomas are the most common of these. Ventricular tumors, such as choroid plexus papillomas of the lateral ventricles, may also affect the hemispheres and diencephalon.

AXIS II

Tumors of the posterior fossa and cerebellopontine angle all produce dysfunction of cerebellar coordination, cranial nerves, and brain stem tracts. Ventricular tumors of this area can produce obstructive hydrocephalus. Medulloblastoma, cerebellar astrocytoma, ependymoma, brain stem gliomas, and acoustic neurinomas (eighth nerve schwannomas) are common tumors of axis II. The poorest prognosis of childhood tumors is associated with the brain stem glioma (Duffner & Cohen, 1992).

AXIS III

Spinal cord tumors are less common than intracranial tumors, constituting only about 15% of central nervous system tumors (Adams & Victor, 1993). The majority do not metastasize and exert their effects by compression of the spinal cord. Spinal tumors can be divided into extramedullary and intramedullary tumors. Extramedullary tumors arise outside the spinal cord, in the vertebral bodies and epidural tissues (extradural) or in the leptomeninges or roots (intradural). Intramedullary tumors arise within the substance of the spinal cord and destroy tracts and central gray structures. People with spinal cord tumors manifest one of three clinical syndromes: sensorimotor loss referable to dysfunction of spinal cord motor and sensory tracts, radicular–spinal cord syndrome referable to involvement of peripheral nerve roots as well as spinal cord tracts, and syringomyelia syndrome referable to loss of central cord function.

Human responses to tumors of axes I, II, and III are of three types: (1) specific symptomatic alterations referable to the portion of the brain, brain stem, or spinal cord affected; (2) responses to the surgical, chemotherapeutic, or radiotherapeutic modality used; and (3) responses related to uncertainty about the future and about residual neurologic deficits. The category of altered human response (e.g., altered communication and cognition) can be inferred from the discussion of the more common locations of brain and spinal cord tumors. All tumor-destructive medical and surgical interventions carry the potential for inflammatory response and local brain swelling. These, in turn, carry the potential for increased intracranial pressure and brain herniation. Corticosteroids reduce cerebral edema related to brain tumors and are often used to minimize the swelling associated with radiotherapy and chemotherapy as well.

AXIS IV (PERIPHERAL NERVE)

There are three types of tumors that affect the peripheral nerves: schwannomas, neurofibromas, and malignant peripheral nerve sheath tumors. All are of nerve sheath origin rather than arising from the nerve itself. Schwannomas and neurofibromas are most often benign, encapsulated tumors, which may or may not be removed surgically depending on symptoms and risk of damage to the nerve. MRI helps distinguish the various types of peripheral nerve tumor.

Neurofibromatosis (NF), the most common genetically transmitted disorder affecting the nervous system (with an estimated prevalence of 1 in 3000), is an autosomal dominant disease due to a mutation on chromosome 17. NF type 1 is characterized by skin discoloration called café-au-lait spots and by neurofibromas, schwannomas, optic nerve gliomas, and characteristic eye lesions in the iris called *Lisch nodules* (Karnes, 1998). Appropriate diagnosis is essential to ensure that genetic counseling is provided for the family.

Like neuropathy, peripheral nerve tumors have the potential to alter responses in all areas of human function except consciousness and cognition. Nursing diagnoses include risk for infection and injury, impaired tissue integrity, and chronic pain.

Responses to the uncertainty of future function and life may create a variety of coping responses for the individual and family. Often a need arises for community support systems for people with terminal central nervous system neoplasms. Chapter 17 illustrates some of these responses.

NEUROMUSCULAR DISORDERS

The neuromuscular disorders are all disorders of axis IV, specifically, the neuromuscular junction or the muscles themselves.

Myasthenia Gravis

Myasthenia gravis (MG) affects adults and children. It is characterized by muscular weakness and easy fatigability. It can also present as a transient syndrome in newborns, manifested by hypotonia and difficulty feeding (Fenichel, 1989). Facial, extraocular, masticatory, deglutitional, and lingual muscles are particularly involved, but respiratory and limb muscles are also affected. The most common symptom experienced by people with MG is double vision (41%), followed by drooping eyelids (24%), difficulty with voice (16%), weak legs (13%), general weakness (11%), difficulty with swallowing (10%), difficulty with chewing (7%), and weak arms and hands (7%).

The fatigability of muscles is traced to a defect at the juncture between nerve and muscle. Specifically, acetylcholine receptors on the muscle fiber are decreased in number, presumably through an autoimmune response to the receptors. In transitory neonatal myasthenia, passive transfer of acetylcholine receptor antibody from the affected mother causes the symptoms. Treatment includes nutritional support until symptoms subside in about 3 weeks.

Epidemiologic studies demonstrate the incidence and prevalence of MG to be much higher in women than in men. A Norwegian study reported an incidence of 5.3 per million population for women, compared with 2.6 per million for men, as well as a prevalence of 127 per million for women and 52 per million for men (Storm-Mathisen, 1984). Two thirds of women develop symptoms before age 40 years, whereas two thirds of men develop symptoms after age 40 years (Kurtzke, 1984). Mortality is related to respiratory insufficiency and is higher than that of the age-matched population (1.5 times that of women younger than 60 years, nearly 5 times that of women older than 60 years, and 1.4 times that of all men) (Storm-Mathisen, 1984). The outlook for a normal life span has improved considerably since the 1970s, however. Formerly, nearly one third of patients died from respiratory complications of the disease; currently, this figure is less than 5% as a result of improvements in intensive care management, respiratory nursing care, and new treatment modalities. Spontaneous remission is said to occur in 10% to 20% of cases, and remission can be induced in 60% to 87% of selected cases by thymectomy (Johns, 1982).

Early in the course of the disease, patients can be managed with anticholinesterase medications: pyridostigmine bromide, neostigmine bromide, or ambenonium chloride four to six times daily. Most patients require further medical or surgical therapy, including corticosteroids, thymectomy, immunosuppressive drugs, plasma exchange, or gamma globulin (Grob, 1981).

Corticosteroid therapy is associated with improvement in a large proportion of patients (Johns, 1982) but carries all the numerous side effects of long-term steroid administration. Immunosuppressive drugs, particularly azathioprine, have been successful in treating symptoms of MG. Compared with those of prednisone, the side effects are mild, consisting of occasional gastrointestinal upset, leukopenia, liver enzyme elevation, and interstitial cystitis. The potential for teratogenesis in women of childbearing age is a concern for many MG patients, and the risk of acquired malignancy is unknown (Hertek, Mertens, Reuther, & Picker, 1979). Plasma exchange temporarily removes antibodies to the acetylcholine receptors and may be effective in myasthenic crisis, but it does not offer long-term remission (Howard, 1982). However, the use of regular plasma exchange to prevent crises is under investigation. Thymectomy is particularly effective in young women and often induces remission or marked improvement.

Botulism

Botulism is an uncommon but frequently fatal disorder caused by a bacterial toxin (*Clostridium botulinum*) that acts at the myoneural junction. Botulinum toxin is produced from the spores of *C. botulinum* and prevents the release of acetylcholine from the presynaptic nerve terminal, thus preventing function of all smooth and skeletal muscle fibers. The organism is ubiquitous in the soil, but its spores are normally destroyed by acidic foods or with pressure cooking in commercial preparation. Improper home-canning techniques may not kill the spores, which will then produce the toxin when the sealed container remains at room temperature. Less frequently, toxin-producing spores may enter the body through wounds contaminated with dirt or may propagate in the infant gastrointestinal tract. Very few cases are reported each year in the United States (e.g., 21 during 1979 and 1980), and most occur in the western United States, particularly Alaska, California, Colorado, Oregon, and Washington (Rubenstein, 1985).

Death may be rapid, depending on the amount of toxin circulating. Improvements in intensive care, particularly in respiratory support, have reduced the death rate from 60% to 20% (Rubenstein, 1985). Symptoms appear within 6 hours to a few days and initially consist of dry mouth, diplopia, difficulty focusing, dysphagia, and dysarthria. Nausea, vomiting, diarrhea, and abdominal cramping are common. Infant botulism frequently begins with constipation and presents as hypotonia (Gay & Bodensteiner, 1990). Descending motor weakness or paralysis and respiratory muscle insufficiency often follow, and sensory involvement is rare.

Treatment is entirely symptomatic, with respiratory support and nursing prevention of immobility complications essential. Antitoxin may be of help if given early. In many cases the disease may mimic Guillain-Barré syndrome, tick paralysis, and a variety of chemical intoxications. The diagnosis is confirmed by excluding other causes. In infants, the organism can be isolated from the stool. Recovery is slow as the patient's body gradually metabolizes the toxin. The prognosis for full recovery is good provided the intercurrent complications of immobility and respiratory insufficiency are prevented. Human responses to this disorder can be expected to be similar to those of patients with other acute immobilizing disorders, such as Guillain-Barré syndrome and acute spinal cord injury.

Myopathies

Chronic myopathies are disorders of the muscle fibers that produce weakness and progressive loss of functional mobility. The two major categories are the muscular dystrophies and the inflammatory diseases, such as polymyositis.

Both categories are characterized by progressive weakness, as well as myopathic changes apparent on electromyography, high serum enzyme levels that reflect muscle damage (creatine kinase levels), and abnormal muscle biopsy findings.

MUSCULAR DYSTROPHIES

The muscular dystrophies are genetic diseases characterized by progressive deterioration of skeletal muscle function without associated pathologic changes in the peripheral nerves or central nervous system. Several types of muscular dystrophy have been identified.

The muscular dystrophies are undergoing rapid changes in definition based on the impact of molecular genetics. Clinical criteria for diagnosis are giving way to DNA analysis, providing greater specificity and more reliable genetic counseling. New concepts of pathogenesis are evolving. Traditional forms of inheritance patterns are undergoing modification as new information emerges (Rowland, 1992).

Duchenne's muscular dystrophy (DMD) is the most common type, a sex-linked recessive disorder, with the DNA abnormality localized to the middle of the short arm of the X (female) chromosome (Kunkel, 1986). The disease is thus carried by the mother on one X chromosome but is manifested only in her male children, who do not have a healthy X chromosome to prevent expression of the disorder. The gene product has been identified to be a protein called dystrophin. Diagnosis is based on testing for the genetic abnormality by blood sampling or dystrophin analysis using a muscle biopsy. Becker's muscular dystrophy, a milder disorder with adult onset and less severe symptoms, shows the same DNA deletion but to a lesser extent.

Symptoms of DMD begin when the child begins to walk. The family will notice frequent falls, a lordotic toe-walking gait, and difficulty climbing stairs and running. By age 10 years, the child usually requires a wheelchair. Other complications include obesity, severe contractures, scoliosis, and occasional learning disabilities. Pulmonary function abnormalities begin in the late teens and early twenties. Without respiratory intervention, survival rarely extends beyond the thirties.

Myotonic muscular dystrophy (MMD) is an autosomal dominant disorder with a DNA expansion present on chromosome 19 (Harley et al., 1992). This finding demonstrates that an excess of DNA, as well as a deletion, can cause disease. MMD is characterized by an abnormality in muscle relaxation, as well as by defects in a variety of specialized and smooth muscle functions, such as cardiac conduction abnormalities, gastrointestinal slowing, and cataracts. Mental retardation is also a frequent finding. The age at onset varies from childhood to early adulthood.

Since the discovery of the dystrophin abnormality in DMD, trials of dystrophin replacement in affected muscle have been attempted. Preliminary reports have not shown substantial or lasting benefit. No medical therapies slow the progressive muscle deterioration seen in muscular dystrophy. Symptomatic therapy, such as bracing of extremities, appropriate exercise, and prescription of functional wheelchairs, remains the primary therapeutic intervention. Genetic counseling is an important component of care for these families.

An emerging cause for disorders of muscle is abnormalities in mitochondrial DNA. The mitochondria are the "power plants" of the cell, an important energy source. Mitochondria have their own circular DNA, which is inherited from the mother. Mitochrondrial dysfunction may also play an important role in Parkinson's disease and aging (Tritschler & Medori, 1993).

INFLAMMATORY DISEASES

The inflammatory myopathies, such as polymyositis and dermatomyositis, have an autoimmune origin. The symptoms include symmetrical proximal muscle weakness, muscle tenderness, reduced mobility, and, in dermatomyositis, a distinctive rash. The disease can be found in all age groups but is most common in childhood and middle age. Treatment with immunosuppressive agents, such as prednisone and azathioprine, has been successful in many cases, suggesting that an autoimmune response to muscle fiber is the source of the disorder. The illness can be lifelong, controlled rather than cured by medication.

NEUROTRAUMA

Trauma to the central nervous system is a major source of disability and death in the United States. The primary types of neurotrauma are head injury and spinal cord injury. The U.S. Department of Health and Human Services estimates that 1 million cases of head and spinal cord injury occur each year. The cost of these injuries totals $4.68 billion.

Both head injuries and spinal cord injuries are largely preventable, because they are caused mainly by motor vehicle accidents and falls. Neuroscience nurses can contribute to improved data collection for national estimates of head and spinal cord injury by carefully documenting the reason for the injury in the medical record. Efforts to prevent nervous system trauma include educational programs targeting youth such as Think First and Feet First; political activism to support legislation to toughen drunk-driving, helmet and seat belt use, and gun control laws; enforcement of the speed limit; separate bicycle lanes; and allowing only provisional licensing for drivers younger than 21 years. Dissemination of information regarding head and spinal cord injury does not in itself change behavior. The combination of legislation, tough enforcement, and information dissemination has been shown to be the most effective.

Head Injury

Head injury is a term for a cluster of diagnostic entities that result from trauma to the cranial cavity. Head injuries affect both axis I and axis II, and the human responses reflect a combination of problems in these axes.

Frankowski (1986) estimated the incidence of fatal and nonfatal head injuries at 200 to 300 cases per 100,000 population in the United States. The peak incidence of head trauma occurs in the late teens (567 cases per 100,000), with a second, smaller peak in the sixth decade of life (Minter-Convery, 1985). Males are more than twice as likely as females to sustain such injuries. The most common cause of head injury is transportation accidents (31% to 49%), followed by falls (20% to 32%), assault (7% to 40%), recreational accidents (3% to 14%), and miscellaneous causes (4% to 23%) (Frankowski, 1986).

The mechanism of injury largely determines the areas of the brain affected. Concussion, a transient alteration in neural function and consciousness, is an example of a minor injury in which recovery is the rule. A postconcussive syndrome may occur, however, characterized by headache, dizziness, and difficulty concentrating.

More severe injuries may result in brain contusion or in bleeding at the site of impact and at distant sites secondary to movement of the brain in the cranial cavity. Tearing of extradural and subdural vessels in the brain coverings may result in hematomas, which compress underlying brain tissue and may lead to brain herniation. Hyperemic responses to injury, coupled with intracranial or extracranial bleeding, may lead to intracranial hypertension, decreased brain perfusion, and transtentorial herniation.

Hematomas can often be removed surgically, providing relief from brain compression. The majority of severe head injuries, however, are characterized by widespread disruption in neuronal function and are not treatable by surgical means. Because the cerebral hemispheres and brain stem integrate all human functions, the range of human responses to head injury potentially encompasses all aspects of living. Patients with head injuries are likely to exhibit many of the alterations in human responses discussed in the sections on consciousness (Chapters 5 through 8), cognition (Chapters 10 through 13), communication (Chapters 14 and 15), affiliative relationships (Chapters 16 and 17), and self-care (Chapters 32 and 33).

Spinal Cord Injury

Spinal cord injury reflects neurotrauma in axis III. The annual incidence rate in the United States is 3 cases per 100,000, about 1% of that of head injury. The prevalence of permanent spinal cord injury is about 50 per 100,000, with an average duration of 18 years (Kurtzke, 1982). As with head injury, males are affected far more than females, with 72% of injuries occurring in males (Griffin, Opitz, Kurland, Ebersold, & O'Fallon, 1985). Sixty percent of spinal cord injuries are incurred on the highway, with another 13% incurred at other outdoor sites, 12% in the home, and 7% at work.

Adams and Victor (1993) divided spinal cord injuries into three groups: fracture-dislocations, fractures, and dislocations. Fracture-dislocations are three times as common as the others. Fractures and dislocations of the vertebral column can cause injury to the cord itself by compression or laceration of the cord. Shearing or compression of the cord results in destruction of white and gray matter by hemorrhage and ischemia. Pathologic processes that result in the death of neurons appear to start at the time of impact and do not seem to be prevented by early decompressive laminectomy if signs of spinal cord trauma are already present. However, a study demonstrated improved neurologic outcome following early administration of methylprednisolone. Immobilization, reduction, and stabilization of the fracture or dislocation are important to prevent further trauma to the cord. Characteristics of acute spinal cord injury and associated human responses are discussed in Chapter 20.

SEIZURES

Epilepsy

Epilepsy (recurrent seizures) is one of the most common neurologic disorders. An estimated 2 million people in the United States are affected by this disorder, with an annual incidence of 50 per 100,000 persons and a prevalence rate of 650 per 100,000 or nearly 1 in 25 (Kurtzke, 1982). Epilepsy is a sudden, intermittent alteration in consciousness or function resulting from excessive discharge of cerebral neurons. It is entirely a disorder of axis I. The causes of seizures include systemic disease (fever, neoplasm, vascular disease), sequelae of head trauma, stroke, or such disorders as MS and hypoxic syndromes. The largest number of cases are idiopathic, that is, these cases have no identifiable cause.

Seizures are currently classified on the basis of their clinical form and electroencephalographic (EEG) features as partial, generalized, unilateral, or unclassified (because of incomplete data) (Gastaut, 1970). *Partial seizures* may be one of three forms: elementary, complex, or secondarily generalized. Those that begin locally with elementary symptoms usually take a simple form (motor, sensory, autonomic, or a mixture of the three) and cause no impairment of consciousness. Complex partial seizures generally cause some impairment of consciousness in that the patient cannot recall events that happened during the seizure but is able to carry on automatic activities that require consciousness. The automatisms of psychomotor seizures are in this classification. Partial seizures may spread secondarily to become generalized seizures. The so-called aura for many people with epilepsy is actually a sensory, motor, or complex partial seizure that precedes a secondary generalization.

Generalized seizures are characterized by bilaterally symmetrical EEG changes and no local onset. Consciousness is impaired for very brief periods (absence) or longer periods (major motor seizures). Generalized seizures may take many forms: absence (formerly petit mal); clonic motor; tonic motor; tonic-clonic (formerly grand mal); atonic; or akinetic, myoclonic, and infantile spasms.

Various antiepileptic drugs specific to the seizure type are used to alter membrane properties and raise the seizure threshold. Therapeutic levels can be monitored in the serum or saliva to help titrate therapy for adequate seizure control. Surgical removal of epileptogenic foci is sometimes possible in cases that are uncontrolled by medication and in which a focus can be found. Vagus nerve stimulation has been found to be effective in controlling certain types of seizures. Human responses to seizures are discussed in Chapter 8.

INFECTIOUS DISORDERS

Bacterial and viral organisms may gain access to the central nervous system either through the blood (as septic emboli or thrombi or in overwhelming bacteremia) or through direct extension from extracranial sources (with traumatic penetrating injuries; from the nose or ear secondary to basal skull fracture; or through direct extension from infections of facial, skull, or spinal bones). Neural tissue appears relatively resistant to direct bacterial and viral infection but is less resistant if there is intercurrent systemic disease and in malnourished, aged, and immunosuppressed patients.

Infectious Disorders of Axes I, II, and III

MENINGITIS

Infections of the brain and spinal cord and their coverings may be caused by bacteria, viruses, or fungi. Meningitis is the most common of these infections and is characterized by inflammation of the meninges.

Bacterial meningitis is reported to have an annual incidence in the United States varying from 3 to 10 cases per 100,000 population. *Streptococcus pneumoniae* is the most common causative agent, accounting for 38% of reported cases. *Neisseria meningitidis* is the second most common causative agent. The attack rate is highest in children younger than 1 year (7.6 per 100,000) and greater in males than females of all ages (3.3 cases versus 2.6 cases, respectively, per 100,000 in one series) (Durand et al., 1993).

Bacterial meningitis accounts for approximately one third of all meningitis cases (Skoch & Waling, 1985), with the remainder being termed aseptic meningitis. A virus can be demonstrated conclusively in approximately 12% of cases of aseptic meningitis (Beghi et al., 1984).

Aseptic meningitis has a seasonal pattern, with the majority of cases occurring in the summer months, whereas bacterial meningitis is more common in the winter. Aseptic meningitis is characterized by influenza-like symptoms, with fever, drowsiness, stiff neck, and often headache and paresthesias. There is no specific therapy, but recovery is usually complete and hospitalization is not commonly required.

In contrast, bacterial meningitis produces purulent exudate that can interfere both with the function of cranial nerves as they exit the meninges and with the flow of cerebrospinal fluid. Medical therapy consists of large doses of intravenous antibiotics specific to the organism. Penicillin G remains the drug of choice for most organisms, with chloramphenicol as a second choice, then cephalosporins. Gram-negative organisms respond to chloramphenicol or aminoglycosides. Among children with *Haemophilus influenzae* meningitis, dexamethasone shortens the duration of fever and reduces the incidence of hearing loss. Monoclonal immunoglobulin M has been used to improve the shock state (Bell, 1992). Immunization to prevent *H. influenzae* meningitis is available.

Potential human responses include brain herniation secondary to swelling or communicating hydrocephalus, airway and visual disturbances as a result of cranial nerve dysfunction, and pain (headache). In infants, feeding abnormalities can occur. Sequelae include death, blindness, spastic paraparesis, and dementia.

ENCEPHALITIS

Encephalitis is inflammation and infection of the brain parenchyma (cortex and white matter) as well as the meninges, and it most commonly has a viral etiology. Herpes simplex virus type I is the most common causative virus, with arboviruses (eastern and western equine), enteroviruses (poliovirus, coxsackie-virus), and viruses that cause systemic illness (measles, mumps) also accounting for some cases. Each year in the United States, about 20,000 cases are reported (Whitley, 1990). Encephalitis is seasonal, with nearly half of cases occurring in spring and summer.

Patients with AIDS show a spectrum of neurocognitive defects due to HIV encephalitis. At autopsy, the brains of patients with AIDS dementia complex show neuropathologic changes, including dendritic and synaptic damage (Masliah et al., 1992). Persons with HIV also experience central nervous system damage secondary to opportunistic infections such as toxoplasmosis.

Viruses gain access to the central nervous system via the blood or peripheral nerves, causing a nonexudative inflammation. Because viruses replicate inside cells, there is often neuronal degeneration, demyelination of axons and dendrites, and subsequent necrosis, hemorrhage, and cavitation. The amount of tissue destruction varies with the organism, but the potential for significant neurologic sequelae is greater for encephalitis than it is for meningitis.

Medical therapy is supportive, because few antiviral agents are available. Acyclovir is effective in herpes encephalitis, but mortality remains high even with the drug (28%, compared with 54% before introduction of the drug). Treatment of HIV- and AIDS-related central nervous system involvement with immunomodulating agents may create adverse effects as a result of the neurotoxic effects of the drugs (Belman, 1993).

Human responses include the potential for brain herniation secondary to swelling; alterations in arousal that range from coma to hyperarousal; and a variety of cognitive problems, particularly memory loss, infection control issues, and, with HIV, stigmatization.

BRAIN ABSCESS

Brain abscess is a localized area of infection usually caused by direct extension of bacteria from an infected wound or sinus. Bacteria also may enter via the blood stream and create a localized, walled-off infection. The abscess acts as a space-occupying lesion and thus may mimic a tumor or hematoma. Medical therapy consists of systemic antibiotics or craniotomy or stereotactic drainage for removal of encapsulated abscesses.

POLIOMYELITIS

Poliomyelitis is rare in developed countries because of widespread preventive immunization but remains common in developing countries. The poliovirus is an enterovirus. In the vast majority of cases, symptoms are nonspecific and influenza-like or the disease may produce a mild aseptic meningitis. In a small percentage of cases, however, the virus gains entry to the central nervous system and is believed to travel along nerve fibers, being particularly attracted to the motor neurons of the brain stem (bulbar polio) or spinal cord. In paralytic cases, the motor neuron is destroyed, producing a flaccid paralysis of the muscles innervated by the portion of the brain stem or spinal cord affected. In mild cases, there may be only localized motor weakness, but in severe cases, the muscles of the limbs, trunk, head, and neck are involved. Years after the initial illness, neurologic deterioration can follow a period of stability. This is called postpolio syndrome. The etiology is unknown. There is no specific medical therapy once the disease is established, and nursing management is identical to that for the patient with severe Guillan-Barré syndrome (see Degenerative Disorders of Axis IV in this chapter).

TETANUS

Tetanus is a rare but life-threatening disease caused by the neurotoxin tetanospasmin that is produced by the bacillus *Clostridium tetani*. The disorder is rare in the industrialized world as a result of widespread use of active immunization. Fewer than 200 cases are reported annually in the United States, and these are in nonimmunized or insufficiently immunized people. The incidence in developing countries, however, is high, with an estimate of more than 1 million deaths annually (Simon & Swartz, 1984).

The organism is commonly introduced through puncture wounds contaminated with dirt. The spores germinate and produce toxin, which then spreads along axons to the spinal cord and may also spread via the general circulation. Tetanus toxin acts on the spinal cord to suppress the reflex inhibition mediated by internuncial neurons. Thus, when a muscle contracts, the contraction of its antagonist is no longer suppressed, and muscle spasm occurs. The disease is characterized by initial spasm at the wound site, with subsequent difficulty opening the mouth (lockjaw), dysphagia related to pharyngeal spasm, and generalized muscular spasm that is both painful and metabolically costly. The sympathetic nervous system is also affected by the toxin, producing labile hypertension, tachycardia, arrhythmias, sweating, and tachypnea.

There is no specific therapy once the toxin has bound to spinal neurons, although antitoxin can neutralize circulating toxin. The primary therapy is supportive: ventilatory support; muscle-relaxing drugs, such as diazepam; paralyzing drugs, such as curare; or pancuronium to reduce the metabolic demand of uncontrolled spasms. Sensation and cognition are not affected by the toxin, so care of these patients requires continual attention to relief of pain and fear as well as respiratory support, autonomic stability, and control of muscle spasm.

Mortality varies with rapidity of onset. It has been reported as 100% when symptoms appear within 1 to 2 days of injury and at 35% to 40% when incubation exceeds 10 days (Simon & Swartz, 1984).

NEUROSURGICAL PROCEDURES

A number of disorders of the nervous system lend themselves to surgical therapy, either to remove the source of the problem, as in tumors, or to provide decompression of the brain for temporary palliation and relief of symptoms, as in intracranial hypertension or invasive tumors. It is beyond the scope of this chapter to discuss the variety of neurosurgical procedures that one may encounter in the care of patients with nervous system disorders. There are some general principles related to care of patients after neurosurgical intervention that suggest common categories of human responses that neuroscience nurses should consider. Classic textbooks of neurosurgery and basic textbooks of neurosurgical nursing should be consulted for information about specific surgical procedures and standard nursing care plans after the procedures (Hickey, 1997; Youmans, 1996).

Surgical procedures subject tissues to controlled trauma, and the response of neural tissues to trauma is some degree of edema. Some potential for tissue swelling always exists, therefore, after any neurosurgical procedure that involves handling or invading the brain, spinal cord, or peripheral nerve tissues. In the case of craniotomy (removal of a part of the cranium to enter the cranial cavity), this potential for tissue swelling creates the potential for brain swelling and subsequent brain herniation. An example of such a situation is described in Chapter 6. Infratentorial craniotomy (below the tentorium, usually to gain access to the brain stem or posterior fossa) carries the additional risk of swelling that will compromise the brain stem nuclei or cranial nerves that serve swallowing and breathing. Particular attention is therefore required for monitoring respiration and airway protection. Laminectomy (removal of part of the vertebrae to gain access to the spinal canal) carries some risk of swelling that can compromise spinal cord function. Careful monitoring for signs of worsening spinal cord function is therefore necessary.

The basic complications of immobility that attend any surgical procedure, for example, thrombophlebitis and atelectasis, are just as likely after neurosurgical procedures. In addition, the lengthy procedures carry additional risk of skin breakdown and peripheral nerve palsies related to prolonged positioning on the operative table. Leg exercises, elastic stockings, and early ambulation are just as important after neurosurgery as after any other type of surgical procedure. In the case of infratentorial craniotomy and laminectomy, however, special support must be given to the operative site during dangling and ambulation to compensate for the lack of integrity of normal bony or muscle support. In the unresponsive patient, frequent repositioning and stimulation to breathe deeply must be used to compensate for the lack of voluntary movement.

SUMMARY

Human responses to any given neurologic disorder will manifest in a combination of the dysfunctions that are related to the area of the nervous system involved and of the coping responses of the individual and family to the prognosis and social meaning of the specific disease. This chapter has briefly described a number of the more common nervous system disorders and human responses that often accompany them. The remaining chapters are organized around the functional human responses, such as arousal and cognition, that may be seen in many different disorders.

References

Adams, R. D, & Victor, M. (1993). *Principles of neurology* (5th ed.). New York: McGraw-Hill.

Alter, M. (1990). The epidemiology of Guillain-Barre syndrome. *Annals of Neurology, 27*(Suppl.), S7–S12.

American Academy of Neurology Task Force. (1989). Human immumodeficiency virus (HIV) infection and the nervous system. *Neurology, 39,* 119–122.

American Heart Association. (1993). *Stroke facts.* Dallas, TX: Author.

Anderson, D. W., Ellenberg, J. H., Leventhal, C. M., Reingold, S. C., Rodriguez, M., & Silberberg, D. H. (1992). Revised estimate of the prevalence of multiple sclerosis in the United States. *Annals of Neurology, 31,* 333–336.

Baillie, V., Norbeck, J. S., & Barnes, L. E. A. (1988). Stress, social support, and psychological distress of family caregivers of the elderly. *Nursing Research, 37,* 217–222.

Beghi, E., Nicolosi, A., Kurland, L. T., Mulder, D. W., Hauser, W. A., & Shuster, L. (1984). Encephalitis and aseptic meningitis, Olmsted County, Minnesota, 1950–1981: I. Epidemiology. *Annals of Neurology, 16,* 283.

Bell, W. E. (1992). Bacterial meningitis in children. *Pediatric Clinics of North America, 39*(4), 651–668.

Belman, A. (1993). AIDS and the child's central nervous system. *Pediatric Clinics of North America, 39*(4), 691–714.

Campbell, L., Potter, A., Ignatius, J., Dubowitz, V., & Davies, K. (1997). Genomic variation and gene conversion in spinal muscular atrophy. *American Journal of Human Genetics, 61,* 40.

Chalk, C. M. (1997). Acquired peripheral neuropathy. *Neurologic Clinics, 15,* 501–511.

Duffner, P. K., & Cohen, M. E. (1992). Changes in the approach to central nervous system tumors in childhood. *Pediatric Clinics of North America, 39*(4), 859–877.

Durand, M. L., Calderwood, S. B., Weber, D. J., et al. (1993). Acute bacterial meningitis in adults. *New England Journal of Medicine, 328,* 21–26.

Farlow, M. R. (1998). Etiology and pathogenesis of Alzheimer's disease. *American Journal of Health-System Pharmacy, 55*(24), 26–40.

Fenichel, G. M. (1989). Myasthenia gravis. *Pediatric Annals, 18*(7), 432–438.

Frankowski, R. F. (1986). Descriptive epidemiologic studies of head injury in the United States: 1974–1984. *Advances in Psychosomatic Medicine, 16,* 153.

Gastaut, H. (1970). Clinical and electroencephalographical classification of epileptic seizures. *Epilepsia, 11,* 102.

Gay, C. T., & Bodensteiner, J. B. (1990). The floppy infant: Recent advances in the understanding of disorders affecting the neuromuscular junction. *Neurologic Clinics of North America, 8*(3), 715–725.

Griffin, M. R., Opitz, J. L., Kurland, L. T., Ebersold, M. J., & O'Fallon, W. M. (1985). Traumatic spinal cord injury in Olmsted County, Minnesota, 1935–1981. *American Journal of Epidemiology, 121,* 884.

Grob, D., Brunner, N. G., & Namba, T. (1981). The natural course of myasthenia gravis and effect of therapeutic measures. *Annals of the New York Academy of Sciences, 377,* 652.

Harding, A. K. (1993). Clinical features and classification of inherited ataxias. In A. K. Harding & T. Deufel (Eds.), *Inherited ataxias* (pp. 1–14). New York: Raven Press.

Harley, H. G., Brook, J. D., Rundle, S. A., Crow, S., Reardon, W., Buckler, A. J., Harper, P. S., Housman, D. E., & Shaw, D. J. (1992). Expansion of an unstable fragment of DNA specific to individuals with myotonic dystrophy. *Nature, 355,* 547–548.

Hertel, G., Mertens, H. G., Reuther, P., & Picker, K. (1979). The treatment of myasthenia gravis with azathioprine. In P. Dan (Ed.), *Plasmapheresis and the immunobiology of myasthenia gravis* (p. 315). New York: Houghton Mifflin.

Hickey, J. (1997). *The clinical practice of neurological and neurosurgical nursing* (4th ed.). Philadelphia: J. B. Lippincott.

Howard, J. F. (1982). Nonsteroidal immunosuppressive therapy for myasthenia gravis. *Seminars in Neurology, 2*(3), 265.

Huntington's Disease Research Collaborative Group. (1993). A novel gene containing a trinucleotide repeat that is expanded and unstable on Huntington's disease chromosomes. *Cell, 72,* 971–983.

IFNB Multiple Sclerosis Study Group. (1993). Interferon beta-1b is effective in relapsing-remitting multiple sclerosis. *Neurology, 43,* 655–661.

Jenner, P., Schapira, A. H. V., & Marsden, C. D. (1992). New insights into the cause of Parkinson's disease. *Neurology, 42,* 2241–2250.

Johns, T. R. (1982). Treatment of myasthenia gravis by thymectomy. *Seminars in Neurology, 2*(3), 271.

Jorm, A. R. & Jolley, D. (1998). The incidence of dementia. *Neurology, 51*(3), 732.

Karnes, P. S. (1998). Neurofibromatosis. A common neurocutaneous disorder. *Mayo Clinic Proceedings, 73,* 1072.

Kunkel, L. M. (1986). Analysis of deletions in DNA from patients with Becker and Duchenne muscular dystrophy. *Nature, 322,* 73–77.

Kurtzke, J. F. (1982). The current neurologic burden of illness and injury in the United States. *Neurology, 32,* 1207.

Kurtzke, J. F. (1984). Neuroepidemiology. *Annals of Neurology, 16,* 265.

Kwentus, J. A., Hart, R., Lingpon, N., Taylor, J., & Silverman, J. J. (1986). Alzheimer's disease. *American Journal of Medicine, 81,* 91.

Lang, A. E., Lozano, A. M. (1998). Parkinson's disease. *New England Journal of Medicine, 339*(16), 1134.

Martin, J. B. (1993). Molecular genetics in neurology. *Annals of Neurology, 34,* 757–773.

Masliah, E., Achim, C. L., Ge, N., DeTeresa, R., Terry, R. D., & Wiley, C. A. (1992). Spectrum of human immunodeficiency virus–associated neocortical damage. *Annals of Neurology, 32,* 321–329.

Max, W. (1993). The economic impact of Alzheimer's disease. *Neurology, 43*(Suppl. 4), 6–10.

McDonald, W. I. (1984). Multiple sclerosis: Epidemiology and HLA associations. *Annals of the New York Academy of Sciences, 436,* 109.

Miller, R. G., Sufit, R., Mitsumoto, H., et al. (1997). ALS standard of care consensus. *Neurology, 48*(Suppl. 4), 536.

Minter-Convery, M. A. (1985). Head injury. *Annual Review of Rehabilitation, 4,* 215.

Norberg, A., Asplund, K., & Waxman, H. (1987). Withdrawing feeding and withholding artificial nutrition from severely demented patients. *Western Journal of Nursing Research, 9,* 348–356.

Page, W. F., Kurtzke, J. F., Murphy, F. M., & Norman, J. E., Jr. (1993). Epidemiology of multiple sclerosis in US veterans: V. Ancestry and the risk of multiple sclerosis. *Annals of Neurology, 33,* 632–639.

Robinson, K. M. (1989). Predictors of depression among wife caregivers. *Nursing Research, 38,* 359–363.

Rosen, D. R., Siddique, T., & Patterson, D. (1993). Mutations in Cu/Zn superoxide dismutase gene are associated with familial amyotrophic lateral sclerosis. *Nature, 362,* 59–62.

Rowland, L. P. (1992). The first decade of molecular genetics in neurology: Changing clinical thought and practice. *Annals of Neurology, 32,* 206–214.

Rubenstein, E. (1985). Botulism. In E. Rubenstein & D. D. Federman (Eds.), *Scientific American medicine: Section 8, II* (p. 1). New York: Scientific American.

Rudick, R. A. (1999). Disease modifying drugs for relapsing-remitting multiple sclerosis. *Archives of Neurology, 56*(9), 1080.

Schlech, W. F., Ward, J. I., Band, J. D., Hightower, A., Fraser, D. W., & Broome, C. V. (1985). Bacterial meningitis in the United States 1978 through 1981. *JAMA, 253,* 1749.

Schneider, L. S. (1993). Clinical pharmacology of amincacridines in Alzheimer's disease. *Neurology, 43*(Suppl. 4), 564–579.

Schulman, E. A., & Silberstein, S. D. (1992). Symptomatic and prophylactic treatment of migraine and tension-type headache. *Neurology, 42*(Suppl.), 16–21.

Simon, H. B., & Swartz, M. N. (1984). Tetanus. In E. Rubenstein & D. D. Federman (Eds.), *Scientific American medicine: Section 7, V* (p. 9). New York: Scientific American.

Skoch, M. G., & Waling, A. D. (1985). Meningitis: Describing the community health problem. *American Journal of Public Health, 75,* 550.

Smith, C., & Sheinberg, L. (1985). Clinical features of multiple sclerosis. *Seminars in Neurology, 5*(2), 122.

Smith, P. F., & Darlington, C. L. (1999). Recent developments in drug therapy for multiple sclerosis. *Multiple Sclerosis, 5*(2), 110.

Storm-Mathisen, A. (1984). Epidemiology of myasthenia gravis in Norway. *Acta Neurologica Scandinavica, 70,* 274.

Tritschler, H., & Medori, R. (1993). Mitochondrial DNA alterations as a source of human disorders. *Neurology, 43,* 280–288.

Weinfeld, F. D., & Baum, H. M. (1984). The national multiple sclerosis survey: Background and economic impact. *Annals of the New York Academy of Sciences, 436,* 469.

Whitley, R. J. (1990). Viral encephalitis. *New England Journal of Medicine, 323,* 242–251.

Wilson, H. (1989). Family caregiving for a relative with Alzheimer's dementia: Coping with negative choices. *Nursing Research, 38,* 94–98.

Youmans, J. R. (1996). *Neurological surgery* (5th ed.). Philadelphia: W. B. Saunders.

Nursing Therapeutics: An Overview

MARIAH SNYDER • YUEH-HSIA TSENG
• WEN YUN CHENG

Nursing actions play a key role in the outcomes of care for persons with both acute and chronic neurologic problems. Although assessing and monitoring patients with neurologic problems are important nursing care activities, the focus of this chapter is the intervention phase of the nursing process. Patients with neurologic conditions provide unique opportunities for nurses to assess, plan, and intervene autonomously.

Only since the 1980s has nursing given attention to specific interventions that are within its realm. *Nursing Interventions* (Bulechek & McCloskey, 1985 & 1992) and *Independent Nursing Interventions* (Snyder, 1985 & 1992; Snyder & Lindquist, 1998) were the first textbooks devoted entirely to independent nursing interventions. Both texts describe the interventions, identify populations for whom the interventions can be used, and provide the scientific basis for the interventions. Considerable research, however, is needed to establish the scientific basis for the effectiveness of the majority of these interventions.

In addition to the two previously noted texts on independent nursing interventions, work on the identification and description of nursing interventions has been done within the Nursing Interventions Classification (NIC) project (McCloskey & Bulechek, 1992). The 336 interventions that have been identified, however, include both nurse-initiated and physician-initiated treatments. A notable outcome of the NIC project is to make nurses aware of the many interventions in which they engage to achieve health outcomes for clients.

According to a number of nursing leaders, it is critical that nurses give attention to the nursing elements of care (Mechanic, 1988; Mundinger, 1980; Snyder, 1993). This is particularly necessary in today's health care system, in which attention is given to the cost-effectiveness of outcomes and the contributions of each profession to these outcomes (Lang & Marek, 1992). Unless nurses can specifically describe the interventions used and document the outcomes from these interventions, the future of nursing may be in jeopardy.

The interventions presented in this chapter are divided into three sections: interventions for the patient, interventions for families and significant others, and interventions for the community. Although each type of intervention is discussed in its own section, in many instances, the intervention would also be appropriate for use with clients discussed in other sections.

INTERVENTIONS FOR THE PATIENT

Movement and Proprioceptive Interventions

Promoting mobility and preventing problems associated with immobility are frequent goals for patients with neurologic problems. Strokes, spinal cord injuries, head trauma, Parkinson's disease, and multiple sclerosis are among the conditions causing mobility problems and for which a number of these interventions would be appropriate. Movement and proprioceptive interventions also are useful in promoting wholeness, improving self-concept, and decreasing stress. These outcomes are frequently seen in nursing care plans for patients with neurologic conditions.

EXERCISE

Exercise is an intervention used often by neuroscience nurses. Active and passive range-of-motion exercises, ambulation, exercises to increase muscle strength, and general exercise to promote well-being are modes that nurses prescribe routinely. Basmajian (1978) defined therapeutic exercise as the movement of the body or its parts to relieve symptoms of pathology or improve the body's function. Exercise has been shown to improve the overall psychophysiologic functioning of persons (Kostrubala, 1984).

Exercise can be classified in several ways: as isotonic, isometric, or isokinetic and as aerobic or anaerobic. Isotonic exercise involves changing the length of muscles; range-of-motion exercises are an example of isotonic exercise. In isometric exercise, the length of the muscle does not change, but contraction of fibers occurs with increase in tension of the muscle; this form is used when a person has a limb immobilized, such as in a cast. Isokinetic contraction involves trying to contract the muscle group against graded resistance; it is used in rehabilitation to increase strength in a muscle group. Minimal oxygen is consumed in anaerobic exercise, whereas considerable oxygen is consumed in aerobic exercise. Efficient functioning of the heart, lungs, and circulatory systems is promoted through aerobic exercise.

For many patients with neurologic problems, exercise must be continued for extended periods or for a lifetime. Hurwitz (1989) found that a home exercise program for persons with Parkinson's disease resulted in improved memory, decreased nausea, lessened urinary retention, and decreased urinary incontinence. Finding ways to make exercise sessions fun so that the person will continue to practice is a challenge. Many patients find group exercises enjoyable; socialization is an added benefit from such sessions. Likewise, the family can be involved in the exercise program. Doing exercises to music, as in aerobic exercise classes, reduces boredom. Altering routines or the sequence of exercises, if possible, provides a newness to the sessions.

Although other disciplines, such as physical therapy, are often involved in the exercise program, nurses play a key role in the success of this intervention. Consistency of doing transfers, range-of-motion exercises, and mobilization is critical to the patient's recovery. Patients with cognitive impairment have difficulty learning when multiple methods are used.

MOVEMENT THERAPY

Movement therapy is closely aligned with exercise. One of the most commonly used forms of movement therapy is dance. Dance places emphasis on the holism of the human being. The person, through the body, externalizes concepts created in the mind. Movements allow people to express themselves nonverbally and to release emotions in this manner. This promotes physical relaxation and increases an awareness of self.

Laban (1984) described dance as

movement, by which I mean the interaction of effort and space through the medium of the body. Our bodily movements make shapes in space and they are charged with effort, that is energy coming from within, springing from a whole range of impulses, intentions, and desires (p. 108).

Schoop (1974) identified four goals of dance therapy:

1. To develop functional patterns for parts of the body that have been inactive or that have been misused

2. To establish unifying relationships between mind and body

3. To bring conflicting emotions into an objective physical form that allows the person to deal with them in a constructive manner

4. To assist the person in adapting to the environment

All these purposes have relevance for patients with neurologic deficits.

Dance has been used with patients with several types of neurologic conditions. Hecox, Levine, and Scott (1976) used dance with patients who had mild to moderately severe physical disabilities. Patients increased awareness of themselves and explored and used abilities that had been dormant. Adaptation of movement therapy has been used with quadriplegic patients to increase physical and mental well-being (Gerhart, 1979). Group dance sessions have been used to facilitate social interaction (Feder & Feder, 1982). Application of the intervention of dance with other patient populations is feasible.

Tai chi is a type of movement therapy that has been used for centuries in China (Downs, 1992). It is often classified as a martial art. In tai chi, a person engages in a sequence of postures, and one movement melts smoothly into the next movement. This martial art technique has been adapted for use with elderly persons or other persons who have reduced energy or restrictions in movement. Engaging in tai chi may assist persons with many chronic neurologic conditions in maintaining functional abilities. Performing tai chi movements can improve balance, flexibility, and well-being (Downs, 1992).

PROGRESSIVE MUSCLE RELAXATION

Progressive muscle relaxation is one of a number of interventions that are labeled as stress management techniques or relaxation techniques. The technique involves tensing and then relaxing successive muscle groups, with the person learning to discriminate between the feelings experienced when the muscle group is tensed and when it is relaxed (Snyder, 1992). Eventually, the person is able to bring about relaxation merely by recalling the image of the muscles being relaxed. Jacobson first publicized the technique in 1938; since that time, many variations of his technique have evolved and have been used in clinical settings.

People with neurologic problems who are faced with new situations, such as surgery, diagnostic tests, or crises, frequently exhibit high levels of stress. Persons with chronic conditions likewise have to make many adaptations. High levels of stress may occur at such times. If patients use interventions such as progressive relaxation, some of the negative effects from sustained high levels of stress may be reduced or avoided.

Brown (1977) noted that a circuitous feedback loop between the muscles and the mind operates in the stress process. The person perceives a situation as threatening; the brain sends a message to the muscles alerting them to prepare for the stressful event. The muscles tense; the proprioceptive status of the muscles is sent to the brain, which interprets this as an impending threat and sends messages to the muscles alerting them to the threat. The muscle tension thus increases. According to Brown, the scientific basis for the use of progressive relaxation in reducing tension is that fewer impulses are sent to the brain from relaxed muscles, so there are fewer stimuli to have an impact on the cerebral cortex and keep it alerted. This, in turn, decreases the cortical action on the brain stem areas that have been maintaining muscle tension.

Physiologic findings resulting from the relaxed state include decreased oxygen consumption, metabolism, respiratory rate, heart rate, muscle tension, premature ventricular contractions, and systolic and diastolic blood pressure and increased alpha waves (Jacobson, 1964). Others have found that progressive relaxation reduces overall anxiety (Borkovec, Grayson, & Cooper, 1978; Woolfolk, Lehrer, McCann, & Rooney, 1982).

To implement progressive muscle relaxation, the nurse creates a quiet environment. A comfortable chair, such as a recliner, is ideal. Tight or binding clothing is loosened, and shoes and glasses are removed. The nurse is seated so that the patient can be viewed while directions for the technique are given. Before beginning the instructions, the nurse provides the patient with the rationale for use of the technique and demonstrates the methods used to tense the various muscle groups. A typical session lasts 20 to 30 minutes.

In Bernstein and Borkovec's technique (1973), 16 muscle groups are alternately tensed and relaxed. These are identified in Figure 4–1, along with the combinations of muscles that are used as the person masters the technique. The patient is asked to tense (for approximately 7 seconds) and then relax each of the 16 groups. Encouragement and directions that assist the patient to concentrate on the muscle groups are provided by the nurse. The nurse assesses the patient to determine if relaxation is being achieved; indications of relaxation include slowed breathing, decreased body movement, and feedback from the patient (Liehstein, 1988). Electromyography may also be used to measure the degree of relaxation of specific muscle groups. To end the training session, the nurse instructs the patient to move the hands and feet and then the arms and legs and finally to open the eyes.

Four to six teaching sessions are usually needed for the patient to master the technique (Borkovec & Sides, 1979). Daily practice is a vital component of the learning process. Some people prefer practicing in the morning because it helps them relax during the day, whereas others prefer practicing in the evening because it calms them and helps promote sleep.

Although progressive relaxation appears to be a benign intervention, certain precautions are necessary. Combining several larger muscle groups (e.g.,

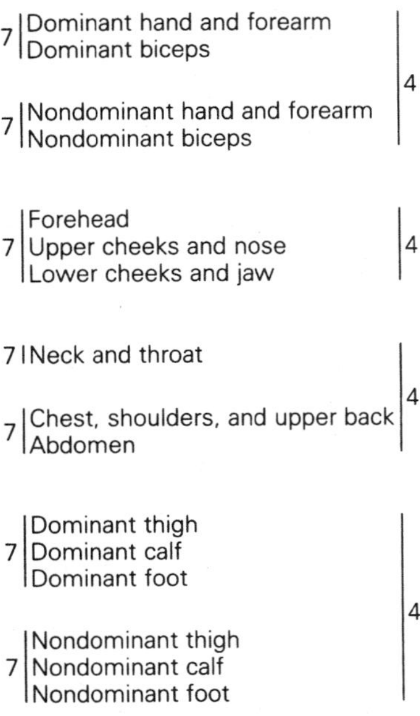

FIGURE 4–1 • Combination of 16 muscle groups in sets of seven (7) and four (4). The muscle groups can be combined into seven large sets, designated by the number 7 at the left of each group, or four larger groups, designated by the number 4 at the right of each group.

those designated 7 and 4 in Fig. 4–1) should never be done by people with hypertension. Relaxing the large muscle groups after they have been tensed often forces a large volume of blood to be returned at one time to the heart, a situation that can tax the vascular system. Some patients with chronic pain find that the technique heightens the experience of pain. Hypotension may occur after total body relaxation is attained; movement in place before rising will help alleviate this problem.

Progressive relaxation has been used with many patient populations. Of particular interest to neuroscience nurses is its use in reduction of seizures (Cabral & Scott, 1976; Whitman, Dell, Legion, Eibhlyn, & Statsinger, 1990), in reduction of hypertension (Pender, 1984), in postoperative pain reduction (Flaherty & Fitzpatrick, 1978; Wells, 1982), in reduction of headaches (Cox, Freundlich, & Meyer, 1978), in reduction of chronic pain (Greziak, 1977), and in lessening of dyspnea (Gift, Moore, & Soeken, 1992).

Cognitive Interventions

Many interventions can be placed in this category. Sensory information, imagery, decisional control, and reminiscence are examples of cognitive interventions that neuroscience nurses can implement. Although cognitive interventions can be used to attain a variety of outcomes, one common goal is to provide the patient with a sense of control over a situation. Patients with neurologic disorders often feel overwhelmed by their conditions and think that there is nothing they can do to change the situation. Cognitive interventions may help decrease these concerns and may improve functional status.

SENSORY INFORMATION

In implementing the intervention of sensory information, an objective description of what the person will see, feel, hear, smell, and taste in a specific situation is provided. Attention to objective sensations rather than to subjective feelings is needed. Findings from research studies have verified that providing the patient with sensory information before a procedure or surgery has, in many instances, decreased anxiety and promoted comfort (Johnson, Christman, & Stitt, 1985; Rice, Sieggreen, Millin, & Williams, 1988; Sime & Libera, 1985). According to Johnson et al. (1985), provision of sensory information reduces the incongruence between the expected and the experienced sensations; this results in lessened emotional responses to the threat situation.

Many patients with neurologic conditions experience heightened anxiety before and during diagnostic and surgical procedures. Sime (1976) reported that preoperative patients with high anxiety who were provided with sensory information before surgery benefited from this information. Sime and Libera (1985) found that providing sensory information to patients with low anxiety may interfere with their ability to cope. Adequate assessment of the patient is needed before giving sensory information.

To develop scripts of objective sensory information relating to specific procedures, the nurse interviews patients who have undergone the procedure. Open-ended questions are best to obtain data about experienced sensations. Only responses reported by more than 50% of the patients should be incorporated into the script to be used (Leventhal & Johnson, 1981). Preparing an audiocassette of the script helps ensure completeness and accuracy. Few scripts have been developed for neurologic diagnostic procedures and tests. Sharing of developed scripts with colleagues is encouraged.

IMAGERY

Imagery, in the form of distraction, has been used extensively by nurses. More formal use of imagery is becoming increasingly familiar to nurses. Imagery is defined as the formation of a mental representation of an object that is usually perceived only through the senses (Sodergren, 1992). Two types of imagery are commonly used: free and guided. In the former, the person formulates his or her own images, whereas in guided imagery the instructor provides specific images to the patient.

Imagery, also called visualization, can be used to achieve several types of outcomes. It is sometimes used to help the patient gain insight into the nature of a problem being experienced. Imagery may also be used to help the patient work out a solution to a problem in a symbolic manner; the nurse then helps the patient apply this to real-life situations. Adjustment to adaptations required by a neurologic condition would be one instance in which imagery could be used. The patient with decreased mobility is asked to visualize getting around at home; barriers and problems can be identified and solutions found before the patient goes home. Imaging or fantasizing has been used to lessen anxiety; providing images of quiet meadows or seashores is often used to promote relaxation.

Imagery can be used as part of a multimodal treatment program for people with chronic pain. According to Korn (1983), its success may be that imagery interferes with the processing of pain information or that imagery enhances the secretion of endorphins and thereby relieves pain. He suggested using visual or auditory images because pain is a kinesthetic experience and images of a kinesthetic nature may be blocked by the pain. McCaffery and Beebe (1989) proposed using imagery to help patients remove themselves from the pain by taking imagery vacations or enjoying other pleasant experiences through imagery.

Imagery has been used to help people relearn lost functions or skills. Korn (1983) described using imagery to help a patient who had a closed head injury to relearn swallowing mechanisms and motor skills. He also used it with a person who had suffered a stroke, to facilitate learning balance and speech and improving memory. The hypothesis for use in these situations is that through imagery the person reexperiences the psychomotor task, activating sensory and neuromuscular mechanisms similar to those involved when doing the task before the accident. This is similar to an athlete mentally rehearsing skills before an event. One nurse used imagery during exercises with a female patient who had severe weakness from Guillain-Barré syndrome. The patient was asked to visualize herself dancing while the movements were performed. Nurses can devise other creative uses for imagery.

DECISIONAL CONTROL

Most people like to be in control of their life and environment. Many illnesses interfere with a person's sense of control. A person who has had a stroke is often unable to communicate requests, to dress, to feed himself or herself, or to control when things will be done. Other neurologic conditions likewise alter a person's life and control over the surrounding environment. Decisional control is one of the three types of control described by Averill (1973). Implementing the intervention of decisional control involves providing the patient with opportunities to choose among various courses of action.

Kallio (1979) compared intensive care unit patients who had been given control over certain activities with those who had not. Patients were given choices regarding where cards, flowers, and other articles would be displayed in their rooms; when they wished to ambulate; and when they wanted their bath. The experimental group had significantly less fatigue, anxiety, anger, and depression than did the control group. The items Kallio allowed patients to control may seem minor, but giving the patients control of these activities improved their mental state. Langer and Roden (1976) reported similar findings in nursing home residents who were offered choices.

Caution must be observed when using strategies for decisional control. It has to be clear to the patients that they are allowed to make these choices but do not have to do so. The options available must be ones that the patient can control and that the nursing staff will honor. The effects of the intervention may be negated if the nurse offers options and then is unable to allow the patient to make the choice. Only a limited number of choices should be provided to the patient; large numbers of options may overwhelm patients, particularly those who have cognitive impairments.

REMINISCENCE

Reminiscence is a planned strategy to help a person recall past events, feelings, and thoughts so that the person can better adapt to the present (Snyder, 1992). Reminiscence is an adaptive mechanism for helping the person compensate for losses that have been experienced and for past inadequacies (Ryden, 1981). Although reminiscence is frequently used with older persons, its use is not restricted to this group. Reminiscence can be used to help orient people who are confused, to orient head-injury patients with short-term memory loss, to assist younger people who are facing death to reconcile past problems, and to improve feelings of self-worth (Chubon, 1980). Borden (1989), using life review with young adults with acquired immunodeficiency syndrome, reported that this intervention assisted the patients in shifting their focus from disability to concern for their health and personal growth.

In implementing reminiscence, the nurse helps the patient recall past events and experiences. Asking open-ended questions assists the patient in exploring the past. Lewis and Butler (1974) used a variety of strategies to help patients explore the past, including developing written or taped autobiographies; making pilgrimages through correspondence; and using scrapbooks, photo albums, and letters. All these strategies help persons to reconcile differences with the past, to establish a continuity with the past, and to build for the future.

Sensory Interventions

Interventions in this category may be used for stimulation, communication, healing, relearning, and stress reduction. Therapeutic touch, music, purposeful touch, massage, and biofeedback are interventions in this category that can be used with patients who have a variety of neurologic conditions.

THERAPEUTIC TOUCH

Krieger (1975) called touch the imprimatur of nursing because nurses use it so often. Therapeutic touch differs from affective touch. In therapeutic touch, energy is transmitted from one person to another for the purpose of potentiating the healing process of one who is ill or injured (Egan, 1992). Implementing the intervention consists of four steps: centering, assessment, unruffling, and transferring energy. First, the nurse relaxes and directs attention inward (centering). In assessment, the nurse moves his or her hands, held several inches away, over the patient's body to determine differences in the quality of energy flow in the patient. Unruffling is done to relieve pressure in areas where the energy is dense. The nurse's hands are moved from the area of density outward with sweeping motions. The last step, transferring energy, requires knowing the types of energy available and introducing the one appropriate to the patient. Blue energy is used to calm or sedate a patient, yellow energy is used to energize, and green energy is used to achieve harmony. To transfer energy, the nurse must intend to help the patient. Nurses wishing to use therapeutic touch should first attend a workshop on the intervention; knowledgeable use is necessary to avoid harmful effects.

Much controversy surrounds the effectiveness of therapeutic touch. However, scientific evidence supports use of therapeutic touch in specific situations (Heidt, 1981; Krieger, 1991). Therapeutic touch has been used to decrease pain, to increase energy, and to decrease anxiety. Neuroscience nurses may find therapeutic touch an appropriate intervention to use for patients with many neurologic problems, particularly persons with pain or high levels of anxiety (Krieger, 1991).

MUSIC

Music has been used since ancient times as a treatment modality for a wide variety of conditions. It has been used as an adjunct to other interventions, such as imagery, exercise, and meditation. Music therapy can involve active patient participation (playing instruments or singing) or listening to musical selections. Both methods are appropriate for use with patients with neurologic problems. Alvin (1975) delineated five elements of music: frequency (pitch), intensity, tone color, interval, and duration and rhythm. The nurse must have an understanding of these elements to choose selections for specific patient populations. Pitch refers to the number of vibrations; rapid vibrations tend to act as a stimulant, whereas a slow pitch induces relaxation. Intensity relates to the amplitude of the vibrations. A person's like or dislike of a selection is often based on the intensity of the piece. Tone color is determined by the harmony of the piece. The psychologic significance of a piece is created by the tone color. The interval creates the melody and harmony. Cultural norms greatly influence a person's perception of what is pleasant to hear. Duration and rhythm are similar; duration is the length of sounds, and rhythm is a time pattern fitted into a certain speed. The rhythm of a piece is a major determinant of when it would be most appropriately used.

Music is appropriate for various patient problems. Music has been used to create internal harmony within the person (Guzzetta, 1988). Therefore, it can be used to help orient confused patients and to decrease agitation in patients with psychiatric problems (Courtright, Johnson, Baumgartner, Jordan, & Webster, 1990). Music with a strong beat helps a person gain an awareness of self; both the auditory and the kinesthetic senses are activated. Mason (1978) used music to decrease tension in elderly people with Parkinson's disease and disseminated sclerosis; thus, persons were able to move more freely. Hoskyns (1982) used music to promote relaxation and decrease choreic movements in people with Huntington's chorea. She also found that speech improved in these patients. Herth (1978) played music during exercises for hemiplegic patients to make the exercises less boring.

Music can be used either to calm or to stimulate patients. Soothing music has been suggested for patients prone to increases in intracranial pressure. Some believe that music familiar to the patient is more calming than unfamiliar music. Selections for stimulation should have a strong beat and intensity. Sisson (1979) used "A Fifth of Beethoven" and "Theme from *Grease*" to stimulate patients who had remained comatose after head injury.

PURPOSEFUL TOUCH

Estabrooks (1989) identified three types of touch: protective, instrumental, and purposeful. An example of protective touch is when a nurse grasps a patient's hand to restrain the patient from removing a nasogastric tube. Instrumental or procedural touch is used when carrying out procedures or in assessing the patient. Purposeful touch, or intentional touch, is touch implemented with the primary purpose of helping the patient. Purposeful touch is one of the most commonly used interventions in nursing, but nurses rarely think about its use or when it can be used therapeutically. Findings from a study by Barnett (1972) showed that nurses touch patients twice as often as do other health personnel.

Examples of types of purposeful touch include handholding, soothing touch, and an application of greater intensity that acts as a stimulant. Knable (1981) found that adult patients in an intensive care unit reported very positive reactions to nurses purposefully holding their hand. Nurses noted that both appropriate timing and intent to help were necessary for the handholding to be therapeutic. Touch is one of the most primitive forms of communication; its use with people who have decreased levels of responsiveness or are confused is one means of conveying care and presence.

Walleck (1982) investigated the impact that soothing touch had on patients with increased intracranial pressure. She reported that touching the patient's hand or face resulted in a decrease in intracranial pressure. Although it is not completely clear if these findings resulted from touch or from the accompanying rest periods, the intervention holds promise as a simple means that nurses and family members can use to bring about beneficial effects.

Touch as stimulation is used early in neurorehabilitation programs (Farber, 1982). Inhibitory techniques are used first to normalize hypersensitive areas. During the inhibitory phase, constant pressure is applied to one spot for a time. Pressure is applied to the perioral region, the abdomen, and the palms of the hands. Facilitory techniques are applied after normalization is established. A moving stimulus is used in facilitory techniques; for example, the nurse moves her or his forefinger caudally from under the patient's nose to the tip of the chin. This movement is repeated a number of times with a short rest period between each repetition. Textured materials and hot and cold frequently are used in stimulation programs for head-injured patients or others recovering from coma to increase tactile stimulation.

MASSAGE

Massage produces effects on multiple body systems: integumentary, musculoskeletal, cardiovascular, lymphatic, and nervous systems. Manipulation of the skin causes it to become more supple, and sebaceous excretion is enhanced (Wakim, 1985). Massage increases or improves movement of the musculoskeletal system by reducing edema, loosening and stretching contracted tendons, and aiding in the reduction of soft-tissue adhesions. Fatigue is lessened, because massage causes a more rapid removal of waste products.

Back rubs, one form of massage, can be easily implemented to reduce anxiety and promote rest. Spending a few minutes giving a thorough back rub can do much to promote the patient's well-being. Longworth (1982) reported a reduction in muscle tension and increases in skin temperature after a 6-minute back rub. Fakouri and Jones (1987) found that back rubs produced relaxation in elderly patients.

In addition to back rubs, massage of other body parts can be used by neuroscience nurses to produce relaxation. Snyder et al. (1993) found that use of hand massage with persons who had dementia produced relaxation. When hand massage was implemented before care, a reduction in the frequency and intensity of agitated behaviors occurred (Burns et al., 1993). Hand massage may also be useful with persons who have had strokes or head injuries and who manifest agitated behaviors.

BIOFEEDBACK

Biofeedback has been used to manipulate functions related to the autonomic, peripheral, and central nervous systems. Katkin and Goldband (1980) defined biofeedback as any technique that uses instrumentation to provide a person with immediate and continuous signals concerning body functions of which the person is not normally conscious. Nurses who wish to use biofeedback need to learn about its instrumentation and the basis for the technique and to understand conditions for which it can be used.

Biofeedback has been used for treating many conditions, including strokes (Tries, 1989), epilepsy, insomnia, pain, headache, chronic lower back pain, Bell's palsy, weaning from respirator (Acosta, 1988), and urinary incontinence (Middaugh, Whitehead, Burigo, & Engel, 1989). Much of the success of the intervention depends on the person's ability to cooperate and his or her commitment to practice. Patients experience a strong sense of personal control in mastering the process and in altering certain body functions.

Other Interventions

Many other independent nursing interventions exist that neuroscience nurses can prescribe. Several of these that have particular relevance for care of patients with neurologic conditions will be discussed.

HUMOR

Cousins (1979) drew attention to the use of humor as an intervention. He attributed his recovery from an illness to laughing while watching a series of comedy movies. Humor is individualistic and even differs for the same person over time. Thus, it is important that nurses determine the type of humor a patient enjoys before implementing this intervention. Mindess, Niller, Turek, Bender, and Corbin (1984) developed a questionnaire for assessing the type of humor that a particular person enjoys.

Humor can be used to aid in establishing relationships, to help relieve anxiety and tension, to release anger and aggression, to avoid feelings that are too painful to face immediately, and to facilitate learning (Robinson, 1970). Kubie (1971) found that humor helped create a relaxed atmosphere that promoted communication. Patients who have been presented with a difficult diagnosis are often unable to discuss its impact on their lives. Many times when a patient jokes about an illness, health professionals interpret this as denial. Humor and laughter can be helpful in alleviating anxiety, fear, and anger (Gaberson, 1991; Simon, 1988). In addition, laughter produces positive physiologic effects.

Patient education is important in the nursing care of patients with neurologic deficits. Clabby (1979) reported that information taught in a humorous manner was retained to a greater extent than was information presented routinely. Humor can be added judiciously to patient teaching to enhance learning.

TIMING

Findings from the field of chronobiology are relevant for neuroscience nurses. A considerable body of research is evolving concerning the impact that the time of administration of medications has on their effectiveness. If therapeutic effects can be maximized by administration at specific times of the circadian cycle, lower dosages could be used and toxic effects and side effects could be lessened. Decreased side effects may increase patient compliance, particularly with antiepileptics, antihypertensives, and other drugs that have notable side effects. Because nurses often establish the times for administration of medications, findings from chronobiology could assist nurses in selecting the times of greatest benefit from the medication.

Blood pressure readings, temperature, and other parameters vary during the circadian cycle. Borderline hypertension, for example, may go undetected for a time if pressure readings are measured during only one time frame. Measurements at varying times are needed to obtain an accurate assessment. It is believed that intracranial pressure also varies during the circadian cycle, and this has implications for selecting when activities are performed. Astute assessments by nurses can add to the body of knowledge related to rhythms.

HOPE

Many people with neurologic problems feel devastated; life and the future hold no meaning. Miller (1991) stated that hope nurtures the person's transition from being weak and vulnerable to functioning as fully as possible. Caregivers have the opportunity to inspire the patient. Hope arises from different sources for each person. Miller suggested the following strategies to be used by nurses to inspire hope:

1. Emphasize sustaining relationships, such as mentioning the names of loved ones to the unresponsive patient.

2. Allow the patient to know if the current situation is a temporary state.

3. Radiate hope by recognizing the person's intrinsic worth and viewing the person's illness as only one facet of the individual.

4. Expand the patient's repertoire of coping mechanisms.

5. Teach reality surveillance by surveying the situation and making contingency plans.

6. Assist the patient in devising and revising goals.

7. Help the patient expand the spiritual self.

8. Help guard against despair; teach the patient to live in the moment.

Providing hope does not mean being unduly optimistic or masking the truth in dealing with the patient's condition, but rather helping the person find meaning in the present situation.

PRESENCE

Presence is closely akin to caring. Liehr (1989) defined presence as "genuinely engaging with another" (p. 7). Presence thus means being there for the patient and conveying this support to the patient. For many patients and their families, this aspect of nursing is greatly valued. To implement presence, the nurse must consciously attend to the moment by centering the self; this enables the nurse to sense the needs of the patient. According to Moch and Schaefer (1992), the nurse's attitude of openness is the most critical factor for implementation of presence. Although it is difficult to define and evaluate presence, it is one intervention that neuroscience nurses can use with all patients.

INTERVENTIONS FOR FAMILIES AND SIGNIFICANT OTHERS

Nurses have placed a major emphasis on viewing the patient as part of a family group. (The term *family* includes all persons who are significant to the patient.) Although nursing has emphasized inclusion of the family in patient care planning, in actual practice the busyness of the hospital and clinic setting has left little time for nurses to provide care to the family. This section presents interventions that have particular relevance for use with families of patients with neurologic conditions.

Groups

Establishing and conducting support groups for families fall within the realm of nursing practice. Groups have been formed to assist families of patients in crisis situations (Halm, 1990), such as with trauma or brain tumors (Wilson, 1982); to help families deal with adjustment problems, such as with post–head-injury patients (Mauss-Clum & Ryan, 1981); and to help families with a member with a chronic condition, such as multiple sclerosis, Parkinson's disease, Alzheimer's disease, or epilepsy. Specific strategies for developing support groups with families are described in Chapter 17.

Counseling

Although group sessions may be extremely helpful for many family members, individual counseling is an intervention that nurses may need to use to help some families or family members. Banks (1985) defined counseling as

> *an interactive helping process between a counselor and a client characterized by the core elements of acceptance, empathy, genuineness, and congruency. This relationship consists of a series of interactions over time in which the counselor, through a variety of active and passive techniques, focuses on the needs, problems, or feelings of the client which have interfered with the client's usual adaptive behavior (p. 105).*

Counseling in this context is formalized. Many times, the counseling provided to family members is more informal and may occur over a cup of coffee or during a walk.

The counselor needs to have a genuine interest in the client and to accept the intrinsic worth of the person. Because of this, the client senses acceptance and trusts the counselor. Caring, a key component of nursing, is felt by families as well as by patients and is one reason that families often seek out the nurse for assistance. If the nurse feels that the time demands for the assistance needed go beyond the time available, referrals to appropriate resources are necessary. Referrals to a social worker, a chaplain, or other health care personnel can be made. Frequently, however, the nurse is able to provide counseling about concerns related to the patient and the impact that these may have on the family.

Journal

Use of a journal is an intervention that may help families in dealing with either the acute or the long-term phase of a family member's illness. A journal is different from a diary in that in the journal the person records not only the event but also feelings and reflections on the event. There is an interplay between the conscious and the unconscious in journal entries. Putting feelings on paper can assist in giving insights into the problem or can serve as a catharsis for the person. Progoff (1975) believed that the journal aids the person in discovering new capabilities.

The nurse can suggest use of a journal to a family member as a means of coping with the situation. Making daily entries is suggested during times of crisis. Later, the person may make less frequent entries. It should be emphasized that what is written is private and need not be shared with anyone else. Some people find it helpful to share insights they have gained or questions that may have arisen when making entries. The nurse can offer to discuss the journal but should make the offer in such a way that the person does not feel obligated to share what has been written.

INTERVENTIONS FOR THE COMMUNITY

The scope of nursing practice has expanded to include involvement in developing policies and regulations that benefit patients, working with community organizations to improve care for people with particular illnesses or conditions, providing education about health conditions, and being an advocate for people with particular problems. Education and advocacy will be elaborated in this section.

Education

Public education is an important nursing function. The public often lacks knowledge about many neurologic conditions. People with epilepsy may be ostracized; people with multiple sclerosis may be thought to be alcoholics; employers generally do not understand the long-term effects of head injuries. These are only examples of the many areas in which nurses can provide valuable information.

Education may consist of scheduling classes for specific groups, such as firefighters or police officers; working to get public service commercials on radio or television; or preparing literature for distribution. Nurses have much knowledge about specific neurologic conditions and are able to put this information into language that the public can understand. This ability is a key ingredient in the success of an education program. Reading, marketing, and media specialists can be helpful in the development of educational materials.

Advocacy

Advocacy has existed since there have been powerless groups in need of a champion (Donahue, 1985). People within the health care system or those in need of health care often feel powerless. Nurses have acted as advocates for patients and have helped patients know their rights. The upsurge of consumerism has put added emphasis on the advocacy role. Introduction of advocates, particularly advocates for certain groups of patients, has resulted.

Advocacy for patient groups can be extended to the political realm. Working to get legislation passed that will provide health care for particular groups is critical. Many patients with neurologic problems are unable to return to their former occupation, yet they are capable of doing some work. If they work, however, they lose their welfare benefits, and the jobs they are able to obtain often do not provide sufficient remuneration on which they can live. Nurses can serve as advocates in the political arena for persons with neurologic conditions who require home care. Many families are unable to receive any assistance if they elect to care for a family member at home. Knowledge of the political process and willingness to become involved are key components of the advocacy role.

SUMMARY

Implementation of independent nursing interventions plays a role in obtaining positive outcomes for persons with neurologic conditions. Not only do the patients benefit from such interventions, but nurses also feel rewarded when selecting and using nursing interventions. Use of nursing interventions constitutes the art of nursing, the caring element of practice.

References

Acosta, F. (1988). Biofeedback and progressive relaxation in weaning the anxious patient from the ventilator: A brief report. *Heart and Lung, 17*(3), 299–301.

Alvin, J. (1975). *Music therapy.* New York: Basic Books.

Averill, J. R. (1973). Personal control over aversive stimuli and its relationship to stress. *Psychological Bulletin, 80,* 286–303.

Banks, L. J. (1985). Counseling. In G. M. Bulechek & J. C. McCloskey (Eds.), *Nursing interventions* (pp. 99–112). Philadelphia: W. B. Saunders.

Barnett, K. (1972). A survey of the current utilization of touch by health team personnel with hospitalized patients. *International Journal of Nursing Studies, 9,* 195.

Basmajian, J. (1978). *Therapeutic exercise.* Baltimore: Williams & Wilkins.

Bernstein, D., & Borkovec, T. (1973). *Progressive relaxation training.* Champaign, IL: Research Press.

Borden, W. (1989, November). Life review as a therapeutic frame in the treatment of young adults with AIDS. *Health and Social Work, 14*(4), 253–259.

Borkovec, T., Grayson, J., & Cooper, K. (1978). Treatment of general tension: Subjective and physiological effects of progressive relaxation. *Journal of Consulting and Clinical Psychology, 46,* 518.

Borkovec, T., & Sides, J. (1979). Critical procedural variables related to the physiological effects of progressive relaxation: A review. *Behaviour and Research Therapy, 17,* 119.

Brown, B. (1977). *Stress and the art of biofeedback.* New York: Bantam Books.

Bulechek, G. M., & McCloskey, J. C. (Eds.) (1985). *Nursing interventions.* Philadephia: W. B. Saunders.

Bulechek, G. M., & McCloskey, J. C. (Eds.) (1992). *Nursing interventions* (2nd ed.). Philadelphia: W. B. Saunders.

Burns, K., Cheng, W. Y., Cho, K. S., Egan, E., St. George, C., & Snyder, M. (1993). Interventions to decrease agitation behaviors associated with care. In *Proceedings of the 17th Annual Midwest Nursing Research Conference* (p. 71). Glenview, IL: Midwest Nursing Research Society.

Cabral, R., & Scott, D. (1976). Effect of two desensitization techniques, biofeedback and relaxation, on intractable epilepsy: A follow-up study. *Journal of Neurology, Neurosurgery and Psychiatry, 39,* 504.

Chubon, S. (1980). A novel approach to the process of life review. *Journal of Gerontological Nursing, 6,* 543–546.

Clabby, J. (1979). Humor: A preferred activity of the creative and humor as a facilitator of learning. *Psychology, 16,* 5.

Courtright, P., Johnson, S., Baumgartner, M. A., Jordan, M., & Webster, J. C. (1990). Dinner music: Does it affect the behavior of psychiatric inpatients? *Journal of Psychosocial Nursing, 28*(3), 37–40.

Cousins, N. (1979). *Anatomy of an illness as perceived by the patient: Reflections on healing and regeneration.* New York: W. W. Norton.

Cox, D., Freundlich, A., & Meyer, R. (1978). Differential effectiveness of electromyography feedback: Verbal relaxation instructions, and medication placebo with tension headaches. *Journal of Consulting and Clinical Psychology, 13,* 892.

Donahue, M. (1985). Advocacy. In G. M. Bulechek & J. C. McCloskey (Eds.), *Nursing interventions* (1st ed., pp. 338–352). Philadelphia: W. B. Saunders.

Downs, L. B. (1992). Tai chi. *Modern Maturity, 35*(4), 60–65.

Egan, E. C. (1992). Therapeutic touch. In M. Snyder (Ed.), *Independent nursing interventions* (2nd. ed., pp. 173–183). Albany, NY: Delmar.

Estabrooks, C. A. (1989). Touch: A nursing strategy in the intensive care unit. *Heart and Lung, 18,* 392–401.

Fakouri, C., & Jones, P. (1987). Relaxation Rx: Slow stroke back rub. *Journal of Gerontological Nursing, 13*(2), 32–35.

Farber, S. (1982). *Neurorehabilitation.* Philadelphia: W. B. Saunders.

Feder, E., & Feder, B. (1982). The therapeutic use of dance and movement. In E. Nickerson & R. O'Laughlin (Eds.), *Helping through action: Action-oriented therapies* (p. 141). Los Angeles, CA: Human Resources Development Press.

Flaherty, G., & Fitzpatrick, J. (1978). Relaxation technique to increase comfort level of postoperation patients: A preliminary study. *Nursing Research, 27,* 352.

Gaberson, R. B. (1991). The effect of humorous distraction on preoperative anxiety. *AORN Journal, 54*(6), 1258–1263.

Gerhart, K. (1979). Increasing sensory and motor stimulation for patients with quadriplegia. *Physical Therapy, 59,* 1518.

Gift, A. G., Moore, T., & Soeken, K. (1992). Relaxation to reduce dyspnea and anxiety in COPD patients. *Nursing Research, 41*(4), 242–246.

Greziak, R. (1977). Relaxation techniques in treatment of chronic pain. *Archives of Physical Medicine and Rehabilitation, 58,* 270.

Guzzetta, C. E. (1988). Music therapy: Hearing the melody of the soul. In B. Dossey, L. Kelgan, C. E. Guzzetta, & L. Kalkmeier (Eds.), *Holistic nursing: A handbook for practice* (pp. 263–288). Gaithersburg, MD: Aspen.

Halm, M. A. (1990). Effects of support groups on anxiety of family members during critical illness. *Heart and Lung, 19,* 62–71.

Hecox, B., Levine, E., & Scott, D. (1976). Dance in physical rehabilitation. *Physical Therapy, 56,* 919.

Heidt, P. (1981). Effect of therapeutic touch on anxiety level of hospitalized patients. *Nursing Research, 30,* 32–37.

Herth, K. (1978). The therapeutic use of music. *Supervisor Nurse, 9*(10), 22–23.

Hoskyns, S. (1982, June). Striking the right cord. *Nursing Mirror, 154*(2), 14–17.

Hurwitz, A. (1989). The benefit of at-home exercise regimen for ambulatory Parkinson's disease patients. *Journal of Neuroscience Nursing, 21*(3), 180–184.

Jacobson, E. (1938). *Progressive relaxation.* Chicago: University of Chicago Press.

Jacobson, E. (1964). *Anxiety and tension control: A physiologic approach.* Philadelphia: J. B. Lippincott.

Johnson, J. E., Christman, N. J., & Stitt, C. (1985). Personal control interventions: Short- and long-term effects on surgical patients. *Research in Nursing and Health, 8,* 131–145.

Kallio, J. T. (1979). *The relationship among perceived control, mood state, and perception of nursing care for a control-induced and comparison group of patients in the critical care setting.* Unpublished master's thesis, University of Minnesota, Minneapolis.

Katkin, E., & Goldband, S. (1980). Biofeedback. In F. Kanfer & A. Goldstein (Eds.), *Helping people change* (p. 537). Tarrytown, NY: Pergamon Press.

Knable, J. (1981). Handholding: One means of transcending barriers to communication. *Heart and Lung, 10,* 1106.

Korn, E. R. (1983). The use of altered states of consciousness and imagery in physical and pain rehabilitation. *Journal of Mental Imagery, 7,* 25–34.

Kostrubala, J. (1984). Running and therapy. In M. Sacks & G. Buffone (Eds.), *Running as therapy: An integrated approach* (pp. 112–124). Lincoln, NE: University of Nebraska Press.

Krieger, D. (1975). Therapeutic touch: The imprimatur of nursing. *American Journal of Nursing, 75,* 784–787.

Krieger, D. (1991). Therapeutic touch: Toward an understanding of unitary human beings. *Cooperative Connnection, 12*(1), 1, 3–4, 7.

Kubie, L. (1971). The destructive potential of humor in psychotherapy. *American Journal of Psychiatry, 127,* 861.

Laban, R. (1984). *Modern educational dance.* London, England: MacDonald Evans.

Lang, N. M., & Marek, K. D. (1992). Outcomes that reflect clinical practice. In *Patient outcomes research: Examining the effectiveness of nursing practice* (NIH Publication No. 93–3411, pp. 27–38). Washington, DC: U.S. Department of Health and Human Service.

Langer, E. J., & Rodin, J. (1976). The effects of choice and enhanced personal responsibility for the aged: A field experiment in an institutional setting. *Journal of Personality and Social Psychology, 34,* 191–196.

Levanthal, H., & Johnson, J. E. (1981). Laboratory and field experimentation: Development of a theory of self-regulation. In P. Woolridge, R. Leonard, & M. Sehmitt (Eds.), *Behavioral science and nursing theory* (pp. 189–262). St. Louis: CV Mosby.

Lewis, M., & Butler, R. (1974). Life-review therapy. *Geriatrics, 11,* 165–173.

Liehr, P. R. (1989). The core of true presence: A loving center. *Nursing Science Quarterly, 2,* 7–8.

Liehstein, K. L. (1988). *Clinical relaxation strategies.* New York: John Wiley & Sons.

Longworth, J. (1982). Psychophysiological effects of slow stroke back massage in normotensive females. *Advances in Nursing Science, 4*(4), 44–61.

Mason, C. (1978). Musical activities with elderly patients. *Physiotherapy, 64*(3), 80–82.

Mauss-Clum, N., & Ryan, M. (1981). Brain injury and the family. *Journal of Neurosurgical Nursing, 13,* 165.

McCaffery, M., & Beebe, A. (1989). *Pain: Clinical manual for nursing practice.* St. Louis: CV Mosby.

McCloskey, J. C., & Bulechek, G. M. (1992). *Nursing interventions classification (NIC).* St. Louis: Mosby–Year Book.

Mechanic, H. F. (1988). Redefining the expanded role. *Nursing Outlook, 36*(6), 280–284.

Middaugh, S., Whitehead, W., Burigo, K., & Engel, B. (1989). Biofeedback in treatment of urinary incontinence in stroke patients. *Biofeedback and Self-Regulation, 14*(1), 3–18.

Miller, J. F. (1991). *Coping with chronic illness: Overcoming powerlessness.* Philadelphia: F. A. Davis.

Mindess, H., Niller, C., Turek, J., Bender, A., & Corbin, S. (1984). *The Antioch sense of humor inventory.* Unpublished manuscript, Antioch University, Los Angeles.

Moch, S. D., & Schaefer, C. C. (1992). Presence. In M. Snyder (Ed.), *Independent nursing interventions* (2nd ed., pp. 238–243). Albany, NY: Delmar.

Mundinger, M. O. (1980). *Autonomy in nursing.* Gaithersburg, MD: Aspen.

Pender, N. (1984). Physiology responses of clients with essential hypertension to progressive muscle relaxation training. *Research in Nursing Health, 7,* 197.

Progroff, I. (1975). *At a journal workshop.* New York: Dialogue House Library.

Rice, V. H., Sieggreen, M., Millin, M., & Williams, J. (1988). Development and testing of an arteriography information intervention for stress reduction. *Heart and Lung, 17,* 23–28.

Robinson, V. (1970). Humor in nursing. In C. Carlson (Ed.), *Behavioral concepts and nursing intervention* (p. 129). Philadelphia: J. B. Lippincott.

Ryden, M. (1981). Nursing intervention in support of reminiscence. *Journal of Gerontological Nursing, 7,* 461–463.

Schoop, T. (1974). *Won't you join in the dance?* Washington, DC: National Press Books.

Sime, A. (1976). Relationship of preoperative fear, type of coping and information received about surgery to recovery from surgery. *Journal of Personality and Social Psychology, 34,* 716.

Sime, A. M., & Libera, M. B. (1985). Sensation information, self instruction and responses to dental surgery. *Research in Nursing and Health, 8,* 41.

Simon, J. M. (1988). Therapeutic humor: Who's fooling who? *Journal of Psychosocial Nursing, 26*(4), 9–12.

Sisson, R. (1979). *The effect of stimuli on patients with closed head injuries.* Unpublished doctoral dissertation, University of Texas, Austin.

Snyder, M. (Ed.) (1985). *Independent nursing interventions* (1st ed). New York: Wiley.

Snyder, M. (1992). Progressive relaxation. In M. Snyder (Ed.), *Independent nursing interventions* (2nd ed., pp. 47–62). Albany, NY: Delmar.

Snyder, M. (1993). Critique: Focus on therapeutics. *Proceedings of the Annual Forum on Doctoral Nursing Education* (pp. 83–93), St. Paul, Minnesota.

Snyder, M., Egan, E., Burns, K., Nelson, J., LaVelle, E., & Lytton, A. (1993). Interventions to decrease disruptive behaviors in persons with dementia. *Proceedings of the 17th Annual Midwest Nursing Research Conference* (p. 72). Glenview, IL: Midwest Nursing Research Society.

Snyder, M., & Lindquist, R. (1998). *Complementary/alternative therapies in nursing*. New York: Springer.

Sodergren, K. M. (1992). Guided imagery. In M. Snyder (Ed.), *Independent nursing interventions* (2nd ed., pp. 95–109). Albany, NY: Delmar.

Tries, J. (1989). EMG feedback for the treatment of upper extremity dysfunction: Can it be effective? *Biofeedback and Self-Regulation, 14*(1), 21–53.

Wakim, K. (1985). Physiologic effects of massage. In J. Basmajian (Ed.), *Manipulation, traction, and massage* (pp. 256–262). Baltimore: Williams & Wilkins.

Walleck, C. (1982). *Effect of touch on intracranial pressure*. Speech at the American Association of Neurosurgical Nurses, Honolulu, Hawaii.

Wells, N. (1982). The effect of relaxation on postoperative muscle tension and pain. *Nursing Research, 31*, 236.

Whitman, S., Dell, J., Legion, V., Eibhlyn, A., & Statsinger, J. (1990). Progressive relaxation for seizure reduction. *Epilepsy, 3*(1), 17–22.

Wilson, L. (1982). How to develop a support group for families of open heart surgery patients. *Dimensions in Critical Care Nursing, 1*, 108.

Woolfolk, R., Lehrer, P., McCann, B., & Rooney, A. (1982). Effects of progressive relaxation and meditation on cognitive and somatic manifestations of daily stress. *Behaviour Research and Therapy, 20*, 461.

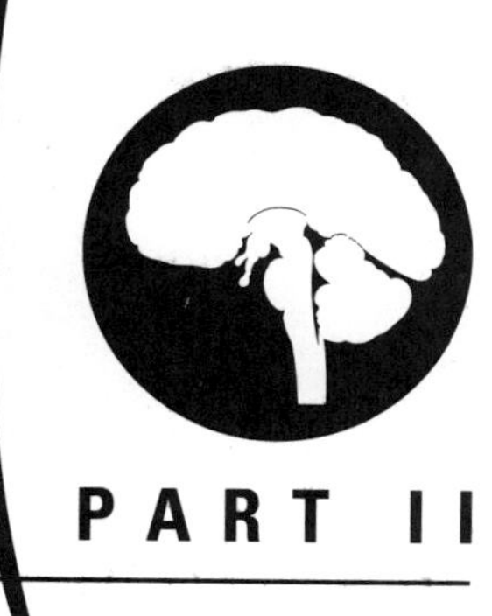

Phenomena Central to Neuroscience Nursing

CONSCIOUSNESS PHENOMENA

5 | Consciousness: An Overview

PAMELA H. MITCHELL

The classic clinical definition of consciousness—*awareness of self and of the environment*—sounds deceptively simple and leads us to think of simple dichotomies: conscious/unconscious, alert/comatose, awake/asleep. Yet, as we shall see, the concept of consciousness is far from simple and leads us from attempts to quantitate the amount of consciousness to metaphysical ventures into the relationships of mind, soul, and brain (Kushner, 1984). A definition from Webster's unabridged dictionary, although old, illustrates the breadth of concepts commonly subsumed under the "simple" term consciousness (*Webster's New International Dictionary*, 1943):

1. Awareness, especially of something within oneself
   The state or fact of being conscious with regard to something

2. Philos. That state of being which is characterized by sensation, emotion, thought or any psychical attribute whatever; mind in the broadest possible sense: that in nature which is distinguished from the physical; that form of existence which, in its full development, is able to distinguish itself from other existence
   a. An attribute or condition of soul, or of spiritual substance, not necessarily consciously
   b. Itself a spiritual substance
   c. One aspect of the real, correlative with the physical as another aspect
   d. An epiphenomenon or dependent accompaniment of physical existence
   e. That which all phenomena, physical as well as psychical, are forms, the ultimate form of existence

3. The totality of conscious states or processes connected with any single organism, as a man, or with any group of mental factors closely interrelated, as one of the personalities in the phenomenon of multiple personality; a mind; a single mental life

4. A particular consciousness or process

5. The normal state of conscious life, as distinguished from sleep, a trance, etc.

6. The upper kind of mental life, as contrasted with unconscious

Clinically, consciousness is considered in terms of responsiveness to the environment and is measured as a reflection of the integrity of the brain as a whole. Some have gone so far as to propose that consciousness is the fundamental substance of brain life (as opposed to brain death) and personhood (Kushner, 1984). This approach serves us well clinically but incorporates only a few aspects of the phenomena of consciousness, as just described. Plum and Posner (1980, p. 11) distinguished two aspects of consciousness: the content (or the sum of cognitive functions) and the arousal component. It is far easier to evaluate arousal (as responsiveness to the environment) than it is to understand and quantitate the content of self-awareness and responsiveness to self as aspects of consciousness.

For the purposes of this chapter, consciousness is considered to be composed of arousal and awareness. It is the substrate of all responsive behavior and, therefore, of the cues necessary to human interaction. Because this book is directed to clinicians caring for people with health problems stemming from the nervous system, the major focus of the chapters in this section is alteration of consciousness related to disorders and conditions of the nervous system. Alterations of consciousness related to such experiences as use of hallucinogens, psi experience, or religious transcendence, for example, are beyond the scope of this book. This chapter focuses on the arousal component of consciousness. The awareness component, as reflected in cognition, is discussed later in the book.

THE PHENOMENON: AROUSAL

Arousal is defined as being awakened from sleep, stimulated to action or to physiologic readiness for activity, or excited (*Webster's Ninth Dictionary*, 1988). Clearly, we cannot know that someone is aroused unless that person exhibits some behavior that communicates arousal to us. Therefore, a more clinically useful definition of arousal is "excitation of behavior by internal or external stimuli" (Daube & Sandok, 1986). Therefore, clinical estimates of arousal are estimates of externally observable responsive behavior. Such behaviors may include simple responses, such as eye opening, head turning, and restless movements, or more complex responses, such as obeying commands or answering questions.

Behaviors that manifest arousal may be characterized as those indicating (1) nonspecific alerting and (2) attention to specific environmental stimuli. *Nonspecific alerting* behaviors are elicited by any novel, uncertain, incongruous, or painful stimulus both in normal humans and animals and in those with pathologic depression of alertness. Nonspecific alerting is characterized by orienting responses (head turning to the source of the stimulus, increased muscle tone, sympathetic nervous system responses preparatory to defense or flight) and by electroencephalogram changes such as decreased amplitude and higher frequency (Magoun, 1963; Norsell, 1986). In normal humans and animals, familiarity with a stimulus or repetition of the stimulus will diminish the nonspecific alerting response, and the person will either ignore the stimulus if it is irrelevant or attend to only its particular properties. This ability to tune out or habituate to such a stimulus is believed to require some degree of higher cortical inhibition (Gulbranson, Kristiansen, & Ursin, 1972).

The second component of arousal behaviors—attention to specific stimuli—has been termed *vigilance* by von Cramon (1977). He considered vigilance to have two components: behavioral arousal, or the nonspecific susceptibility to stimuli described earlier, and reactivity to the specific stimulus. This specific reactivity is characterized behaviorally by directional movements of the body and by obeying of simple and complex commands. These behavioral components of arousal form the basis for much of our clinical evaluation of degree of consciousness.

Neuroanatomic Basis of Arousal

Our knowledge of the neuroanatomic basis for arousal stems from extensive study of animals with respect to brain structures associated with changes in arousal behavior. Our knowledge of clinical states associated with altered arousal is a result of observation of human injury and disease, complemented by lesion studies in animals.

It is useful to consider the phenomenon of arousal as dependent on an integrated neural system, rather than on isolated consciousness centers. In order for behavior to occur that allows us to infer arousal, information must be received through the sensory structures, perceived in the reticular activating system (RAS), and acted on by the language and motor systems. A defect in any portion of this overall system will alter the behavioral output that we call arousal.

This systemic view of consciousness becomes important when we consider the dangers of inferring lack of arousal or consciousness in persons for whom brain processing is intact but sensory input or motor output is altered. It becomes necessary to use a wide range of sensory stimuli as input and to recognize special cases in which the absence of motor output should not be accepted as evidence for absence of arousal or content of consciousness (see Assessing Arousal and Awareness in this chapter for examples).

INPUT

We receive information constantly from both our external and our internal environments. Visual, auditory, tactile, and thermal stimuli are examples of the kind of information we receive from the external world. The sensory systems for vision, hearing, touch, and temperature sensing serve as transducers of physical information contained in those stimuli to transmit them to the central nervous system (CNS) for processing.

Internal stimuli consist of the sensations from viscera, muscles and joints, heartbeat, and respiration, for example. These physical signals are also transmitted from the peripheral nervous system to the CNS for processing.

PROCESSING

Some sensory information is processed at the segment of the spinal cord where it enters. This processing is part of the reflex arc systems that regulate homeostasis or vegetative functions, such as muscle tension, among other functions. However, the information that is translated into observable arousal must reach the RAS to be processed in such a way as to produce the behaviors we term arousal.

The RAS is a physiologic concept rather than a discrete, dissectible structure. It consists of a reticular core and its projections. The reticular core is a diffuse collection of neurons extending from the medulla headward toward the midbrain (Fig. 5–1). The projections of this core ascend to the structures that activate behavioral arousal. Medially, the reticular core projects fibers to

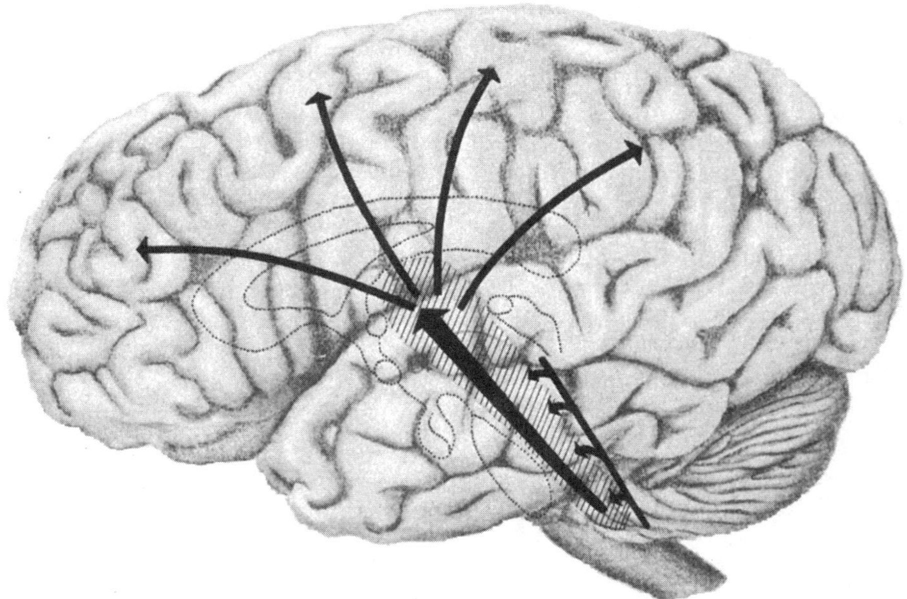

FIGURE 5–1 • Reticular activating system. The thick arrow represents the reticular formation, with diffuse projections to the cortex indicated by thin arrows. Sensory input to the reticular formation is indicated by connected small arrows. (From Mitchell, P. H., Cammermeyer, M., Ozuna, J., & Woods, N. F. (1984). *Neurological assessment for nursing practice.* New York: Appleton and Lange.)

the thalamus and from the thalamus to the cerebral cortex. Presumably, this set of projections serves the integration of the cognitive or content aspects of arousal. Laterally, the fibers from the reticular core project to the hypothalamus and from there to the autonomic nervous system and the motor reflex systems. These systems serve the more basic or vegetative responses seen in arousal.

Our understanding of the key role of the RAS in the maintenance of arousal stems from a series of investigations beginning in the late 1930s. In 1937, Bremer (1977) found that a very small area or core of the midbrain was critical for maintenance of the awake state in the cat. This area was subsequently named the reticular core. If a lesion was made in the cat's midbrain (upper portion of the core), the animal remained in persistent sleep. If, however, the lesion was made in the midpons, the animal remained persistently awake. Lesions in the medulla allowed normal cycling between asleep and awake. These findings suggested to Bremer that animals (and presumably people) fall asleep unless sensory stimuli from the body travel through the brain stem to reach the cerebral hemispheres. Moruzzi and Magoun's later discovery that electrical stimulation of midbrain reticular formation could activate arousal clearly showed arousal to be a nonspecific but active process, dependent not only on the reticular core but also on the ascending projection fibers linking midbrain to thalamus and cortex (Moruzzi & Magoun, 1949). The term *ascending reticular activating system* (ARAS) was derived from their work.

In humans, the smallest lesions capable of causing impaired arousal occur in the brain stem central area (paramedian tegmentum), often from hemorrhage or infarction in the pons or midbrain. Isolated lesions of the medulla have not been reported to impair arousal. Diencephalic lesions from stroke or traumatic injury can also impair arousal, particularly in bilateral paramedian areas of the hypothalamus and subthalamus. Lesions in a cerebral hemisphere generally do not impair consciousness unless both hemispheres are involved. Plum and Posner (1980), however, cited several cases of greater clouding of consciousness with massive left hemisphere infarct, compared with similar right hemisphere lesions (Daube & Sandok, 1986). More recent ability to correlate consciousness with computed tomographic and magnetic resonance imaging studies has shown that lateral brain shift of as little as 3 to 4 mm is associated with decreasing levels of arousal in acute mass lesions (Reich et al., 1993; Ropper, 1986; Ross, Olsen, Ross, Andrews, & Pitts, 1989). Such brain shifts can occur with brain swelling or rapid expansion of a mass lesion such as tumor, infarct, or hemorrhage. More chronic mass lesions (such as with slowly growing tumors or obstruction of cerebrospinal fluid pathways) do not show such clear correlation of clinical alteration in consciousness or other neurologic signs with lateral or downward brain shift. In such chronic mass lesions, studies often showed anatomic herniation well before the appearance of clinical signs (Feldmann et al., 1988; Reich et al., 1993). These studies suggest that unilateral cerebral lesions can indeed alter consciousness if they are of rapid onset and cause lateral shift of brain structures in the upper reticular system or downward displacement of hemisphere onto brain stem structures. The various types of lesions that impair consciousness are shown in Figure 5–2.

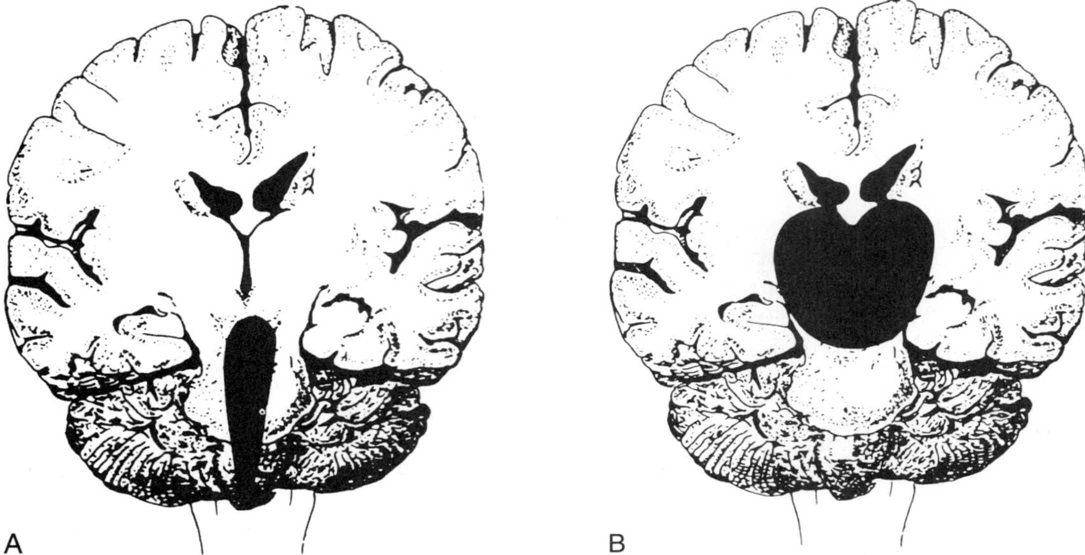

FIGURE 5–2 • Diencephalic and brain stem areas serving consciousness. *A*, The smallest lesions that can alter consciousness, those in the reticular core of the brain stem (shown in black). *B*, Diencephalic lesions that may impair consciousness (shown in black). (From Mitchell, P. H., Cammermeyer, M., Ozuna, J., & Woods, N. F. (1984). *Neurological assessment for nursing practice.* New York: Appleton and Lange.)

Developmental Variations in Processing. As mammals and humans develop from fetus to newborn to adult, the ability of the nervous system to integrate multiple stimuli increases. Newborns, for example, require more stimulus for arousal from sleep than do adults and may become more behaviorally aroused if presented with too many stimuli when awake. These variations in arousal are defined as behavioral states in infants and consist of deep sleep, light sleep, drowsy, quiet alert, active alert, and crying (Brazelton, 1984). Operational definitions of these states are presented in Table 5–1. In infants, knowing the initial behavioral state is an important condition for evaluating subsequent behavior (Apkarian, Mirmiran, & Tijssen, 1991; Brazelton, 1984). Ability to modulate the behavioral state increases with nervous system maturity. Similarly, parents' assessments of subtle changes in the behavioral state of their infant or child are an important clue to change in arousability that may not yet be detectable by clinical assessment tools. Brain damage can alter this feedback modulation, making a chronologically mature individual respond to external stimuli much as a more neurologically immature person might.

OUTPUT

Fibers from the reticular core pass through the diencephalon to end diffusely at the cerebral cortex. Not only do RAS fibers project to the cortex, presumably

TABLE 5–1 • INFANT BEHAVIORAL AROUSAL STATES

Behavioral State	Behavioral Indicators
Sleep states	
1. Deep sleep	• Regular breathing • Eyes closed, no eye movement • No spontaneous activity (except startles or regular jerky movement) • Startles produced by external stimuli, with some delay • Rapid suppression of startles
2. Light sleep	• Irregular respirations • Eyes closed, often with rapid eye movements • Possible brief eye opening • Low activity, random movements and startles • Smoother movements than in state 1
Awake states	
3. Drowsy, semidoze	• Eyes open (heavy lidded) or closed (eyelids fluttering) • Variable activity level: mild startles, reaction to sensory stimuli with delay, state change after stimulation • Smooth movements • Dazed look, as if not "available"
4. Quiet alert	• Bright look • Attention focusing on source of stimulation • Some delay in response • Minimal motor activity
5. Active alert	• Eyes open • Considerable motor activity, spontaneous startles • Reaction to stimuli difficult to identify discretely because of general motor activity • Brief fussy vocalizations
6. Crying	• Intense crying that is difficult to interfere with by stimulation • High motor activity

Adapted from Brazelton, T. B. (1984). *Neonatal behavioral assessment scale* (2nd ed., p. 19). Philadelphia: J. B. Lippincott.

stimulating response to arousing stimuli, but cortical fibers project back to the RAS. It is assumed that this cortical feedback is part of the mammalian ability to modulate arousal responses depending on the psychologic qualities or interpretation of the meaning of the stimulus at the specific areas of the cerebral cortex that serve movement, language, and integrated thought.

Further projections within the diencephalon pass through hypothalamic structures that serve the autonomic nervous system and then project onto the basal forebrain and the limbic system, which serves basic emotional response. Because of the diffuse innervation of the limbic cortex and neocortex, we can infer that pathways exist for behavioral output of three types: movement, language, and vegetative response. The assessment and inference of this behavior are discussed under Assessing Arousal and Awareness.

Neurochemical Basis of Arousal

The anatomic structures described provide a framework by which information can travel from one area of the CNS to another. The transmission of information from the ascending RAS to the cortex and back, however, requires chemical messengers to alter the membrane potential of neurons and thus stimulate or inhibit the action potentials that actually transmit information in the CNS. Two types of chemical substances are required to maintain consciousness and arousal. First are the basic metabolic substrates necessary for cellular function of neurons. Glucose, enzymatic cofactors, and oxygen are the elements essential for synthesis of adenosine triphosphate (ATP), the essential energy supply of the neuron. Second are the neurotransmitters elaborated and used by the ARAS and its projections. These neurotransmitters are believed to be acetylcholine, monoamines, glutamate, and gamma-aminobutyric acid (GABA) (Kuhar, De-Souza, & Unnerstall, 1986; Plum & Posner, 1980, p. 22; Yamamoto, 1988).

METABOLIC SUBSTRATES

Neurons, like all cells, require nutrients and enzymes to catalyze the basic chemical reactions necessary to maintain cellular respiration and energy production. These basic processes of energy production and cellular respiration underlie the specific functions of neurons and glial cells in the CNS. Neurons must maintain electrochemical gradients at the cell membrane to generate action potentials in the transmission of information, to manufacture and recover chemical neurotransmitters, to manufacture cytoplasm, and to repair themselves through protein and lipid synthesis. Glial cells (oligodendroglia and astrocytes) manufacture myelin, regulate the ionic environment of the neurons, and maintain the capillary endothelial blood-brain barrier.

The energy requirements of these functions exceed those of any other organ function of the body and depend entirely on a constant supply of glucose and oxygen. In addition to glucose and oxygen, the brain requires enzymatic cofactors, such as the B vitamins (thiamine, pyridoxine, cyanocobalamin, and niacin), to catalyze energy production through cellular respiration. Unlike cells of other organs of the body, the brain cells do not store alternative energy sources, and alternate energy sources, such as fatty acids, cannot pass through the capillary endothelium into the brain tissue. Loss of these metabolic substrates, which might result from such disorders or clinical situations as hypoglycemia, hypoxia, or cofactor deficiency, can lead to general disorders of arousal as the result of generalized brain dysfunction. Brain injury from trauma, for example, leads to a cascading set of changes initiated by microhemorrhage and hypoxia-ischemia that ultimately lead to failure of cells to maintain energy through oxidative phosphorylation to produce ATP in focal and general areas of the brain. Hypoxia-ischemia results in anaerobic metabolism (glycolysis), which is inadequate to meet the energy needs of the brain. ATP cannot then be renewed sufficiently to maintain the cellular machinery, and the cellular ion pump fails, disrupting the electrochemical gradient at the cell membrane and thus the cellular signaling ability. Free fatty acids and byproducts of prostaglandin breakdown accumulate, including oxygen free radicals (oxygen molecules with an uneven number of electrons). The latter attack the lipid portion of the cell membrane itself and contribute to lasting damage to the cell wall. Liberation of free iron from microhemorrhage is postulated to enhance the liberation of free radicals. The end result of this injury cascade of events is release of vasoactive substances that spread the area of ischemia beyond the initial injury through vasospasm and instability or destruction of the cell membrane, leading to cell malfunction or cell death. The studies of calcium channel blockers (e.g., nimodipine), 21-aminosteroids (e.g., tirilazad) and buffering agents (e.g., tromethamine) in acute brain injury were attempts to prevent the spread of hypoxic-ischemic injury beyond the initial focus (Hall, 1989; Marmarou, 1992; Murdoch & Hall, 1990; Vannucci, 1990).

CENTRAL NEUROTRANSMITTERS

The number of known and putative neurotransmitters in the CNS continues to grow immensely. Research techniques allow mapping of nerve fibers served by the monoamine transmitters, detection of enzymes that serve the cholinergic system, and dynamic mapping of metabolic activity of transmitter systems (Kuhar et al., 1986; Yamamoto, 1988).

Acetylcholine is found widely throughout the CNS. It is difficult to map precisely the location and fibers for this transmitter because its presence must be inferred from the activity of its enzymatic activators or inactivators or from the change in behavioral or neurophysiologic activity when cholinergic drugs or their antagonists are given systemically. A variety of indirect evidence supports the existence of cholinergic neuronal fiber systems that correspond to the reticular formation–thalamic projections and to the reticular formation–basal forebrain pathways. These pathways receive fibers from the monoamine pathways in the locus ceruleus in the brain stem and project diffusely to the parietal and frontal cortex (Bartus, Dean, Beer, & Lippa, 1982; Shute & Lewis, 1967; Whitehouse, Price, Struble, Clark, & Coyle, 1982). Pontine cholinergic activity is associated with profound inhibition of postural motor reflexes and eye opening in experimental models (Katayama, Young, Dunbar, & Hayes, 1988).

The monoamines found in the brain (norepinephrine, dopamine, and serotonin) play an important role in consciousness through their function in regulating waking and sleeping. Because a substantial number of people in long-term states of decreased arousal (persistent vegetative states) appear to recover normal sleep-wake cycles, it is clear that sleep-wake components of consciousness are at least partly independent of systems that maintain high-level vigilance behavioral arousal. Given the anatomic connections between the brain stem monoamine pathways and the forebrain cholinergic pathways, it is possible that disorders that result in persistent vegetative states with preserved sleep-wake cycles represent a disconnection of two components of an integrated consciousness system. Observations that increased levels of norepinephrine and serotonin metabolites correlate with failure to recover from coma in a variety of traumatic and metabolically induced coma states suggest a major role for monoamines, particularly norepinephrine and serotonin, in mediating arousal in brain injury (Ali, Jairaj, Newport, Lipe, & Slikker, 1990; Bergeron, Reader, Layrargues, & Butterworth, 1989; Markianos, Seretis, Kotsou, Baltas, & Sacharogiannis, 1992).

GABA is an inhibitory neurotransmitter found widely throughout the brain. A relative decrease in GABA has been implicated in generalized seizures, which are characterized by loss of consciousness with excessive firing of neurons in the RAS (Bosman, Van Den Buijs, De Haan, Maas, & Chamuleau, 1991). In addition, some metabolically induced alterations in consciousness, such as hepatic encephalopathy, are associated with increased GABA (inhibitory transmitter) and decreased glutamate (excitatory transmitter) activity. At least temporary restoration in consciousness has been achieved in animal models of hepatic encephalopathy with administration of benzodiazepine receptor inverse agonists, drugs that reduce the ability of GABA to bind to receptors presumably important in decreasing wakefulness (Bosman et al., 1991).

Alterations in Arousal

Sleep as described more fully in Chapter 8 represents a normal alteration in arousal and consciousness. As noted previously, normal cycles of sleep and waking can exist in people who have intact brain stems yet have injuries that impair their ability to respond to stimuli from the environment; that is, people in persistent vegetative states. Variants of normal sleep that represent pathologic alterations in arousal and their attendant nursing diagnoses are discussed in Chapter 8.

ABNORMAL ALTERATIONS IN AROUSAL

Hypoarousal or hyperarousal can result from three main sources:

1. Damage to structures of the ARAS and its projections—this includes destructive lesions and mass lesions as well as diffuse damage to connecting structures.

2. Loss of metabolic substrates for brain metabolism—this may be related to oxygen deprivation, hypoglycemia, or other metabolic disorders.

3. Disruption of neurotransmitter synthesis, uptake, or release—this is generally related to seizures or drugs that affect neurotransmitters.

Resulting conditions may involve more than one source; for example, a person with a diffuse axonal brain injury may become hypoglycemic or hypoxic. Table

5–2 summarizes disorders that impair consciousness (arousal) in these three categories. Nursing diagnoses that may accompany these disorders are considered in subsequent chapters.

ASSESSING AROUSAL AND AWARENESS

Arousability (susceptibility to stimuli) and attention (reactivity to stimuli) are the two dimensions of the assessment of *vigilance* as described by von Cramon (1977). Although many tools and terminologies have been developed in an attempt to quantify consciousness, all implicitly contain measurement of the amount and kind of stimulus required and the nature of the response to the stimulus. Initially, one observes the person's response to general environmental stimuli and to specific verbal stimuli. Only if no response to auditory stimuli

TABLE 5–2 • CLASSIFICATION OF DISORDERS THAT IMPAIR AROUSAL

Damage to Structures

Destructive lesions

- Thalamic lesions
- Pontine (other brain stem) lesions
- Massive hemispheric infarct

Mass lesions

- Hemorrhage (subdural, epidural, intracerebral, pituitary, cerebellar)
- Tumors (abscesses, supratentorial, cerebellar)

Diffuse damage to connecting structures

- Head injury with diffuse axonal injury

Loss or Alteration in Brain Metabolites

Oxygen deprivation

- Hypoxia (pulmonary disease, anemia, carbon monoxide poisoning, inadequate atmospheric oxygen)
- Ischemia (decreased cardiac output, hypovolemic shock, small vessel occlusion)

Hypoglycemia

- Acid-base and ion abnormalities (acidosis, alkalosis, water intoxication, hypernatremia)
- Cofactor deficiency (thiamine, niacin, folic acid)
- Systemic disorders—the toxic metabolites (uremia, hepatic encephalopathy, Reye's syndrome)

Disruption of Neurotransmitters Central to Arousal

- Poisons (barbiturates, ethanol, opiates, street drugs)
- Anticholinergic excess (scopolamine)
- Psychotropic drugs (antihistamine excess)
- Generalized seizures

Adapted from Plum, F., & Posner, J. (1980). *The diagnosis of stupor and coma* (3rd ed.). Philadelphia: F. A. Davis.

occurs is the use of painful stimuli appropriate. The kinds of responses to be observed include eye opening, movement of the head or body toward the stimulus, verbalizations, and more complex responses, such as obeying commands.

At a minimum, one attempts to distinguish the patient who is comatose (does not open the eyes) from the patient who is awake (opens the eyes) and the patient who is both awake and aware (opens the eyes and follows commands) (Reich et al., 1993). Such a minimal distinction, however, does not allow the clinician to detect subtle changes in arousal status or to determine differences in awareness or vigilance functions of the many patients who are awake and aware but vary in the degree to which they can sustain self-care activity. A variety of coma tools and cognitive assessment tools have been developed in an attempt to grade more accurately a patient's progress from truly comatose to fully conscious.

The Glasgow Coma Scale (GCS) is the best known of the scales that attempt to quantitate arousability in the acute and critical care settings (Mitchell, Ozuna, & Bolles, 1983; Teasdale, 1975; Teasdale & Galbraith, 1975; Teasdale & Jennett, 1974; Teasdale, Knill-Jones, & Van de Sande, 1978). It was developed to standardize initial observations of acutely head-injured persons in an international study of the consequences of head injury. It is one of the few coma scales for which testing of interrater reliability has been reported (Murray et al., 1993). As with all observational tools, specific training is required to achieve a high degree of reliability among observers.

Three parameters of behavioral response observed in the GCS are eye opening, verbalization, and movement (Table 5–3). The initial stimulus is the examiner's voice (asking the patient to obey a command); if no response occurs, fingertip or supraorbital pressure is applied as a painful stimulus. In each category, the patient's best response is recorded. The developers of the GCS found that observers could better agree on the best of a series of responses than on the worst. The scoring system ranges from a score of 3 (no response in any category) to a score of 15 (response in all categories or awake and aware). Numerous clinical studies have supported the interpretation that the lower the GCS score the deeper the coma and the higher the associated mortality and morbidity. Clearly, such situations as endotracheal intubation, administration of paralyzing agents with ventilator therapy, and aphasia alter the ability to accurately score and interpret the GCS.

The GCS was developed primarily to predict outcome from head injury based on initial severity of neurologic injury. Although it is reasonably specific as a predictor of outcome in such injury (Murray et al., 1993), there are valid criticisms of its relative insensitivity to significant clinical change in the early postinjury period as well as its insensitivity to subtle change in function in severely injured patients who are recovering (Crosby & Parsons, 1989; Price, 1986; Stewart-Amidei, 1991). The developers of the GCS have emphasized the need to incorporate neurologic evaluation of brain stem and overall motor function with use of the GCS in the acute phase. The Glasgow-Liege Scale (GLS) is a variant of the GCS that does incorporate more extensive neurologic evaluation. It has also undergone testing of the reproducibility of multiple

TABLE 5–3 • GLASGOW-LIEGE SCALE SCORING*

Parameter	Observation	Score
Brain stem reflexes	Fronto-orbicular	5
	Vertical oculovestibular	4
	Pupillary light	3
	Horizontal oculovestibular	2
	Oculocardiac	1
	No response	0
Eye opening	Spontaneously	4
	To voice	3
	To pain	2
	None	1
Best verbal response	Oriented	5
	Confused	4
	Inappropriate words	3
	Incomprehensible sounds	2
	None	1
Best motor response	Obeys commands	6
	Localizes	5
	Flexion withdrawal	4
	Abnormal flexion	3
	Abnormal extension	2
	None	1

Range of possible scores for the Glasgow-Liege combination is from 3 to 30 (from no response in any category to maximal response in all categories, including all reflexes present).

* The Liege addition to the Glasgow Coma Scale scores brain stem reflexes.
Adapted from Born, J. D. (1987). Assessment of impaired consciousness. *Acta Anaesthesiologica Belgica, 38,* 381–386; Born, J. D., Hans, P., Albert, A., & Bonnal, J. (1987). Interobserver agreement in assessment of motor response and brain stem reflexes. *Neurosurgery, 20,* 513–517.

observers, showing that areas of interrater disagreement are greatest in the motor and brain stem reflex areas (Born, 1987; Born, Hans, Albert, & Bonnal, 1987). The GLS essentially adds a quantification of brain stem reflexes to the GCS; researchers claim better prediction of ultimate outcome from head injury when the brain stem reflexes are included in the total score (Born, 1987; Born, Hans, Albert, & Bonnal, 1987). The brain stem reflexes scored are the following:

1. Fronto-orbicular—also called the glabellar reflex; the reflex is present when the orbicularis oculi muscle contracts with percussion of the glabella.

2. Vertical oculocephalic or oculovestibular—also called the cold caloric test; rapid flexion and extension of the neck, or iced-water irrigation of the external auditory canal if the patient has suspected cervical spinal cord injury; a positive response consists of vertical deviation or movement of at least one eye; both eyes usually move.

3. Pupillary light reflex—this is scored if the pupil in at least one eye constricts on exposure to light.

4. Horizontal oculocephalic or oculovestibular—doll's eye test using rapid lateral rotation of the head (in the absence of cervical spine injury); a positive response is the lateral deviation of at least one eye, but both eyes should move.

5. Oculocardiac reflex—this is the slowing of the heart rate with pressure on the eyeball.

Scores on the GCS and GLS are shown in Table 5–3.

Other scales that incorporate evaluation of consciousness and general neurologic function include the Glasgow-Pittsburgh Coma Score (Teasdale et al., 1988), the Pinderfield Scale (Price, 1986; Williams, 1992), the Edinburgh-2 Coma Scale (Sugiura, Muraoka, Chishiki, & Baba, 1983), the Clinical Neurological Assessment (CNA) tool (Crosby & Parsons, 1989), and pediatric versions of the GCS and Pinderfield scales (Reilly, Simpson, Sprod, & Thomas, 1988; Williams, 1992).

The Reaction Level Scale (RLS85) was developed for assessment of arousal in acute injury and differs from the GCS in that the RLS85 has eight mutually exclusive categories based on behavioral manifestations of arousal (Table 5–4) (Starmark, Stalhammar, & Holmgren, 1988). Thus one knows immediately from

TABLE 5–4 • REACTION LEVEL SCALE (RLS85)

Level	Label	Operational Description of Behavior
1	Alert	Oriented; if intubated reacts quickly, if sleeping arouses quickly
2	Drowsy or confused	Responds to light stimuli; delayed reactions; may be disoriented to time and place
3	Very drowsy or confused	Responds to strong stimuli such as loud noise, shaking, or pain; may respond verbally or by attempting eye contact, warding off pain, or obeying commands
4	Unconscious, localizes	On painful stimulation of fingertips, other hand moves to push stimuli away
5	Unconscious, withdraws	On painful stimulation of fingertips, pulls stimulated hand away
6	Unconscious, flexion response	Does not localize or withdraw, flexes arms and wrists to stimuli
7	Unconscious, extension response	Does not localize or withdraw, arms and legs extend to stimuli (if both flexion and extension are noted, best response is recorded)
8	Unconscious, no response to pain	With repeated strong stimulation, no movement noted in face, arms, or legs

Adapted from Starmark, J. E., Stalhammar, D., & Holmgren, E. (1988). The Reaction Level Scale (RLS85): Manual and guidelines. *Acta Neurochirurgica, 91,* 12–20; Stewart-Amidei, C. (1991). Assessing the comatose patient in the intensive care unit. *AANN Clinical Issues in Critical Care Nursing, 2*(4), 613–622.

the score what behaviors the patient is manifesting, whereas in the GCS several possible combinations of behavior might yield the same score. International comparisons have shown the RLS85 to correlate highly, to achieve higher agreement among examiners, and to have greater ability to classify all patients than is true with the GCS (Stalhammar et al., 1988; Tesseris, Pantazidis, Routsi, & Fragoulakis, 1991). On the basis of this evidence, the RLS85 was recommended to replace the GCS in Sweden (Starmark et al., 1988).

All the scales used as prognostic indicators in acute brain injury are relatively insensitive to the subtleties of changing arousal and behavioral response seen in the recovering patient. The CNA tool (Crosby & Parsons, 1989), the Munich Coma Scale (MCS) (Brinkman, von Cramon, & Schulte, 1976), the MCS Scale of Reactivity (Smith, Smith, & Speirs, 1986), and the Rancho Los Amigos Levels of Cognitive Functioning Scale (Malkmus, Booth, & Kodimer, 1980) all attempt to quantify these more complex and subtle behaviors over time.

The MCS has been used more in research than for clinical monitoring (Schuri & von Cramon, 1979, 1980, 1981) but has several attractive features in that it grades the type of stimulus used and is more responsive to variations in motor response than is the GCS. This ability to detect more subtle change is desirable when patients with altered arousal become more stable with respect to physiologic function but are still in a state of decreased arousal. Some of the original MCS stimuli, such as brief electric shock or use of a loud siren, are not clinically acceptable but have been appropriately replaced in one adaptation by stimuli such as bells, a telephone's ring, and pinpricks (Smith et al., 1986). More complex and potentially variable stimuli and more complex behavioral indicators of arousal, however, are likely to require more training on the part of observers to consistently grade responses. The MCS Scale of Reactivity is shown in Table 5–5.

The Rancho Los Amigos Levels of Cognitive Functioning Scale has also been used extensively to evaluate levels of awareness in patients who are awake but have varying levels of awareness (Malkmus, 1980). Dowling has shown that a reasonably high level of interrater consistency occurs with this tool, even in untrained individuals (Dowling, 1985). Levels 3 and 4 yielded the most ambiguous results, perhaps because study participants overinterpreted behavior from videotaped stimuli. This scale is reproduced in Chapter 7.

SUMMARY

Consciousness is a complex concept, comprising arousal and self-awareness. The anatomic substrate for arousal consists of brain stem reticular formation, input from sensory systems, and projections to the thalamus, hypothalamus, limbic system, and neocortex. Damage to these structures, loss of substrates necessary for brain metabolism, or interference with the function of CNS neurotransmitters can all act separately or together to alter arousal. Arousal can be detected only by observing behavioral indicators of the aroused awakened state, such as eye opening, verbalization, and simple to complex movements.

TABLE 5–5 • MUNICH COMA SCALE

Scale of Susceptibility to Stimulation	
MCS stimulus	**Clinical stimuli used by Smith et al**
Electrical (1–10 mA shock)	Olfactory (ammonia, fruit, vinegar)
Tactile (2 cm nylon hair)	Tactile (sharp, dull, varying texture)
Acoustic (90 dB siren)	Acoustic (bell, car sounds, telephone)
Optical (4000 lux flashlight)	Visual (lights, mirrors)
	Kinesthetic (range of motion)
MCS Scale of Reactivity	
Category of reactivity	**Response definition**
1	Any body movement; movement of head without clear-cut directional component in relation to stimulus
2	Any orofacial movements (e.g., frowning), single or repeated contraction of eyelids with closed or open eyes; any movements of perioral muscles, of tongue, or of muscles for swallowing
3	Unequivocal turning of head toward or away from stimulus; opening of eyes or state of open eyes
4	Unequivocal looking at stimulus or examiner; understandable verbal utterance

Adapted from Brinkman, R., von Cramon, D., & Schultz, H. (1976). The Munich Coma Scale (MCS). Journal of *Neurology, Neurosurgery and Psychiatry, 39,* 788; Smith, C., Smith, J., & Speirs, J. 1986). *Coma stimulations: An interdisciplinary approach for treatment of the coma patient.* Unpublished paper, Speech-Language Pathology Department, Regency Rehabilitation Center, Denver, CO.

References

Ali, S. F., Jairaj, K., Newport, G. D., Lipe, G. W., & Slikker, W., Jr. (1990). Thallium intoxication produces neurochemical alterations in rat brain. *Neurotoxicology, 11,* 381–390.

Apkarian, P., Mirmiran, M., & Tijssen, R. (1991). Effects of behavioural state on visual processing in neonates. *Neuropediatrics, 22*(2), 85–91.

Bartus, R. T., Dean, R. L., Beer, B., & Lippa, A. S. (1982). The cholinergic hypothesis of geriatric memory dysfunction. *Science, 217,* 408–414.

Bergeron, M., Reader, T. A., Layrargues, G. P., & Butterworth, F. R. (1989). Monoamines and metabolites in autopsied brain tissue from cirrhotic patients with hepatic encephalopathy. *Neurochemical Research, 14,* 853–859.

Born, J. D. (1987). Assessment of impaired consciousness. *Acta Anaesthesiologica Belgica, 38,* 381–386.

Born, J. D., Hans, P., Albert, A., & Bonnal, J. (1987). Interobserver agreement in assessment of motor response and brain stem reflexes. *Neurosurgery, 20,* 513–517.

Bosman, D. K., Van Den Buijs, C. A. C. G., De Haan, J. G., Maas, M. A. W., & Chamuleau, R. A. F. M. (1991). The effects of benzodiazepine-receptor antagonists and partial inverse agonists on acute hepatic encephalopathy in the rat. *Gastroenterology, 101,* 722–781.

Brazelton, T. B. (1984). *Neonatal behavioral assessment scale* (2nd ed.). Philadelphia: J. B. Lippincott.

Bremer, F. (1977). Cerebral hypnogenic centers. *Annals of Neurology, 2,* 1–6.

Brinkman, R., von Cramon, D., & Schultz, H. (1976). The Munich Coma Scale (MCS). *Journal of Neurology, Neurosurgery and Psychiatry, 39,* 788.

Crosby, L., & Parsons, L. C. (1989). Clinical neurological assessment tool: Development and testing of an instrument to index neurologic status. *Heart and Lung, 18,* 121–129.

Daube, J. R., & Sandok, R. A. (1986). *Medical neurosciences* (2nd ed.). Boston: Little, Brown.

Dowling, G. A. (1985). Levels of cognitive functioning: Evaluation of interrater reliability. *Journal of Neuroscience Nursing, 17,* 129–134.

Feldmann, E., Gandy, S. E., Becker, R., Zimmerman, R., Thaler, H. T., Posner, J., & Plum, F. (1988). MRI demonstrates descending transtentorial herniation. *Neurology, 38,* 697–701.

Gulbranson, G., Kristiansen, K., & Ursin, H. (1972). Response habituation in unconscious patients. *Neuropsychology, 10,* 313.

Hall, E. D. (1989). Free radicals and CNS injury. *Critical Care Clinics, 5*(4), 793–805.

Katayama, Y., Young, H. F., Dunbar, J. G., & Hayes, R. L. (1988). Coma associated with flaccidity produced by fluid-percussion concussion in the cat. II: Contribution of the activity in the pontine inhibitory system. *Brain Injury, 2,* 51–66.

Kuhar, M. J., DeSouza, E. B., & Unnerstall, J. R. (1986). Neurotransmitter receptor mapping by autoradiography and other methods. *Annual Review of Neuroscience, 9,* 27–59.

Kushner, T. (1963). Having a life versus being alive. *Journal of Medical Ethics, 10,* 5–8.

Magoun, H. W. (1963). *The waking brain* (2nd ed.). Springfield, IL: Charles C Thomas.

Malkmus, D., Booth, B., & Kodimer, C. (1980). *Rehabilitation of the head injured adult.* Downey, CA: Professional Staff Association of the Rancho Los Amigos Hospital.

Markianos, M., Seretis, A., Kotsou, S., Baltas, I., & Sacharogiannis, H. (1992). CSF neurotransmitter metabolites and short-term outcome of patients in coma after head injury. *Acta Neurologica Scandinavica, 86,* 190–193.

Marmarou, A. (1992). Intracellular acidosis in human and experimental brain injury. *Journal of Neurotrauma, 9*(Suppl. 2), S551–S562.

Mitchell, P. H., Ozuna, J., & Bolles, J. (1983). *Evaluating the comatose patient* [Videotape]. Seattle, WA: Health Sciences Center for Learning Resources, University of Washington.

Moruzzi, G., & Magoun, H. (1949). Brainstem reticular formation and activation of the EEG. *Electroencephalography and Clinical Neurophysiology, 1,* 455–473.

Murdoch, J., & Hall, R. (1990). Brain protection: Physiological and pharmacological considerations. Part I: The physiology of brain injury. *Canadian Journal of Anaesthesia, 37,* 663–671.

Murray, L. S., Teasdale, G. M., Murray, G. D., Jennett, B., Miller, J. D., Pickard, J. D., Shaw, M. D., Achilles, J., Bailey, S., & Jones, P. (1993). Does prediction of outcome alter patient management? *Lancet, 341,* 1487–1491.

Norsell, U. (1986). Awareness, wakefulness and arousal. *Acta Neurochirurgica, 36*(Suppl.), 86–88.

Plum, F., & Posner, J. (1980). *The diagnosis of stupor and coma* (3rd ed.). Philadelphia: F. A. Davis.

Price, D. J. (1986). Factors restricting the use of coma scales. *Acta Neurochirurgica, 36*(Suppl.), 106–111.

Reich, J. B., Sierra, J., Camp, W., Zanzonico, P., Deck, M. D., & Plum, F. (1993). Magnetic resonance imaging measurements and clinical changes accompanying transtentorial and foremen magnum brain herniation. *Annals of Neurology, 33,* 159–170.

Reilly, P. L., Simpson, D. A., Sprod, R., & Thomas, L. (1988). Assessing the conscious level in infants and young children: A paediatric version of the Glasgow Coma Scale. *Child's Nervous System, 4,* 30–33.

Ropper, A. H. (1986). Lateral displacement of the brain and level of consciousness in patients with an acute hemispheral mass. *New England Journal of Medicine, 314,* 953–958.

Ross, D. A., Olsen, W. L., Ross, A. M., Andrews, B. T., & Pitts, L. H. (1989). Brain shift, level of consciousness and restoration of consciousness in patients with acute intracranial hematoma. *Journal of Neurosurgery, 71,* 498–502.

Schuri, U., & von Cramon, D. (1979). Autonomic responses to meaningful and nonmeaningful auditory stimuli in coma. *Archives of Psychological and Neurological Sciences, 227,* 143–149.

Schuri, U., & von Cramon, D. (1980). Autonomic and behavioral responses in coma due to drug overdose. *Psychophyiology, 17,* 253–258.

Schuri, U., & von Cramon, D. (1983). Electrodermal responses to auditory stimuli with different significance in neurological patients. *Psychophysiology, 18,* 248–251.

Shute, C. C. D., & Lewis, P. R. (1967). The ascending cholinergic reticular system: Neocortical, olfactory and subcortical projections. *Brain, 90,* 497.

Smith, C., Smith, J., & Speirs, J. (1986). *Coma stimulations: An interdisciplinary approach for treatment of the coma patient.* Unpublished paper, Speech-Language Pathology Department, Regency Rehabilitation Center, Denver, CO.

Stalhammar, D., Starmark, J. E., Holmgren, E., Eriksson, N., Nordstrom, C. H., Fedders, O., & Rosander, B. (1988). Assessment of responsiveness in acute cerebral disorders: A multicentre study on the Reaction Level Scale (RLS85). *Acta Neurochirurgica, 90*, 73–80.

Starmark, J. E., Stalhammar, D., & Holmgren, E. (1988). The Reaction Level Scale (RLS85): Manual and guidelines. *Acta Neurochirurgica, 91*, 12–20.

Stewart-Amidei, C. (1991). Assessing the comatose patient in the intensive care unit. *AACN Clinical Issues in Critical Care Nursing, 2*(4), 613–622.

Sugiura, K., Muraoka, K., Chishiki, T., & Baba, M. (1983). The Edinburgh-2 coma scale: A new scale for assessing impaired consciousness. *Neurosurgery, 12*, 411–415.

Teasdale, G. (1975). Acute impairment of brain function. 1: Assessing conscious level. *Nursing Times, 71*, 914–917.

Teasdale, G., & Galbraith, S. (1975). Acute impairment of brain function. 2: Observation record chart. *Nursing Times, 71*, 972–973.

Teasdale, G., Knill-Jones, R., & Van de Sande, J. (1978). Observer variability in assessing impaired consciousness and coma. *Journal of Neurology, Neurosurgery and Psychiatry, 41*, 603–610.

Teasdale, G., & Jennett, B. (1974). Assessment of coma and impaired consciousness: A practical scale. *Lancet, 2*, 81–85.

Teasdale, G., Safar, P., & Smyder, J. (1988). Brain resuscitation clinical trial II, 1984–1989 (Glasgow-Pittsburgh scoring method). In P. Safar & N. G. Bircher (Eds.), *Cardiopulmonary cerebral resuscitation* (3rd ed., p. 262). Philadelphia: W. B. Saunders.

Tesseris, J., Pantazidis, N., Routsi, C. R., & Fragoulakis, D. (1991). A comparative study of the Reaction Level Scale (RLS85) with Glasgow Coma Scale (GCS) and Edinburgh-2 Coma Scale (Modified) (E2CS(M)). *Acta Neurochirurgica, 110*, 65–76.

Vannucci, R. C. (1990). Experimental biology of cerebral hypoxia-ischemia: Relation to perinatal brain damage. *Pediatric Research, 27*, 317–326.

von Cramon, D. (1977). The structure of vigilance. *Archives of Psychiatric and Neurologic Sciences, 225*, 201–209.

Webster's new international dictionary of the English language (2nd ed.) (1943). Springfield, MA: GC Merriam.

Webster's ninth new collegiate dictionary (1988). Springfield, MA: Merriam-Webster.

Whitehouse, P. J., Price, D. L., Struble, R. G., Clark, A. W., & Coyle, J. T. (1982). Alzheimer's disease and senile dementia: Loss of neurons in the basal forebrain. *Science, 215*, 12–37.

Williams, J. (1992). Assessment of head injured children. *British Journal of Nursing, 1*(2), 82–84.

Yamamoto, J. (1988). Roles of cholinergic, dopaminergic, noradrenergic, serotonergic and GABAergic systems in changes of the EEG power spectra and behavioral states in rabbits. *Japanese Journal of Pharmacology, 47*, 123–134.

Decreased Behavioral Arousal

PAMELA H. MITCHELL

Arousal is a component of consciousness. As discussed in Chapter 5, level of arousal can be detected only through evaluation of *responsiveness*, or behavioral responses to a variety of stimuli. We therefore infer the degree of arousal from the nature of the behavioral response. Technologies that evaluate neurophysiologic functioning after central nervous system (CNS) injury may make it possible to evaluate internal behavior—that is, *physiologic responses*—in people with decreased behavioral arousal and thus enable us to make more accurate inferences about the arousability and awareness of such people.

The focus of this chapter is the phenomenon of decreased arousal in people with neurologic disease and injury. Disorders that produce decreased arousal are presented briefly, categorized by their effect on input, processing, or behavioral output of the arousal system. Nursing diagnoses commonly seen in such patients are discussed in two categories: those that stem from the pathophysiologic processes that produce the decreased arousal and those that stem from the diminished ability to interact with the environment.

DISORDERS PRODUCING DECREASED AROUSAL

Coma is the most profound clinical state manifested by decreased arousal and can be defined behaviorally as the absence of opening of the eyes, intelligible verbalization, and following of commands (Jennett & Teasdale, 1981). Disorders that produce coma can be classified as structural and metabolic (Plum & Posner, 1980). Structural disorders include tumors, intracranial bleeding, and abscesses that alter consciousness by distorting the neuroanatomic structures that serve consciousness. Metabolic disorders affect overall brain function by altering the supply of nutrients and metabolic substrates (e.g., oxygen, glucose, enzymatic cofactors) required by brain cells to produce energy. Hypoglycemia, hypoxia, and hyperammonemia are examples of metabolic states that can produce decreased arousal and coma.

As discussed in Chapter 5, arousal requires sensory input into the reticular activating system; central processing of that input by the reticular formation, limbic system, and cortex; and behavioral output, or the motor and verbal behaviors that indicate responsiveness. Table 6–1 shows disorders that produce decreased arousal and coma, categorized by their effect on input, processing, or behavioral output.

Diminished Input

The CNS must receive sensory input to maintain arousal. Sensory input can be diminished either by an impoverished sensory environment or by profound alteration in the sensory pathways that transmit information to the CNS. Either of these conditions produces a state of *sensory deprivation*—alteration in the pattern or meaning of sensory information. Confusion, lethargy, and diminished brain activation are well-documented effects of both experimental and clinical conditions of sensory deprivation (Slade, 1984; Wolanin & Phillips, 1981). When there is structural or metabolic injury, one might expect diminished

TABLE 6–1 • DISORDERS THAT ALTER AROUSAL

Diminished Input	Impaired Central Nervous System Processing	Diminished Behavioral Output
Isolation	**Structural disorders**	Locked-in syndrome
Impoverished sensory environment	• Tumors (supratentorial, infratentorial)	Paralysis
Deafness	• Hemorrhage (subarachnoid, intraventricular, diencephalic, subdural, epidural)	
Profound sensory neuropathy	• Abscesses (large hemispheric, small infratentorial)	
	• Meningitis, encephalitis	
	• Infarcts (central brain stem, diencephalic, large hemispheric)	
	• Diffuse axonal degeneration (traumatic head injury)	
	• Diffuse gray matter degeneration (Creutzfeld-Jakob syndrome, late Alzheimer's disease, subacute combined degeneration)	
	Metabolic disorders	
	• Oxidative (hypoxia, anoxia, ischemia, hypercarbia)	
	• Metabolic substrate (hypoglycemia, thiamine deficiency)	
	• Metabolic poisons (hyperammonemia [hepatic encephalopathy, Reye's syndrome], hyperuremia [renal encephalopathy], drug overdose)	

external sensory input to compound the problem (Le Winn & Dimanescu, 1978; Mitchell, Bradley, Welch, & Britton, 1990; Walsh, 1981).

Impaired Central Nervous System Processing

The most frequent sources of decreased arousal observed by the neuroscience nurse are those diseases and conditions that impair processing of sensory input in the brain. As described in Chapter 5, structural lesions of the central brain stem, diencephalon, or bilateral cerebral hemispheres can impair arousal and produce coma. In addition, systemic processes that impair metabolism of the whole CNS can cloud consciousness and produce coma.

Structural disorders, such as tumors, abscesses, and hemorrhage, produce alterations in consciousness by displacing and distorting brain tissue. Tumors or hematomas that cause a shift of one hemisphere across the midline of the brain produce bilateral hemispheric damage and thus decreased arousal. Hemorrhage, tumor, or abscesses in the diencephalon decrease the ability of the reticular activating system to send information along the diffuse projection systems from thalamus to cortex. Tumor, infarct, or compression of the brain stem produces coma by direct action on the reticular formation. It is possible for certain brain stem infarcts to impair the motor output necessary for behavioral evidence of arousal without impairing arousal itself (see Diminished Behavioral Output in this chapter).

Disorders that impair the metabolic processes necessary for whole brain function can also alter consciousness. Exogenous poisons or drugs act to depress consciousness either by interfering with the cellular oxidative metabolic processes (e.g., carbon monoxide, cyanide) or by depressing overall cellular function (e.g., barbiturates, narcotics, sedatives). A variety of systemic disorders alter consciousness by depriving the brain of necessary metabolic substrates (e.g., glucose in the case of profound hypoglycemia, the enzymes necessary to use glucose in the case of thiamine deficiency). Other systemic diseases produce metabolic waste products that act as cellular poisons in the brain (e.g., urea in acute renal failure, hyperammonemia in Reye's syndrome or in acute hepatic encephalopathy).

Diminished Behavioral Output

The final category of disorders that alter consciousness includes conditions that create diminished ability to produce the behavioral output (motor and verbal behaviors) from which we infer responsiveness. These disorders do not impair consciousness but the person's ability to communicate consciousness to the world.

Disorders that impair motor output so profoundly that the patient appears to be unresponsive compose this category. For example, patients with high cervical cord injuries may have intact shoulder and neck muscles. Thus, no one confuses lack of verbalization by the person who is quadriplegic and on a ventilator with lack of consciousness, because the person is still capable of blinking the eyes and nodding the head. However, the person who has Guillian-Barré syndrome (ascending polyneuropathy) that has affected the cranial nerves may have great difficulty communicating consciousness. These patients, however, usually retain the ability to open and close the eyes.

A disorder of motor output that can easily be confused with coma is the locked-in syndrome, a relatively uncommon form of brain stem stroke in which the anterior brain stem is infarcted, usually at the base of the pons. Any anterior infarction from the midbrain to the lower pons can produce this syndrome. This portion of the brain stem carries all the motor fibers from the lower cranial nerves (those that serve phonation and facial expression) as well as those from the cortex to the limbs. It is anterior to the reticular formation, and thus consciousness is spared. However, all motor output is disconnected between the cortex and the effector cranial and spinal nerves that serve verbal and motor output. Usually, at least vertical eye movements are preserved, and the patient may be capable of communication through eye movement.

HUMAN RESPONSES ASSOCIATED WITH DECREASED CONSCIOUSNESS

People with decreased consciousness have responses, and thus nursing diagnoses, that are specifically related to the pathophysiologic states that produce diminished responsiveness, and they have nursing diagnoses that stem directly from lack of volitional movement and from which we infer loss of consciousness. The nursing diagnoses related to the basic pathology commonly are clinical problems that must be managed collaboratively by nurses and other health professionals (collaborative problems), whereas the diagnoses related to lack of movement are usually managed independently by nurses (nursing diagnoses). The following case studies are used to illustrate nursing diagnoses often found in patients with coma from a variety of sources.

• C A S E   S T U D Y   1

Decreased Arousal After Neurosurgery

Mr. P was a 50-year-old man admitted to an acute care hospital for craniotomy to remove a left frontal brain mass. Over the 4 months before admission, he had experienced constant and stabbing frontoparietal headaches, associated nausea without vomiting, and loss of appetite. The headaches had no apparent precipitators and were not relieved by aspirin, acetaminophen, or ibuprofen. His family had encouraged him to seek medical attention when he began to have weakness and pain in his right shoulder, arm, and leg. In retrospect, his family also noted that he seemed to have difficulty finding words and hesitancy initiating speech.

The physician's initial examination noted the following abnormalities: difficulty initiating sentences and pronouncing words with an initial ''n'' sound; decreased strength of the right proximal arm muscles (3/5 compared with 5/5 in the left arm and both legs), pronator drift in the right arm, deep tendon reflexes 3+ on the right compared with 2+ on the left, Babinski's reflex present bilaterally. The patient was alert, oriented, and without cranial nerve deficits. A magnetic resonance imaging (MRI) scan of the head revealed a probable tumor in the left frontal lobe, with left-to-right brain shift.

Mr. P underwent a left frontal craniotomy, with removal of a grade III astrocytoma. Postoperatively, he was on bedrest, with the head of the bed elevated 30 degrees. Other medications included intravenous (IV) fluids to maintain normovolemia, IV dexamethasone 4 mg every 6 hours, and cimetidine 300 mg every 6 hours.

Immediately after surgery, Mr. P's Glasgow Coma Scale (GCS) score was recorded at 14: his eyes opened spontaneously, his verbal response was confused ("I'm at home"), and he obeyed commands. His pupils were equal at 4 mm and reactive to light, and eye movements were conjugate. The right-hand grasp was weaker than that of the left hand. Respirations and cardiovascular status were unremarkable. The assessment remained much the same for about 6 hours, when the nurses' notes indicated that commands were followed slowly, that the patient was "lethargic," and that the right-hand grasp was markedly weaker than that of the left hand. The GCS score was not reported in the nurses' notes at this time. Vital signs and pupils remained unchanged.

The patient was judged by the night nurses to be stable, and the frequency of assessment was decreased to every 4 hours. At noon the next day, Mr. P was noted to be difficult to arouse and "sleeping at times," and his right arm was flaccid, with flexion withdrawal to painful stimuli. The ability to obey commands was inconsistent. At this point, the neurosurgeon was called. He instituted intracranial pressure (ICP) monitoring and mannitol. ICP was 25 mm Hg, but it decreased rapidly to 8 to 10 mm Hg with therapy. A computed tomography (CT) scan showed brain swelling in the left hemisphere but no postoperative hemorrhage, and the brain swelling was brought under control with mannitol. Mr. P regained his previous level of arousal within 12 hours and regained motor function on the right side to his preoperative level. The remainder of his postoperative course was uneventful, and he was discharged to home with plans for a course of radiation therapy.

Collaborative Problems Related to Arousal for Case Study 1

Mr. P's case illustrates several collaborative problems that stem from the pathophysiologic state accompanying supratentorial craniotomy. The overall category of collaborative problems is high risk for secondary brain injury, with specific risks including the following (Mitchell, 1994):

- Potential for brain herniation secondary to brain swelling or postoperative hemorrhage
- Potential for intracranial hypertension and cerebral ischemia secondary to brain swelling
- Potential for inadequate cerebral oxygenation related to impaired gas exchange (postoperative atelectasis)

In addition, several highly probable independent nursing diagnoses relate to Mr. P's and his family's cognitive, motor, and coping responses to the residual physical disabilities and to the meaning Mr. P and his family attribute to the diagnosis of brain tumor. These diagnoses, however, are not manifested by and do not stem from his decreased arousal. Therefore, diagnoses related to cognitive, self-care, communication, and coping responses are more appropriately illustrated in the case studies in other chapters in this book.

Potential for intracranial hypertension and potential for brain herniation are two clinical problems that stem directly from the pathophysiologic state—brain swelling—that commonly follows manipulation of the brain during craniotomy. Brain swelling is the net increase in volume of any one of the brain fluid compartments (vascular, intracellular, extracellular). *Hyperemia* (acute vasodilation of cerebral vessels) is the most immediate cause of brain swelling in acute head injury or brain insult and may be caused by a combination of hypoxemia and release of vasoactive substances from injured cells. Vasodilation as a source of brain swelling is to be distinguished from cerebral edema, a more slowly developing process of accumulation of extracellular or intracellular water. Cerebral edema results in a net increase in the water content of the cranial cavity 24 to 72 hours after injury (Langfitt, 1983; Miller, 1985, 1993). In Mr. P's case, the postoperative deterioration was most likely a manifestation of early brain swelling surrounding the operative site, although the possibility of mass effect from postoperative hemorrhage was also entertained; this was ruled out by the CT scan.

Brain swelling can produce decreased arousal and coma by (1) acting as a whole brain depressant, (2) displacing tissues across the midline or onto the diencephalic and midbrain arousal structures, or (3) producing rapidly increasing ICP.

Potential for Brain Herniation

The potential for brain herniation is a risk for all patients who undergo either supratentorial or infratentorial craniotomy. It is further compounded by the risk of postanesthesia complications that impair pulmonary gas exchange and thus the delivery of oxygen to the brain. The defining characteristic of brain herniation is CT or MRI evidence of such (Feldmann et al., 1988; Reich et al., 1993; Ropper, 1986; Ross, Olsen, Ross, Andrews, & Pitts, 1989); however, it would be highly impractical to conduct serial scanning for all patients at risk. Thus, clinically evident defining characteristics of brain herniation are decreasing level of consciousness, asymmetry of motor response, and signs of brain stem dysfunction (abnormal or absent extraocular movement; pupillary asymmetry; abnormal breathing patterns; and, if allowed to progress, Cushing's phenomenon—bradycardia, increased systolic blood pressure, and widening pulse pressure).

The most prominent aspect of altered arousal in Mr. P's case is the decrease in responsiveness within the first 12 hours after surgery. Although the nurses caring for him recognized the need for neurosurgical intervention relatively early in the course of probable brain herniation, subtle signs of decreased arousal appeared even earlier. Had the terminology of the GCS been used consistently throughout the early postoperative course, it is possible that the "lethargy" reported at 6 hours after surgery would have been manifested by a lack of spontaneous eye opening and confusion and thus a measurable decrease in level of responsiveness. Because either lateral brain shift or downward brain herniation would affect proximal motor function before distal function, the use of hand grips (distal motor strength) to test motor function failed to detect increasing proximal motor weakness that might also have shown early progression of a motor deficit. Because this patient did obey commands, he should have been asked to hold his arms in front of him while the nurse observed for downward drift and pronation of either arm (weakness of the proximal upper arm muscles).

Nursing assessment of this potential problem consists of serial monitoring for signs of brain herniation, with the goal of earliest possible detection of brain herniation. At a minimum, the monitoring protocol requires assessment of level of consciousness and brain stem functions that indicate the status of the arousal system. The GCS is the most widely used assessment tool for level of consciousness, but it cannot be relied on as the sole indicator for brain herniation because it does not include assessment of brain stem and symmetry of motor function. One must therefore include serial assessment of the following:

- Symmetry of motor response to verbal and painful stimuli, including deep tendon and superficial reflexes
- Eye signs—extraocular movements, pupillary responses
- Protective reflexes—lash (corneal), gag, or swallow
- Vital signs—pulse, blood pressure, respiratory pattern

In tertiary care and trauma centers, one may also have the benefit of serial measures of cerebrovascular status including ICP, cerebral perfusion pressure (CPP), and cerebral blood flow velocity (CBV) obtained through transcranial Doppler ultrasonography. Changes in patterns of waveforms and autoregulatory status may signal impending brain shift or herniation before clinical signs become evident (see Intracranial Hypertension: Potential for Decreased Adaptive Capacity and Secondary Brain Injury later in this chapter).

Nursing intervention is prompt referral for neurosurgical management if signs of herniation are detected. Neurosurgical intervention consists of management of intracranial hypertension, if it coexists with the impending brain herniation, and diagnosis and control of the pathophysiologic state causing the brain herniation. Brain swelling and postoperative hemorrhage are the most common causes of brain herniation after craniotomy. Many neurosurgeons will therefore institute measures to reduce hyperemia and brain swelling as immediate management and then obtain a CT scan for definitive diagnosis. Mannitol or other osmotic diuretics are used to reduce total brain water volume.

In Mr. P's case, osmotic diuretics were adequate to reduce brain water volume sufficiently to reverse the impending brain herniation and to prevent concomitant increase in ICP until the postoperative brain swelling had resolved. Had this therapy not been sufficient, more aggressive measures to control ICP might have been necessary. As expected, the CT scan did not show any signs of postoperative hematoma.

Potential for Intracranial Hypertension

Any patient with significant brain injury, including craniotomy as a form of controlled trauma, is at risk for intracranial hypertension. Intracranial hypertension is defined as resting sustained ICP equal to or greater than 20 mm Hg. Although some nursing textbooks continue to describe a variety of clinical signs as indicators of intracranial hypertension, the only valid indicator is direct measurement of ICP. Research since the 1970s has shown clearly that the traditional clinical signs of increased ICP have poor correlation with the actual level of ICP. Even the level of arousal may not change in clear relationship to the measured level of ICP; that is, arousal may decrease at low levels of ICP or be unchanged until ICP is quite high. It is inappropriate, therefore, to define intracranial hypertension in terms of clinical signs alone.

In Mr. P's situation, ICP was measured after surgery and found to be high at some point after his decrease in level of arousal. Because he also showed signs of early brain herniation, it is impossible to determine if his decreased arousal was a manifestation of intracranial hypertension, early brain shift, or both. Medical intervention is designed to maintain CPP (by reducing ICP, supporting systemic arterial pressure, or both) and to correct the underlying pathologic state if possible. Hyperventilation to control hyperemia and osmotic diuretics were used. Nursing therapies to reduce activity-related transient elevations are described in Case Study 2.

Once Mr. P's ICP was found to be elevated, it was important to monitor CPP continually to determine that brain cells were being adequately perfused. Because an arterial pressure monitoring catheter was in place, the monitoring was simple. CPP is calculated at the bedside by subtracting mean ICP from mean arterial blood pressure (ABP). The goal is to maintain CPP at around 70 mm Hg (Chesnut & Marshall, 1993; Miller, 1993). Mr. P's CPP remained at 70 to 90 mm Hg.

Mr. P's brain herniation and intracranial hypertension were detected relatively early and were able to be reversed by neurosurgical intervention. His right-sided motor deficits were not resolved completely by removal of the tumor and probably complicated the postoperative assessment for the nurses. Those who discounted his lethargy and tested only hand grips may have assumed that the asymmetry between right and left motor function was the same as had been noted preoperatively. This case illustrates the importance of serial assessment of brain stem and motor function, as well as of arousal (or level of consciousness).

• C A S E   S T U D Y   2

Sudden-Onset Coma

Alex was a 24-year-old man employed as an automobile mechanic who lived with his family in Alaska. He arrived home from a party at 3 AM and was noted by his father to be still resting at 6 PM that day. By 11 PM, Alex's parents had called the rescue squad to the home because Alex would not respond and seemed "stiff and strange."

In the emergency department, Alex was noted to have no spontaneous opening of the eyes, although his eyes did open to painful stimuli. Pupils were fixed in midposition, and spontaneous gaze was dysconjugate. The ocular fundi were remarkable for venous engorgement, although the optic disks were sharp and pale. He did not respond to verbal commands or verbalize intelligibly. His teeth were clenched, and there was fecal-smelling material at his mouth. Painful stimulation produced extension at both elbows, internal rotation of the shoulders, and extension at the wrist. The legs were also extended. CT scanning equipment was not available, and there was no capacity for ICP monitoring. The local physician noted that Alex had had a "major intracranial event"; intubated the patient; instituted furosemide and mannitol; and had the patient airlifted to a major trauma center for further evaluation and care.

On arrival at the trauma center, Alex had no spontaneous opening of the eyes and no verbal response and exhibited flexion withdrawal to painful stimulation. Corneal reflexes were absent bilaterally, pupils were fixed in midposition, and slight conjugate movement of the eyes was present on oculovestibular (cold caloric) testing. A CT scan showed intraventricular clots and dilated ventricles thought to be secondary to hemorrhage from a left posterior cerebral artery arteriovenous malformation (AVM).

A Camino catheter was placed to monitor ICP, and a right frontal ventriculostomy was performed to drain cerebrospinal fluid. Arterial pressure monitoring, cardiac monitoring, and assisted ventilation were instituted. Cardiac arrhythmias (premature ventricular contractions [PVCs] and inverted T waves) were evident during the first 48 hours. The ICP initially was 25 mm Hg, decreasing to 8 to 10 mm Hg with intermittent ventriculostomy drainage. Dexamethasone 4 mg was given intravenously every 6 hours initially. Tube-feeding was instituted because adequate bowel tones were present, with feedings of 3000 kilocalories daily and 100 mL/hr free water.

Over the course of the next 4 weeks, ICP stabilized as hydrocephalus resolved. Oxygenation was adequate with spontaneous breathing. Spontaneous opening of the eyes and opening of the eyes to painful stimuli were present, but opening of the eyes was not consistently present with verbal stimulation. No verbal response was present to any stimulus, and motor response remained flexion withdrawal to painful stimuli. Gaze was conjugate with spontaneous eye movements, but no orienting or tracking of objects occurred. The patient tended to gaze to the left when undisturbed. Facial grimacing was present both spontaneously and to painful stimuli; it occurred regularly when family members spoke to him. Spontaneous swallow was present, but gag was markedly diminished. Deep tendon reflexes were hyperactive in all extremities, and the plantar reflex was present on the right.

Tube-feeding was necessary for nutritional intake. Although Alex was no longer hypermetabolic, the earlier hypermetabolic state had resulted in loss of weight, primarily muscle. Pressure hyperemia was evident on the hips and sacrum and did not resolve rapidly with turning from the affected areas. Elimination of urine was controlled with a condom catheter; Alex was incontinent of loose stool one or more times daily. Aspiration pneumonia had been present during the early hospitalization but was resolved.

Although the possibility of surgical embolization of the AVM had been entertained early in the course of the illness, Alex's continued functioning at a subcortical level suggested that irreversible and massive brain damage had occurred with the initial hemorrhage. The physicians and family decided, therefore, to forego surgery and to place the patient in an extended care facility when his physical condition was stabilized. No facilities were available near the family home that offered specialized care for the brain-damaged patient, and Alex was transferred to a nursing home that could provide tube-feeding and basic physical care. He died 6 months later of aspiration pneumonia, having never manifested signs of arousal beyond spontaneous opening of the eyes and facial grimacing.

Alex's case illustrates a greater variety of collaborative problems and nursing diagnoses than does the case of Mr. P. See Table 6–2 for a summary of Alex's problems. Although the particular pathology in Alex's case was AVM, the clinical problems illustrated are found in a wide variety of severe brain injuries, including closed head injury.

TABLE 6–2 • SUMMARY OF NURSING DIAGNOSES FOR CASE STUDY 2: SUDDEN-ONSET COMA

Diagnoses Stemming from the Pathophysiologic Process

For the individual

- Physiologic instability related to impaired central nervous system integrative functions: cardiovascular, respiratory, temperature regulation
- Intracranial hypertension: potential for decreased adaptive capacity and secondary brain injury
- Nutritional deficit related to hypermetabolism
- Potential for infection related to invasive monitoring devices

For the family

- Potential for knowledge deficit concerning nature and prognosis of coma

For the community

- Potential for knowledge deficit regarding prevention of pathology

Diagnoses Stemming from Reduced Ability to Interact with Environment

For the individual

- Self-care deficit: protective reflexes related to lack of volitional responsiveness
- Impaired mobility, level 4: potential for disuse syndrome and immobility complications
- Potential for skin breakdown related to nutritional deficit and self-care deficit
- Potential for psychologic responses to external environmental stimuli

For the family

- Potential for impaired family coping

For the community

- Inadequate resources for care of people with prolonged unawareness

DIAGNOSES RELATED TO THE PATHOPHYSIOLOGIC STATE

The sudden onset of a massive hemorrhage from the AVM precipitates a number of problems that must be managed collaboratively by nurses and physicians. These problems include multisystem physiologic instability, intracranial hypertension, and potential nutritional and infection problems that stem from the medical therapies.

Physiologic Instability Related to Impaired Central Nervous System Integrative Functions

Cardiovascular, respiratory, temperature regulation, and fluid balance homeostatic functions are all regulated at the level of the hypothalamus (see Chapter 34 for further discussion). The regulatory functions of the hypothalamus can be altered in severe and generalized insult to the CNS (as in head injury or massive intracranial bleeding), global ischemia from systemic low perfusion states or severe intracranial hypertension, or focal ischemia in the diencephalon (as may occur with some strokes or in diffuse axonal injury). Systemic problems may be evident, particularly in cardiovascular, pulmonary, temperature regulation, and fluid-electrolyte balance systems. This was the case for Alex and was manifested in cardiac arrhythmilas, spontaneous hyperventilation, possible non–aspiration-related ventilation-perfusion abnormalities, and initial *poikilothermy* (tendency to take on the environmental temperature). There was no evidence of hyperosmolar or hypo-osmolar states (fluid-electrolyte regulatory disturbance).

The defining characteristic for this class of collaborative problem is abnormal systemic function in the absence of systemic disease. Examples are cardiac arrhythmias in a young person with head injury and no history of cardiac disease, ventilation-perfusion abnormalities with no evidence of pneumonia or primary respiratory disease, fever with no evidence of infection, or hyperosmolar or hypo-osmolar plasm and urinary laboratory values in the absence of diabetes, primary pituitary dysfunction, or inappropriate parenteral fluid management. Aspiration pneumonia, nosocomial infection, and inappropriate parenteral fluid management are by far the most common sources of pulmonary, temperature, and fluid balance problems in patients with CNS disorders and must be ruled out before it is assumed that the problems stem from disordered diencephalic regulation (Miller, 1993; Ropper, 1993).

In the case of Alex, only the cardiac arrhythmias (PVCs and inverted T waves) can be assumed to stem from hypothalamic regulatory dysfunction. His pulmonary problems were likely the result of aspiration of gastric contents during the prehospitalization period. Some degree of shunt (ventilation-perfusion mismatch) has been shown in experimental head injury and may be present to compound the altered ventilation stemming from aspiration pneumonia. Both a hyperosmolar state (diabetes insipidus)and a hypo-osmolar state (syndrome of inappropriate antidiuretic hormone) can occur in brain injury that is sufficient to cause coma and can be a direct result of hypothalamic ischemia or injury.

A hyperosmolar state results from the inability to produce antidiuretic hormone or from nonketotic hyperglycemia. This leads to osmotic diuresis, which is manifested by urine output in excess of fluid intake, hypotonic urine (specific gravity 1.001 to 1.005, urine osmolarity 50 to 150 mOsm/kg), and normal or increased serum sodium (the latter is particularly likely if the patient is not able to drink to compensate for water loss). A hypo-osmolar state is caused by excess production of antidiuretic hormone and thus retention of excess free water. This state is manifested by low urine output compared with urine intake, hypertonic urine (increased urinary sodium, urine osmolarity higher than serum osmolarity), and decreased sodium and serum osmolarity (<280 mOsm/kg) (Diringer, Borel, & Hanley, 1993; Saul, 1983).

Nursing management of these neurally induced systemic states consists of (1) monitoring and surveillance to detect the specific system problem and (2) collaborative implementation of medical therapy for the specific systemic clinical problem. Careful monitoring of cardiac, pulmonary, temperature, and fluid-balance systems is essential. There is considerable evidence that the cardiac arrhythmias seen after head injury and subarachnoid hemorrhage are manifestations of microinfarcts of the myocardium stimulated by neurally induced excessive sympathetic activity (Samuels, 1993). Many recommend that patients who manifest these cerebrally induced arrhythmias be treated as if they had a myocardial infarction, implementing a plan of bedrest and graded resumption of activity consistent with the activity capabilities of patients with decreased levels of consciousness (McCarthy, 1986). Interruption of the sympathetic-ischemic cascade shortly after the acute neurologic event with beta blockers has shown some clinical promise (Cruickshank et al., 1987).

Monitoring of ventilation (blood gases, respiratory response to activity) and temperature is important both in following the course of pulmonary and infectious problems and in estimating the demands of such clinical problems on the patient's metabolic capacities. Increasing activity and mobility creates demands on the patient's ability to expend energy and may create a demand greater than the ability to respond in patients with compromised ventilation and excess metabolic demand of fever. The patient with diminished consciousness cannot tell us that he or she is exhausted after sitting up for 30 minutes, for example. Therefore, changes in heart rate, respiratory rate, and blood pressure must be used as rough estimates of the person's ability to tolerate increased activity.

Monitoring intake and output and the specific gravity of urine is warranted in any patient with severe CNS insult because of the potential for either neurally or iatrogenically induced fluid balance problems. Thirst is our most important signal for self-regulation of fluid intake. Although we cannot know if people with decreased consciousness experience thirst, we are certain that they cannot communicate thirst to us. We must rely on indicators of intake and output of osmolarity to detect hyperosmolar and hypo-osmolar problems. Alex's fluid balance remained normal. With manifestation of the hyperosmolar state, the usual medical treatment is to replace urinary losses plus insensible losses with dextrose and water rather than saline. Supplementary vasopressin (antidiuretic hormone) may be necessary to control diuresis. The hypo-osmolar state is treated with fluid restriction (1000 to 1500 mL daily) and adequate salt intake, if possible. When this is not possible, as in persons with multiple injuries, rapid correction is advocated, titrating urine and serum osmolarity with hypertonic saline administered through a central IV line (Diringer et al., 1993; Saul, 1983).

Intracranial Hypertension: Potential for Decreased Adaptive Capacity and Secondary Brain Injury

A clinical problem directly related to the pathophysiology of Alex's massive intracranial hemorrhage is intracranial hypertension. ICP is normally between 0 and 10 mm Hg when the volumes of brain, blood, and cerebrospinal fluid in the cranial cavity are in their normal proportions. When the volume of any of these components increases, compensatory changes occur to maintain ICP at a normal level. These compensatory changes include a shift of a larger proportion of cerebrospinal fluid to the spinal sac, a slight increase in venous outflow, and a slight compression of brain tissue. If the volume of one of the components continues to increase, ICP will eventually rise.

In Mr. P's case, brain swelling was the source of increased intracranial volume that manifested as increased ICP. In Alex's case, the clots from the intraventricular hemorrhage blocked the flow of cerebrospinal fluid and produced noncommunicating hydrocephalus, thus increasing the volume of cerebrospinal fluid in the cranial cavity. Because the cerebrospinal fluid could not flow out of the cranial cavity by the usual route through the ventricles and basal cisterns, the normal ability to compensate by shifting cerebrospinal fluid to the spinal sac was lost. In the case of head injury, intracranial hypertension often results from a combination of reflex hyperemia (increased intracranial blood volume), brain swelling, and cerebrospinal fluid obstruction.

A nursing diagnosis sometimes coexisting with intracranial hypertension is decreased intracranial adaptive capacity. The cause of the diagnosis is failure of normal intracranial compensatory mechanisms, resulting in the defining characteristic: repeated, disproportionate increases in ICP (more than 10 mm Hg over baseline for more than 5 minutes) in response to a variety of noxious and nonnoxious stimuli (Mitchell, 1986, 1999). This means that a patient whose ICP increases 10 mm Hg for 5 minutes or longer with repeated episodes of turning or suctioning, for example, is manifesting decreased adaptive capacity. Because CPP is a function of ICP and systemic blood pressure, these increases in ICP would also threaten CPP unless there was a corresponding increase in mean ABP. Thus patients with resting CPP less than 60 to 70 mm Hg are at even greater risk of secondary cerebral hypoperfusion if they exhibit decreased adaptive capacity. Characteristics of patients at high risk for disproportionate increase in ICP are those with resting ICP greater than 20 mm Hg, resting CPP less than or equal to 50 mm Hg, wide amplitude ICP tracing, elevated P_2 segment of the ICP waveform, abnormal CBV (as measured by transcranial Doppler techniques), or repeated spiking of ICP in response to nursing maneuvers (March, Mitchell, Grady, & Winn, 1990; Mitchell, 1986, 1999; Mitchell & Ackerman, 1992; Rauch, Mitchell, & Tyler, 1990).

Nursing interventions for this diagnosis consist of measures to decrease environmental demands on the intracranial system or measures to increase the intracranial adaptive capacity. Measures designed to reduce the demand of rapid changes in posture include turning patients with head held in midline, using turning sheets, turning slowly, or using mechanical turning beds. Prevention of constipation (and thus straining at stool), reduction of coughing with endotracheal tube suctioning, and avoidance of loud noises and sudden tactile stimuli are other examples of activities that reduce demand on the cardiovascular system and thus prevent adding transient additional vascular volume to the intracranial cavity. Increases in systemic blood pressure can increase cerebral blood volume, and Valsalva's maneuver associated with coughing and straining acts to reduce cerebral venous outflow (and thereby increase net cerebral blood volume).

Many of the medical therapies described for intracranial hypertension—for example, osmotic diuresis—act to increase adaptive capacity. Mechanical drainage of cerebrospinal fluid reduces the volume of cerebrospinal fluid in the cranial cavity and thus temporarily increases intracranial adaptive capacity. In Alex's case, the nurses implemented the medical protocol to drain a small amount of cerebrospinal fluid from the ventriculostomy before initiating such activities as suctioning, turning, and chest physiotherapy. This provided sufficient intracranial adaptive capacity so that resting ICP was maintained at 8 to 10 mm Hg and he never showed a peak pressure beyond 15 mm Hg in response to activities that initially produced an ICP of 30 to 40 mm Hg. CPP remained adequate during and after all nursing care activities. As the intraventricular clots and the blood products in the subarachnoid space were reabsorbed, the hydrocephalus resolved, and ICP remained within normal limits without ventricular drainage.

Nutritional Deficit Related to Hypermetabolism

Patients who are sufficiently unresponsive to be unable to take oral food and fluids are at risk for nutritional deficits because parenteral fluids alone cannot supply enough calories to meet basal metabolic needs. Compounding this relatively simple supply problem is the fact that significant trauma, including CNS trauma or injury, results in a hypermetabolic state (Chesnut & Marshall, 1993; Deutschman, Konstantinides, Raup, Thienprasit, & Cerra, 1986; Young, Ott, Phillips, & McClain, 1991). The caloric and protein needs of such patients can be approached only by hyperalimentation, preferably enteral. There is growing evidence that enteral hyperalimentation provides better control of hyperglycemia and protection to both the gut and the immune system in severely traumatized patients (Chesnut & Marshall, 1993; Moore, Moore, Jones, McCroskey, & Peterson, 1989; Young et al., 1991). Such nutritional supplementation needs to be carefully monitored to avoid hyperglycemia, which may act to increase brain damage in an already injured mature nervous system. The detrimental effect of glucose on the injured neonatal or immature brain is not as clear (Kraft et al., 1990; Longsteth & Inui, 1984; Vannucci, 1990).

Alex had bowel tones and was fed enterally via nasogastric tube, with a high-protein nutritional prescription tailored to 140% of his estimated basal metabolic needs. The nutritional prescription is best managed collaboratively by nutritionist, physician, and nurse. The nutritionist's assessment of nutritional deficit includes serial monitoring of weight, fluid intake and output, serum sodium, albumin, glucose, lymphocyte count, and urine creatinine and urea as markers of protein loss. The laboratory monitoring of markers of nutritional status is primarily a collaborative endeavor of nutritionist and physician. It is often the nursing staff, however, that recognizes the need for nutritional intervention from patterns of weight loss. If hyperalimentation is delivered parenterally, a high risk for infection of the hyperalimentation line exists, and nursing interventions consist of scrupulous aseptic technique and monitoring of the aseptic technique of others. If enteral hyperalimentation is used, the risk of aspiration of nasogastric tube-feeding or reflux is present. Nursing interventions consist of monitoring the tube placement before each feeding by testing for pH consistent with gastric placement (pH ≤6.0, in contrast to pulmonary aspirate with a pH of >6.5), monitoring the respiratory status for signs of silent aspiration (sudden fever, atelectasis, respiratory distress), and monitoring the pulmonary secretions for signs of the dye marker that is added to the enteral formula (Metheny et al., 1993). Because the patient cannot complain of thirst if free water in the feeding is insufficient, the nurse should monitor serum sodium, urinary output, and urine specific gravity for signs of extracellular volume deficit. This is manifested by increasing serum osmolarity (estimated by doubling the serum sodium) as serum water volume decreases and decreasing urine output as the body seeks to conserve free water. If long-term tube-feeding is required, esophagostomy or gastrostomy decreases the risk of aspiration of tube-feeding that is inherent in nasogastric feedings (Olivares, Segovia, & Revuelta, 1974). Further information on the hypermetabolic state and nutritional support is detailed in Chapter 34.

Potential for Infection Related to Invasive Monitoring Devices

Early in Alex's hospitalization, several invasive monitoring devices were used to diagnose and track the pathophysiologic problems underlying the coma. ICP monitoring, intra-arterial pressure monitoring, and parenteral delivery of medications all carry the risk of nosocomial infection. The depressed immune response characteristic of severe injury compounds this risk. Assessment consists of monitoring for signs of infection and fever, lymphocyte count, and local inflammation. Intervention consists of scrupulous aseptic technique whenever the system is opened to the air (e.g., for calibration or removal of cerebrospinal fluid or blood specimens), faithful handwashing, and changing of tubing every 48 hours as recommended by the Centers for Disease Control and Prevention. Some centers use antibacterial agents for daily cleansing and dressing of the proximal point of entry, and some continue to use prophylactic antibiotics, although such use is controversial in light of concern about increasing antibiotic resistance of organisms (Barnett, 1993).

Potential for Family Knowledge Deficit Concerning Nature and Prognosis of Coma

At the time of Alex's transfer to the medical center hospital, his family hoped that the cause of the coma would be discovered and removed and that he would be the same person he had been before the catastrophic illness. Although the attending neurosurgeon told them early that people with this kind of hemorrhage often do not wake up or are left with severe deficits, they could not believe that Alex would not recover. Their hopes were particularly buoyed when he began to open his eyes and make facial grimaces when they were in the room. As the weeks wore on, however, they began to believe that the physician had been correct after all, and they reached out for the support and help with long-term placement that had been offered earlier.

Assessment and intervention for family knowledge deficit about the nature and implications of the patient's pathophysiologic state must be a collaborative effort of physician, nurse, and often such support people as social worker and chaplain. The goal of increasing family knowledge is to provide an adequate information base on which the family may make decisions about future care.

Only since the 1970s has sufficient evidence accumulated to make reasonably accurate prognoses from early neurologic status for patients with traumatic and nontraumatic coma. In both head injury and nontraumatic causes of coma, the presence or absence of specific combinations of neurologic signs on admission or in the first few days of hospitalization is a more accurate prognosticator of survival and the extent of recovery than is the specific disease process. However, the relative insensitivity of clinical signs creates a situation in which it is far easier to predict who will not be likely to recover than to predict the quality of recovery of the larger number with a greater chance of recovery. Nevertheless, knowing that a given patient has essentially no chance of a satisfactory recovery can prompt the family and the caregiving team to provide supportive rather than inappropriately heroic care. Similarly, knowledge that a patient has, for example, a 50% chance of meaningful recovery allows one to support honestly the family's hope and provide appropriately aggressive intensive care.

On the basis of clinical signs in traumatic head injury, the bulk of evidence suggests that there is less than a 5% chance of satisfactory recovery in the patient who does not open the eyes, does not make intelligible sounds, does not make localizing movements to pain, and has absent pupillary or oculocephalic responses at any point in the hospitalization. By 6 hours after the onset of coma, abnormal flexor or extensor motor responses are associated with 80% to 100% mortality if abnormal eye signs are present and 60% mortality if eye signs are normal (Jennett & Teasdale, 1981; Plum & Posner, 1980). Significantly depressed cerebral metabolic rate for oxygen or electrophysiologic monitoring parameters (such as electroencephalogram compressed spectral array and brain evoked potentials) may add precision to the prognostication of poor outcome obtained with clinical signs alone (Chiappa & Hoch, 1993; Jaggi, Obrist, Gennarelli, & Langfitt, 1990).

Nontraumatic coma is caused by drug overdose, cerebral vascular disease (infarct and hemorrhage), CNS infection, spontaneous subarachnoid hemorrhage, cardiac arrest, and such metabolic disorders as hepatic encephalopathy and renal encephalopathy. The prognostic indicators for this group of disorders is built on a multivariate analysis of 500 patients in coma from medical causes. This study showed that if coma lasted longer than 6 hours and was accompanied by abnormal neuro-ophthalmologic signs on admission (absence of any two of the following responses: corneal, oculocephalic, oculovestibular, or pupillary), chance of survival was less than 1%, regardless of the disease state. Conversely, even if coma lasted longer than 6 hours, comprehending of words, obeying of commands, orienting eye movements, or localizing of response during the first week after admission correlated with a 60% to 80% change of at least a moderately disabled or good outcome (Levy et al., 1981; Plum & Posner, 1980). Similar findings have been shown in cardiac arrest and are comparable in predicting poor outcome with somatosensory evoked potentials but better in predicting intermediate outcomes (Levy et al., 1985; Maise & Caronna, 1993).

The prognosis offered to Alex's family clearly was based on the grim signs on admission to the medical center: absence of pupillary response, absence of corneal response, and abnormal motor responses. Although he did regain spontaneous eye movements and eye opening, he never regained comprehension of sounds, eye movements that clearly tracked objects, or ability to obey commands. He was in a state that some have termed *prolonged unawareness* and others have called *persistent vegetative state* (Plum & Posner, 1980; Sazbon & Groswasser, 1991).

The intensive care team was faced with the assessment the family's readiness to hear the prognostic information as well as with the intervention of providing information. Nursing assessment in such situations consists of listening to the family's questions for change in emphasis (for example, change from "When will he wake up?" to "Do you think he will wake up?") and eliciting the family's understanding of and reaction to the information provided by the physician. In some situations, nursing intervention with the physician may be needed to encourage provision of prognostic information when the family is ready to hear it. Ways in which the nurse can facilitate family support during acute hospitalization are discussed in Chapters 16 and 17.

Potential for Community Knowledge Deficit Regarding Prevention of Pathology

Although Alex's pathology (AVM) was a congenital one for which there is no known prevention, a great many of the disorders that result in prolonged states of decreased arousal are largely preventable. Examples include traumatic head injury from motor vehicle accidents and cerebral hemorrhage from hypertension, drug overdose, and alcoholic hepatic encephalopathy (McGuire, 1986). Nurses can and should be vitally involved in community organizations, such as the National Head Injury Foundation and the American Heart Association, that seek to assess community knowledge and behavior and bring about changes in health behaviors.

DIAGNOSES STEMMING FROM REDUCED ABILITY TO INTERACT WITH THE ENVIRONMENT

The diagnoses under this heading are independent nursing diagnoses that have as their cause the patient's inability to communicate or to meet voluntarily his or her own basic physiologic and psychosocial needs. The diagnoses may be present for variable lengths of time, depending on whether or how rapidly the patient regains responsive awareness.

Self-Care Deficit: Protective Reflexes Related to Lack of Volitional Responsiveness

As discussed in Chapter 33, a continuum of self-care deficits ranges from complete deficits, including loss of protective reflexes, to deficits in one or more aspects of daily living. In Alex's case, the initial assessment demonstrated absence of corneal reflexes, pupillary responses, and presumably gag and cough reflexes (based on his prior aspiration and the loss of cranial nerve reflexes located higher in the brain stem). Intervention consists of basic nursing care that is protective of all the vital functions usually served by these reflexes. Loss of corneal reflex implies high risk of corneal abrasion, with secondary infection and loss of eyesight should there be functional recovery of consciousness. Careful application of artificial tears and use of eyepads or eyelid taping is indicated to protect eyes. Alex later regained the corneal reflex but still required regular eye care, because he had no ability to remove lint, dried secretions, or other material that might lodge in the eyes.

Initially, protection against the loss of gag and cough reflexes was managed medically by endotracheal tube and suctioning. When spontaneous breathing returned and the tube was removed, nursing assessment was crucial in determining Alex's ongoing ability to swallow his secretions and avoid aspiration. Methods of assessing swallowing are described in Chapter 22.

Impaired Mobility, Level 4: Potential for Disuse Syndrome and Immobility Complications

Movement and change of posture relative to gravity are activities that are automatic and frequent enough to maintain normal ventilation through periodic full expansion of the lungs and normal cardiovascular compensation for change to upright posture. The patient with absent volitional movement depends on the nursing staff for position change and stimulation of orthostatic vascular reflexes. Position change (turning and sitting upright) is an intervention that is useful for many diagnoses for patients with decreased arousal: prevention of inadequate gas exchange, prevention of skin breakdown, promotion of sensory stimulation, and prevention of orthostatic hypotension. In the early days of Alex's care, the nurses had to reduce ICP by ventriculostomy drainage before turning Alex, because the position change acted as an adaptive demand. Once his ICP stabilized, he could be safely turned to any position, including prone and sitting positions. Further assessment and intervention measures for problems induced by immobility are discussed in Chapter 20.

Potential for Skin Breakdown Related to Nutritional Deficit and Self-Care Deficit

The combination of Alex's inability to respond to sensations of pressure by moving and his loss of body protein from the hypermetabolic response to injury put him at high risk for breakdown of skin and underlying tissues and development of pressure sores.

For clinical purposes, pressure sores can be classified as one of two types: superficial friction lesions (sheet burn) and deep, pressure- and shearing-induced tissue necrosis. If superficial redness and friction lesions do not heal, they may progress to ulcerations of the skin and underlying tissues. The costs to the patient are severe, both in monetary costs of treatment and of extra days in the acute care hospital and in terms of pain and discomfort. The time taken by staff to treat active pressure ulcers is far greater than the minutes needed to prevent them (Panel for the Prediction and Prevention of Pressure Ulcers in Adults, 1992).

Shannon (1982) reviewed the literature and identified the major factors associated with development of pressure ulcers, a set of prognostic factors that have been confirmed and expanded in a set of guidelines from the Agency for Health Care Policy and Research. Patient factors include degree of immobility, state of the sensorium, chronologic age, nutritional status, kind of diagnosis, presence of major surgical procedure, type of medication, presence of infection, musculoskeletal alterations, soft-tissue changes, and presence of bowel or bladder incontinence. Environmental factors include situations that result in unrelieved external pressure (e.g., confinement to bed or chair that increases pressure at the interface of the supporting surfaces and the skin), inadequate supervision of patient mobility, restriction of patient movement by external devices, increased friction, shearing forces exerted when the patient is moved, lack of adequate nutritional management, and failure to maintain a dry environment. Those at highest risk are patients with paralyzing conditions, and the second highest risk group comprises those patients with decreased consciousness (Shannon, 1982).

Alex had 12 of the patient and environmental factors identified by Shannon (1982). Patient factors were immobility produced by neurologic injury, unconsciousness, hypoproteinemia, cachexia, neurologic diagnosis, loss of muscle mass, steroid therapy, bowel and bladder incontinence, and sustained elevated body temperature from this pulmonary infection. Environmental risk factors included confinement to bed, shearing damage when turned, and movement without clearing body off the mattress. As staff became discouraged about his prognosis, it is possible that he was repositioned less frequently than required when other patients' care assumed higher priority.

The goal of nursing management for the diagnosis of high risk of pressure sores is prevention of skin breakdown. Assessment has two components: assessment for risk factors and assessment for signs of beginning skin breakdown in patients at risk. Those assessed to be at high risk require continual monitoring of skin surfaces for signs of friction or pressure lesions. The nurse inspects the skin for redness that does not disappear with relief of pressure, excoriation or blistering of skin, and open abrasions. Simultaneously, the nursing staff uses a variety of preventive interventions such as repositioning the patient frequently to prevent prolonged pressure on any body part, ensuring that the patient's body clears the mattress when he or she is repositioned to prevent shearing of underlying tissues, providing enteral or parenteral hyperalimentation as prescribed while monitoring weight and serum protein to maintain nutritional status at adequate levels, and changing bed linens promptly when they are wet to maintain a dry environment.

Potential for Psychophysiologic Responses to External Environmental Stimuli

One of the dilemmas faced by staff who care for unresponsive patients is the inability to gauge if the patient is influenced by events in the environment that might be either distressful or positively stimulating to people with overt awareness and responsiveness. Nearly everyone who has worked in clinical neuroscience for any length of time has had one or more experiences of patients recalling events that occurred during a time when the patient appeared unresponsive to the environment and is aware of anecdotal accounts in the literature of similar situations. These anecdotes suggest potential for processing complex environmental stimuli even when overt signs of awareness are not present, at least in some patients.

The dilemma posed by these observations is this: are such observations merely of passing interest, an epiphenomenon of no particular meaning, or is it possible that the internal, not readily observable response to environmental stimuli is potentially harmful or helpful to the recovery of patients with absent or decreased responsiveness? This question can be examined from two perspectives: (1) the impact of environmental stimuli on physiologic stability in the acute phase of injury and (2) the impact on recovery of psychophysiologic overt responsiveness in later phases of illness (e.g., "coma stimulation" programs).

Environmental Stimuli and Physiologic Stability in the Acute Phase of Illness. Several investigators have documented clear and reproducible responses of the autonomic nervous system to a variety of auditory and somatosensory stimuli in neurologic patients with varying degrees of arousal. The findings may be summarized as follows:

1. Autonomic responses to new stimuli were of the alarm response nature—increased heart rate, skin conductance, and electroencephalogram activation, sometimes but not predictably concomitant with behavioral activity (grimacing, change in spontaneous movement) (Evans, 1976; Pfurtscheller et al., 1986; Schuri & von Cramon, 1979, 1981).

2. Stimulus intensity is more important in eliciting an alarm autonomic response than is the type or meaningfulness of the stimulus. Ability to

habituate or decrease the response to repeated instances of the same stimulus was evident in patients who made eye contact or followed simple commands (Schuri & von Cramon, 1980, 1981).

This alarm autonomic response has the potential to be harmful during the acute phase of illness or during intercurrent illness when physiologic instability is present. For example, increased respiratory rate, pulse, or blood pressure could be translated into increased demand on the intracranial compensatory system if autoregulation was impaired. Therefore, during periods of physiologic instability, the nurse should assess both the source of environmental stimuli (voices, noises, alarms, abrupt contact with the patient) and the patient's physiologic response to such stimuli (heart rate, ICP, blood pressure, respiratory rate). If all remain stable, no intervention is necessary. If instability occurs, the nurse may intervene to reduce the frequency and intensity of the particular environmental stimulus until such time as the patient becomes more physiologically stable.

Deliberative Sensory Stimulation in the Stable Phase of Reduced Responsiveness. Although the alarm or activation response may be potentially harmful when physiologic instability is present, there is also evidence that some positive physiologic responses are associated with environmental stimuli. Booth (1982) and Weber (1984) both used compressed spectral array to demonstrate electroencephalographic changes in response to differing sensory stimuli (voice versus music and sensorimotor therapy, respectively). Similarly, a few investigators have noted decreases in ICP (but not in CPP) in patients with GCS scores less than 8, associated with the sensory input of stroking and talking, particularly by family members (Hendrickson, 1987; Mitchell, Johnson, Habermann-Little, 1986A, 1986B; Pollack & Goldstein, 1981; Walleck, 1983). Coma stimulation protocols are based on enhancing the patient's physiologic and behavioral responses to environmental stimuli (Le Winn & Dimanescu, 1978; Mitchell et al., 1990). Such arousal can be helpful in restoring responsiveness in longer-term unconsciousness. Such stimulation programs provide planned stimuli to each of the senses—visual, auditory, olfactory, tactile, gustatory, and kinesthetic—in varying orders and for varying times.

Formal evaluation of the efficacy of such programs in shortening the duration of unresponsiveness and improving the quality of functional recovery has been plagued by lack of consistency in identification of the target patients, lack of control for spontaneous recovery, and inconsistency in specifying just what constitutes recovery (Wilson, Powell, Elliott, & Thwaites, 1991; Wood, 1991). Although a small body of controlled study provides evidence that duration of coma (defined as time to first recovery of obeying commands) is shorter in patients who have coma arousal procedures begun as soon as clinical stability is evident (Kater, 1989; Mitchell et al., 1990), other controlled studies do not show such effects (Johnson, Roethig, & Richards, 1993; Pierce et al., 1990). Because there is a fairly high level of misdiagnosis (Child, Mercer, & Child, 1993) and because it is so difficult to predict which patients in prolonged coma will eventually recover spontaneously, the claims purporting to show improved responsiveness with coma stimulation in patients in a persistent vegetative state are more controversial (Wood, 1991).

Potential for Impaired Family Coping

Traumatic brain injury and prolonged unresponsiveness after medical sources of coma strain both financial and psychosocial family resources. Although Alex was an adult, the fact that he had been living with his parents and the long period between his arrival home and his subsequently being found unresponsive produced strong feelings of guilt and responsibility in his parents. Because there are many similarities in family responses to a variety of devastating neurologic diseases, the discussion in Chapters 16 and 17 is applicable to Alex's case as well.

Inadequate Resources for Care of People with Prolonged Unawareness

The final diagnosis related to Alex's state of decreased arousal is lack of adequate community resources for care of patients with prolonged unawareness or with sufficient inability to interact with the environment such that they require total care for their most basic needs. The terminology to characterize patients who do not recover responsiveness rapidly continues to evolve. Because surviving but otherwise unresponsive persons tend to recover eye opening and apparent sleep-wake cycles within 24 weeks after insult, the term *coma* is no longer accurate, so the terms *vegetative state* (Jennett & Plum, 1972) or *prolonged postcomatose unawareness* (Bricolo, Turazzi, & Feriotti, 1980; Sazbon & Groswasser, 1991) are used instead. Characteristics of this state of apparent unawareness are open eyes in response to verbal stimuli but absence of visual tracking of objects, sleep-wake cycles with periodic spontaneous eye opening, and maintenance of vegetative functions (heart rate, respiration, blood pressure). Such patients have abnormal motor responses, do not utter comprehensible sounds, and do not obey commands (Jennett & Plum, 1972; Jennett & Teasdale, 1981). Given the variable and as yet not well predicted recovery for many of these patients, several recommend that the term "persistent" vegetative state not be used until at least 1 year of prolonged unawareness has passed (Berrol, 1986; Bricolo, Turazzi, & Feriotti, 1980).

Although such patients compose only a relatively small percentage of those surviving various sources of brain injury, estimates range from 3% to 14% of head-injured patients and from 5% to 20% of those surviving medical coma (Jennett & Plum, 1972; Jennett & Teasdale, 1981; Levin et al., 1991). These, plus the unknown number of people with disabilities severe enough to require total custodial care, tax the resources of home care and extended care facilities. In many cases, the inability of extended care facilities to take such patients requires many extra days of acute hospitalization until placement can be found.

The very poor prognosis for productive life gives rise to a number of legal and ethical dilemmas for providers of care (McIntyre, 1993). Several nurses have identified the many sources of psychological stress on nurses who care for these patients and some of the means nurses use to cope (Flaherty, 1982; Loen & Snyder, 1979, 1980). The questions of when or whether to treat intercurrent illness, to withdraw nutritional and fluid support, or even to consider such patients as organ donors have become important ethical considerations as prognostication has become more precise (Fox & Stocking, 1993; Mitchell, Kerridge, & Lovat, 1993). In the United States, some jurisdictions explicitly allow families to withhold any form of treatment, including nutrition, from patients in such hopelessly ill situations (Bernat, 1993).

The majority of patients with severe neurologic deficits who require extended care placement are not in persistent vegetative states and have a chance for meaningful recovery. Nurses as well as other community activists are important to monitoring patients and to lobbying for higher standards of care in these facilities and for adequate funding to provide such care.

SUMMARY

People with decreased arousal exhibit a complex array of human responses to their neurologic insult. Because the disorders that alter arousal also alter integration of body systemic function in the cerebral hemispheres, the care of such people requires a high degree of skillful nursing monitoring of all functions, not just neurologic status. Although the basic pathology cannot be altered, a key set of nursing interventions concerns manipulating the environment, initially to reduce demands on the patient's ability to respond, and later to increase the level of stimulation that the patient can tolerate.

References

Barnett, G. H. (1993). Intracranial pressure monitoring devices: Principles, insertion and care. In A. H. Ropper (Ed.), *Neurological and neurosurgical intensive care* (3rd ed., pp. 53–68). Lancaster, CA: Raven.

Bernat, J. L. (1993). Ethical aspects of withdrawing treatment from patients with severe brain damage. In A. H. Ropper (Ed.), *Neurological and neurosurgical intensive care* (3rd ed., pp. 481–490). Lancaster, CA: Raven.

Berrol, S. (1986). Evolution and the persistent vegetative state. *Journal of Head Trauma Rehabilitation, 1,* 7–13.

Booth, K. (1982). *Responses of unconscious patients to auditory stimuli: An electroencephalographic study.* Unpublished master's thesis, University of Washington, Seattle.

Bricolo, A., Turazzi, S., & Feriotti, G. (1980). Prolonged post-traumatic unconsciousness. Therapeutic assets and liabilities. *Journal of Neurosurgery, 52,* 625–634.

Chesnut, R. M., & Marshall, L. F. (1993). Management of severe head injury. In A. H. Ropper (Ed.), *Neurological and neurosurgical intensive care* (3rd ed., pp. 203–246). Lancaster, CA: Raven.

Chiappa, K. H., & Hoch, D. B. (1993). Electrophysiologic monitoring. In A. H. Ropper (Ed.), *Neurological and neurosurgical intensive care* (3rd ed., pp. 147–183). Lancaster, CA: Raven.

Child, N. L., Mercer, W. N., & Child, H. W. (1993). Accuracy of diagnosis of persistent vegetative state. *Neurology, 43,* 1465–1467.

Cruickshank, J. M., Neil-Dwyer, G., Degaute, J. P., Hayes, Y., Kuurne, T., Kytta, J., Vincent, J. L., Carruthers, M. E., & Patel, S. (1987). Reduction of stress/catecholamine-induced cardiac necrosis by beta 1-selective blockage. *Lancet, 2,* 585–589.

Deutschman, C. S., Konstantinides, F. N., Raup, S., Thienprasit, P., & Cerra, F. B. (1986). Physiological and metabolic response to isolated closed-head injury. *Journal of Neurosurgery, 64,* 89–98.

Diringer, M. N., Borel, C. O., & Hanley, D. F. (1993). Metabolic derangements in critically ill neurologic patients. In A. H. Ropper (Ed.), *Neurological and neurosurgical intensive care* (3rd ed., pp. 133–144). Lancaster, CA: Raven.

Evans, B. M. (1976). Patterns of arousal in comatose patients. *Journal of Neurological and Neurosurgical Psychiatry, 39,* 392–402.

Feldmann, E., Gandy, S. E., Becker, R., Zimmerman, R., Thaler, H. T., Posner, J., & Plum, F. (1988). MRI demonstrates descending transtentorial herniation. *Neurology, 38,* 697–701.

Flaherty, M. J. (1982). Care of the comatose patient: Problems faced alone. *Nursing Management, 13*(19), 44–46.

Fox, E., & Stocking, C. (1993). Ethics consultants recommendations for life-prolonging treatment of patients in a persistent vegetative state. *JAMA, 270,* 2578–2582.

Hendrickson, S. L. (1987). Intracranial pressure changes and family presence. *Journal of Neurosurgical Nursing, 19,* 14–17.

Jaggi, J. L., Obrist, W. D., Gennarelli, T. A., & Langfitt, T. W. (1990). Relationship of early cerebral blood flow and metabolism to outcome in acute head injury. *Journal of Neurosurgery, 72,* 176–182.

Jennett, B., & Plum, F. (1972). Persistent vegetative state after brain damage. *Lancet, 1,* 734.

Jennett, B., & Teasdale, G. (1981). *Management of head injuries.* Philadelphia: F. A. Davis.

Johnson, D. A., Roethig, J. K., & Richards, D. (1993). Biochemical and physiological parameters of recovery in acute head injury: Response to multisensory stimulation. *Brain Injury, 7,* 491–499.

Kater, K. M. (1989). Response of head-injured patients to sensory stimulation. *Western Journal of Nursing Research, 11,* 20–33.

Kraft, S. A., Larson, C. P., Shuer, L. M., Steinberg, G. K., Benson, G. V., & Pearl, R. G. (1990). Effect of hyperglycemia on neuronal changes in a rabbit model of focal cerebral ischemia. *Stroke, 21,* 447–450.

Langfitt, T. W. (1983). CT, NMR and emission tomography in the diagnosis and management of brain swelling and intracranial hypertension. *Intracranial Pressure, 5,* 54–55.

Le Winn, E. B., & Dimanescu, M. D. (1978). Environmental deprivation and enrichment in coma. *Lancet, 2,* 156–157.

Levin, H. S., Saydjari, C., Eisenberg, H. M., Foulkes, M., Marshall, L. F., Ruff, R. M., Jane, J. A., & Marmarou, A. (1991). Vegetative state after closed-head injury. A Traumatic Coma Data Bank report. *Archives of Neurology, 48,* 580–585.

Levy, D. E., Bates, D., Caronna, J. J., Cartlidge, N. E., Knill-Jones, R. P., Lapinski, R. H., Singer, B. H., & Shaw, D. A. (1981). Prognosis in nontraumatic coma. *Annals of Internal Medicine, 94,* 293–301.

Levy, D. E., Caronna, J. J., Singer, B. H., Lapinski, R. H., Frydman, H., & Plum, F. (1985). Predicting outcome from hypoxic-ischemic coma. *JAMA, 253,* 1420–1426.

Loen, M., & Snyder, M. (1979). Psychosocial aspects of care of the long-term comatose patient. *Journal of Neurosurgical Nursing, 11,* 235–237.

Loen, M., & Snyder, M. (1980). Care of the long-term comatose patient. *Journal of Neurosurgical Nursing, 12,* 134–137.

Longsteth, W. T. J., & Inui, T. S. (1984). High blood glucose level on hospital admission and poor neurological recovery after cardiac arrest. *Annals of Neurology, 15,* 59–63.

Maise, K., & Caronna, J. J. (1993). Coma after cardiac arrest: Clinical features, prognosis, and management. In A. H. Ropper (Ed.), *Neurological and neurosurgical intensive care* (3rd ed., pp. 331–349). Lancaster, CA: Raven.

March, K., Mitchell, P., Grady, S., & Winn, R. (1990). Effects of backrest position on ICP and CPP. *Journal of Neuroscience Nursing, 22,* 375–381.

McCarthy, E. (1986). Cardiovascular complications of intracranial disorders. In D. Nikas (Ed.), *The critically ill neurosurgical patient* (p. 53). New York: Churchill Livingstone.

McGuire, A. (1986). Issues in the prevention of neurotrauma. *Nursing Clinics of North America, 21,* 549–554.

McIntyre, K. M. (1993). Legal aspects of decision making in neurologic intensive care. In A. H. Ropper (Ed.), *Neurological and neurosurgical intensive care* (3rd ed., pp. 467–479). Lancaster, CA: Raven.

Metheny, N., Reed, L., Wiersema, L., McSweeney, M., Wehrle, M. A., & Clark, J. (1993). Effectiveness of pH measurements in predicting feeding tube placement: An update. *Nursing Research, 42,* 324–331.

Miller, J. D. (1985). Head injury and brain ischaemia—Implications for therapy. *British Journal of Anesthesia, 57,* 120–130.

Miller, J. D. (1993). Head injury. *Journal of Neurological and Neurosurgical Psychiatry, 56,* 440–447.

Mitchell, K. R., Kerridge, T. H., Lovat, T. J. (1993). Medical futility, treatment withdrawal and the persistent vegetative state. *Journal of Medical Ethics, 19*(2), 71–76.

Mitchell, P. H. (1986). Decreased adaptive capacity, intracranial: A proposal for a nursing diagnosis. *Journal of Neurosurgical Nursing, 18,* 170–175.

Mitchell, P. H. (1999). Decreased adaptive capacity: Intracranial. In B. J. Ackley & G. B. Ludwig (Eds.), *Nursing diagnosis handbook* (4th ed.) (pp. 395–400). St. Louis, C. V. Mosby.

Mitchell, P. H. (1994). Central nervous system I: Closed head injuries. In V. D. Cardona (Ed.), *Trauma nursing* (2nd ed., pp. 365–418). Philadelphia: W. B. Saunders.

Mitchell, P. H., & Ackerman, L. (1992). Secondary brain injury reduction. In G. M. Bulechek & J. C. McCloskey (Eds.), *Nursing interventions* (2nd ed., pp. 558–573). Philadelphia: W. B. Saunders.

Mitchell, P. H., Johnson, F. B., & Habermann-Little, B. (1986A). Nursing and ICP: Studies of two clinical problems. In J. D. Miller, G. M. Teasdale, J. O. Rowan, S. L. Galbraith, & A. D. Mendelow (Eds.), *Intracranial pressure VI* (p. 702). New York: Springer-Verlag.

Mitchell, P. H., Johnson, F. B., & Habermann-Little, B. (1986B). Promoting physiologic stability: Touch and ICP. *Community Nursing Research, 18,* 93.

Mitchell, S., Bradley, V. A., Welch, J. L., & Britton, P. G. (1990). Coma arousal procedure: A therapeutic intervention in the treatment of head injury. *Brain Injury, 4,* 273–279.

Moore, F. A., Moore, E. E., Jones, T. N., McCroskey, B. L., & Peterson, V. M. (1989). TEN versus TPN following major abdominal trauma-reduced septic mortality. *Journal of Trauma, 29,* 916–922.

Olivares, L., Segovia, A., & Revuelta, R. (1974). Tube feeding and lethal aspiration in neurological patients: A review of 720 autopsy cases. *Stroke, 5,* 654–657.

Panel for the Prediction and Prevention of Pressure Ulcers in Adults (1992). *Pressure ulcers in adults: Prediction and prevention. Clinical practice guideline number 3* (DHHS Publication No. 92–0047). Rockville, MD: Agency for Health Care Policy and Research, U.S. Department of Health and Human Services.

Pfurtscheller, G., Schwarz, G., & List, W. (1986). Long-lasting EEG reactions in comatose patients after repetitive stimulation. *Electroencephalography and Clinical Neurophysiology, 64,* 402–410.

Pierce, J. P., Lyle, D. M., Quine, S., Evans, N. J., Morris, J., & Fearnside, M. R. (1990). The effectiveness of coma arousal intervention. *Brain Injury, 4,* 191–197.

Plum, F., & Posner, J. (1980). *The diagnosis of stupor and coma* (3rd ed., p. 11). Philadelphia: F. A. Davis.

Pollack, L. D., & Goldstein, G. W. (1981). Lowering of intracranial pressure in Reye's syndrome by sensory stimulation [Letter to the editor]. *New England Journal of Medicine, 304,* 732.

Rauch, M., Mitchell, P. H., & Tyler, M. (1990). Validation of risk factors for the nursing diagnosis of decreased intracranial adaptive capacity. *Journal of Neuroscience Nursing, 22,* 173–178.

Reich, J. B., Sierra, J., Camp, W., Zanzonico, P., Deck, M. D., & Plum, F. (1993). Magnetic resonance imaging measurements and clinical changes accompanying transtentorial and foremen magnum brain herniation. *Annals of Neurology, 33,* 159–170.

Ropper, A. H. (1986). Lateral displacement of the brain and level of consciousness in patients with an acute hemispheral mass. *New England Journal of Medicine, 314,* 953–958.

Ropper, A. H. (Ed.) (1993). *Neurological and neurosurgical intensive care* (3rd ed.). Lancaster, CA: Raven.

Ross, D. A., Olsen, W. L., Ross, A. M., Andrews, B. T., & Pitts, L. H. (1989). Brain shift, level of consciousness and restoration of consciousness in patients with acute intracranial hematoma. *Journal of Neurosurgery, 71,* 498–502.

Samuels, M. A. (1993). Cardiopulmonary aspects of acute neurologic disease. In A. H. Ropper (Ed.), *Neurological and neurosurgical intensive care* (3rd ed., pp. 103–119). Lancaster, CA: Raven.

Saul, T. (1983). Intensive care of the brain-injured patient. *Critical Care Quarterly, 5*(4), 82.

Sazbon, L., & Groswasser, Z. (1991). Time-related sequelae of TBI in patients with prolonged postcomatose unawareness (PC-U) state. *Brain Injury, 5,* 3–8.

Schuri, U., & von Cramon, D. (1979). Autonomic responses to meaningful and nonmeaningful auditory stimuli in coma. *Archives of Psychiatric and Neurologic Science, 227,* 143–149.

Schuri, U., & von Cramon, D. (1980). Autonomic and behavioral responses in coma due to drug overdose. *Psychophysiology, 17,* 253–258.

Schuri, U., & von Cramon, D. (1981). Electrodermal responses to auditory stimuli with different significance in neurological patients. *Psychophysiology, 18,* 248–251.

Shannon, M. L. (1982). Pressure sores. In C. Norris (Ed.), *Concept clarification in nursing* (p. 357). Gaithersburg, MD: Aspen.

Slade, P. D. (1984). Sensory deprivation and clinical psychiatry. *British Journal of Hospital Medicine, 32,* 256–260.

Vannucci, R. C. (1990). Experimental biology of cerebral hypoxia-ischemia: Relation to perinatal brain damage. *Pediatric Research, 27,* 317–326.

Walleck, C. (1983). The effects of purposeful touch on intracranial pressure. *Heart and Lung, 12,* 428.

Walsh, R. (1981). Sensory environments, brain damage and drugs: A review of interactions and mediating mechanisms. *International Journal of Neuroscience, 14,* 129–137.

Weber, P. L. (1984). Sensorimotor therapy: Its effect on electroencephalograms of acute comatose patients. *Archives of Physical Medicine and Rehabilitation, 65,* 457–462.

Wilson, S. L., Powell, G. E., Elliott, K., & Thwaites, H. (1991). Sensory stimulation in prolonged coma: Four single case studies. *Brain Injury, 5,* 393–400.

Wolanin, M. O., & Phillips, L. (1981). *Confusion: Prevention and care.* St. Louis: C. V. Mosby.

Wood, R. L. (1991). Critical analysis of the concept of sensory stimulation for patients in vegetative states. *Brain Injury, 5,* 401–409.

Young, B., Ott, L., Phillips, R., & McClain, C. (1991). Metabolic management of the patient with head injury. *Neurosurgery Clinics of North America, 2*(2), 301–320.

7 Abnormally Increased Behavioral Arousal

MICHAELENE PHEIFER MIRR

The term *altered level of consciousness* makes most people immediately think of decreased levels of arousal. Abnormally increased behavioral arousal is a category that few people consider. A possible reason is that minimal attention has been given to this area in nursing research and publications. The questions proposed by Meleis (1991) for studying nursing phenomena are helpful in exploring the phenomenon of abnormally increased behavioral arousal:

1. When does the phenomenon occur?
2. Why does it occur?
3. How do we deal with it?
4. How do we prevent it?
5. What other conditions occur at the same time?

This chapter attempts to answer these questions in relation to abnormally increased behavioral arousal in patients with neurologic problems.

MANIFESTATIONS

Aggressive behavior, severe agitation, rage, and acting out are human responses that are difficult for the caregiver and the patient's family. The threat of the person's behavior both to the caregiver and to the patient increases anxiety in most caregivers. The behavior is often viewed as being "less than human." Unconsciously, we hope that the person will regain composure and behave like other human beings. Some of these feelings result from a lack of understanding of the underlying mechanisms associated with aggressive behavior. Aggressive behavior and delirium are two states that can be considered indicators of abnormally increased behavioral arousal and are discussed in this chapter. It is important to realize that both conditions are controllable and potentially reversible.

Many definitions of aggression exist. Aggressive behavior has been defined as "a behavioral response resulting from a highly agitated state. The aggression may be verbal or physical" (Plylar, 1989). This definition is more applicable to patients who are hyperarousable because of neurologic conditions than are definitions that include conscious intent to harm. Inaccurate interpretation of stimuli precipitates the aggressive behavior. Often, the person views the situation as a threat and uses aggressive behavior to decrease anxiety created by the threat. Accompanying autonomic nervous system findings include decreased salivation, decreased gastrointestinal activity, and increased heart rate and perspiration.

Delirium is characterized by reduced ability to maintain attention to external stimuli, disorganized thinking, and at least two of the following: reduced level of consciousness, perceptual disturbances, disturbance of sleep-wake cycle, increased or decreased psychomotor activity, disorientation to time, and memory impairment (American Psychiatric Association, 1994). People classified as delirious often have complex and protracted delusions—a dreamlike state during which the person is out of contact with the environment. Characteristic of delirium is alteration between lucid periods and times of confusion; during the lucid periods, people are frightened by their inability to control their mental functioning and actions (Carpenito, 1999; Snyder, 1991). Delirium often lasts a relatively short time, usually about 36 to 48 hours.

Table 7–1 lists conditions in which the hyperarousal state may be found. Whether abnormally increased arousal occurs because of misperceptions from defects in the sensory system, because of inability to integrate new stimuli with old because of memory problems, or as a partial result of an association with the person's premorbid personality is not fully known. In this chapter, particular attention is given to delirium and the aggressive state found in recovery from brain injury. The former state may be observed in patients who have alcohol suddenly withdrawn from them. Delirium may also be found in patients with encephalitis.

TABLE 7–1 • POSSIBLE ETIOLOGIES OF ABNORMALLY INCREASED BEHAVIORAL AROUSAL

Withdrawal from drugs, such as alcohol and barbiturates
Acute encephalitis
Head trauma, particularly during resolution of coma
Epilepsy (some forms of complex partial seizures)
Metabolic disorders (electrolyte imbalance)
Intracranial space-occupying lesions
Alzheimer's disease
Rabies
Strokes, particularly right hemispheric lesions
Multiple sclerosis

ANATOMIC BASIS

The four anatomic areas primarily associated with hyperarousal are the limbic system, the hypothalamus, the temporal lobes, and the frontal lobes. Phylogenetically, limbic structures are among the oldest parts of the brain, whereas the frontal and temporal lobes are classified as neocortex. There is some disagreement among scientists as to the total list of structures that compose the limbic system, although most would include the cingulate and parahippocampal gyri, the hippocampal formation, the amygdala, and the septal area (Nolte, 1993). These areas and their interconnections with the hypothalamus produce emotional behavioral responses. Figure 7–1 shows the components of the limbic system.

The amygdala, part of the limbic system, is a collection of nuclei that lie under the uncus of the temporal lobe. It has connections with the hypothalamus, the preoptic area, the septum, and the thalamus. The amygdala receives input directly and indirectly from the sensory systems, particularly from the olfactory system. The amygdala may be involved in integrating environmental cues with appropriate affective states that govern behavior. It is believed that the amygdala influences aggression through its role as coordinator of sensory input from the cortex. Lesions and stimulation of the amygdala produce a variety of effects on autonomic responses and emotional behaviors (Fox, 1999; Kupfermann, 1991). Therefore, the amygdala is considered more of a modulator of behavior rather than a primary source of aggressive behavior (Allison, 1993).

The hippocampus is located in proximity to the lateral ventricle. Afferent pathways connect it with sensory areas of the cortex. A main efferent connection is the subiculum, which has numerous links with many areas of the brain including the neocortex (Kandel, 2000). Although numerous anatomical studies

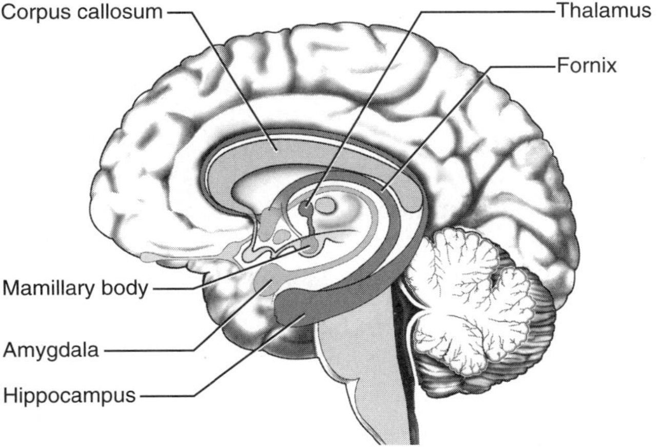

FIGURE 7–1 • Cerebrum: Mesial view. Limbic system and structures.

have been conducted on the hippocampus, a single function or set of functions has not been determined. The major role of the hippocampus in humans has to do with memory and learning (Nolte, 1993).

The hypothalamus integrates and coordinates the behavioral expression of emotional states and is believed to play a key role in mitigating aggressive behavior (Fox, 1999). The hypothalamus has control over some visceral, autonomic, and endocrine functions. It has multiple connections with other parts of the brain and limbic system. Nolte (1993) stated, "Many of the hypothalamic sites associated with particular behaviors may really be trigger points that, when stimulated, initiate neural activity in other parts of the CNS [central nervous system], which in turn causes the behavior pattern" (p. 271).

Animal studies have provided some knowledge about the functions of specific regions of the hypothalamus. Stimulation of the lateral hypothalamus causes autonomic and somatic responses characteristic of anger (Kandel, 2000). Observations from animal studies demonstrate that the hypothalamus is not a motor nucleus for the autonomic nervous system, but more of an integration center that produces a well-organized, coherent, and appropriate set of autonomic and somatic responses.

The septal complex lies under the corpus callosum. It is believed to have both an inhibitory and a facilitory influence on the hypothalamus. Septal lesions can reduce the rage or fear precipitated by hypothalamic lesions.

The temporal lobe is in close proximity to components of the limbic system and has many connections with the structures of this system. Injury to the temporal lobe often includes damage to these underlying structures. One function of the temporal lobe is memory. Interference with memory can cause problems with perception and integration of new stimuli. Lowered frustration tolerance that may result from memory impairment may manifest itself in aggressive behaviors (Hogan, 1988). At times, a minor event can elicit a major aggressive response.

The prefrontal area of the frontal lobe is associated with higher intellectual functions and is important for conscious expression of emotion. This area also suppresses emotional response to trivial and inconsequential stimuli (Kandel, 2000). Personality changes, lack of initiative, poor judgment, and inappropriate sexual behavior occur when the frontal lobes are damaged. These manifestations are usually seen with bihemispheric rather than unilateral involvement. The bifrontal area is readily damaged in brain injury; impact thrusts the lobes down against the orbital roof of the skull. People who have suffered bifrontal damage have a poor prognosis for full recovery of functions located in this area. These individuals often have permanent behavioral problems. Often, patients know what they need to do but are unable to do it because of deficits in planning and executing a sequence of behaviors to attain a goal. This deficit can be misinterpreted by others as resistance or lack of motivation (Hart & Harvey, 1993).

A fifth area of the brain may also be involved in modifying aggressive behavior. In addition to its role of controlling motor activity, the cerebellum also may be involved in higher-order behavior such as aggression (Allison, 1993; Schmahmann, 1991).

Research has also been conducted on the left and right hemispheres of the brain. Two hypotheses are popular although not supported by research (Gianotti, 1991). The first hypothesis posits specialization of the left hemisphere for positive emotions (e.g., happiness, affection) and of the right hemisphere for negative emotions (e.g., anger, hostility). The second hypothesis posits that there is an overall dominance of the right hemisphere for emotional behavior. Therefore, with injury to the right cerebral hemisphere, emotional stability and control are disrupted. More recent study suggests a complex interaction among the nervous system, the immune system, and the endocrine system, all of which modulate behavior as well as health. Thus, endocrine responses may also play a role in aggressive behavior. The interactions between physical and psychologic systems are studied in the emerging field of psychoneuroimmunology (Fox, 1999).

CASE STUDIES

Two case studies are presented to typify the responses in people who manifest abnormally increased behavioral arousal: aggression after brain injury and delirium resulting from alcohol withdrawal. The latter example was chosen because of the high incidence of trauma resulting from alcohol intoxication.

• C A S E   S T U D Y   1

Aggression after Traumatic Brain Injury

Andy, 30 years old, suffered a traumatic brain injury in a motorcycle accident. The computed tomography (CT) scan showed a subdural hematoma in the right temporoparietal area causing a shift of the midline structures, small areas of contusion in the right temporal lobe, and a nondepressed fracture of the left occipital bone. The subdural hematoma in the right temporal lobe area was evacuated, and part of the temporal lobe from the temporal gyrus to the tentorial notch was also removed. After surgery, Andy had a left hemiparesis, which gradually lessened.

His postoperative course was characterized by severe behavioral problems. Behaviors included wandering aimlessly, spitting out pills, yelling, taking off his clothes in the hall, striking out at or biting staff, kicking and hitting people, and speaking incoherently. Many episodes of severe agitation and violence occurred. In addition, slight conductive aphasia, poor orientation, and poor short-term memory were present. Lithium, haloperidol, physostigmine, and lecithin were administered at various times during his recovery to help subdue the violent behavior. At the end of 3 months, Andy was less violent but still manifested aggressive behavior, poor short-term memory, and difficulty interacting.

Andy fell into level 4 of the Rancho Los Amigos Levels of Cognitive Functioning Scale (Table 7–2) (Malkmus & Booth, 1980) for traumatic brain injury (TBI) patients and stage 2 of Sbordone's Stages of Recovery in TBI (Table 7–3) (Sbordone, 1990). Not all TBI patients pass through an agitated phase, and, for those who do, the length of time varies. A few, like Andy, never progress beyond this level. Nursing care needs to focus on decreasing agitation to enable the patient to process external stimuli rather than internal stimuli. Therefore, nursing interventions include channeling excess energy constructively as well as promoting simple gross motor activity and automatic self-care tasks (Malkmus & Booth, 1980).

TABLE 7–2 • RANCHO LOS AMIGOS LEVELS OF COGNITIVE FUNCTIONING SCALE AFTER HEAD TRAUMA

Level	Response	Description
1	None	Completely unresponsive to any stimulus
2	Generalized	Reacts inconsistently and nonpurposefully to stimuli; may respond with physiologic changes, gross body movements, or utterances
3	Localized	Reacts specifically but inconsistently to stimuli; responds directly to a stimulus; shows vague awareness of self and body; may pull at tubes and react to discomfort
4	Confused Agitated	Heightened state of activity but unable to process information correctly; reacts to internal confusion; nonpurposeful behavior with confabulation present; cries, screams, and manifests aggressive behavior; cannot discriminate among people; performs gross motor activities but not self-care activities
5	Confused Inappropriate	Follows simple commands; may show agitated behavior from inability to cope with external demands; gross inattention to environment, easily distracted; impaired memory and inappropriate verbalization; cannot initiate tasks; often uses things incorrectly
6	Confused Appropriate	Displays goal-directed behavior but requires direction from others; follows simple commands; shows carryover of information from previously learned tasks; memory problems persist; inconsistently oriented to time and place; increased awareness of self and others
7	Automatic Appropriate	Oriented in hospital and home settings; performs tasks in robotlike manner; superficial awareness of own condition but lacks good problem-solving abilities; carryover for new learning; independent in self-care activities; needs structure but can initiate tasks of interest
8	Purposeful Appropriate	Alert and oriented; few memory problems; can begin vocational rehabilitation; carryover for new learning; social, emotional, and intellectual capacities may be decreased from pretrauma level

From Malkmus, D., Booth, B., & Kodimer, C. (1980). *Rehabilitation of the head injured adult—Comprehensive cognitive management.* Downey, CA: Professional Staff Association of the Rancho Los Amigos Hospital.

TABLE 7–3 • SELF-CARE DEFICIT SCALE

Numerical Index	Definition
0	Independent, able to perform activity with no one present
1	Requires use of equipment or device
2	Requires help from another person for assistance, supervision, or teaching
2.2	Supervision—may include verbal reinforcement or standby assistance
2.4	Minimal assistance, patient does 75% of work
2.6	Moderate assistance, patient does 50% of work
2.8	Maximal assistance, patient does 25% of work
3	Requires help from another person and equipment or device
4	Dependent, does not participate in activity

From Baer, C., Delorey, M., & Firzmaurice, J. (1984). A study to evaluate the validity of the rating system for self-care deficit. In M. Kim, G. McFarland, & A. McLane (Eds.), *Classification of nursing diagnoses.* St. Louis: C. V. Mosby.

Delirium from Alcohol Withdrawal

Paul was a 40-year-old businessman who was hospitalized after being involved in a motor vehicle accident in which he sustained a fractured femur and a mild concussion. Paul was alert when he was admitted to the emergency department. In response to questioning about alcohol, he stated that he was a social drinker. Two days after admission, the nurses noted that Paul was extremely restless, picking at the bed sheets, and jumping from one topic to another during conversations. He would begin to answer a question but after a few words would shift to other topics. Paul talked constantly. The nurses noted that he had difficulty holding eating utensils and his electric razor because of a tremor. Vital signs revealed a heart rate of 112, a temperature of 100°F, and a systolic blood pressure slightly elevated from that at admission.

When his wife came to visit in the afternoon, Paul believed that she was his mother. Paul was unable to rest or sleep and was in constant motion. He reached for objects in the air and hit staff who tried to measure vital signs or provide care. He perspired profusely. His heart rate increased to 130 and his temperature to 101°F. The severe delirium phase lasted 24 hours. After this had subsided, Paul was exhausted and slept a great deal of the time.

Medical treatment included administering chlorpromazine, lorazepam for sedation, and phenytoin to decrease the likelihood of seizures (Segatore, 1999). Intravenous fluids were begun, and vitamins were given. The primary nursing concern focuses on safety. Measures to minimize the risk of self-injury or accidental injury to others are essential.

HUMAN RESPONSES ASSOCIATED WITH ABNORMALLY INCREASED BEHAVIORAL AROUSAL

In this section, nursing diagnoses appropriate for patients who manifest abnormally increased behavioral arousal are presented, along with assessments and interventions that nurses can use to meet outcomes for these diagnoses.

Diagnoses for the Patient

The nursing diagnoses that pertain to the patient include the following:

1. High risk for injury (trauma)
2. Alterations in nutrition: less than body requirements
3. Self-care deficits
4. Sensory-perceptual alterations
5. Sleep pattern disturbance (particularly in delirium)
6. Alteration in thought processes
7. High risk for violence

Other diagnoses may be appropriate in some situations, but those listed are common for patients with abnormally increased behavioral arousal.

HIGH RISK FOR INJURY (TRAUMA)

This diagnosis is defined as the "presence of risk factors for bodily injury" (Carpenito, 1999; Gordon, 1993). Defining characteristics or risk factors of this diagnosis include disorientation, impaired judgment, muscle weakness, paralysis, incoordination, mobility impairment, and sensory-perceptual deterioration. People in the abnormally increased behavioral arousal state are prone to injury because they are unable to make correct judgments about their own capabilities, they misperceive items in the environment, or they act impulsively.

Assessment includes surveying the environment for objects that could be harmful to the patient, determining the patient's cognitive state, and evaluating the staff's and family's knowledge of the condition. The goal for the patient with this diagnosis is that the patient remain free of injury.

Although it may seem simplistic to list removal of harmful objects from the immediate environment as a nursing intervention for this diagnosis, many nurses who do not routinely care for hyperarousal patients do not remember to survey the environment for such objects. All glass objects, items that have sharp edges, and substances that can be consumed must be removed from the patient's immediate territory. Rubbing alcohol, lotion, and other skin care materials are items in the last category that are often at the bedside and could be harmful to the patient.

Restraints may be necessary to prevent the patient from removing tubes or from getting out of bed, but they should be used sparingly. Some rehabilitation specialists believe that alternatives to restraints, such as a sitter or a controlled activity (e.g., walking the agitated patient), have a better therapeutic outcome. If restraints are used, sites under the restraints need frequent assessment to determine the integrity of the underlying tissue and any nerve or circulatory impairment resulting from the high level of patient activity. Providing periods when restraints can be removed helps reduce agitation. Most institutions have restraint policies that conform to hospital and federal guidelines.

The presence of tubes and catheters often increases agitation. Whenever possible, these stimuli should be removed. Hand mitts are useful to help prevent dislodgment of tubes and catheters if it is necessary to keep them in place. People who are delirious must be monitored frequently because of the severity of their condition and the strain of the high level of activity on the heart.

A floor bed (Brigman, Dickey, & Zegeer, 1983) may be useful for patients in the confused-agitated phase of recovery following TBI (Fig. 7–2). Such a bed eliminates the need for restraints to keep the patient in bed, and patients can move about, which helps dissipate energy and aggression. Feeding tubes and tracheostomies pose no care problems on floor beds. It is not possible, however, to use an indwelling catheter because the urine will not drain, so an external catheter is needed. Frequent assessment of this patient population must be part of the care plan. It is easy to forget this on a busy unit, and injuries can occur very quickly unless there is adequate supervision.

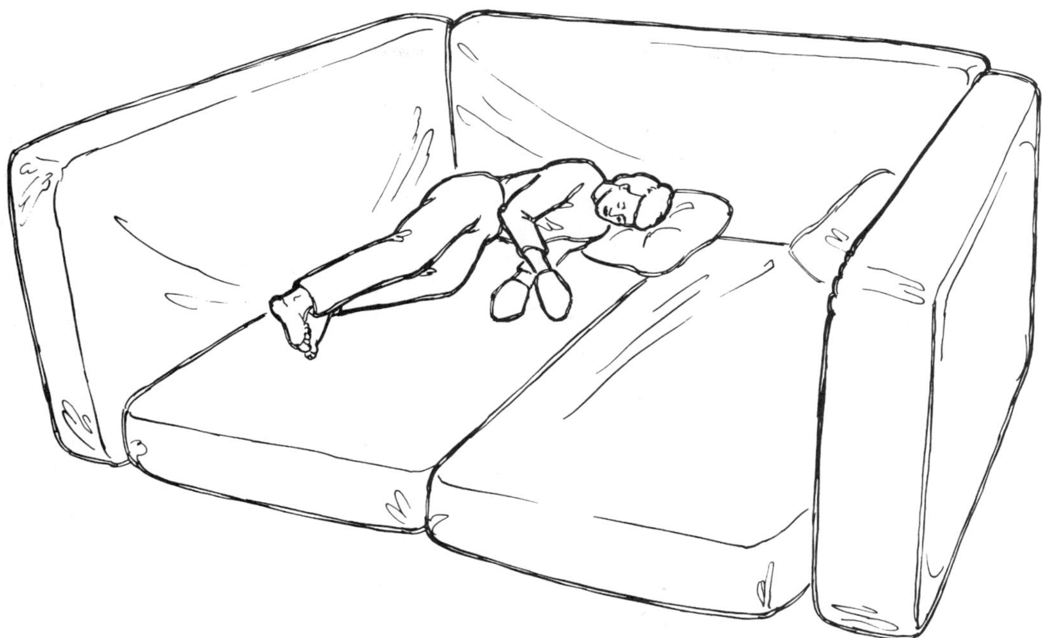

FIGURE 7–2 • A floor bed used for head-injured patients who are hyperactive. Mattresses are placed on the floor and as padding on the sides. Patients can move about without fear of injury.

ALTERATIONS IN NUTRITION: LESS THAN BODY REQUIREMENTS

The nursing diagnosis, as accepted by the North American Nursing Diagnosis Association (NANDA), includes among the defining characteristics people who require additional nutrients because of their high level of activity (Carpenito, 1999). Many people in the hyperarousal state, particularly those in delirium, manifest signs of inadequate nutritional and fluid intake. They also lack the ability to concentrate and thus forget the food placed before them. Patients in delirium frequently have elevated temperature, which places an added demand on their nutritional status.

Assessment includes determining the patient's needed caloric level in relation to his or her activity level by observing the patient and using charts for energy expenditure associated with exercise. The patient's temperature is noted in determining the number of calories required. The nurse must consider the patient's past nutritional status, such as having been given intravenous fluids for protracted periods. The development of institutional multidisciplinary nutrition teams has been helpful in assessing and determining nutritional needs for high-risk patients. The goal of this diagnosis is that the patient will have sufficient intake of nutrients to meet energy expenditure.

Safety measures must be considered in providing interventions for nutritional needs. Sturdy plastic glasses are preferred for patients who can hold them, because glass utensils are easily broken and patients may use the broken pieces to harm themselves. Styrofoam or paper cups collapse if the patient grasps them tightly. Covered, untippable cups or plastic sports bottles are practical. These are especially helpful for people who also have a tremor, incoordination, or hemiparesis. Small, frequent feedings are best because of the person's short attention span. Meals served at room temperature prevent burn injuries. Eating meals in a group setting, such as a dining area, is preferred not only to encourage socialization at mealtime but also to provide role-modeling behavior. Promoting participation in simple, automatic self-care activities such as eating finger foods facilitates nutritional needs. Food items such as cheese, fruits, vegetables, hard cookies, and crackers are desirable finger foods. "Junk food" items such as potato chips and candy should be avoided. If the patient has muscle wasting, protein supplements may be needed. Collaboration between the dietitian or nutrition team and the nurse is needed to plan and implement a nutrition program that will provide an adequate supply of nutrients for the hyperactive patient.

SELF-CARE DEFICITS

People in the abnormally increased behavioral arousal state will manifest various levels of self-care deficits, from the completely dependent state to the ability to perform much of their own care. The self-care deficits may be a result of the use of restraints to prevent injury, of the person's inability to concentrate, or of the presence of associated problems.

Assessment includes noting the capabilities of the patient so that these can be incorporated into the plan of care. Self-care deficits in hygiene, grooming, elimination, and eating are of particular concern. The goals for this diagnosis are that the patient's basic needs will be met and that the patient will progress, as his or her condition permits, toward independence.

Interventions include using automatic, familiar, gross motor activities to help the person regain motor coordination. Such activities place few demands on the patient (McNeny, 1990). Some of these are self-care activities, such as combing the hair and washing the face. The nurse initiates the activity, because the person would most likely only look at the utensils or use them for other purposes. Emphasis is not placed on completing the task; at this stage of recovery, that would only increase agitation.

Hygiene requires close attention. For the patient with an elevated temperature, frequent bathing and skin care are required. If the person is incontinent, care is needed to prevent incontinence; tub baths may prove both relaxing and helpful in promoting skin integrity. Chapters 32 and 33 provide additional information on self-care activities.

SENSORY-PERCEPTUAL ALTERATIONS

The etiology for this diagnosis includes environmental complexity that may be either excessive or insufficient (Carpenito, 1999; Gordon, 1993). Delirium can originate from sensory overload or from sensory deprivation. Isolation, socially restricted environment, impaired communication, and uncompensated visual or hearing deficit are other possible etiologies of this diagnosis. Defining characteristics include irritability, anxiety, restlessness, disorientation, sleeplessness, decreased problem-solving ability, increased muscle tension, change in usual response to stimuli, and, possibly, hallucinations (Carpenito, 1999; Gordon, 1993). All of these may be observed in people with abnormally increased behavioral arousal.

Assessment is aimed at determining the extent of the alteration. Elderly patients need to be assessed closely because decreased sensory function is part of the aging process and may influence the assessment of this alteration (Drury & Akins, 1991). In people in delirium, the type and extent of the hallucinations must be evaluated. Whereas the medical diagnosis seeks to determine the underlying pathology resulting in the alterations in perception, the nurse is concerned with identifying the problems that interfere with the patient's functional ability and safety. The goal for this diagnosis is that the patient will be able to interpret the immediate environment correctly.

Interventions vary depending on whether the etiology is excessive stimuli or inadequate stimuli. If it is excessive stimuli, interventions to decrease stimuli are indicated. Placing the patient in a quiet atmosphere, reducing activity, and avoiding loud noises and sudden changes will help the person to interpret the environment correctly. A structured environment is also helpful (Sbordone, 1991). A calm manner, a soothing voice, and playing quiet, restful music are other interventions that can be used. A quiet room for patients who seem to become agitated from too much stimulation may also be helpful. The staff usually makes this determination for the patient because the person is usually unaware of his or her need for decreased stimulation. Care must be taken, however, to prevent sensory deprivation, which may occur if too much stimulation is removed for a long period of time.

In patients having hallucinations, the nurse does not support or encourage the patient's misperceptions. The nurse may ask the patient to describe his or her surroundings without arguing with the patient. Providing reassurance that the patient is safe decreases the patient's anxiety and lessens restlessness. Whispers and muffled conversations should be avoided, because they can be misinterpreted by the patient and serve to increase anxiety.

SLEEP PATTERN DISTURBANCE

This diagnosis is made frequently in people with delirium. Lack of sleep contributes to the symptoms found. Chapter 9 provides a discussion of the phenomenon of sleep.

ALTERATION IN THOUGHT PROCESSES

This diagnosis is common to all people with abnormally increased behavioral arousal and accounts for many of the other problems found. Defining characteristics of this diagnosis include impaired attention span, inappropriate behavior, impaired recall ability, decreased ability to conceptualize ideas, impaired judgment or decision making, increased self-concern, and hypo- or hypervigilance (Carpenito, 1999).

The goal for this diagnosis is to increase the person's ability to process information correctly. Patients in a hyperarousal state or an agitated state cannot be held accountable for their behavior because they are not yet capable of producing thought-out actions (Sbordone, 1991). Patients experience inner confusion originating from cognitive disruption and are unable to process information from the environment correctly. This is often manifested in agitated behaviors.

Chapters 10 and 11 provide additional interventions that are useful in caring for people with alteration in cognitive processes.

HIGH RISK FOR VIOLENCE

Aggressive behavior is a frequent finding in people manifesting abnormally increased behavioral arousal. Some of the defining characteristics include body language or facial expression, clenched fists, rigid posture, and tautness; increased motor behavior, such as pacing; overt aggressive acts; rage; self-destructive behavior; suspicion of others; and hostile, threatening verbalizations. Some other characteristics are increased anxiety, fear of self or others, hypersexual behavior, argumentative behaviors, and antisocial character disturbance (Carpenito, 1999).

The goal for this diagnosis is that the patient will not harm self or others. Family members may become frequent targets of aggressive behavior. A number of interventions can be used to achieve this goal, but one of the most important considerations is the knowledge nurses, families, and others have about techniques they can use to protect themselves from assaultive and aggressive behaviors. If the nurse or family member feels secure, it is communicated to the patient, which helps decrease the patient's anxiety and aggressive behavior. Because many of the nurses and families have little knowledge about techniques that are effective in dealing with potentially violent patients, education is indicated. A calm, quiet, but firm approach conveys to the patient that the nurse or family member is in control. This helps alleviate the fear the patient has of losing control and striking out at those present.

Working with patients who have aggressive tendencies taxes the nursing staff and family. A multidisciplinary approach with consistent response and reaction by all team members will best benefit the patient. Care conferences are useful in that fears and concerns can be voiced along with suggestions for modifying the plan of care. It has been demonstrated that aggressive patients are less confused when cared for by a consistent group of staff persons (Tomberlin, 1990).

Interventions that serve to calm the patient are appropriate. These include the use of soothing music and tapes of familiar voices when the patient must be left alone. The patient should be left alone as little as possible, because human contact tends to reduce the fright of these patients. It is important to avoid sudden changes or surprises, and attention should be directed away from sources of agitation. Activity is alternated with rest. Activities such as throwing a soft foam ball and other gross motor actions help lessen aggressive actions. Activities should be geared to the patient's level of cognitive functioning to avoid insulting the person's intelligence by using activities deemed childish. Allowing freedom of movement as much as possible is desirable because restraints tend to increase agitation. Because the patient's cognitive abilities are extremely limited in this stage of recovery, minimal demands should be placed on the patient. The goal is to have the patient progress through this phase rather than acquire any specific skills.

It is important to speak directly to the patient in a calm voice. All care activities are explained to the patient so that the element of surprise is decreased. Information is repeated as often as seems necessary to ensure understanding. If the patient appears to be becoming agitated, the amount of stimulation is lessened.

McKinlay and Hickox (1988) developed an effective method of working with family members to decrease aggressive behavior. Treatment is usually implemented in the home and involves assertiveness training along with a behavior management program. The program stresses identification of situations likely to trigger aggressive behavior, increasing the families' sensitivity to these signals and responding with relaxation procedures. The patient's attention span and cognitive abilities are important points to assess in implementing a behavior modification program; the expectations should not exceed the patient's abilities.

It is recommended that medications to lessen agitation be used sparingly and only when other measures have proven ineffective, because the use of medications prolongs the time spent in this stage of recovery (O'Shadick & Zasler, 1990; Segatore, 1999). Aggression, hallucinations, and potential for harming self or others are reasons to institute pharmacologic control (Adis International, 1997). Three categories of drugs are given most often in the treatment of aggressive behavior: beta blockers, serotonin agonists, and antiepileptics (Adis International, 1997; Hirsh, 1993; Inoye et al., 1999; Rose, 1988). Beta blockers prevent the sympathetic response to various stimuli. Serotonin agonists may also be given based on the theory that aggressive behavior results from imbalances in the serotonergic system. Antiepileptics have proven effective in decreasing aggressive behavior, supporting the belief that the behavior is the result of seizure activity (Yatham & McHale, 1989). Other medications that may be used include haloperidol or lithium. Medications are more often used in treating delirium because of the extreme agitation present. Benzodiazepines, such as lorazepam, diazepam, oxazepam, and alprazolam, may be given to reduce the agitation from delirium (Adis International, 1997). These drugs have a rapid onset but a short duration and may cause more sedation than haloperidol causes. Low doses of haloperidol can also be given for severe agitation.

Diagnoses for the Family and Significant Others

The diagnoses that relate to the family include the following:

1. Knowledge deficit regarding the condition
2. Ineffective family coping: compromised

KNOWLEDGE DEFICIT REGARDING THE CONDITION

Behaviors found in the increased arousal state can be very frightening to the patient's family. A number of etiologies suggested by NANDA for lack of knowledge are applicable for families of patients who manifest abnormally increased behavioral arousal: inability to seek information, such as not knowing about resources; lack of readiness for reception of information; cognitive limitation; and lack of external support and resources. Defining characteristics include verbalization of lack of knowledge, inappropriate behaviors, and inaccurate follow-through of previous instruction (Carpenito, 1999). Assessment may reveal high anxiety because of lack of understanding about the condition, undue expectations of the patient, and denial. The goal for families with this diagnosis is that the family will express an understanding and acceptance of the patient who is manifesting abnormally increased arousal behavior.

Kreutzer, Zasler, Camplair, and Leininger (1990) suggested several interventions for families that increase the knowledge level for dealing with an agitated or aggressive individual. These strategies include family education, family support groups, family networking, family advocacy, family therapy, marital therapy, and sexual counseling. Although all these interventions are useful at various points in time, the use of family support groups and family networking may initially be the most helpful.

Support groups provide a variety of sources of information. Knowledge about the cause of the behavior manifested, the length of time that such behavior can be expected to exist, and the ways the family can assist the patient are presented. Information provides the family with a sense of control. Knowledge can lead to a reduction in anxiety. Support can be gained from hearing others relate the process that their relative has gone through and the ways they have dealt with the condition. A more detailed discussion of support groups and networks is found in the chapters on affiliative relationships.

Parents of brain-injured children have special needs. Education and information regarding the injury and the recovery process, as well as resources, are often needed. Perceived support and control of life events are major predictors of an injured child's outcome. Very few families are prepared to deal with a child's behavioral changes and physical needs following a traumatic brain injury (Waaland, 1990). In addition to meeting educational needs of families, periodic individual and family counseling may be needed to address concerns as they arise over time. Support through special education programs from the school system may also be of benefit.

Role modeling is another intervention nurses can implement in helping families of patients acquire knowledge about the hyperarousal state. Just as nurses may at first be frightened by aggressive behavior, family members may also be afraid. Being present with the family members when they visit is one method for instructing them in techniques that can be used to improve interaction with the patient. Sensitivity to family members' reactions to the condition is needed; they should never be pushed into staying with the patient if they feel insecure or afraid.

INEFFECTIVE FAMILY COPING: COMPROMISED

For family members, aggressive behavior by the patient is very trying. Seeing a loved one unable to control behavior or even striking out and hitting staff and family members is extremely difficult. Behavioral indicators of ineffective coping include crying, avoiding the patient and the care setting, denial, being critical of care and caregivers, blaming self, expressing anger, becoming overprotective, and performing actions associated with high levels of anxiety (Kreutzer et al., 1990). Etiologies related to ineffective family coping may be inadequate information or disability progression that exhausts the supportive capacity of family members as well as causes emotional conflicts. Defining characteristics include the significant other's preoccupation with personal reactions to the patient's condition, the family member's attempt at supportive behaviors being less than adequate, and withdrawal from the situation. Understanding and acceptance of the patient's behavior, an outcome given for the preceding diagnosis, Knowledge Deficit, is appropriate for meeting this goal.

Other resources may be needed to assist the family to cope with the patient's condition. Providing time and opportunities for the family members to discuss their concerns is helpful. This is especially necessary if the patient has been abusive to family or staff members. Offering realistic hope is another intervention that can be used. Knowing that most patients are in this state—be it post trauma or delirium—for a limited period of time provides the family with an end goal. Interacting with a loved one who is abusive or aggressive is very taxing. Suggesting that family members take time away—a free day or free weekend—can do much to renew their energies. If the family seems anxious about doing this, giving them a telephone number and a specific nurse to call will help ease their fears about not being present all the time. The availability of respite care is also an important aspect of any discharge planning.

Ineffective family coping may be more evident in families where the injured family member is a child. Although research is lacking on long-term follow-through with brain-injured children, there is evidence to suggest that the full extent of cognitive impairment may not manifest itself until adolescence. Therefore, the connection between an early traumatic brain injury and later behavioral problems is frequently missed (Waaland, 1990). This leads to unnecessary stress and frustration for all family members. Children with severe traumatic brain injury have more difficulty with memory and attention, creating significant learning and parenting challenges. Children younger than 6 years are more vulnerable to expressive language and motor dysfunctions.

Diagnosis for the Community

KNOWLEDGE DEFICIT

The nursing diagnosis related to abnormally increased behavioral arousal that is found in the community is knowledge deficit. Knowledge is lacking about the long-term effects of trauma and about the seriousness of delirious states associated with withdrawal from drugs such as alcohol (Segatore, 1999). Public education is needed to alert the public to means that can be used to prevent TBI. Control of the environment, such as continued seat belt legislation, strict drunk driving laws, mandatory insurance for license renewal, and safety in all sports, can do much to alleviate the cause of the underlying problem. People who have not had close interaction with anyone who has suffered a severe TBI are often unaware of the behavioral problems present in the recovery phases. Society is now being forced to look at management for severely disabled TBI patients; in the past, these people rarely survived the trauma. Making the public more knowledgeable about the serious implications of TBI and the often-permanent effects may assist in decreasing trauma in our society.

Although many brain injury rehabilitation programs are available throughout the United States, few have programs specifically designed for behaviorally challenging patients (Lucas, 1993). Therefore, patients with aggressive behaviors are likely to be placed in brain-injury rehabilitation programs, in psychiatric units, or even in prison. Placement of behaviorally challenging patients in programs that specialize in neurobehavioral dyscontrol can result in stabilization of behavior and successful reintegration into community settings. These programs combine behavior therapy, cognitive therapy, and neuropsychiatry. The lack of adequate facilities for patients with aggressive behaviors may be due to the lack of knowledge of brain injury and recovery in the general population. However, the success of rehabilitation programs specifically designed for behaviorally challenging patients has led to programs that offer a continuum of services from secured environments to community-based neurobehavioral programs (Lucas, 1993).

SUMMARY

Abnormally increased behavioral arousal can be manifested as aggressive behavior or as delirium. Whereas both conditions are potentially reversible, delirium is considered a temporary state. Aggressive behavior resulting from traumatic brain injury may be long term or permanent. Specific physiologic mechanisms of aggressive behavior have not yet been determined, although it is known that the limbic system, hypothalamus, temporal lobes, and prefrontal cortex are involved. Human responses associated with abnormally increased behavioral arousal provide challenges for nursing care. Careful assessment and family-centered nursing interventions are critical for the multiple health deviations that result.

References

Adis International. (1997). Drug-induced delirium. *Drugs and Therapeutic Perspectives, 10,* 5–9.
Allison, M. (1993). Exploring the link between violence and brain injury. *Headlines, 4,* 12–15.
American Psychiatric Association (1994). *Quick reference to the diagnostic criteria from DSM-IV-R.* Washington, DC: Author.

Brigman, C., Dickey, C., & Zegeer, L. (1983). Agitated aggressive patient. *American Journal of Nursing, 83,* 1409–1412.

Carpenito, L.J. (1999). *Handbook of nursing diagnosis* (8th ed.). Philadelphia: J.B. Lippincott.

Drury, J., & Akins, J. (1991). Sensory/perceptual alterations. In M. Maas, K.C. Buckwalter, & M. Hardy (Eds.), *Nursing diagnoses and interventions for the elderly* (pp. 369–386). Reading, MA: Addison-Wesley.

Fox, S., Shephard, T., McCain, N. (1999). Neurologic mechanisms in psychoneuroimmunology. *Journal of Neuroscience Nursing, 31,* 87–96.

Gianotti, G. (1991). Frontal lobe damage and disorders of affect and personality. In M. Swash & J. Oxbury (Eds.), *Clinical neurology* (vol. 1, pp. 71–81). Philadelphia: Churchill Livingstone.

Gordon, M. (1993). *Manual of nursing diagnosis, 1993–1994.* St. Louis: Mosby–Year Book.

Hart, T., & Harvey, E.J. (1993). Rehabilitation and management of behavioral disturbance following frontal lobe injury. *Journal of Head Trauma Rehabilitation, 8*(1), 1–12.

Hirsh, J. (1993). Promising drugs for neurobehavioral treatment. *Headlines, 4,* 10–11.

Hogan, R.T. (1988). Behavior management for community reintegration. *Journal of Head Trauma and Rehabilitation, 3*(4), 62–71.

Inoye, S.K., et al. (1999). A multicomponent intervention to prevent delirium in hospitalized older adults. *New England Journal of Medicine, 340,* 669–672.

Kandel, I., Schwartz, J., & Jessell, T. (2000). *Principles of neural science.* New York: McGraw-Hill.

Kreutzer, J.S., Zasler, N.D., Camplair, P.S., & Leininger, B.E. (1990). A practical guide to family intervention following adult traumatic brain injury. In J.S. Kreutzer & P. Wehman (Eds.), *Community integration following traumatic brain injury* (pp. 249–273). Baltimore, MD: Brookes Publishing.

Lucas, B. (1993). Community re-entry programs for behavioral patients. *Headlines, 4,* 16.

Malkmus, D., Booth, B., & Kodimer, C. (1980). *Rehabilitation of the head injured adult—Comprehensive cognitive management.* Downey, CA: Professional Staff Association of the Rancho Los Amigos Hospital.

McKinlay, W., & Hickox, A. (1988). How can families help in the rehabilitation of the head injured. *Journal of Head Trauma Rehabilitation, 3*(4), 64–72.

McNeny, R. (1990). Daily living skills. The foundation of community living. In J.S. Kreutzer & P. Wehman (Eds.), *Community integration following traumatic brain injury* (pp. 105–113). Baltimore, MD: Brookes Publishing.

Meleis, A. (1991). *Theoretical nursing: Development and progress* (2nd ed). Philadelphia: J.B. Lippincott.

Nolte, J. (1993). *The human brain* (3rd ed.). St. Louis: Mosby–Year Book.

O'Shadick, G.J., Zasler, N.D. (1990). Neuropsychopharmacological approaches to traumatic brain injury. In J.S. Kreutzer & P. Wehman (Eds.), *Community integration following traumatic brain injury* (pp. 15–27). Baltimore, MD: Brookes Publishing.

Plylar, P.A. (1989). Management of the agitated and aggressive head injury patient in an acute hospital setting. *Journal of Neuroscience Nursing, 21*(6), 353–356.

Rose, M. (1988). The place of drugs in the management of behavior disorders after traumatic brain injury. *Journal of Head Trauma Rehabilitation, 3*(3), 7–13.

Sbordone, R.J. (1990). Psychotherapeutic treatment of the client with traumatic brain injury. In J.S. Kreutzer & P. Wehman (Eds.), *Community integration following traumatic brain injury* (pp. 139–153). Baltimore, MD: Brookes Publishing.

Sbordone, R.J. (1991). Overcoming obstacles in cognitive rehabilitation of persons with severe traumatic brain injury. In J.S. Kreutzer & P. Wehman (Eds.), *Community integration following traumatic brain injury* (pp. 105–116). Baltimore, MD: Brookes Publishing.

Schmahmann, J. (1991). An emerging concept. The cerebellar contribution to higher function. *Archives of Neurology, 48,* 1078–1087.

Segatore, M., Adams, D., Lange, S. (1999). Managing alcohol withdrawal in the acutely ill hospitalized adult. *Journal of Neuroscience Nursing, 31,* 129–141.

Snyder, M. (1991). Potential for violence. In M. Snyder (Ed.), *A Guide to neurological and neurosurgical nursing* (2nd ed., pp. 555–570). Albany, NY: Delmar.

Tomberlin, J. (1990). Physical therapy in community reentry: Assessment and achievement of physical fitness. In J.S. Kreutzer & P. Wehman (Eds.), *Community integration following traumatic brain injury* (pp. 29–46). Baltimore, MD: Brookes Publishing.

Waaland, P.K. (1990). Family response to childhood brain injury. In J.S. Kreutzer & P. Wehman (Eds.), *Community integration following traumantic brain injury* (pp. 225–247). Baltimore, MD: Brookes Publishing.

Yatham, L.N., & McHale, P.A. (1989). Carbamazepine in the treatment of aggression: A case report and review of literature. *Acta Psychiatrica Scandinavica, 78*(2), 188–190.

Intermittent Loss of Arousal

JUDY OZUNA

Arousal is the aspect of consciousness that is behaviorally linked to the appearance of wakefulness (Plum & Posner, 1980). It is characterized by the person's eyes being open and, in most cases, by some degree of interaction by the person with the environment. Intermittent loss of arousal poses unique problems in daily living and social interaction. People with this problem can function normally between episodes of loss of arousal but are incapacitated during the episodes. Because the episodes are generally unpredictable, individuals are at risk for injury during an episode. This risk limits their ability to work in certain jobs, to drive a motor vehicle, and to enjoy certain types of recreational activities. In addition, the unpredictability and intermittent nature of these episodes, especially those of epilepsy, contribute to a social stigma unmatched by other chronic and more visible disorders.

SOURCES OF INTERMITTENT LOSS OF AROUSAL

Intermittent loss of arousal can occur in several ways. Among these are alteration of circulation to the brain, excessive electrical discharge of neurons in the brain, and psychogenic phenomena. The most common types of intermittent loss of arousal are syncope and seizures.

Syncope

Syncope, or faint, involves an episodic interruption of consciousness, usually of abrupt onset and brief duration. Recovery from syncope is usually complete. The physiologic causes of syncope fall under two categories: decreased blood flow to the brain and altered oxygen-carrying capacity of blood. Clinical states in the latter category include hypoxia and anemia. Conditions commonly leading to decreased blood flow to the brain include vasovagal syncope, which results from vasodilation of peripheral resistance vessels (Adams & Victor, 1993). It can be induced by physical injury, strong emotion (these may occur together), or a hot, crowded environment. A vagal response, which includes bradycardia, perspiration, nausea, salivation, and increased peristaltic activity, may accompany the faint. Postural (orthostatic) hypotension occurs in people with unstable or defective vasomotor reflexes from a variety of causes—for example, prolonged bedrest, drug effects, peripheral nerve dysfunction, hypovolemia, and autonomic insufficiency.

Syncope of cardiac origin is due to a sudden reduction in cardiac output, usually because of a dysrhythmia. Pulse rates of fewer than 40 beats per minute impair cerebral circulation and can lead to syncope. The cardiac condition most frequently causing syncope is complete atrioventricular block. Carotid sinus syncope is due to an overly sensitive carotid sinus. In this condition, fainting can occur when slight pressure is applied to the neck area where the carotid sinus is located. A person with this condition may faint when turning the head while wearing a tight collar or even when shaving over the region of the carotid sinus.

Seizures

Certain types of seizures produce intermittent loss of arousal, and some of these may closely resemble syncope. The pathophysiology of seizures, however, arises within the brain itself rather than in the circulation to the brain. A seizure is a paroxysmal, uncontrolled, excessive firing of hyperexcitable neurons within the brain. Causes of neuronal hyperexcitability include metabolic imbalance, trauma, tumor, hemorrhage, infection, genetic predisposition, degenerative disease, and adverse drug effects. Epilepsy is defined as a condition of recurring seizures, regardless of cause, and is treated with chronic use of antiepileptic medication. Seizures owing to reversible causes, such as metabolic imbalance and adverse drug effects, are not usually considered epileptic because once the underlying cause is corrected, the seizures do not recur.

The most common seizure resulting in loss of arousal is the generalized tonic-clonic seizure. It is characterized by sudden loss of consciousness that is followed by stiffening of the body for several seconds (tonic phase) and subsequent jerking of the extremities (clonic phase). Some people experience only tonic or only clonic seizures. Clonic seizures involve loss of consciousness, whereas in tonic seizures consciousness is only impaired.

Recovery of consciousness after a tonic-clonic seizure is gradual, unlike recovery from syncope, which is usually rapid once the blood supply to the brain has been restored. The time for recovery after a seizure depends on how quickly the neurons regain normal functioning from their exhausted state. This may take up to several hours.

Two other types of seizure involve an alteration in consciousness rather than a complete loss of consciousness. The more common of these two types is the complex partial seizure. This seizure type has a wide range of duration (seconds to minutes) and of manifestations, from simple staring and relatively few motor signs to very complex behaviors despite lack of awareness of one's surroundings. The second seizure type is the generalized (both typical and atypical) absence spell. In this seizure, there is alteration in consciousness and sometimes minor movements of the face and limbs, but return to normal arousal is usually more rapid than in a complex partial seizure. Table 8–1 shows the International Classification of Epileptic Seizures.

Seizures in elderly people may be mistaken for other disorders (Lannon, 1993). Seizures involving speech arrest or postictal Todd's paralysis may be mistaken for a stroke. Postictal confusion, which can last several days in older people, may be attributed to dementia. Epileptic seizures may be misdiagnosed as cardiac syncope, transient ischemic attacks, Meniere's disease, or psychiatric disorder.

HUMAN RESPONSES TO INTERMITTENT LOSS OF AROUSAL

A variety of behavioral and physical responses to intermittent loss of arousal form the basis for nursing diagnoses related to the individual, the family, and the community.

Diagnoses for the Individual

Nursing diagnoses in people who experience intermittent loss of arousal include fear, high risk for injury, ineffective denial, social isolation, altered role performance, noncompliance, knowledge deficit, and impaired memory.

FEAR

Fear is the state in which an individual or group experiences a feeling of physiologic or emotional disruption related to an identifiable source that is perceived as dangerous (Carpenito, 1997). People prone to episodes of intermittent arousal manifest the defining characteristics of feelings of dread, fright, and apprehension about several factors. Fear of danger to oneself, in the form of injury and even death, has been mentioned by some patients with seizures. Etiologies include fear of death, fear of rejection or prejudice, fear of losing a job, and fear of bearing children. Fear of death also occurs in people with syncope. The following episodes illustrate how and why fears may arise:

A man blacked out while driving but fortunately was unhurt when his car ran into a ditch. Both he and his family feared he would not be so lucky if another blackout occurred while he was driving. He was eventually diagnosed as having carotid sinus syndrome, and, after a pacemaker was inserted, he had no more blackouts.

TABLE 8–1 • INTERNATIONAL CLASSIFICATION OF EPILEPTIC SEIZURES*

I. Partial (focal, local) seizures
   A. Simple partial seizures (consciousness not impaired)
      1. Motor (abnormal movement of an arm, leg, or both; jacksonian march)
      2. Somatosensory or special sensory (gustatory, olfactory, auditory)
      3. Autonomic (tachycardia, respiration, flushing)
      4. Psychic (deja vu, fearful feeling)
   B. Complex partial seizures (with impairment of consciousness)
      1. Beginning as simple partial seizure and progressing to impairment of consciousness
         a. No other symptoms
         b. Motor, somatosensory, special sensory, autonomic, or psychic symptoms
         c. Automatisms
      2. With impairment of consciousness at onset
         a. No other symptoms
         b. Motor, somatosensory, special sensory, autonomic, or psychic symptoms
         c. Automatisms
   C. Partial seizures evolving to secondarily generalized seizures
      1. Simple partial leads to generalized seizures
      2. Complex partial leads to generalized seizures
      3. Simple partial leads to complex partial leads to generalized seizures
II. Generalized seizures (convulsive or nonconvulsive—all associated with loss of consciousness)
   A. Absence (petit mal)
      1. Onset in childhood; approximately 50% ending in adolescence and 50% supplanted by tonic-clonic
      2. Symptoms include altered awareness or attention and blank stare, may include eye blinking lasting 5 to 30 sec
      3. Can be mistaken for learning disabilities or behavior problems if unrecognized
   B. Myoclonic
      1. Characterized by short, abrupt muscular contractions of arms, legs, or torso
      2. Symptoms include symmetrical or asymmetrical, synchronous or asynchronous single or multiple jerks; possible brief loss of consciousness
   C. Clonic
      1. Symptoms include muscle contraction and relaxation usually lasting several minutes
      2. Distinct phases may not be easily observable
   D. Tonic
      1. Symptoms include an abrupt increase in muscle tone (contraction), loss of consciousness, and autonomic signs, lasting from 30 sec to several minutes
   E. Tonic-clonic (grand mal)
      1. Tonic—may begin with a shrill cry caused by secondary expulsion of air due to abrupt closure of the epiglottis; rigidity, opisthotonos, extension of arms and legs; jaw may snap shut; temporary (up to 1 min) cessation of respiration; nonreactive, dilated pupils; decreased heart rate
      2. Clonic—begins suddenly and ends gradually; characterized by quick, bilateral, severe jerking movements; stertorous respirations; autonomic symptoms; lasts 2 to 5 min
      3. Postictal—muscle flaccidity; gradual return of consciousness; amnesia related to the seizure; patient may need ½ to 1 hr of sleep
   F. Atonic
      1. Characterized by abrupt loss of muscle tone followed by postictal confusion; injury likely if seizure uncontrolled
III. Unclassified epileptic seizures—cannot be classified because of inadequate or incomplete data. Data include some neonatal seizures, eg, rhythmic eye movements, chewing, and swimming movements.

* See Table 1 in Santilli, N., & Sierzant, T. L. (1987). Advances in the treatment of epilepsy. *Journal of Neuroscience Nursing, 19*(3), 142. International League Against Epilepsy. (1981). *Epilepsia, 22,* 489–501.

Adapted from Commission on Classification and Terminology of the International League Against Epilepsy. (1981). Proposal for revised clinical and electroencephalic classification of epileptic seizures. *Epilepsia, 26,* 268–278.

An elderly woman was known to have blackout spells, supposedly from cardiac arrhythmia. Her fears and her family's fears of injury were realized when she blacked out, fell, and broke her hip. In retrospect, her new doctor decided that she had probably been taking higher than necessary dosages of her cardiac and antihypertensive medications based on her age (90 years) and her weight (100 lb).

People who have syncopal attacks or seizures also fear how others might perceive them if they have an attack in public. Our society affirms people who are "normal" and conform to the expectations of society. Society rejects those who deviate from the norm, who display abnormal behavior, or who lack self-control (Bagley, 1971). The person who has a syncopal attack, especially in public, however unwillingly, acts well outside the expected norms of society. The person with uncontrolled episodes of intermittent loss of consciousness is understandably fearful of rejection.

Prejudice against people with epilepsy exists in modern industrial society (Bagley, 1972). A well-known businessman in a medium-sized community expressed strong fear of others' learning that he had epilepsy and even greater fear of their seeing him in a tonic-clonic seizure. He had had one seizure in the past several years, but because of fear he withdrew from his social contacts and retired from his job as owner and operator of an automobile sales business.

There are other sources of fear in people with epilepsy. Women with epilepsy may fear the effects of epilepsy and of medications on a fetus. They may fear bearing children who will develop epilepsy.

In assessment, the nurse must comprehensively explore the patient's fears to identify the real source of the fear. Once this is determined, appropriate interventions can be implemented. Often, information about the disease can help alleviate fear when the source of the fear is lack of knowledge (see Knowledge Deficit for the individual in this chapter).

Interventions should include assessment of the type and frequency of attacks, the conditions under which they occur, the treatment regimen if there is one, and the compliance with that regimen. A move toward self-management of seizures (Legion, 1991) suggests that people with epilepsy can take more control over their seizures by measures other than just taking medication. Individuals can be taught to avoid situations that tend to precipitate their particular seizures, such as loss of sleep, fatigue, seizure-inducing stimuli, use of recreational drugs and alcohol, and, most importantly, stress. Stress is a well-recognized and common precipitator of seizures. Studies have shown progressive relaxation training to be an effective, easily learned adjunctive therapy that encourages people to take an active role in controlling their seizures (Whitman, Dell, Legion, & Hermann, 1990).

Infrequent (one or two per year) partial seizures may not require any special limitations, but more frequent partial seizures, syncopal spells, or generalized tonic-clonic seizures require that the person be accompanied while climbing in high places, swimming, or working around dangerous machinery.

If seizures occur only when a person is very tired, regular rest periods can be planned so that seizures are less likely. Assessment of compliance with a medication regimen is very important because noncompliance is a significant factor in breakthrough seizures (see Noncompliance in this chapter). The fear of seizures and of injury during a seizure may subside significantly with improved compliance and subsequent seizure control.

People with epilepsy who fear rejection by others present a challenge to health care providers and caregivers from both patient care and community perspectives. Although public attitudes toward people with epilepsy have improved greatly over the years (Caveness & Gallup, 1980), some people still react negatively to those with epilepsy. Often this is because of lack of knowledge about the disorder. Thirty-nine percent of the general public surveyed in a poll in 1979 said that they did not know the cause of epilepsy (Caveness & Gallup, 1980).

Identify the source of the patient's fear of rejection. If it is family members, assess their fears and concerns, correct misconceptions, and encourage family counseling if necessary. If the person feared is an employer, refer the patient to a vocational counselor. If the people feared are classmates in school, ask the school nurse or the teacher to educate the students about epilepsy. The Epilepsy Foundation (EF) has an excellent resource for school nurses and teachers (Santilli, Dodson, & Walton, 1991). Parents and teachers are role models for children, and if adults treat the epileptic child as they treat any other child, classmates will most likely do the same.

For those who have fears about bearing children, determine exactly what is feared. Is it fear of the effects of pregnancy on seizure frequency, or is it fear of a bad outcome of pregnancy (e.g., malformations or epilepsy in the child)? In the majority of women with epilepsy, the frequency of seizures does not increase during pregnancy. From 17% to 37% will experience an increase, mostly owing to sleep deprivation or to willful noncompliance because of concerns about effects of antiepileptic medication on the fetus (Delgado-Escueta & Janz, 1992). Although children of epileptic mothers have a twofold to threefold higher risk of malformations than do children of mothers without epilepsy, this risk is still small (4% to 6% versus 2%) (Delgado-Escueta & Janz, 1992). Children of a person with typical absence epilepsy have approximately a 6% to 12% risk of having seizures, whereas siblings or children of persons with true idiopathic epilepsy have a 2% to 14% chance of having seizures by age 40 years (Bird, 1992). If parents are especially concerned about the effect of a parent's epilepsy on their offspring, it is best to refer them to a genetic counselor.

HIGH RISK FOR INJURY

Any time there is loss of awareness or an alteration in consciousness, the potential for injury exists. Both syncope and seizures, with the exception of simple partial seizures and some myoclonic seizures, present a risk for injury because of alteration in consciousness. Injuries encountered include head trauma, burns, bone fractures, aspiration, and multiple traumas. Head trauma occurs if sudden loss of consciousness leads to a fall. The head may strike furniture or other objects during the fall or may hit the ground, resulting in scalp or facial lacerations or even skull fracture and hematoma. Burns may result from falling onto a heating element of a stove, onto a heater, or into a fire, or if the person is smoking. Burns may also occur if the person is in the shower or bathtub with hot water running. Bone fractures are usually associated with falls but can result when jerking limbs strike adjacent objects. Aspiration can occur if a person is not properly positioned during a generalized tonic-clonic seizure. Some people have drowned while in the bathtub or while swimming. Multiple traumas can result from a fall or an automobile accident precipitated by an epileptic or syncopal attack.

Assessment for potential for injury includes determining frequency of seizure or syncopal episodes, adequacy of seizure control, and type of activities commonly performed. The patient, family, and caregivers need to understand the risk for injury, and the patient should be allowed to participate in as many activities as are within reason. As an intervention, people who experience episodes of loss of consciousness should be advised not to go swimming alone, not to climb high places (both at recreation and at work) without safety lines, and not to work around dangerous machinery (although some machines can be adapted so that they run only if the operator applies constant pressure to a footpedal or a button). People should be advised of the legal restrictions for driving a motor vehicle. The specific seizure-free interval required to qualify for a driver's license varies among states. It is usually between 6 months and 2 years.

All who come in contact with a person with seizures should have knowledge of first aid management of seizures to minimize the risk of injury. Care of a person during a generalized tonic-clonic seizure is twofold: protection from injury and prevention of aspiration. Remove furniture and other large objects in the immediate surroundings so that the person's limbs do not strike them. Cradle the head, either on someone's lap or on soft padding. Do not attempt to prevent limb movement or to place anything between the person's teeth once the jaws are tightly clenched. The jaws generate 1000 pounds of pressure per square inch, and no amount of human force can open them during a seizure. In addition, injuries caused by forcing objects into the mouth are far greater than local oral mucosal and tongue trauma caused by clenching of the jaws. Table 8–2 lists guidelines on first aid management of generalized tonic-clonic seizures.

Once the seizure is over, gently turn the person on the side so that saliva that has accumulated during the seizure can drain from the mouth. Someone should remain with the person until he or she regains consciousness.

First aid care for older people may require variations in traditional interventions (Lannon, 1993). If someone is confined to a wheelchair, it may be better to leave the person in the chair. The nurse can stand behind the chair, slip his or her arms under the person's arms to support the body, and support the person's chin to maintain an open airway. Once the seizure is over, the person can be placed in bed. The nurse should remain with the person until he or she has fully recovered.

TABLE 8–2 • FIRST AID FOR SEIZURES

Generalized Tonic-Clonic Seizures

1. Keep calm and reassure other people who may be nearby.
2. Clear the area around the person of anything hard or sharp.
3. Loosen ties or anything around the neck that may make breathing difficult.
4. Put something flat and soft, like a folded jacket, under the head.
5. Turn the person gently onto the side to help keep the airway clear. Do *not* try to force the mouth open with any hard implement or with fingers. A person cannot "swallow the tongue."
6. Do not hold the person down to try to stop the seizure movements.
7. Do not attempt artificial respiration except in the unlikely event that the person does not start breathing again after the seizure has stopped.
8. Stay with the person until the seizure ends naturally.
9. Offer to call a taxi, friend, or relative to help the person get home if he or she seems confused or unable to get home alone.

Adapted from Epilepsy Foundation. (1994). *Questions and answers about epilepsy* [Pamphlet]. Landover, MD: Author.

Care of a person having a complex partial seizure primarily involves close observation. The witness should remain with the person throughout the seizure and not attempt to restrain him or her, even if the person tries to walk away. The person's behavior is being driven by the seizure activity, and he or she may become combative if restraint is attempted. General goals for first aid management of seizures are to provide physical safety, emotional support, and privacy.

INEFFECTIVE DENIAL

Ineffective denial is the state in which the individual minimizes or disavows symptoms or a situation to his or her detriment of health (Carpenito, 1997). Among people with epilepsy, the ability to cope can vary greatly. Some people whose seizures are relatively minor and infrequent have a surprisingly difficult time adjusting to their condition, whereas others cope well with more severe epilepsy.

Several aspects of epilepsy make adjusting to epilepsy more difficult than adjusting to syncope. Epilepsy is a chronic condition, with the likelihood of seizures occurring throughout a lifetime. Epilepsy is incurable. Although seizures can be controlled for a period, the condition is rarely cured. Epilepsy is invisible. It is not apparent to others unless a seizure occurs. People tend not to understand epilepsy because they rarely witness actual seizures. Epilepsy is unpredictable. Witnesses are never prepared when a seizure occurs. Epilepsy requires that medications be taken regularly and for many years to control seizures, which forces a kind of dependency that some reject. Epilepsy means restrictions on driving, alcohol consumption, occupation, and recreation even though the person with epilepsy may not be ill between seizures. Epilepsy carries a stigma because of ongoing misconceptions.

Among people with epilepsy, ineffective denial may occur when the diagnosis is first made and may continue for several years. Defining characteristics of ineffective denial of epilepsy include poor medication compliance, continuation of activities known to precipitate seizures, or continuing to drive a car despite a history of recent seizures.

Denial of epilepsy has a variety of causes: fear of being labeled epileptic, with its negative connotations; any of the fears discussed in the section on fear in this chapter; and loss of independence. The following episode illustrates an instance of denial resulting from a possible misconception:

A passenger on an airplane stated that he was on his way to see a neurologist for another opinion about his blackouts. He had already seen five physicians. He said that he was taking phenytoin (Dilantin), but when asked if he had epilepsy, he said, "Oh no, I just have blackouts, but I let them think I have epilepsy so I can get Workers' Compensation. I pop these pills just before I go to the doctor so it will show up in my blood." On further questioning, he said that he had been injured in a construction accident 2 years previously, which resulted in a depressed skull fracture. The blackouts began shortly after that injury.

He said that he was having these spells a few times a week. He continued to drive a car and fly an airplane. When asked why he did not think he had epilepsy, he could not really answer. He said, "I just don't think I have it." When it was explained to him that epilepsy simply means recurring seizures and that many people develop seizures after a severe head injury because of damage to brain cells, he said, "Really? You're the first person who's ever told me that." He may have been denying his epilepsy because of misconceptions that only retarded or severely brain-damaged people have epilepsy.

Some people deny the prognosis that epilepsy is likely to continue throughout their lifetime. This is particularly true if they have not had a seizure for several months or years. Some patients may decide to discontinue medication, only to be shocked by the occurrence of another seizure. Denial of epilepsy by family members is discussed in the sections on ineffective family coping in this chapter.

As with other psychosocial problems, the nurse should explore the patient's feelings and assess the patient's conception of epilepsy and its connotations. The preceding case illustrates that correcting misconceptions can reverse denial in some people. Ascertain how the patient perceives the treatment regimen and how it affects her or his lifestyle, and determine if noncompliance is willful or is a result of forgetfulness, because interventions for these two situations differ (see Noncompliance in this chapter).

SOCIAL ISOLATION

Social isolation is the state in which an individual or group experiences a need or desire for contact with others but is unable to initiate that contact (Carpenito,

1997). Stated another way, social isolation can be defined as a lack of societal fulfillment, a condition in which individuals set themselves apart from the societal whole with which they could be expected to interact and affiliate (Beniak & Beniak, 1983). Social isolation is not an unusual consequence of having epilepsy. In some cases, fear of or actual rejection by others may lead an otherwise socially adroit person into seclusion. In other cases, the condition of epilepsy removes an already socially unskilled person even farther from the mainstream of social interactions.

Social isolation's defining characteristics are withdrawal from social contacts, activities, and responsibilities; lack of genuine interest in other people; little, if any, development of vocational or recreational pursuits; lack of social poise; poor communication skills; and general aloofness (Beniak & Beniak, 1983). The onset of epilepsy in childhood can make it doubly hard to develop social skills because the child may be denied early opportunities for socialization. The denial may come from the family, who unknowingly overprotect the child, or it may come from the child's classmates, friends, and siblings, who ridicule and ostracize the child.

Antiepileptic medications can cause emotional and physical adverse effects (e.g., irritability, depression, aggression, sleepiness, dizziness, clumsiness) that are etiologic factors in social isolation. Legal, vocational, and activity restrictions on people with epilepsy also add to the likelihood that some will decrease their social interactions.

Beniak and Beniak (1983) propose the following assessments and interventions for people with epilepsy manifesting social isolation. One should first assess the person's level of cognitive and intellectual functioning, because this helps determine the form of therapy that might be most helpful. Formal personality assessment (Minnesota Multiphasic Personality Inventory and Washington Psychosocial Seizure Inventory) (Dodrill, Batzel, Queisser, & Temkin, 1980) can provide additional data. One should note the person's routine behavior and how and under what circumstances the person interacts with others. Establish individualized goals, such as (1) a specific number of social interactions with staff or other patients, (2) participation in a novel social activity, and (3) patient responsibility for some aspects of care. In settings where there are several people who experience seizures, formal group interactions can be arranged. Group discussions about common problems can help establish socialization among all the members. Role-playing can help members practice social interactions such as greeting a stranger, asking an agent for tickets to an event, and inviting someone to a function.

Relaxation training has been used with some success (Snyder, 1983). This method enhances psychic comfort, thereby enabling a person to interact more openly and spontaneously.

ALTERED ROLE PERFORMANCE

Altered role performance is the state in which an individual experiences or is at risk of experiencing a disruption in the way he or she perceives his or her role (Carpenito, 1997). In the author's view, altered role performance is an internal conflict based on a discrepancy between what a person wants her or his role to be and what the role actually is. This problem can develop particularly in the adult years when certain roles have been established or at least planned for and a diagnosis of epilepsy or syncope requires changes in these roles. A person may manifest the defining characteristics of role disturbance by expressing frustration and feelings of inadequacy related to loss of job, inability to find work, loss of independence, or inability to participate in previous activities (e.g., child care, work, recreation). The person may perceive and grieve the loss of such roles as breadwinner, parent, homemaker, or athlete.

Interventions for role disturbance depend on assessment of the role involved. Vocational counseling and social services are in order for the person who has employment difficulties. Family counseling can help the person with role disturbance regarding parenting and providing child care. For the person who is worried about his or her role as a procreator, genetic counseling may be helpful. Recreation therapists can offer ideas for those who need to choose alternative diversional activities. Local EF affiliates sponsor self-help groups.

NONCOMPLIANCE

Noncompliance with a prescribed antiepileptic medication regimen is a common problem among people with epilepsy and is the most frequent cause of poor seizure control (Leppik, 1993). Certain features of epilepsy contribute to the likelihood of noncompliance: the need for long-term compliance to a medical regimen, the requirement that medication be taken regardless of the presence of symptoms (seizures) and often during symptom-free periods, the need for change in the patient's lifestyle, and the fact that the drug regimen may produce adverse effects (Green & Roter, 1977). Psychologic and financial factors, such as denial and rebellion against dependency on medications and cost of medications (especially in elderly people [Lannon, 1993] and others on fixed incomes), can contribute to noncompliance. Medications that come in childproof safety containers may be too difficult to open, especially by elderly people. These are factors of willful noncompliance, a situation in which a person makes a conscious decision not to take medication as prescribed. There are, however, people who do not comply with a medication regimen because of simple forgetfulness. These people need different interventions than those needed by people who exhibit willful noncompliance.

The defining characteristic of noncompliance, whatever the reason, is a lower-than-expected antiepileptic drug serum level—that is, a level below what would be expected for a given patient on a given dosage. Because most patients are taking sufficient dosages to achieve a therapeutic level, the drug level usually will be subtherapeutic if the person is noncompliant. However, one must rule out other causes of a subtherapeutic level before making this assumption. These include altered drug metabolism (some people are fast or slow metabolizers), altered drug utilization (as a consequence of disease), altered physiologic state (e.g., pregnancy), age (children utilize drugs at a faster rate, elderly people at a slower rate), and drug interactions.

Assessment of noncompliance should include both examination of the drug serum level and direct questioning of the patient. When questioned, up to half of noncompliers will admit their noncompliance (Sackett, 1977), and this group responds most positively to compliance-improving strategies (Sackett, 1979). Once noncompliance has been determined, the reasons for noncompliance should be assessed. These include but are not limited to forgetfulness, misunderstanding of the medication schedule, adverse drug effects, complexity of the medication schedule, hesitation at taking medications in front of others (at school or work), attitude toward illness, family problems, financial problems, poor social support, poor patient–health care provider interaction, denial, and rebellion (Haynes, 1979A; Marston, 1970; Shope, 1982).

The Health Belief Model (Rosenstock, 1966) is a useful model on which to base a compliance counseling approach. The model suggests that people are not likely to take a health action (e.g., take medication) unless (1) they believe themselves susceptible to the disease, (2) they believe the disease would have serious effects on their lives, (3) they are aware of actions and treatments and believe they will help, and (4) they believe the risk of taking action is less serious than the illness itself. A prerequisite of each belief is the preceding belief in the hierarchy; for example, a person who does not believe his illness is serious is not likely to follow a treatment regimen for that illness. The nurse can evaluate the health beliefs of his or her patients and use the information to guide his or her compliance-improving interventions. The Health Belief Model is also a useful guide for general patient and family education (see Knowledge Deficit for the individual in this chapter) (Ozuna & Cammermeyer, 1982).

Discussion of interventions for each of the cited reasons for noncompliance is beyond the focus of this chapter; however, interventions for a few of the major reasons are presented. For those who are forgetful, several methods are helpful. Provide the patient with written instructions for taking medication and have him or her record each dose taken on a calendar. Encourage the use of pillboxes or containers that have compartments for every day of the week. The MediSet (manufactured by Apothecary Products, 11750 12th Avenue South, Burnsville, Minnesota, 55337-1295) has four compartments for each day of the week, for patients who take several doses a day. Suggest that the patient associate taking medication with a routine daily activity, such as use of the bathroom, daily hygiene activities, meals, and so on. The following case is an example of noncompliance as a result of forgetfulness:

A young man was referred by his private physician because of inability to control his seizures. After attempts by the referral physician to raise the patient's serum levels by increasing the medication dosage were unsuccessful, the author asked the young man about his medication-taking habits. He said that he was somewhat irregular in taking his medication because he worked late hours some days and would forget to take it. When asked where he kept his medication, he said, "In the kitchen cupboard." He was asked if he always went to the kitchen after coming home from work, and he said, "No." The author suggested that it would be easier for him to remember taking his medication if he associated it with a routine daily activity, but he said that he did not have any routine, especially when he worked such late hours. When asked, ''Do you use the bathroom every night before you go to bed?'' the patient responded affirmatively. The author suggested that he keep the medication in the bathroom and put a note on the bathroom mirror to remind himself to take his medication. He accepted these suggestions readily and was able to obtain therapeutic serum phenytoin levels and seizure control. (Note: This suggestion is not advisable for people taking carbamazepine because its potency can be affected by humidity.)

For people who exhibit willful noncompliance, ask why this is their choice. Many times, misconceptions about antiepileptic therapy or denial of epilepsy is the reason. (Refer to the section on ineffective denial in this chapter.) Try to correct misconceptions. Because many patients lack understanding of antiepileptic drugs, the nurse can do much to improve compliance by providing information about the action of the drugs and their pharmacokinetics (e.g., why some drugs can be taken once a day) and a realistic perspective of their side effects. Through discussions with the primary provider, the number of medications can be kept to a minimum, the frequency of doses can be lowered, and the complexity of the medication regimen can be simplified.

Many patients respond well to increased supervision (Haynes, 1979B). Regular feedback to them about their drug levels and regular discussions about their seizure control and medication-taking habits can provide positive reinforcement of compliant behavior. The increased attention also gives the patient a favorable impression of her or his relationship with the health care provider, a factor known to influence compliance behavior (Shope, 1982).

Contributions by nurses in advanced practice and specialty roles of nurses in promoting compliance have been particularly important in chronic disease, partly because of their supportive role functions and, in some situations, because of their ability to provide greater continuity of care (Hogue, 1979). Hogue suggests that nurses employ several strategies to improve compliance: use clear, concise information when instructing patients; help the patient feel competent to manage the treatment regimen; encourage use of natural support systems (family, friends); and facilitate teamwork with others interested in the patient's progress.

KNOWLEDGE DEFICIT

Knowledge deficit is the state in which an individual or group experiences a deficiency in cognitive knowledge or psychomotor skills concerning the condition or the treatment plan (Carpenito, 1997). Knowledge deficits among people with epilepsy can occur in several areas: the disorder of epilepsy, the diagnostic procedures and rationale, the medications and the medication regimen, the follow-up care, the legal restrictions, and the community resources.

Because of the relatively high percentage of people who lack knowledge about epilepsy (Caveness & Gallup, 1980) and the persistence of misconceptions about what epilepsy is, basic teaching in layperson's language about the pathophysiology of epilepsy should be a priority not only for newly diagnosed patients but for long-term patients as well. A useful way to assess patients' knowledge is to ask them to describe what epilepsy is and why they think they have it. For some, the first step is to acknowledge that they have epilepsy (see Ineffective Denial in this chapter). Some physicians tell patients they have a seizure disorder, and the patients are shocked to learn that this term is synonymous with epilepsy. In addition to offering verbal explanations of epilepsy, the nurse can provide the patient and family with educational pamphlets published by the EF.

Nursing interventions must include information that epilepsy is not a curable condition but one that can be controlled in most cases with regular use of antiepileptic medication and self-management behaviors. The patient should know his or her seizure type and its manifestations. Incorrect labeling of seizure type could lead to improper treatment because most medications used to treat partial seizures are not useful in treating generalized nonconvulsive seizures and vice versa. Patients should know what they do during seizures so that they can tell loved ones and coworkers what to expect should a seizure occur. Although some people choose not to reveal their epilepsy to their employers because of a sometimes valid fear of losing their jobs, many of the frightening aspects of a seizure can be lessened by knowing what to expect.

Patients should know what kind of first aid care will be needed. Patients and their families should be reminded that unless an injury results from a seizure or the seizure is prolonged, there is no need to summon medical help. Lack of this information often leads to unnecessary and very expensive medical bills. Table 8–3 offers a teaching plan based on the Health Belief Model.

When a person is undergoing a diagnostic work-up for epilepsy, the nurse should explain both the value and the limitations of the electroencephalogram and brain imaging, such as computed tomographic or magnetic resonance imaging scans. Explain that much of the diagnosis still depends on the history and witness descriptions of the seizure.

Once the diagnosis is made and the medication regimen is started, provide information about the prescribed drugs, including the mechanism of action of the drugs, their adverse effects, their interactions with other drugs, and the need for routine assessment of serum drug levels. Instruct the patient to report any adverse effects or changes in well-being. Remind the patient not to change the dosage of medication without first consulting the health care provider or to discontinue medications abruptly because this can precipitate seizures and even lead to status epilepticus.

Elderly people need special considerations regarding medication (Lannon, 1993). Drug absorption, distribution, metabolism, and elimination are generally reduced in this population. This means they require less drug to achieve a therapeutic level. In addtition, many older people are taking several other medications, which means they have a greater risk for drug interactions.

The nurse in the inpatient setting should include information about follow-up care in discharge planning of newly diagnosed patients. Follow-up visits are needed to ascertain drug efficacy and to discuss side effects and overall

TABLE 8–3 • TEACHING PLAN BASED ON HEALTH BELIEF MODEL

Outcome Criteria	Teaching Plan	Evaluation
Patient and family state that patient is likely to have another seizure (acknowledge susceptibility)	**Review with patient and family** • Anatomy and physiology of recurring seizures, nerve impulse transmission • Probable cause of patient's seizure • Body functions governed by specific brain regions and how patient's seizures relate to these functions	**Patient and family regularly indicate susceptibility to recurring seizures**
Patient and family recognize possible consequences of seizures on patient's life • More seizures, less likely to be controlled • Risk of physical injury during seizure • Difficulty finding employment • Inability to legally drive if not seizure free	**Review with patient and family** • Seizures beget more seizures • Physical danger if patient loses consciousness, falls, drives during seizure • Benefits and risks of telling employer about having epilepsy • State driving law	**Evidence that patient has adjusted to his or her epilepsy** • Demonstrates acceptance of epilepsy • Admits having seizures • Is gainfully employed according to abilities • Does not drive illegally
Patient and family demonstrate positive actions toward controlling patient's seizures • Identify names of prescribed medications, dosage, time schedule, side effects • State understanding of difference in dosage needs for individuals • List factors that precipitate seizures —Sleep deprivation —Fatigue —Intercurrent illness —Menses —Stress —Certain sensory stimuli in susceptible individuals • State understanding of need for follow-up by health provider	**Review with patient and family** • All aspects of medication regimen • Use of serum level determinations • How to avoid or better handle precipitating factors • Need for regular follow-up visits	**Evidence that patient is taking health action for his or her epilepsy** • Obtains maximal seizure control with minimal side effects • Maintains therapeutic serum drug levels • Gives no history of activities or situations that precipitate seizures • Returns regularly for follow-up visits

Table continued on following page

TABLE 8–3 • TEACHING PLAN BASED ON HEALTH BELIEF MODEL *Continued*		
Outcome Criteria	**Teaching Plan**	**Evaluation**
• State advantages and disadvantages of identification tags • Demonstrate appropriate first aid procedures for all seizure types • Express psychosocial concerns	• Pros and cons of identification tags • First aid procedures • Review with patient and family —Progressive relaxation training —Stress management techniques —Self-help/support groups	• Has made logical decision about wearing identification tag • Shows minimal, if any, physical injury after a seizure • Gives feedback that patient and family are coping well

adjustment. The nurse should supply information about community resources (both educational and vocational), state driving laws, and home safety. Home safety tips are based on seizure type and frequency. People who have frequent seizures involving loss of consciousness or impaired consciousness should take precautions in several areas. They should not bathe unattended to avoid the risk of drowning. They should be warned about the risk of being burned by touching a hot stove or spilling boiling water. Childrearing practices may need modification. Infants and toddlers should be placed on the floor or in some other safe place when diapers need changing. Children should be bathed either with supervision or by someone else. Older children should be taught to recognize seizures and to provide appropriate first aid or at least to call for help.

Similar patient education topics should be addressed when advising people with syncope. Inform patients about the cause and treatment of syncope and tell them about the legal restrictions for driving. Advise them about activities that put them at risk for injury if they lose consciousness (e.g., climbing, swimming, working with dangerous machinery).

IMPAIRED MEMORY

Impaired memory is the state in which an individual experiences a temporary or permanent inability to recall bits of information or behavioral skills (Carpenito, 1997). Disruption of short-term memory is a frequent complaint among patients with epilepsy. Memory problems have several causes. They can be a result of antiepileptic medication overdose (Thompson, 1992), of the disorder itself (Binnie & Marston, 1992), and of the patient's reaction to it (e.g., anxiety, depression) (Thompson & Corcoran, 1992). The degree of memory impairment can range from relatively benign forgetfulness to severe cognitive dysfunction. In addition, the memory disturbance can affect medication compliance adversely (see Noncompliance in this chapter).

Many patients with a memory problem recognize it themselves. They complain of forgetting such things as conversations they had recently, what their spouse asked them to do, what they were supposed to get at the store, or what they had intended to do at work on a given day. In other situations, a family member or an employer notes the memory deficit. The nurse can assess a memory deficit by testing immediate and recent recall, although these test results may be normal.

Overdosage of antiepileptic medication should not be overlooked as a cause of memory disturbance. In some cases, reduction of medication dosage can improve memory problems without adversely affecting seizure control. In other cases, a different medication should be tried. If a patient is taking two or more drugs, the regimen could be reduced to a single drug.

The following interventions are for minor verbal memory disturbance. Interventions for those more severely impaired are discussed in Chapter 12. Advise the patient to use memory aids, such as written reminders and daily or weekly calendars. Because memory problems can influence medication compliance, encourage the patient to associate medication taking with routine daily activities, to keep a written log, and to use pill containers (see Noncompliance in this chapter).

Patients will have less difficulty if their daily routine is structured and unchanged from day to day. This kind of repetition, as well as repetition of new information, can improve memory and provide a sense of comfort and security to the person with minor memory disturbance. Memory problems have significant implications for patient education and discharge planning. Any new information that is to be given to a person with impaired memory should be written down and shared with family members or significant others.

Diagnoses for the Family and Significant Others

INEFFECTIVE FAMILY COPING: COMPROMISED

Ineffective family coping: compromised is the state in which a usually supportive primary person is providing insufficient, ineffective, or compromised support, comfort, assistance, or encouragement that may be needed by the client to manage or master adaptive tasks related to a health challenge (Carpenito, 1997). Epilepsy, syncope, and many other health conditions can generate ineffective coping: compromised within certain families and close friendships. Problems in coping with intermittent loss of arousal are addressed from two perspectives: that of a child with the disorder and that of an adult with the disorder.

When a child develops epilepsy, one of several alterations in coping can occur in one parent or both parents. One alteration is denial. The parents may refuse to believe that their child has epilepsy, that a product of themselves is imperfect. Some parents who are fearful about epilepsy and deny its existence are unable to assist the child with her or his own fears (Voeller & Rothenberg, 1973). This denial may have serious consequences if the parents refuse to give the child his or her antiepileptic medication. Once epilepsy is accepted by the parents, feelings of guilt may result from unconscious rejection of the "imperfect" child. The parents may blame themselves for the child's disorder. They may overprotect the child and severely limit his or her activities, or they may overindulge and spoil the child to avoid causing aggravation and therefore causing a seizure. The child then learns to manipulate the parents and get whatever she or he wants. This may lead to an alteration in the family process. If the child's demanding personality carries over into adulthood, the child may have difficulty getting along with others and may suffer rejection (see Social Isolation in this chapter).

Siblings may have difficulty coping with an epileptic child. If the child gets most of the parental attention, siblings may become jealous and exclude him or her from their activities. They may reject their brother or sister as a source of embarrassment, or they may use the child as a scapegoat when altercations occur.

When epilepsy develops in an adult, different stresses on the family occur. The spouse of the patient may be faced with new responsibilities, such as getting a new job or obtaining a driver's license. If the spouse cannot face these challenges, he or she may blame the person with epilepsy for disrupting their lifestyle. Fear and denial may be evident, along with blame, overprotection, and scapegoating. The children of a parent with epilepsy may have difficulty coping. The author is aware of several cases in which the children were afraid that their parent was going to die when she or he had a seizure. An exploratory study of children's adaptation to epilepsy in a parent revealed four major problems that occurred in families: children's learning about the disorder, children's fear of abandonment, overresponsibility of children for their parents, and children's fear of developing epilepsy (Lechtenberg & Akner, 1984). The study concluded that children who adjusted most poorly to epilepsy in a parent were those from whom the seizure disorder had been concealed.

Ineffective family coping: compromised may be detected during an encounter with family members in either an inpatient or an outpatient setting. Comments and behaviors of children, spouses, and friends provide valuable clues in the assessment of family coping. The nurse should explore feelings that are expressed. Use reflective listening to bring out more detailed aspects of the coping pattern. Once the coping problem is identified, interventions can be planned.

If denial is present in a family member, further exploration of the reason for the denial may help in determining how to intervene. For instance, if the family member exhibits lack of knowledge or misconceptions, providing accurate information about epilepsy may help, assuming the person is ready to learn. If parents are overprotecting their child, one may offer information demonstrating that it is in the child's best interest to be treated like any other child. If parents or siblings are blaming the child for their problems, formal family counseling may be needed.

Lack of information about epilepsy is an important cause of coping problems among family members. The least disruptive approach to children of epileptic parents is frank discussion of what epilepsy is and what is being done to control it, because parental efforts to conceal the problem breed distrust in the children (Lechtenberg & Akner, 1984).

INEFFECTIVE FAMILY COPING: DISABLING

Ineffective family coping: disabling is a state in which a family demonstrates destructive behavior in response to an inability to manage internal or external stressors resulting from inadequate resources (Carpenito, 1997). This problem often is an outgrowth of compromised coping problems. If the mother and the father have different perceptions of epilepsy in their child, controversy over childrearing can develop. One may blame the other for the child's epilepsy, ultimately causing the child to suffer. The child begins to lose self-esteem and withdraws. In some families, the parents may blame the epileptic child for the family's difficulties. This maladaptive coping can cause the child to lose self-esteem and the ability to develop relationships with others, thereby leading to social isolation. In addition, Austin, Risinger, and Bechett (1992) found that children who were experiencing behavioral problems tended to have poorer seizure control and to be in troubled families in which mothers were receiving less than needed support from relatives.

For children of epileptic parents, family process alterations may include children taking on responsibilities for family functioning beyond the responsibilities of other children of the same age. Some children may function successfully in these responsibilities, but it may prove to be too great a burden for others. The child may miss normal opportunities for growth and development because of self-imposed or parent-imposed responsibilities for the epileptic parent.

Assessment necessitates further data gathering. Speak to family members individually to allow them to express frank, uninhibited feelings. If both parents agree that they need help, offer the following simple guidelines as nursing interventions:

Discipline of the affected child should be no different from that of the other children in the family. Suggested limitations on the child's activities can be obtained from the child's primary health care provider and should be followed by both parents in a consistent manner. Responsibility for the child's medication should be assumed by one or both parents until the child is old enough to take responsibility. In situations where disagreements between parents are too great, refer parents to family counseling or to a parent support group. Interventions designed to address behavior problems in children with epilepsy should be both family centered and focused on reducing family strain (Austin et al., 1992). Support groups are sponsored by children's hospitals and by local chapters of the EF.

KNOWLEDGE DEFICIT

The previous discussions about family problems demonstrate that lack of knowledge is an important component. Lack of knowledge and misconceptions may become apparent during interviews with family members, and some members may admit openly their lack of knowledge. Teaching approaches are determined based on the type of knowledge deficit, the readiness of the learner, and the age of the learner.

Diagnoses for the Community

STIGMA RELATED TO KNOWLEDGE DEFICIT

Misconceptions and prejudice about people with epilepsy still exist despite improvement in public attitudes toward epilepsy since the 1950s (Bagley, 1972; Caveness & Gallup, 1980). Many patients report that well-meaning bystanders call an ambulance when a seizure occurs, regardless of its severity. Patients are then faced with expensive and unnecessary emergency medical care. Others suffer injuries from witnesses who use improper first aid procedures. On one occasion, a bystander who witnessed a seizure forced a plastic pen into the person's mouth. The cap broke off and was aspirated into a bronchus. The person complained of an irritating chronic cough for several weeks before the offending object was detected on a chest radiograph. Other people with epilepsy suffer ridicule and embarrassment from uninformed bystanders, coworkers, and classmates. The author is aware of one occasion when a teacher ran out of the room in a state of fear when a child had a seizure in the classroom.

Articles about and letters from people who have difficulty with employment because of their epilepsy can be found in almost every issue of *Epilepsy USA* (the EF's newsletter). A national survey of people with epilepsy found that 44% reported limitations in working. Those whose seizures were not well controlled were least likely to be employed and most likely to have been dismissed from a job (Roper Organization, 1992).

Employers and schoolteachers may have misconceptions that all people with epilepsy are mentally deficient, have poor attendance, and perform not as well as nonepileptic people. They may fear that a seizure will disrupt the performance of coworkers or schoolmates. Occupational health nurses and school nurses have an obligation to correct these misconceptions and to educate people about epilepsy so that witnesses can treat the person with epilepsy as an equal and provide appropriate first aid if needed.

Professionals who care for people with epilepsy need to provide the intervention of education about epilepsy to people in the community, including teachers, employers, police officers, firefighters, airline attendants, and the general public. A resource for public education is the EF, which sponsors nationwide programs on many aspects of epilepsy. Local chapters of the EF sponsor educational programs and support groups. The EF publishes a number of educational brochures that are available for a fee and can be used for patient and family teaching and also offers educational program packages for both lay and professional audiences. Information about these resources should be shared with teachers, librarians, physicians, and employers.

KNOWLEDGE DEFICIT REGARDING HEALTH PROMOTION, DISEASE PREVENTION, AND COMMUNITY RESOURCES

Community members can become involved in health promotion behaviors related to epilepsy. By being educated about seizures and proper first aid management, they can help avoid costly emergency transport and emergency department care bills by properly identifying and providing first aid for seizures. People with epilepsy should be encouraged to wear medical identification tags or bracelets or to carry medical information about their condition in a wallet or purse so that a passerby can readily ascertain their condition if a seizure occurs.

Head trauma is one of the most preventable causes of acquired epilepsy. Campaigns to make the public aware of measures to prevent head trauma should include advocating wearing of seat belts and helmets and safe participation in sports (e.g., avoiding diving in shallow water, wearing protective helmets when participating in such sports as football, baseball, hockey, or cycling).

Stroke is to some extent another preventable cause of acquired epilepsy. The public should be educated about the risk factors of stroke, including smoking and hypertension.

For many people with epilepsy, the psychosocial problems far outweigh the physiologic problems of seizures. Knowledge of community resources for employment, financial assistance, housing, child care, transportation, patient advocacy, and social skills improvement should be shared with all health care providers who assist people with epilepsy. Agencies that can assist with these issues include local affiliates of the EF, local comprehensive epilepsy centers, and state departments of vocational rehabilitation, social services, and assistance of developmentally disabled persons.

NURSING ROLES IN MANAGEMENT OF INTERMITTENT LOSS OF AROUSAL AND AWARENESS

Ensuring patient safety is a primary responsibility of the nurse generalist. Patients with syncope or epilepsy are at great risk for injuring themselves during loss of arousal and, therefore, require preventive measures. The nurse must be knowledgeable about the frequency of patients' spells, their precipitating factors, and their warning signs so that appropriate safety measures can be instituted for patients with poorly controlled seizures. In the hospital, bed siderails should be padded. No objects should be forced between the patients' teeth during a seizure. Patients with either uncontrolled syncopal episodes or seizures should never ambulate or transfer unassisted. The nurse generalist is responsible for ensuring that the patients know about their disorder. Pamphlets from the EF or other written resources can be given to patients to enhance retention of information.

The nurse generalist should be knowledgeable about the patients' medication regimens, including mechanisms of action, pharmacokinetics, usual adult and child dosages, and therapeutic ranges of the drugs. Discharge planning should include patient and family teaching of the drug regimen—dose, frequency, and side effects.

The nurse specialist is accountable for assisting in the management of complex patient problems in an inpatient setting and, in some cases, is responsible for directly managing patient care in an outpatient setting. The nurse specialist may help a multidisciplinary team treat complex behavioral or pathophysiologic responses. He or she may become involved in the identification and management of compliance problems. The specialist has a responsibility to educate the public about epilepsy—what it is, how it can be prevented, and why it should not carry a stigma. Hartshorn and Byers (1992) provide a model describing the relationship between the variables of health; family life; social, community, and civic activities; economics; personal development; and quality of life. This model organizes a comprehensive nursing approach to the patient with epilepsy. All nurses who care for patients with epilepsy should consider these variables in providing care.

SUMMARY

Intermittent loss of arousal, especially epilepsy, can produce a range of physical, psychologic, and social human responses. Although the risk of physical injury is great during a seizure, these moments are relatively infrequent and short lived. Psychosocial issues are usually the most common concerns, and they can have a devastating effect on a person's self-concept, family dynamics, and employability. Nurses can play a pivotal role in identifying and treating these human responses, referring people and their families to community agencies, and providing much-needed public education.

References

Adams, R., & Victor, M. (1993). *Principles of neurology* (5th ed.). New York: McGraw-Hill.

Austin, J. K., Risinger, M. W., & Bechett, L. A. (1992). Correlates of behavior problems in children with epilepsy. *Epilepsia, 33*(6), 1115–1122.

Bagley, C. (1971). *The social psychology of the child with epilepsy.* Miami, FL: University of Miami Press.

Bagley, C. (1972). Social prejudice and the adjustment of people with epilepsy. *Epilepsia, 13,* 33–45.

Beniak, J. A., & Beniak, T. E. (1983). Social isolation. In M. Snyder (Ed.), *A guide to neurological and neurosurgical nursing* (pp. 268–290). New York: John Wiley & Sons.

Binnie, C. D., & Marston, D. (1992). Cognitive correlates of interictal discharges. *Epilepsia, 33*(Suppl. 6), S11–S17.

Bird, T. D. (1992). Epilepsy. In R. A. King, J. I. Rotter, & A. G. Motulsky (Eds.), *The genetic basis of common diseases* (pp. 731–752). New York: Oxford University Press.

Carpenito, L. J. (1997). *Handbook of nursing diagnosis* (7th ed.). Philadelphia: J. B. Lippincott.

Caveness, W. F., & Gallup, G. H. (1980). A survey of public attitudes toward epilepsy in 1979 with an indication of trends over the past thirty years. *Epilepsia, 21,* 50–58.

Delgado-Escueta, A. V., & Janz, D. (1992). Consensus guidelines for preconception counseling, management, and care of the pregnant woman with epilepsy. *Neurology, 42*(Suppl. 5), 150–160.

Dodrill, C., Batzel, L., Queisser, H., & Temkin, N. (1980). An objective method for the assessment of psychologic and social problems in epileptics. *Epilepsia, 21,* 123–135.

Green, L., & Roter, D. (1977). The literature on patient compliance and implications for cost-effective patient education programs in epilepsy. In Commission for the Control of Epilepsy and Its Consequences (Ed.), *Plan for nationwide action on epilepsy* (Vol. 11, Part 1, Sections I–IV). Washington, DC: Department of Health, Education, and Welfare.

Hartshorn, J. C., & Byers, V. L. (1992). Impact of epilepsy on quality of life. *Journal of Neuroscience Nursing, 24*(1), 24–29.

Haynes, R. B. (1979A). Determinants of compliance: The disease and the mechanics of treatment. In R. B. Haynes, D. W. Taylor, & D. W. Sackett (Eds.), *Compliance in health care* (pp. 49–62). Baltimore, MD: Johns Hopkins University Press.

Haynes, R. B. (1979B). Strategies to improve compliance with referrals, appointments, and prescribed medical regimens. In R. B. Haynes, D. W. Taylor, & D. W. Sackett (Eds.), *Compliance in health care* (pp. 121–143). Baltimore, MD: Johns Hopkins University Press.

Hogue, C. C. (1979). Nursing and compliance. In R. B. Haynes, D. W. Taylor, & D. W. Sackett (Eds.), *Compliance in health care* (pp. 247–259). Baltimore, MD: Johns Hopkins University Press.

Lannon, S. L. (1993). Epilepsy in the elderly. *Journal of Neuroscience Nursing, 25*(5), 173–282.

Lechtenberg, R., & Akner, L. (1984). Psychologic adaptation of children to epilepsy in parent. *Epilepsia, 25*(1), 40–45.

Legion, V. (1991). Health education for self-management by people with epilepsy. *Journal of Neuroscience Nursing, 23*(5), 299–305.

Leppik, I. E. (1993). Compliance in the treatment of epilepsy. In E. W. Wyllie (Ed.), *The treatment of epilepsy: Principles and practices* (pp. 810–816). Malvern, PA: Lea & Febiger.

Marston, M. V. (1970). Compliance with therapeutic regimens: A review of the literature. *Nursing Research, 19*(4), 312–323.

Ozuna, J., & Cammermeyer, M. (1982). Learning needs of the epilepsy patient. In M. J. VanMeter (Ed.), *Neurologic care: A guide for patient education* (pp. 133–151). Paramus, NJ: Appleton-Century-Crofts.

Plum, F., & Posner, J. B. (1980). *The diagnosis of stupor and coma.* Philadelphia: F.A. Davis.

Roper Organization (1992). *Living with epilepsy: A quality of life survey.* New York: Author.

Rosenstock, I. M. (1966). Why people use health services. *Milbank Memorial Fund Quarterly, 44*(3), 95–127.

Sackett, D. (1977). Why don't patients take their medicine? *Canadian Family Physician, 23,* 462–464.

Sackett, D. (1979). A compliance practicum for the busy practitioner. In R. B. Haynes, D. W. Taylor, & D. W. Sackett (Eds.), *Compliance in health care* (pp. 286–294). Baltimore, MD: Johns Hopkins University Press.

Santilli, N., Dodson, E. W., & Walton, A. V. (1991). *Students with seizures: A manual for school nurses.* Landover, MD: Epilepsy Foundation of America.

Shope, J. T. (1982). The patient's perspective. In R. B. Black, B. P. Hermann, & J. T. Shope (Eds.), *Nursing management of epilepsy* (pp. 43–62). Gaithersburg, MD: Aspen.

Snyder, M. (1983). Effect of relaxation on psychosocial functioning in persons with epilepsy. *Journal of Neurosurgical Nursing, 15*(4), 250–254.

Thompson, P. (1992). Antiepileptic drugs and memory. *Epilepsia, 33*(Suppl. 6), S37–S40.

Thompson, P. J., & Corcoran, R. (1992). Everyday memory failures in people with epilepsy. *Epilepsia, 33*(Suppl. 6), S18–S20.

Voeller, K. K., & Rothenberg, M. B. (1973). Psychosocial aspects of the management of seizures in children. *Pediatrics, 51*(6), 1072–1082.

Whitman, S., Dell, J., Legion, V., & Hermann, B. (1990). Progressive relaxation training as adjunct therapy for seizure reduction. *Journal of Neuroscience Nursing, 22*(4), 250–251.

Rhythmic Alterations in Consciousness: Sleep

ANN E. ROGERS

The rhythmic nature of sleep and wakefulness has fascinated humans from antiquity to the present. Attempts to uncover the mysteries of sleep have led to the observation and measurement of the sleep-wake cycle under various conditions. Many variables are known to influence the sleep-wake cycle, such as neurochemical, physiologic, psychologic, developmental, and temporal factors. As humans have searched for the mechanisms responsible for sleep, many theories have been proposed to account for the necessity of this time-consuming behavior. These theories describe the purpose of sleep as restorative, energy conserving, protective, instinctive, or ethologically adaptive. This chapter reviews the physiologic, psychologic, anatomic, and biochemical correlates of sleep, describes human responses to disordered sleep, and offers appropriate nursing interventions.

PHYSIOLOGIC AND BEHAVIORAL MANIFESTATIONS

By 30 to 32 weeks of gestational age, a regular sleep-wake cycle is established in the human fetus that will continue throughout the life span. The timing and periodicity of sleeping and waking states are modified by maturation and environmental influences. Sleep itself has a cyclical organization and can be divided into two main parts: rapid eye movement (REM) sleep and non-REM (NREM) sleep. Thus, the human body alternates among three states: wakefulness, NREM sleep, and REM sleep. Certain biochemical, physiologic, and behavioral changes are associated with each stage of sleep.

Wakefulness

The electroencephalogram (EEG) of a person who is awake but relaxed is characterized by spontaneous, low-voltage, rapid, electrical activity. Various waveforms may be noted; beta waves (13 cycles per second or 13 Hz), theta waves (4 to 7 Hz), and alpha activity (sinusoidal waves between 8 and 13 Hz). Alpha activity is blocked by eye opening, sudden alerting, attention to stimuli, and mental concentration. Electro-oculogram (EOG) recordings during wakefulness show numerous rapid eye movements and eye blinks. Measurement of submental electromyogram (EMG) activity reveals a baseline level of tonic muscle activity (Parkes, 1985; Riley, 1985).

EEG recordings and performance testing indicate that there are rhythmic fluctuations in vigilance during the waking state (Broughton, 1989). Some fluctuations occur at approximately 24-hour intervals (circadian rhythms), others at approximately 12-hour intervals (circasemedian rhythms), and others at very short intervals (ultradian rhythms). Subjective alertness, objective alertness as measured by the Multiple Sleep Latency Test (MSLT), and performance on most tasks improve throughout the day, peaking during the early evening hours. It should be noted, however, that memory function peaks during the morning and then declines throughout the day (Baddeley, Hatter, Scott, & Snashall, 1970), and that alertness does not increase in a linear fashion until the early evening hours. Subjective alertness declines during the midafternoon and then increases to its highest level during the early evening hours. Daytime napping is most likely to occur between noon and 6 PM (especially between 2 and 4 PM) (Tune, 1968) and has nothing to do with the ingestion of food at midday (Blake, 1967). Finally, vigilance is also influenced by ultradian rhythms, which are quite similar in duration to the period of the within-sleep NREM-REM cycle (72 to 120 minutes).

Non–Rapid Eye Movement Sleep

NREM sleep is also subdivided into four stages (stages 1 to 4) based on each stage's characteristic EEG, EOG, and EMG patterns (Rechtschaffen & Kales, 1990). With the onset of stage 1 sleep, the alpha rhythm of relaxed wakefulness disappears, giving way to low-voltage theta activity (Fig. 9–1). Slow, rolling eye movements replace the rapid eye movements associated with wakefulness. EMG activity continues but is decreased compared to wakefulness. Stage 1 is a transitional phase between full wakefulness and sleep, lasting 30 seconds to 7 minutes (Parkes, 1985). If aroused from stage 1 sleep, individuals usually report having been drowsy or even that they were awake (Riley, 1985). Although individuals may not be aware of a change in their alertness during stage 1 sleep, tests have shown that responses to stimuli are slower and that intellectual acuity is decreased (Riley, 1985).

Stage 2 is characterized by the intermittent appearance of two relatively low-amplitude EEG patterns on the background of theta waves: sleep spindles and K complexes (Fig. 9–2). The slow, rolling eye movements of stage 1 sleep disappear, and eye movement is negligible during stages 2, 3, and 4. If awakened from stage 2 sleep, most persons will recognize that they have been sleeping (Riley, 1985). A stronger stimulus is required to awaken someone from stage

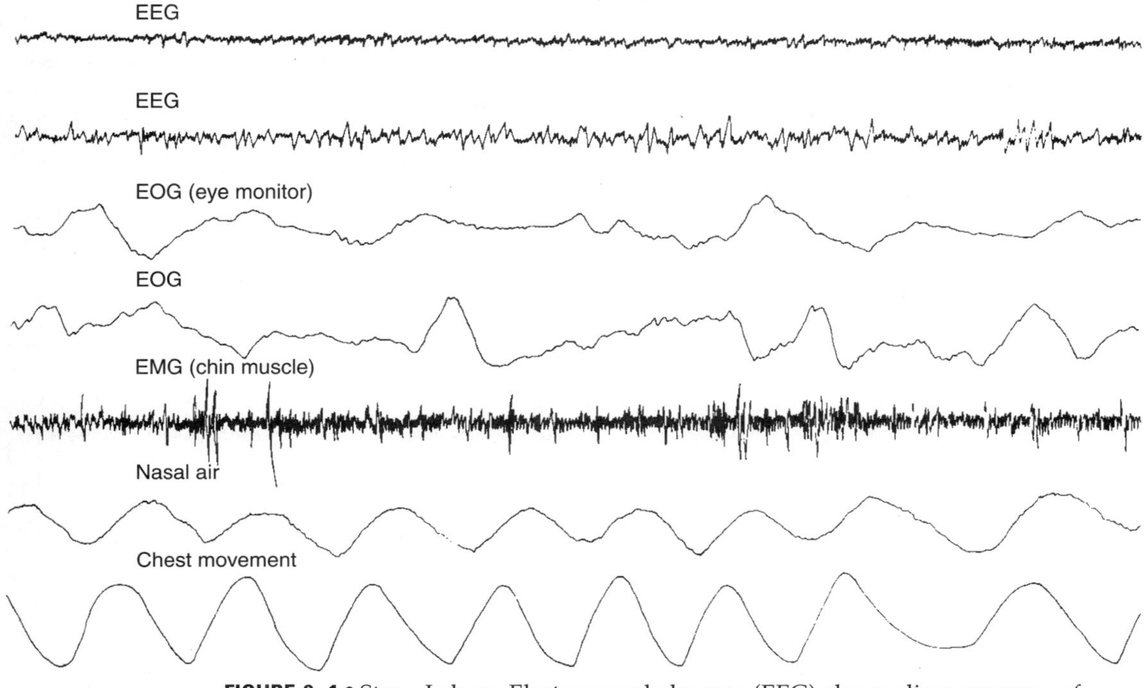

FIGURE 9–1 • Stage I sleep. Electroencephalogram (EEG) shows disappearance of alpha rhythm, gradual development of theta waves, and voltages of 50 to 100 μV (first two lines). Slow, rolling eye movements appear (channels 3 and 4), and respirations are usually regular and unlabored. (From Riley, T. L. [1985]. *Clinical aspects of sleep and sleep disturbance.* Stoneham, MA: Butterworth Publishers.)

2 sleep; however, meaningful stimuli such as a baby's cry or an alarm clock will easily arouse a sleeper from any sleep stage.

Slow wave sleep (SWS) or delta sleep are terms often used to refer to sleep stages 3 and 4 (Fig. 9–3). Both names refer to the appearance of large (greater than 75 μV), rather synchronized, low-frequency (1 to 2 Hz) waves called delta waves. Only the percentage of delta waves present in the EEG record differentiates stage 3 from stage 4 sleep; stage 4 sleep consists of more than 50% delta activity compared to 20% to 50% delta activity for stage 3 sleep. Somatosensory evoked responses are diminished during SWS; this is compatible with the decreased cerebral responsiveness accompanying the slower, high-voltage, synchronous EEG activity of deep sleep. Eye movements are minimal or absent, and EMG activity is low.

Many physiologic changes occur during NREM sleep. Blood pressure, cardiac output, and heart rate decrease during NREM sleep (Mancia & Zanchetti, 1980). The lowest heart rate and blood pressure levels are reached during SWS. Respiration rate and minute ventilation also decrease during NREM sleep (Orem & Keeling, 1980). Breathing is quite regular during NREM sleep,

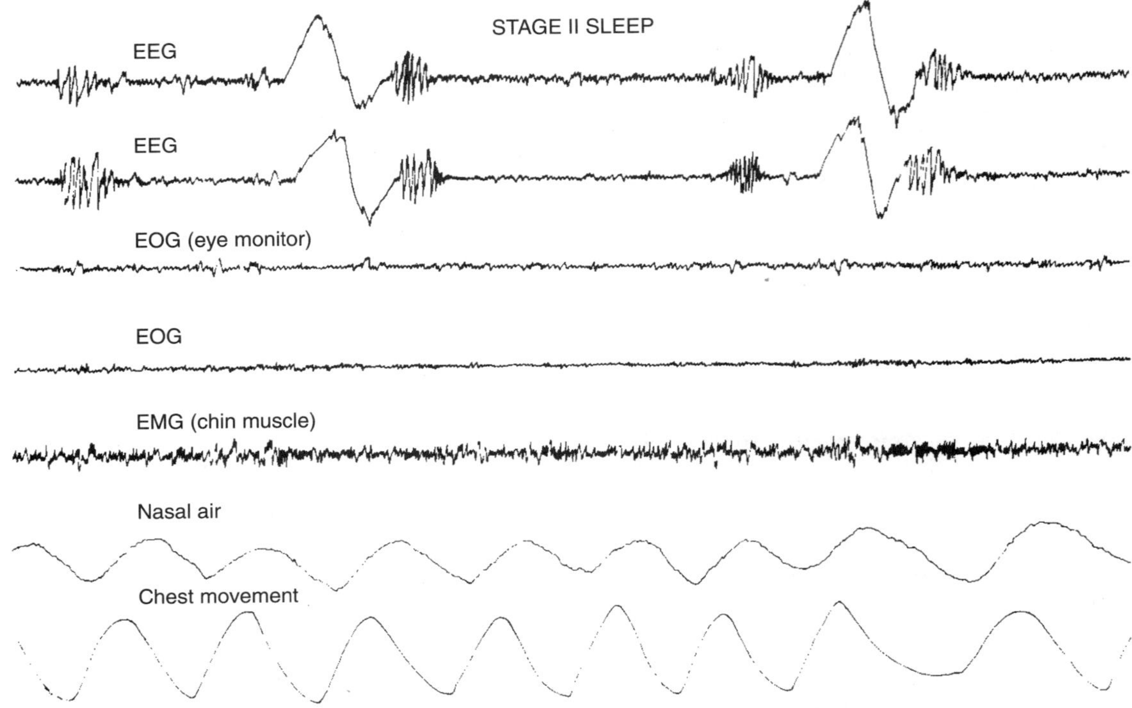

FIGURE 9–2 • Stage 2 sleep. Sleep spindles (sharp 12 to 16 Hz waveforms) are seen four times in electroencephalogram (EEG) channels. K complexes, which are high-voltage (sometimes >200 μV) biphasic waveforms, and also illustrated in channels 1 and 2. Eye movements are usually quiet during stage 2 sleep, and respirations remain regular and often more shallow than during stage I sleep. (From Riley, T. L. [1985]. *Clinical aspects of sleep and sleep disturbance.* Stoneham, MA: Butterworth Publishers.)

especially during SWS. However, some periodic breathing is not uncommon during light sleep (stages 1 and 2). Regional cerebral blood flow to the hemispheres decreases during NREM sleep despite a slight elevation in partial pressure of carbon dioxide (pCO$_2$) (Sakai, Meyer, Karacan, Derman, & Yamamoto, 1980). Carbon dioxide is a potent vasodilator during normal wakefulness. Cerebral vasomotor responsiveness to carbon dioxide thus appears to be decreased during NREM sleep.

Rapid Eye Movement Sleep

REM sleep is sometimes called paradoxical sleep. The fast, asynchronous, cortical EEG activity (generally associated with wakefulness) is present along with the diminished muscle tone associated with deep sleep. The EEG during REM sleep includes low-voltage, fast activity (15 to 20 Hz) mixed with theta activity

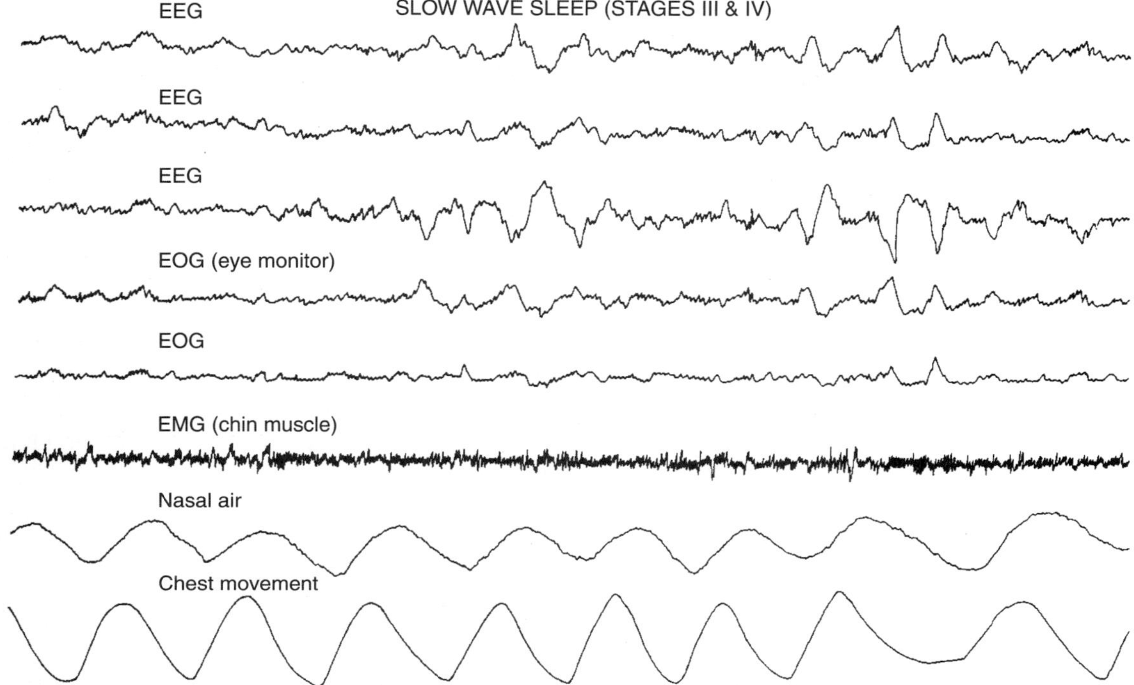

FIGURE 9–3 • Slow wave sleep. Sleep spindles disappear, and large slow waves appear during sleep stages 3 and 4. Eye movements may be absent, although some frontal delta activity may be recorded as artifact in the electro-oculogram (EOG) channels. Respirations remain slow and regular, and muscle tone is unchanged. (From Riley, T. L. [1985]. *Clinical aspects of sleep and sleep disturbance.* Stoneham, MA: Butterworth Publishers.)

plus sawtooth waves that are unique to REM sleep (Fig. 9–4). Although EEG activity during REM sleep may resemble EEG activity recorded during stage 1 sleep (Agnew, Webb, & Williams, 1967), dramatic changes in EOG and EMG activity make this stage unmistakable. Characteristic rapid, conjugate eye movements occur in bursts along with phasic muscle twitches. With the exception of these isolated muscle twitches, skeletal muscle tone is very low or absent during REM sleep. Although thoughts and dreamlike images may occur during any sleep stage, the most vivid and elaborate dreams are associated with REM sleep.

Thermoregulation is impaired; sweating, shivering, and thermoregulatory vasomotor functions do not occur during REM sleep (Parmeggiani, 1980). Total body consumption of oxygen increases, and the arousal response to airway occlusion, hypoxia, hypercapnia, and laryngeal irritation is slowed (Orem & Keeling, 1980). Despite a decrease in cerebral vasomotor responsiveness (vasodilation) to carbon dioxide, regional cerebral blood flow increases in both hemispheres of the brain (Ingvar, 1979). These changes do not influence intra-

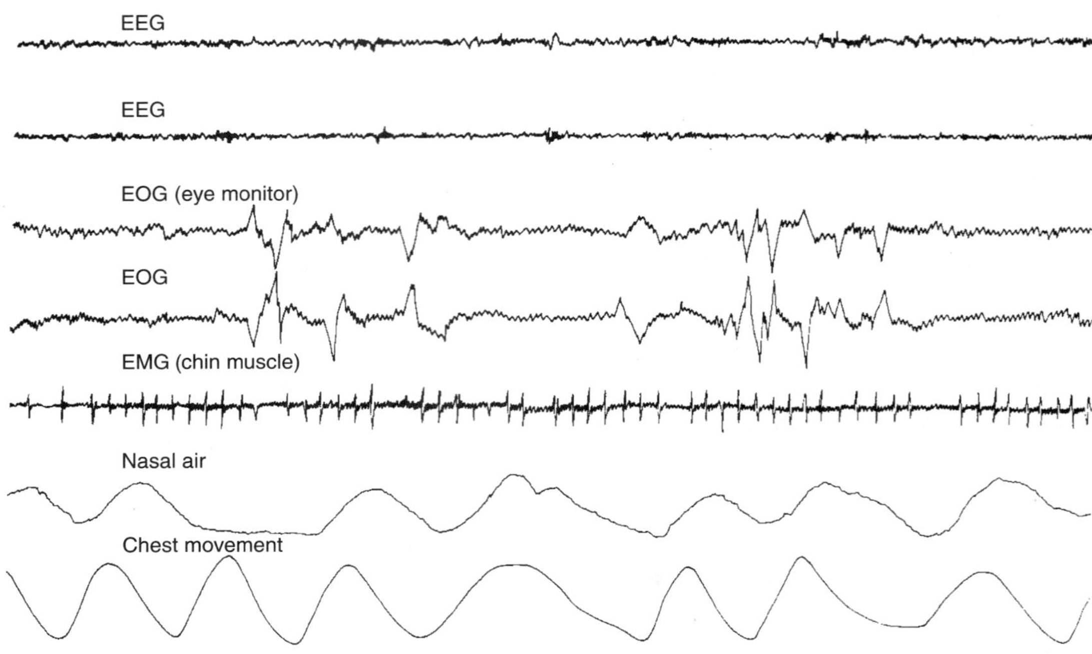

FIGURE 9–4 • REM sleep. Electroencephalogram (EEG) patterns resemble either wakefulness or stage 1 sleep. Eye movements occur in quick, conjugate bursts at intervals of 4 to 10 seconds. The electromyogram (EMG) is flat, reflecting the absence of muscle tone during REM sleep. The irregular spikes noted in the EMG (Channel 5) on this recording are due to pulse artifact. Respirations and pulse may be irregular during REM sleep. REM, rapid eye movement. (From Riley, T. L. [1985]. *Clinical aspects of sleep and sleep disturbance.* Stoneham, MA: Butterworth Publishers.)

cranial pressure (ICP) under normal conditions. In people with intracranial pathology, however, REM sleep can precipitate large elevations in ICP (Ross, Maira, & Vignati, 1975).

Other physiologic changes associated with REM sleep occur during either tonic or phasic events but not throughout REM sleep. Phasic events are transient activities such as rapid eye movements, whereas tonic events are continuous activities such as the muscle atonia associated with REM sleep. Phasic events associated with REM sleep include conjugate eye movements; muscle twitches of the limbs and face; penile tumescence and clitoral-vaginal engorgement; increased brain temperature; and, in some experimental animals, high-voltage EEG spikes in the pons, lateral geniculate nucleus, and occipital cortex (PGO spikes). Minute ventilation, tidal volume, and pCO_2 approach waking levels during phasic REM sleep (Sullivan, 1980). Increases in blood pressure with transient elevations up to 40 mm Hg, tachycardia, and vasoconstriction also occur (Mancia & Zanchetti, 1980).

The tonic or continuous events of REM sleep include desynchronization of the cortical EEG, hippocampal theta waves, diminished or absent deep tendon reflexes, and greatly diminished or absent skeletal muscle tone, especially in the neck and chin (also known as postural atonia). Physiologic changes are less dramatic than they are during phasic REM. Hypotension, bradycardia, and general vasodilatation occur during tonic REM events. Diaphragmatic activity persists, ventilatory responses to hypercapnia and hypoxia remain intact, and there is decreased tone in the smooth muscles of the airway (Orem & Keeling, 1980).

NORMAL SLEEP PATTERNS

Sleep patterns across the 24-hour period are significantly influenced by ontogeny and, to a certain extent, by culture. All aspects of sleep are affected by maturation: its amount, structure, and timing are all influenced by age (Fig. 9–5). Culture also colors our perceptions of both normal sleep patterns and what we define as problems with sleep. For example, in the United States and many other western industrialized countries, infants are put to sleep in their own beds and are expected to rapidly learn to sleep through the night. Although parent-child cosleeping is the predominant sleep arrangement for infants and young children throughout the first few years of life in most nonwestern cultures, (Munroe, Munroe, & Whitting, 1980) it is often viewed as a cause of an infant's nocturnal arousals in the United States (Richman, 1987). The acceptance of napping during the day and the importance of sleep at night also varies across cultures. Daytime napping is widespread between latitudes of 20 degrees north and 20 degrees south and is more common in agricultural societies than in industrialized societies (Webb & Dinges, 1989). In contrast, napping appears to be proscribed by many nomadic groups, even in tropical areas. Other cultural groups, particularly nomadic tribes living in the polar regions, often have very irregular sleep-wake patterns (Webb & Dinges, 1989).

Infant Sleep

Rather than being broken down into several stages, the sleep of newborn infants is classified as either quiet sleep or active sleep (Anders, Emde, & Parmlee, 1971). Periods of sleep that fail to meet the scoring criteria for active REM or quiet NREM sleep are called periods of indeterminate sleep. In a full-term infant, indeterminate sleep is most frequent at sleep onset, during the transition from active REM to quiet NREM, and just before awakening. As the nervous system matures, the amount of indeterminate sleep decreases.

The EEG during active REM sleep includes either a low-voltage irregular (LVI) pattern, a mixed (M) pattern or, less frequently, a high-voltage sleep (HVS) pattern. The EOG shows rapid eye movements and an absence of muscle activity on EMG (Anders et al., 1971). Observation reveals considerable movement during active REM sleep, particularly of the extremities, trunk, head, and

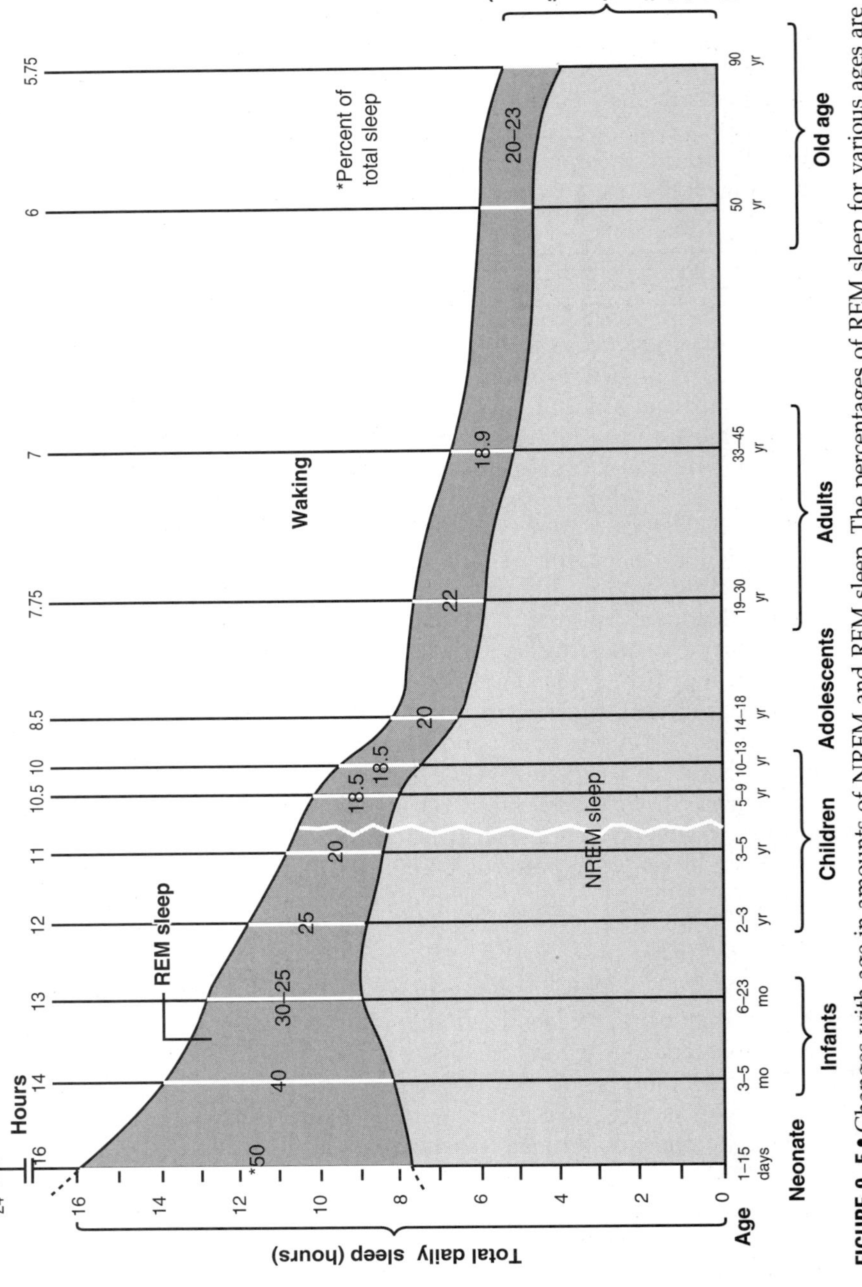

FIGURE 9–5 • Changes with age in amounts of NREM and REM sleep. The percentages of REM sleep for various ages are also included. NREM, non-REM; REM, rapid eye movement. (From Roffwarg, H. P., Muzio, J. N., & Dement, W. C. [1966]. Ontogenetic development of the human sleep-dream cycle. *Science, 152,* 604–619.)

neck. The eyes may be partially open, and the infant may occasionally cry or whimper (Agnew et al., 1967). The EEG during quiet NREM sleep includes an HVS pattern, tracé alternant (TA), or an M pattern. There are no eye movements, and the EMG is elevated (Anders et al., 1971). Observations during quiet NREM sleep reveal that the infant's eyes are closed, that respirations are relatively slow and abdominal in nature, and that motor activity is limited to occasional startles (Thoman, 1975).

Although newborns spend about three quarters of their time asleep, sleeping an average of 17 to 18 hours out of 24 hours, this sleep is not consolidated into one period at night. Instead, sleep and waking periods are distributed in equal amounts around the clock, with the infant awakening every 3 to 4 hours for brief periods to eat. Infants frequently have sleep-onset active REM periods, something seen only in adults with certain pathologic conditions. The ratio of active sleep to quiet sleep is related to maturation. At term, more than 50% of the newborn's sleep consists of active REM sleep. The percentages of active sleep and indeterminate sleep are also elevated in premature infants born before 36 weeks. However, if premature infants are compared to term infants of similar gestational ages, there are no differences in their sleep patterns (Anders et al., 1971).

By 3 months, an infant's sleep is beginning to resemble that of an adult. Spindle activity associated with stage 2 sleep has developed (Metcalf, 1969), and most infants begin sleeping through the night (defined as midnight to 5 AM) between 3 and 6 months. By 6 months, quiet sleep exceeds active sleep in almost all infants. Instead of being evenly distributed throughout the night as it was at birth, quiet NREM sleep becomes predominant in the early part of the night, whereas active REM sleep is increased during the later part of the night. Sleep duration also changes with maturation; infants sleep approximately 16 hours out of 24 at 6 months, 2-year-olds sleep approximately 12 hours per day, and by 4 years, sleep duration has dropped to 10 or 11 hours (Agnew et al., 1967). Between 3 and 5 years, children stop napping during the day.

Sleep During Childhood and Adolescence

Until puberty, nighttime sleep is deep and restorative (Fig. 9–6). In prepubertal children, nighttime sleep durations range from 8.5 to 10 hours, with the sleep time decreasing as the child matures. Elementary school children have a sleep latency (time it takes to fall asleep) quite similar to that of adults (approximately 20 to 25 minutes), and average only 1 to 3 brief awakenings during the night (Coble, Kupfer, Reynolds, & Houck, 1987). As the amount of stage 4 sleep gradually declines between ages 6 and 12 years (from 18% to 14%), stage 2 sleep increases. Although the REM latency gradually declines from 142 minutes to 124 minutes, it still remains higher than that of an adult (Coble et al., 1987). The total duration of REM sleep has declined to 20% to 25% and will remain stable throughout childhood. The length of each period of REM sleep tends to

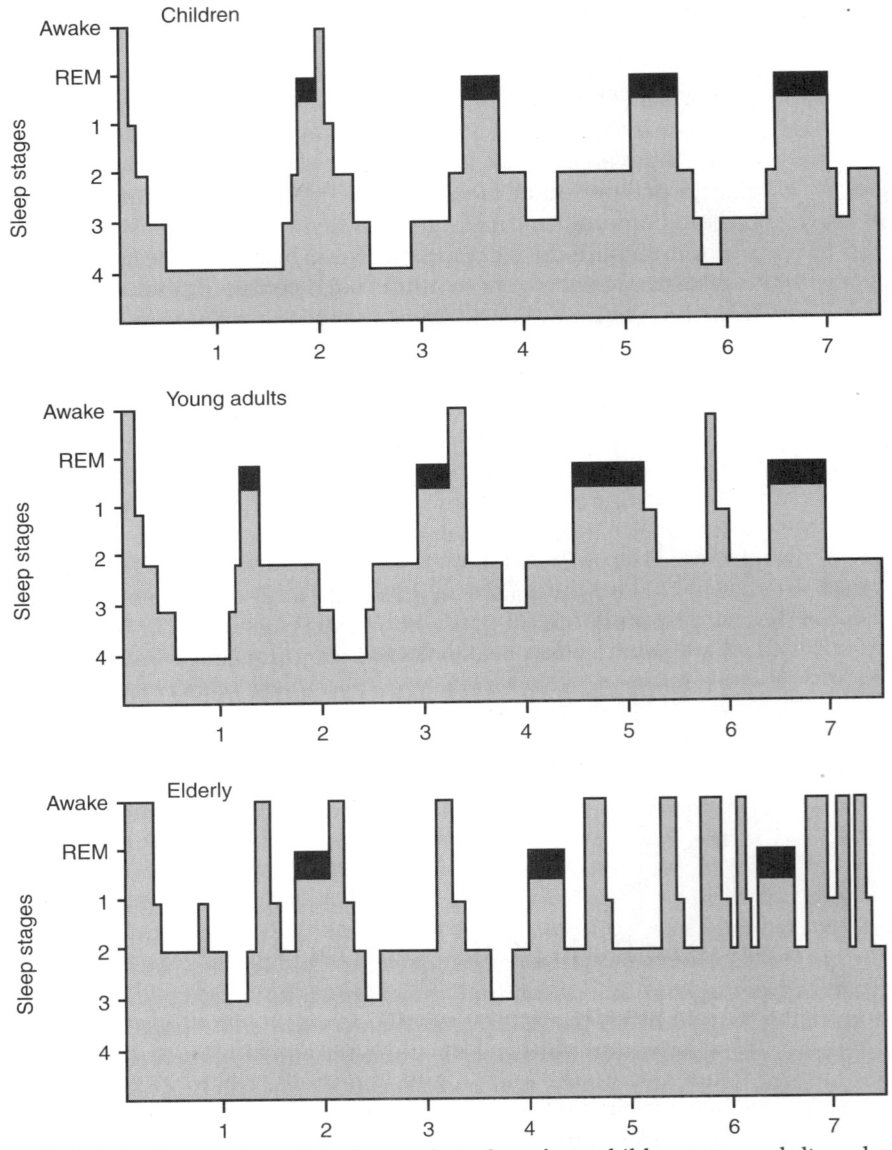

FIGURE 9–6 • Comparison of typical night's sleep for a child, a young adult, and an elderly person. (From Kales, A., & Kales, J. D. [1974]. Sleep disorders: Recent findings in the diagnosis and treatment of disturbed sleep. *New England Journal of Medicine, 290,* 487.)

increase throughout the night, a pattern that will be maintained throughout adulthood (Coble et al., 1987; Williams, Karacan, & Hursch, 1974).

Although there is a significant decline in the amount of SWS during adolescence (Carskadon & Dement, 1987), the most striking change in the sleep of adolescents is its shortened duration. Although it is widely believed that teenagers need less sleep than younger children need, research shows that the need for sleep does not decline during adolescence and may actually increase. Self-reported sleep times decline from approximately 10 hours before puberty, to 8.5 hours at age 13 years, and finally to 7 hours between the ages of 18 and 22 years. Yet, when given the opportunity to sleep either in the sleep laboratory or at home on weekends, teenagers average more than 9 hours of sleep per night (Carskadon & Dement, 1987). After age 13 years, significant increases in daytime sleepiness occur, with daytime sleepiness sometimes reaching pathologic levels. Excessive daytime sleepiness is particularly common among older teenagers, who obtain the fewest hours of sleep (Carskadon & Dement, 1987).

Sleep During Adulthood

On average, adults sleep about 7 to 8 hours per day, with 5% to 10% of their sleep time spent in stage 1 sleep, 50% to 60% in stage 2 sleep, 10% to 20% in SWS, and the remaining 10% to 20% in REM sleep (Kales & Kales, 1984). For an adult, a typical night of sleep begins with a brief period of stage 1 followed by stage 2 sleep and then SWS (see Fig. 9–6). The first deep sleep of the night is usually obtained 30 to 45 minutes after sleep onset in young adults. Within a few minutes or up to an hour later, there is often a brief episode of stage 2 sleep before the first appearance of REM sleep. This first REM period is usually quite short, lasting only about 5 minutes. Adults usually fall asleep within 10 to 20 minutes and enter REM sleep 80 to 90 minutes after falling asleep (Williams et al., 1974).

This sequence of sleep stages (beginning with stages 1 to 4 of NREM and ending with an REM period) is called a sleep cycle. Periods of NREM and REM sleep are alternated 4 to 6 times each night, depending on the total length of time spent sleeping (total sleep time). The first sleep cycle is usually the shortest sleep cycle of the night, and the second cycle the longest, for an average duration of 90 minutes (Agnew et al., 1967). SWS continues to predominate in the first two sleep cycles of the night, with REM and stage 2 sleep being predominant during the later sleep cycles. REM periods lengthen with each successive sleep cycle and can be up to an hour in duration during the early morning hours (Agnew et al., 1967).

Sleep Patterns Associated with Aging

Although the time it takes to fall asleep (sleep latency) does not change with aging (Bliwise, 1989), older persons report more difficulties with their sleep than do younger adults. Elderly persons awaken more often at night and stay awake longer than younger persons, sleeping only 70% to 80% of the time that they are in bed (Prinz, 1977). Sleep architecture also changes with aging (see Fig. 9–6). One of the most consistent changes seen in the sleep of the aged person is a progressive reduction in and, in some cases, the total disappearance of the deepest levels of sleep (stages 3 and 4). The percentage of stage 1 sleep almost doubles during old age, increasing from 8% to 15% of nocturnal sleep time (Bliwise, 1989).

Although it is often presumed that elderly persons need less sleep than do younger persons, numerous studies, including those using animal models and 24-hour recordings, as well as the measurement of recovery sleep following sleep deprivation, suggest that there is no change in the amount of sleep needed by persons as they age. However, after age 70 years, sleep may not remain consolidated into a single nighttime period. Although elderly persons may deny napping during the daytime, all healthy elderly subjects who participated in a recent study napped at least once during the 48-hour monitoring period (Evans & Rogers, 1994).

CIRCADIAN RHYTHMS ASSOCIATED WITH SLEEP

Human beings live in a rhythmic world and are exposed to many external periodicities. These rhythmic influences range from events occurring on a time scale of years (e.g., sunspot cycles) to annual, monthly, and daily oscillations. The dominant rhythm in humans shows a period of 24 hours in synchrony with the light-dark cycle of the solar day. Rhythms that follow this periodicity of about 24 hours are termed circadian. Most behavior (e.g., activity, food intake, rest, sleep) and almost all physiologic phenomena (e.g., body temperature, endocrine secretions, cellular proliferation, pain, responsiveness to drugs) exhibit rhythmic fluctuations across a 24-hour period.

Temperature Rhythm

Sleep duration and structure are closely related to the circadian temperature rhythm. Body temperature fluctuates with circadian rhythmicity around a mean of 36.8°C. Nurses have used their awareness of this rhythmic variation in body temperature to guide practice; they frequently schedule daily measurements of body temperature for during the late afternoon hours. Normally, temperatures are lower during sleep, particularly in the early morning hours; begin to rise just before awakening; and peak in the late afternoon.

Sleep onset usually occurs approximately 6 hours before the lowest body temperature unless the sleep and temperature rhythms have become uncoupled as a result of shift work, travel across several time zones, or temporal isolation. Sleep duration depends more on the circadian phase of body temperature than on the prior amount of wakefulness (Czeisler, Zimmerman, Ronda, Moore-Ede, & Weitzman, 1980). Sleep periods beginning as body temperature is rising tend to be shorter than sleep periods starting when body temperature is falling.

Because most night-shift workers start their major sleep period in the morning when the body temperature is rising, this may be a partial explanation for why night-shift workers obtain less sleep in a 24-hour period than do day-shift workers (Agnew et al., 1967).

The composition of sleep changes with temperature fluctuations; the propensity for REM sleep is increased when sleep occurs after the low point of the temperature cycle (Czeisler, Weitzman, Moore-Ede, Zimmerman, & Knauer, 1980; Czeisler, Zimmerman et al., 1980). Thus, REM sleep is frequent during the early morning hours. Changes in daytime body temperature can also affect sleep cycles. Passive body heating (90-minute water bath at 41°C) in the late afternoon (2:30 to 5:30 PM) produces an increase in presleep tiredness and SWS (Horne & Reid, 1985). The amount of body heating during exercise, rather than the amount of energy expended, appears to be important in causing increases in total NREM sleep time and SWS (Horne & Reid, 1985). When body cooling accompanies exercise, there is no increase in SWS. The number and duration of awakenings increase when sleep is accompanied by a fever or an elevated ambient temperature. Fever also decreases the amount of REM and SWS (Karacan, Thornby, Anch, Williams, & Perkins, 1978; Karacan, Wolff, Williams, Hursch, & Webb, 1968).

Hormone Release During Sleep

Almost all neuroendocrine secretions are released in an episodic, rhythmic fashion. The release of some hormones, like cortisol, adrenocorticotropic hormone (ACTH), melatonin, renin, thyrotropin, and aldosterone may peak during the night when most people are asleep, but their release is not tied to the sleep-wake cycle (Parkes, 1985; Reinberg & Smolensky, 1983). In fact, these rhythmic peaks in secretion occur even during sleep deprivation or during a shift in the timing of the major sleep period. The release of other hormones, however, is rhythmic only because sleep occurs in a rhythmic fashion. The onset of sleep triggers the release of growth hormone (GH), with peak plasma concentrations of GH occurring 30 to 60 minutes later during the first SWS period of the night. After the initial large pulse of GH, additional GH is secreted in smaller bursts throughout the night. Although GH secretion is often thought to occur only during SWS, studies have shown that it is released during all sleep stages (Parkes, 1985; Sakai et al., 1980).

Even though males have lower prolactin levels than do females, both sexes experience episodic, pulsatile releases of prolactin during sleep. Secretion of prolactin begins to increase 60 to 90 minutes after sleep onset and peaks in the last hour or two of sleep, then falls to lower levels on waking (Sassin, Franz, Weitzman, & Kapen, 1972). Daytime napping can also produce a surge in prolactin secretion (Parker, Rossman, & Van der Laan, 1973). Partial or complete inversion of the sleep-wake cycle produces an immediate shift in the secretion of both growth hormone and prolactin (Parker et al., 1973) but does not alter the secretion of ACTH, cortisol, and other hormones listed previously.

The gonadotrophic hormones are released on an episodic basis throughout the 24-hour period during childhood and adulthood. However, just before and during puberty, large surges of luteinizing hormone (LH) and follicle-stimulating hormone (FSH) occur during sleep. Testosterone release in males occurs mainly at night, with maximum concentrations of testosterone tending to occur at about 7 to 8 AM (Piro, Fraioli, Sciarra, & Conti, 1973; Rose, Kreuz, Holaday, Sulak, & Johnson, 1972).

ANATOMIC AND BIOCHEMICAL CORRELATES OF SLEEP

The states of sleep and wakefulness have reciprocal, interacting, complementary mechanisms; both states are active rather than passive physiologic and biochemical processes. The state of wakefulness is maintained by intact cerebral hemispheres interacting with the thalamus, hypothalamus, and brain stem. An activated ascending reticular activating system (ARAS), as well as intact neuroanatomic structures, is required for wakefulness. However, decreased ARAS activity with low levels of sensory, motor, or mental input does not automatically cause sleep onset. Deactivation of the ARAS is required, along with active initiation of the sleep process. This hypnogenic or sleep-producing system consists of neuronal areas in the bulbar part of the lower brain stem, the median raphe nuclear complex of the middle brain stem, the ventromedian central thalamus, and the preoptic region of the anteromedian hypothalamus (Monnier, 1983). The neuronal systems that regulate sleep and wakefulness are functionally interacting.

The anatomic neuronal pathways required for sleep and wakefulness are also subject to biochemical regulation. Neurotransmitters alter the excitability of postsynaptic nerve cells (depolarize or hyperpolarize). Other chemical substances have a more general effect on neurons by altering or modulating the baseline metabolic activity or response to other neuronal input. The transmitters and modulators involved in the biochemical regulation of sleep and wakefulness include serotonin, norepinephrine, dopamine, acetylcholine, amino acids (e.g., tryptophan, L-glutamate, glycine, aspartate, taurine, gamma-aminobutyric acid), steroid hormones, neuropeptides, and related factors (e.g., beta-endorphin, enkephalin, angiotensin, somatostatin).

Two major groups of theories attempt to describe the phenomenon of sleep: the *monoamine theory* of sleep and the *general interaction chemical theory* of sleep. The monoaminergic theory of Jouvet (1969) attempts to correlate specific behavioral states, biochemical activity, and neuroanatomic sites of activity. In this theory, the sleep-wake cycle is postulated to be modulated by the balance between serotonergic neuron activity and catecholaminergic neuron activity. The catecholaminergic systems and cholinergic systems are involved in the behavioral and cortical activation of tonic arousal and the execution of

REM sleep (Bremmer, 1977; Monnier & Gaillard, 1980). The serotonergic median raphe nuclei in the midbrain, pons, and medulla are involved with sleep induction, the maintenance of SWS, and the priming of the brain for transition to REM sleep. REM onset is associated with the secretion of norepinephrine by the locus ceruleus.

In the monoamine theory, specific neurotransmitters and neuroanatomic sites are considered responsible for active mechanisms that initiate and maintain wakefulness (acetylcholine, norepinephrine, dopamine), NREM sleep (serotonin), and REM sleep (norepinephrine). A large number of research findings, however, challenge this mechanistic view and propose a general interaction chemical theory of sleep (Jones, 1979; Morgane, 1981; Ramm, 1979). These researchers describe sleep and wakefulness as the result of multiple independently converging influences involving all areas of the nervous system. The discharge rate, timing, and input-output organization of neurons are studied. Reciprocal interactions between specialized brain stem cells are used to build integrative models of sleep and waking (McCarley & Hobson, 1975; Pompeiano & Valentinuzzi, 1976).

Sleep-inducing or hypnogenic factors, including factor S (Pappenheimer, 1979), delta sleep–inducing peptide (Monnier, Schoenenberger, Dudler, & Herkert, 1975) and an REM-triggering protein substance R (Drucker-Colin & Espejel, 1980) have been isolated in animals. Peptides and humoral factors are postulated sleep-producers in humans, but as yet no endogenous sleep factor has been discovered. Until the late 1980s, when L-tryptophan was withdrawn from the market, nocturnal administration of L-tryptophan, a precursor of serotonin, was often recommended for use as a soporific. Despite anecdotal reports of its effectiveness, researchers found that even in large doses (up to 1 g), L-tryptophan was not effective in inducing sleep in humans (Adam & Oswald, 1979; Small, Milstein, & Golay, 1979). If L-tryptophan in large amounts could not induce sleep, it is very unlikely that foods high in tryptophan (i.e., dairy products) ingested just before bedtime will induce sleep.

HUMAN RESPONSES TO ALTERED SLEEP-WAKE PATTERNS

Human sleep is influenced by many endogenous and environmental factors. Modern sleep-wake problems are further exacerbated by changing lifestyles, work patterns, noise, pollution, stress, and many other environmental conditions. Although sleep disorders and sleep disturbances affect as many as one third of all adults in the United States, the significance of sleep disruptions and sleep disorders is underestimated in clinical areas, in educational programs for nurses and other health care professionals, and in research (National Commission on Sleep Disorders Research, 1992). There are more than 70 distinct sleep disorders described in the *International Classification of Sleep Disorders* (Diagnostic Classification Steering Committee, 1990), with consequences ranging from annoying to potentially life-threatening.

Age Factors in Responses

The type and frequency of sleep disturbances vary with age. About 20% to 30% of children in the first 4 years of life have regular sleeping difficulties (e.g., bedtime fears or struggles, night waking, enuresis). Frequently, these difficulties are transient, developmental, or a result of inappropriate parental management. However, sleep problems that continue for a year or more can be quite disruptive to family life and may signal more pervasive disturbances in the child or the family (Lazoff, Wolf, & Davis, 1985; National Commission on Sleep Disorders Research, 1992).

By the elementary school years, difficulties with going to bed and waking during the night have usually been resolved. However, maturational changes can also be associated with the development of somnambulism (sleepwalking) and sleep terrors. Both these parasomnias have characteristic ages of onset (sleepwalking, ages 4 to 8 years; sleep terrors, ages 4 to 12 years), usually resolve spontaneously within a year, and often seem to run in families. Obstructive sleep apnea, caused by enlarged tonsils or adenoids, may also develop before puberty. As discussed earlier, adolescents may be excessively sleepy during the daytime as a result of reduction in their nocturnal sleep. Daytime sleepiness in the late teen years may also be caused by narcolepsy, as well as by drug and alcohol use. Finally, nocturnal sleep during adolescence can be disrupted by the development of depression, mania, and schizophrenia.

Early adulthood brings situational stressors such as caring for a newborn infant, sleeping in a new environment, and performing shift work that may disrupt sleep. Difficulties falling asleep are more common than are difficulties maintaining sleep. Sleep is subjectively and objectively disrupted during menopause (Shaver, Giblin, & Paulsen, 1991). After middle adulthood, the quality and temporal organization of sleep appear to be much more easily disrupted. There is an increase in the number of awakenings after sleep onset, as well as greater difficulty returning to sleep after waking. Complaints of less restful sleep increase. Affectively charged or mood-disturbing events can modify REM sleep characteristics (Czeisler, Zimmerman et al., 1980). The incidence of obstructive sleep apnea, nocturnal myoclonus, and other sleep disorders increases markedly with age.

Disorders of Sleep-Wake Patterns

In 1990, the American Sleep Disorders Association (ASDA) revised its diagnostic classification of sleep and arousal disorders (Table 9–1). More complex than the first classification scheme, which divided sleep disorders into disorders of initiating and maintaining sleep (DIMS), disorders of excessive daytime sleepiness (DOES), parasomnias, and disorders of the sleep-wake schedule, this new classification scheme divides sleep disorders into four categories: dyssomnias, parasomnias, medical-psychiatric sleep disorders, and proposed sleep disorders. Dyssomnias are the major, or primary, sleep disorders that are associated with disturbed sleep at night or impaired wakefulness. These disorders have characteristic alterations in sleep and are different from medical and psychiatric disorders that can exist without the sleep disturbance being a fundamental part of the disorder. There are three subtypes of dyssomnias: intrinsic sleep disorders, extrinsic sleep disorders, and circadian rhythm sleep disorders. Parasomnias are disorders of arousal, partial arousal, and sleep-stage transition and are not primarily disorders of sleep and wake states per se. These disorders are manifestations of central nervous system activation usually transmitted through skeletal muscle or autonomic nervous system channels. The third category, sleep disorders associated with medical-psychiatric disorders, represents sleep disruptions or excessive daytime sleepiness as a result of a specific medical or psychiatric condition. The final category, proposed sleep disorders, includes newly described sleep disorders that currently lack sufficient evidence for inclusion as recognized sleep disorders.

The *International Classification of Sleep Disorders* (Diagnostic Classification Steering Committee, 1990) also includes a differential diagnosis of insomnia, excessive sleepiness, and other sleep disturbances (Table 9–2) that retains the emphasis on the client's presenting complaint as well as the more familiar categorization of sleep disorders into disorders of initiating and maintaining sleep, disorders of excessive sleepiness, and other sleep disturbances. This classification is more precise than the one category regarding sleep problems in the North American Nursing Diagnosis Association (NANDA) classification (i.e., sleep pattern disturbance). It separates problems underlying difficulty falling asleep from those associated with lack of feeling rested and excessive sleepiness, and it guides the nurse to more precise and appropriate interventions than are possible using the NANDA classification of sleep pattern disturbance. Certainly, many sleep disorders included in the *International Classification of Sleep Disorders* require medical diagnosis and treatment. However, nurses can be instrumental in casefinding and referral as well as important sources of information after diagnosis of these disorders. Finally, many of these disorders can be appropriately managed within the scope of nursing practice. Only selected disorders are discussed in this chapter. A full description of the structure and guidelines for diagnoses is given in the *International Classification of Sleep Disorders* (Diagnostic Classification Steering Committee, 1990).

Disorders of Initiating and Maintaining Sleep

Insomnia refers to the perception of inadequate or nonrestorative sleep of any duration or severity. Difficulties sleeping are quite common among adults. In fact, the National Commission on Sleep Disorders Research (1992) estimated that 60 million adults in the United States have frequent or chronic insomnia. Forty percent of insomniacs also use either over-the-counter medications or alcohol in an inappropriate attempt to alleviate their sleep problem. Women are affected more than men, and elderly persons are affected more than younger persons. The direct costs of treating persons with insomnia in 1990 was estimated to be $15.4 billion. In addition to these direct costs attributable to insom-

Text continued on page 183

TABLE 9–1 • INTERNATIONAL CLASSIFICATION OF SLEEP DISORDERS

1. Dyssomnias
   A. Intrinsic sleep disorders
      1. Psychophysiologic insomnia
      2. Sleep state misperception
      3. Idiopathic insomnia
      4. Narcolepsy
      5. Recurrent hypersomnia
      6. Idiopathic hypersomnia
      7. Posttraumatic hypersomnia
      8. Obstructive sleep apnea syndrome
      9. Central sleep apnea syndrome
      10. Central alveolar hypoventilation syndrome
      11. Periodic limb movement disorder
      12. Restless legs syndrome
      13. Intrinsic sleep disorders not otherwise specified
   B. Extrinsic sleep disorders
      1. Inadequate sleep hygiene
      2. Environmental sleep disorder
      3. Altitude insomnia
      4. Adjustment sleep disorder
      5. Insufficient sleep syndrome
      6. Limit-setting sleep disorder
      7. Sleep-onset association disorder
      8. Food allergy insomnia
      9. Nocturnal eating (drinking) syndrome
      10. Hypnotic-dependent sleep disorder
      11. Stimulant-dependent sleep disorder
      12. Alcohol-dependent sleep disorder
      13. Toxin-induced sleep disorder
      14. Extrinsic sleep disorders not otherwise specified
   C. Circadian sleep disorders
      1. Time zone change (jet lag) syndrome
      2. Shift work sleep disorder
      3. Irregular sleep-wake pattern
      4. Delayed sleep phase syndrome
      5. Advanced sleep phase syndrome
      6. Non–24-hour sleep-wake disorder
      7. Circadian rhythm sleep disorders not otherwise specified
2. Parasomnias
   A. Arousal disorders
      1. Confusional arousals
      2. Sleepwalking
      3. Sleep terrors
   B. Sleep-wake transition disorders
      1. Rhythmic movement disorder
      2. Sleep starts
      3. Sleep talking
      4. Nocturnal leg cramps
   C. Parasomnias usually associated with REM sleep
      1. Nightmares
      2. Sleep paralysis
      3. Impaired sleep-related penile erections
      4. Sleep-related painful erections

TABLE 9–1 • INTERNATIONAL CLASSIFICATION OF SLEEP DISORDERS *Continued*

     5. REM sleep-related sinus arrest
     6. REM sleep behavior disorder
  D. Other parasomnias
     1. Sleep bruxism
     2. Sleep enuresis
     3. Sleep-related abnormal swallowing syndrome
     4. Nocturnal paroxysmal dystonia
     5. Sudden unexplained nocturnal death syndrome
     6. Primary snoring
     7. Infant sleep apnea
     8. Congenital central hypoventilation syndrome
     9. Sudden infant death syndrome
    10. Benign neonatal sleep myoclonus
    11. Other parasomnias not otherwise specified
3. Sleep disorders associated with medical or psychiatric disorders
  A. Associated with mental disorders
     1. Psychoses
     2. Mood disorders
     3. Anxiety disorders
     4. Panic disorders
     5. Alcoholism
  B. Associated with neurologic disorders
     1. Cerebral degenerative disorders
     2. Dementia
     3. Parkinsonism
     4. Fatal familial insomnia
     5. Sleep-related epilepsy
     6. Electrical status epilepticus of sleep
     7. Sleep-related headaches
  C. Associated with other medical disorders
     1. Sleeping sickness
     2. Nocturnal cardiac ischemia
     3. Chronic obstructive pulmonary disease
     4. Sleep-related asthma
     5. Sleep-related gastroesophageal reflux
     6. Peptic ulcer disease
     7. Fibrositis syndrome
4. Proposed sleep disorders
     1. Short sleeper
     2. Long sleeper
     3. Subwakefulness syndrome
     4. Fragmentary myoclonus
     5. Sleep hyperhidrosis
     6. Menstrual-associated sleep disorder
     7. Pregnancy-associated sleep disorder
     8. Terrifying hypnogogic hallucinations
     9. Sleep-related neurogenic tachypnea
    10. Sleep-related laryngospasm
    11. Sleep choking syndrome

REM, rapid eye movement.

TABLE 9–2 • DIFFERENTIAL DIAGNOSIS

A. Insomnia (difficulty initiating or maintaining sleep)
  1. Associated with behavioral or psychophysiologic disorders
      a. Adjustment sleep disorder
      b. Psychophysiologic insomnia
      c. Inadequate sleep hygiene
      d. Limit-setting sleep disorder
      e. Sleep-onset association disorder
      f. Nocturnal eating (drinking) syndrome
      g. Other
  2. Associated with psychiatric disorders
      a. Psychoses
      b. Mood disorders
      c. Anxiety disorders
      d. Panic disorders
      e. Alcoholism
      f. Other
  3. Associated with environmental factors
      a. Environmental sleep disorder
      b. Food allergy insomnia
      c. Toxin-induced sleep disorder
      d. Other
  4. Associated with drug dependency
      a. Hypnotic-dependent sleep disorder
      b. Stimulant-dependent sleep disorder
      c. Alcohol-dependent sleep disorder
      d. Other
  5. Associated with sleep-induced respiratory impairment
      a. Obstructive sleep apnea syndrome
      b. Central sleep apnea syndrome
      c. Central alveolar hypoventilation syndrome
      d. Chronic obstructive pulmonary disease
      e. Sleep-related asthma
      f. Altitude insomnia
      g. Other
  6. Associated with movement disorders
      a. Sleep starts
      b. Restless legs syndrome
      c. Periodic limb movement disorder
      d. Nocturnal leg cramps
      e. Rhythmic movement disorder
      f. REM sleep behavior disorder
      g. Nocturnal paroxysmal dystonia
      h. Other
  7. Associated with disorders of the timing of the sleep-wake pattern
      a. Short sleeper
      b. Time zone change (jet lag) syndrome
      c. Shift work sleep disorder
      d. Delayed sleep phase syndrome
      e. Advanced sleep phase syndrome
      f. Non–24-hour sleep-wake disorder
      g. Irregular sleep-wake pattern
      h. Other

TABLE 9–2 • DIFFERENTIAL DIAGNOSIS *Continued*

    8. Associated with parasomnias (not otherwise classified)
      a. Confusional arousals
      b. Sleep terrors
      c. Nightmares
      d. Sleep hyperhidrosis
      e. Other
    9. Associated with the central nervous system (not otherwise classified)
      a. Parkinsonism
      b. Dementia
      c. Cerebral degenerative disorders
      d. Sleep-related epilepsy
      e. Fatal familiar insomnia
      f. Other
   10. Associated with no objective sleep disturbance
      a. Sleep state misperception
      b. Sleep choking syndrome
      c. Other
   11. Idiopathic insomnia
   12. Other causes of insomnia
      a. Sleep-related gastroesophageal reflux
      b. Fibrositis syndrome
      c. Menstrual-associated sleep disorder
      d. Pregnancy-associated sleep disorder
      e. Terrifying hypnogogic hallucinations
      f. Sleep-related abnormal swallowing syndrome
      g. Sleep-related laryngospasm
      h. Other
B. Excessive sleepiness
    1. Associated with behavioral or psychophysiologic disorders
      a. Inadequate sleep hygiene
      b. Insufficient sleep syndrome
      c. Limit-setting disorder
      d. Other
    2. Associated with psychiatric disorders
      a. Mood disorders
      b. Psychosis
      c. Alcoholism
      d. Other
    3. Associated with environmental factors
      a. Environmental sleep disorder
      b. Toxin-induced sleep disorder
      c. Other
    4. Associated with drug dependency
      a. Hypnotic-dependent sleep disorder
      b. Stimulant-dependent sleep disorder
      c. Other
    5. Associated with sleep-induced respiratory impairment
      a. Obstructive sleep apnea syndrome
      b. Central sleep apnea syndrome
      c. Central alveolar hypoventilation syndrome
      d. Sleep-related neurogenic tachypnea
      e. Other

Table continued on following page

TABLE 9–2 • DIFFERENTIAL DIAGNOSIS *Continued*

6. Associated with movement disorders
   a. Periodic limb movement disorder
   b. Other
7. Associated with disorders of the timing of the sleep-wake pattern
   a. Long sleeper
   b. Time zone change (jet lag) syndrome
   c. Shift work sleep disorder
   d. Delayed sleep phase syndrome
   e. Advanced sleep phase syndrome
   f. Non–24-hour sleep-wake syndrome
   g. Irregular sleep-wake pattern
   h. Other
8. Associated with the central nervous system (not otherwise classified)
   a. Narcolepsy
   b. Idiopathic hypersomnia
   c. Posttraumatic hypersomnia
   d. Recurrent hypersomnia
   e. Subwakefulness syndrome
   f. Fragmentary myocology
   g. Parkinsonism
   h. Dementia
   i. Sleeping sickness
   j. Other
9. Other causes of excessive sleepiness
   a. Menstrual-associated sleep disorder
   b. Pregnancy-associated sleep disorder

C. Other sleep disorders
1. Associated with behavioral or psychophysiologic disorders
   a. Nocturnal eating (drinking) syndrome
   b. Other
2. Associated with psychiatric disorders
   a. Panic disorder
   b. Other
3. Associated with sleep-induced respiratory impairment
   a. Primary snoring
   b. Obstructive sleep apnea syndrome
   c. Central sleep apnea syndrome
   d. Central alveolar hypoventilation syndrome
   e. Sleep-related asthma
   f. Chronic obstructive pulmonary disease
   g. Sleep-related neurogenic tachypnea
   h. Other
4. Associated with movement disorders
   a. Sleep starts
   b. Sleepwalking
   c. Sleep terrors
   d. Sleep bruxism
   e. Periodic limb movement disorder
   f. Restless legs syndrome
   g. Rhythmic movement disorder
   h. Sleep paralysis
   i. Nocturnal leg cramps
   j. REM sleep behavior disorder
   k. Nocturnal paroxysmal dystonia
   l. Other

TABLE 9–2 • DIFFERENTIAL DIAGNOSIS *Continued*

  5. Associated with parasomnias (not otherwise classified)
     a. Nightmares
     b. Sleep talking
     c. Sleep enuresis
     d. Sleep-related painful erections
     e. Other
  6. Associated with central nervous system (not otherwise classified)
     a. Sleep-related epilepsy
     b. Electrical status epilepticus of sleep
     c. Fragmentary myoclonus
     d. Other
  7. Other causes of sleep disturbances
     a. Sleep-related gastroesophageal reflux
     b. Sleep-related sinus arrest
     c. Sleep-related abnormal swallowing syndrome
     d. Sleep-related laryngospasm
     e. Sleep choking syndrome
     f. Terrifying hypnagogic hallucinations
     g. Other

REM, rapid eye movement.

nia, persons with chronic insomnia reported 2.5 times as many fatigue-related traffic accidents as noninsomniacs, as well as more difficulties with concentration, memory problems, and interpersonal difficulties (National Commission on Sleep Disorders Research, 1992). Finally, it is important to remember that insomnia is a presenting complaint or a symptom, not a unique disorder.

The 56 sleep disturbances classified as DIMS are varied and include disturbances ranging from transient problems lasting one or two nights to sleep disturbances that may last for several decades. Difficulties initiating and maintaining sleep may result from behavioral and psychophysiologic factors, psychiatric disorders, environments that are incompatible with sleep, drug dependency, sleep-induced respiratory impairments, movement disorders, alterations in the timing of sleep, parasomnias, and central nervous system diseases. Sleep may also be disrupted by pain, angina, and nocturnal asthma attacks.

An adjustment sleep disorder refers to a sleep disturbance temporally related to acute stress or environmental changes causing emotional arousal. Unfamiliar sleeping environments, stressful life events, acute anxiety, or the threat of loss can produce difficulties falling asleep or premature awakenings. The individual is usually aware of and able to identify the stressor that precipitated the sleeping difficulties (e.g., the death of a loved one, a divorce, an upcoming examination). Once the stressor is removed or the level of adaptation increases, the person's sleep returns to normal. Although a sharp increase in alcohol intake or the use of nonprescription sleep aids or stimulants may occur, serious medical or psychologic complications are rare. Only reassurance that sleep loss does not cause bodily harm may be needed.

An adjustment sleep disorder usually resolves within a few days or weeks, whereas psychophysiologic insomnia may last for years or decades if not treated. Although a stressful life event may have precipitated the original sleeping problem, sleep does not return to normal after removal of the stressor. Patients with psychophysiologic insomnia typically react to stress by denying or repressing the meaning of a stessful event. Increased physiologic arousal coupled with learned sleep-preventing associations exacerbates the person's difficulty obtaining "a good night's sleep." A maladaptive conditioned wakefulness may arise from frequent episodes of lying awake in bed. A poor night of sleep triggers fear of insomnia, which becomes a self-fulfilling prophecy. Bedtime rituals (e.g., toothbrushing) and the physical bedroom environment may be associated with feelings of anxiety, frustration, and anger. A vicious cycle develops; as the person tries harder to fall asleep and becomes more agitated, the less likely it is that sleep will occur. Over time, concerns about obtaining a good night's sleep increase, often becoming the person's major focus. Excessive use of hypnotics or alcohol is often found, plus the daytime use of tranquilizers to reduce somatized tension. Caffeine or other stimulants may also be used to combat daytime fatigue. Polysomnographic recordings reveal increased sleep latency, increased wakefulness, and decreased sleep latency or, in some cases, a reverse first-night effect; that is, the patient sleeps better in the sleep laboratory than at home (Diagnostic Classification Steering Committee, 1990).

Research has shown that stimulus control therapy, described by Bootzin and Nicassio (1978), is particularly effective for patients with psychophysiologic insomnia. This technique has been demonstrated to be more effective than relaxation training and the use of sedative or hypnotic drugs (Bootzin & Perlis, 1992; McClusky, Milby, Switzer, William, & Wooten, 1991). Because patients with psychophysiologic insomnia often associate the bed with staying awake, stimulus control therapy attempts to reassociate the bed with sleep. This is accomplished using the behavioral techniques recommended by Bootzin and Nicassio (1978):

1. Go to bed only when you are sleepy.

2. Use the bed only for sexual activity and sleeping; do not do anything else in the bedroom (no reading, listening to music, or watching television). If you are unable to fall asleep in about 15 minutes, get up, go to another room, and do something relaxing until you are sleepy.

3. Return to bed only when you are sleepy; if sleep still does not come easily, get up again.

4. Turn the clock toward the wall, because concern for time will only exacerbate the problem. The goal is to associate lying in bed with rapid sleep onset.

5. With nocturnal wakefulness, return to bed only when you feel sleepy. Awake at the same time every day, and do not take daytime naps.

In order to maintain this pattern of behavior, most people need the support of and regular contact with a therapist or nurse. A daily sleep log and graph of sleep behavior are helpful to reinforce the behavior pattern and to provide tangible evidence of improvement (Lacks, 1987).

Inadequate sleep hygiene refers to a sleep disorder caused by performance of activities of daily living that are inconsistent with the maintenance of good quality sleep and full daytime alertness (Diagnostic Classification Steering Committee, 1990). Nicotine, caffeine, and other central nervous system stimulants disturb sleep, and the presence of caffeine is pervasive and often unrecognized (e.g., coffee, tea, colas, chocolate, many over-the-counter medications, and some prescription medications all have caffeine). The long-term use of tobacco and the ingestion of caffeinated beverages after lunchtime disturbs sleep, even in those who believe their sleep is not disturbed (Hauri et al., 1982). A single drink of alcohol is sometimes used as self-medication to relieve tension and permit sleep onset. Alcohol, however, does not increase total sleep time. After alcohol consumption, sleep is fragmented, and the numerous partial awakenings cause a decrease in total sleep time. REM periods are fragmented and reduced, and the person more frequently awakens early and feels unrested. The repeated use of a "nightcap" may cause rather than alleviate poor sleep. Regular heavy physical exercise, in an adapted individual, increases total sleep duration and the amount of SWS (Montgomery, Trinder, & Paxton, 1982). The effects of sudden, short-term, or intermittent heavy exercise, however, are variable and difficult to predict. Moderate exercise, if done consistently, may extend and deepen sleep. However, exercise should be avoided in the late evening hours before bedtime.

Environmental factors such as noise, ambient temperature, and early morning light in the bedroom can also increase wakefulness. Reducing nighttime noise results in an overall improvement in sleep organization, subjective sleep quality, and morning performance. There is no long-term physiologic adaptation to nighttime noise (Vallet & Mouret, 1984), isolated noises (e.g., airplane overflight, trucks) produce greater arousal from sleep than does constant background noise of comparable magnitude (e.g., air conditioner). Intermittent intense noise produces increased nocturnal awakenings and stage 1 sleep. Sleep is disturbed even in people who do not remember the event in the morning. The awakening threshold of a noise varies with the sleep stage and the personal sensitivity of the individual. Women and elderly people tend to be more sensitive to environmental noise. The meaning attached to a specific noise is as important as the noise intensity in producing arousal. Sleep may be improved in noisy environments by sound attenuation measures, noise screening by providing constant background noise, and wearing earplugs.

The preferred ambient sleep temperature for humans is around 19°C, with a microclimate temperature inside the bed (provided by pajamas, sheets, and blanket) of 28.6°C to 30.9°C (Muzet, Libert, & Candas, 1984). Increases or decreases in ambient temperature from this thermal comfort zone result in more frequent and longer awakenings, more body movements, and decreased REM cycle length.

These behaviors often lead to disrupted nocturnal sleep by increasing arousal or fragmenting sleep. Other practices do not increase arousal but rather interfere with the regular timing and duration of sleep and waking periods.

Individuals who are distressed by sleep loss and daytime fatigue, sleepiness, or moodiness will often attempt to improve their nighttime sleep by altering their behavior (going to sleep earlier, staying in bed later, napping, and lying down to rest during the day). Although these alterations may occasionally lead to increased sleep, they also lead to increased variability in the timing of sleep and weaken the self-sustaining properties of a regular sleep-wake cycle. Sleep may become disrupted or variable when too much time is spent in bed; when there are large day-to-day variations in bedtime, arising time, and amount of sleep; and when naps are taken during the day (Diagnostic Classification Steering Committee, 1990).

Inadequate sleep hygiene may be the sole cause of a person's disturbed sleep or it may be a contributing factor in the maintenance of another sleep disorder. Therefore, any time a patient complains of insomnia lasting more than a few days, the nurse should assess the adequacy of the sleep hygiene practices. Data should be obtained about the amount (e.g., number of cups of coffee, ounces of cola) of caffeinated beverages consumed per day, as well as the number of cigarettes smoked and the amount of alcohol intake on a daily and weekly basis. Data should also be obtained from the patient and his or her spouse or partner about sleep and napping behaviors. It is important to remember that a single regular daytime nap does not necessarily interfere with nocturnal sleep (Diagnostic Classification Steering Committee, 1990; Dinges, 1989). Instead, the nurse needs to determine if the frequency, duration, proximity to nighttime sleep, or variable timing of naps suggests an impact on sleep.

Once the diagnosis of inadequate sleep hygiene is made, nurses can assist the patient in modifying his or her behavior. Although the patient's behavior may be having a deleterious effect on sleep, the patient may need assistance in recognizing the impact of his or her behavior on sleep and in making the necessary modifications in behavior or sleeping environment (e.g., reducing caffeine intake, stopping smoking, reducing noise, consolidating sleep into one block of time at night). If a person's sleep is nocturnal, sleep is fragmented, or the person is taking numerous daytime naps, sleep restriction can be very effective in consolidating sleep into one period at night (Friedman, Bliwise, Yesavage, & Salom, 1991; Spielman, Saskin, & Thorpy, 1983). The following approach is used:

1. Have the patient determine a time when she or he will get up each morning. Once this time for awakening is set, stress that the patient should get out of bed every morning at that time even if she or he has not slept at all the night before.

2. Point out that having a regular time for arising will help entrain the sleep-wake pattern. Ask the patient how much sleep he or she needs at night to function during the day.

3. Subtract 30 to 60 minutes from this amount (e.g., if the patient reports needing 7.5 hours of sleep at night, allow only 7 hours in bed) to determine how much time the patient is allowed to be in bed at night.

4. Set the patient's bedtime by counting back the required number of hours from the designated arising time. Instruct the patient not to go to bed before that time even if he or she is sleepy.

5. Napping during the day is not allowed even if the patient feels tired and sleepy. In the case of an elderly patient, one short afternoon nap (less than 60 minutes) is allowed. Encourage the patient to substitute physical activity for napping if she or he has difficulty remaining awake during the day.

6. Remind the patient that sleep at night will usually improve within a few days if the sleep restriction schedule is followed correctly. Give the patient a phone number where a clinician can be reached if she or he becomes excessively sleepy or unable to follow through on the sleep restriction schedule.

Again, a daily sleep log and graph of sleep behavior is often helpful to reinforce the behavior pattern and provide tangible evidence of improvement (Lacks, 1987).

Although almost all psychiatric disorders can produce an associated sleep disturbance (sleep disorder associated with mental disorders), patients are most likely to complain about problems sleeping if they have a psychosis, a mood disorder, an anxiety disorder, or panic attacks or are alcoholic. Agitation and hallucinations, particularly during an acute psychotic decompensation, may prevent sleep onset in schizophrenic patients. During an acute exacerbation of symptoms, the patient may also have decreased total sleep time, increased waking after sleep onset, decreased SWS, shortened REM latency, variability in REM time, and increase in REM density. During remission, sleep efficiency may be normal, but sleep architecture may show persistent alterations such as a reduction in SWS (Diagnostic Classification Steering Committee, 1990). Mood disorders refer to bipolar disorders, cyclothymia, major depressive disorders, and dysthymia. Two types of sleep disturbances are common: the short sleep duration and sleep-onset insomnia associated with mania and the difficulty falling asleep and "early morning" (premature) awakenings associated with depression. Waking up too early and not being able to fall asleep are considered cardinal symptoms of depression. In fact, the characteristic insomnia associated with depression is frequently an early sign of mood change, often beginning before the clinical depression is noticed (Diagnostic Classification Steering Committee, 1990). The severity of insomnia is also correlated with the severity of the mood disturbance, with the most severe insomnia associated with a psychotic depression (Diagnostic Classification Steering Committee, 1990). The ingestion of alcohol produces increased sleepiness about 30 minutes after consumption, reduces wakefulness for the first 3 to 4 hours of sleep, but increases wakefulness during the later 2 to 3 hours of sleep. Within a few days of regular consumption, however, sleep becomes fragmented, with frequent brief arousals or periods of restlessness. Abstinence following chronic use of alcohol causes profound sleep disruption and an increase in nightmares and other anxiety dreams. Not only is sleep disrupted, its duration is significantly shorter. This profound sleep loss is quite distressing and may be a contributing factor to the development of delirium tremens and the resumption of drinking (Bates, 1972; Diagnostic Classification Steering Committee, 1990). Sleep continuity gradually improves and both nightmares and anxiety dreams begin to decrease within the first 2 weeks of abstinence. In addition, the number of awakenings gradually decreases over a long period of abstinence (up to 2 years). However, some patients' sleep remains disrupted even after years of abstinence (Diagnostic Classification Steering Committee, 1990).

Because most psychiatric disorders can produce sleep disruptions, it is very important for nurses to inquire about current or past psychiatric problems. All patients should also be asked about the use of recreational substances and alcohol. Information about the amount and frequency of use should be recorded. If a psychiatric-related sleep disorder is suspected, the nurse should refer the patient to a therapist or psychiatrist for further treatment of the underlying psychiatric problem. Once the underlying psychiatric disorder is appropriately treated, the sleep problem usually disappears or is greatly reduced in severity. Behavioral approaches may be used in conjunction with psychotropic medications if inappropriate sleep hygiene is exacerbating the sleep disruption.

An environmental sleep disorder is a sleep disturbance resulting from a disturbing environmental factor that causes a complaint of either insomnia or excessive sleepiness. The onset time, course, and termination of the sleep problem are directly related to the causative environmental condition. Sleep immediately or gradually improves once the disturbing factor is ameliorated or removed from the environment (Diagnostic Classification Steering Committee, 1990). This disturbance is not due to stress, but to measurable environmental stimuli such as heat, cold, noise, movements of a bed partner, or necessity to remain alert when caring for an infant or an invalid. Although medical procedures, discomfort from various drainage tubes, and abnormal sleep-wake schedules imposed on a person during hospitalization may result in a sleep disturbance with insomnia, it is important to remember that a diagnosis of an environmental sleep disturbance is made only after the condition has been present for at least 3 weeks (if disturbance is present for less than 3 weeks, it is categorized as an adjustment sleep disorder); initially, the patient may report a mild mood disturbance, daytime fatigue, concentration problems, irritability, and a preoccupation with the loss of sleep. Over time, symptoms of chronic sleep deprivation (depressed mood, reduced work performance, malaise, chronic daytime sleepiness, and lethargy) may develop, and patients may adopt sleep patterns that further disrupt their sleep (e.g., inadequate sleep hygiene).

An environmental sleep disorder produces partial but not total deprivation of sleep. It also refers to a curtailment in total sleep time, not the selective deprivation of certain sleep stages (NREM or REM). Laboratory studies have shown that restricting sleep to fewer than 4 hours of sleep per night results in reduced amounts of stage 2 and REM sleep; the amount of SWS is usually unaltered (Akerstedt & Torsvall, 1985). Vigilance, mood, and performance of more difficult cognitive tasks decrease rapidly in the first 4 days of sleep curtailment (4 hours of total sleep), and then level out (Haslam, 1984). Physical fitness remains adequate.

A less severe reduction in sleep time appears to be more easily tolerated. Horne and Wilkinson (1985) report that chronic moderate sleep reduction (reduced from 8 hours per night to 6) can be easily learned and tolerated by young, healthy adults. Overall, subjects accomplished this reduction by strictly adhering to bed and arising times for 6 weeks; daytime mood and performance were unaffected. Because most participants in these studies were healthy college students, it is unknown whether middle-aged or older adults can also tolerate reductions in their sleep time. Nor is there any information about the effects of partial sleep deprivation on persons who are ill.

Selective deprivation of sleep stages rarely occurs outside the laboratory setting, unless a patient has taken certain drugs that suppress REM sleep (tricyclic and monoamine oxidase inhibitor antidepressants and certain hypnotic medications). When REM-deprived individuals are allowed to sleep, REM sleep latency is reduced and the intensity of REM phenomena is increased. Large individual differences in the degree of REM rebound are seen (Antonioli et al., 1981), and the selective deprivation of REM sleep appears to affect mood and motivational behavior (Vogel, 1975). Most common are reports of agitation, hyperactivity, emotional liability, and decreased impulse control (Naitoh, Pasnau, & Kollar, 1971). In contrast, people with selective NREM sleep deprivation tend to be hyporesponsive, withdrawn, and more physically uncomfortable (Agnew et al., 1967). Delta sleep (SWS) deprivation also produces a delta rebound, which is less intense and intrusive than REM rebound.

Researchers have found that after 48 to 72 hours of total sleep deprivation, it is impossible to prevent sleep completely. Episodes of "microsleep," which last a few seconds, begin to intrude on wakefulness. Lapses of attention accompany microsleep. As the total sleep deprivation time increases, the frequency and duration of microsleep periods increase. Sleep-deprived individuals complain of fatigue and sleepiness (which follows a diurnal rhythm). They may appear irritable, serious, or listless. However, patients with endogenous depression often experience an elevation in mood after a night of total sleep deprivation (Van de Burg & Van den Hoofdakker, 1975).

After 24 to 48 hours of deprivation, cognitive task performance, vigilance, mood, and motor skills deteriorate (Haslam, 1984; Opstad, Ekanger, Nummestad, & Raabe, 1978), and people report that it takes greater effort to perform tasks requiring speed or perseverance. The behavioral and psychologic effects of sleep deprivation can diminish performance measurably, although recovery to baseline performance levels usually occurs after only 4 hours of sleep. The performance of simple, well-learned physical tasks appears to be unaffected by sleep deprivation (Haslam, 1984; Kolka, Martin, & Elizonda, 1984). In preparation for a period of total sleep deprivation, relatively short periods of sleep (about 4 hours) have been shown to have a beneficial effect on subsequent performance, even in the absence of a prior sleep debt (Nicholson et al., 1985).

Some investigators report that total sleep deprivation disturbs metabolic indices and elevates corticosteroid and catecholamine levels (Kant, Genser,

Thorne, Pfalser, & Mougey, 1984), whereas others found no significant biologic effects with total sleep deprivation (Ahnve, Theorell, Akerstedt, Frogberg, & Halberg, 1981; Horne, 1978). The psychologic stage of the individual (e.g., frustration, anxiety, situational or anticipatory uncertainty) may be responsible for many of the changes seen with sleep deprivation (Francesconi, Stokes, Banderet, & Kowal, 1978).

Periodic limb movements (PLMs) can also disrupt sleep. PLMs are repetitive and highly stereotyped movements of the legs (or arms) that produce partial or complete arousals. Patients may complain of fragmented, restless sleep or may be completely unaware of their frequent arousals. There is often significant night-to-night variability in the frequency and severity of PLMs. These movements may occur as discrete episodes lasting a few minutes to several hours or may be present throughout most of the night. PLMs appear with the onset of stage 1 sleep, are frequent during stage 2 sleep, decrease during stages 3 and 4, and usually disappear during REM sleep. As with other types of chronic insomnia, patients may become depressed or anxious about their sleep.

PLMs are associated with advanced age (up to 35% of persons older than 60 years have PLMs) and with other disorders that produce fragmented sleep (e.g., sleep apnea, narcolepsy). PLMs can also be evoked by or associated with many medical disorders such as chronic uremia and other metabolic disorders. Ingestion of drugs such as tricyclic antidepressants, monamine oxidase inhibitors, and alcohol may also induce or aggravate PLMs. In addition, withdrawal from medications such as anticonvulsants, benzodiazepines, barbiturates, and other hypnotic drugs can cause PLMs (Diagnostic Classification Steering Committee, 1990).

PLMs should be suspected in elderly persons complaining of insomnia and in persons with metabolic disorders who complain about restless and unrefreshing sleep, as well as those taking or being withdrawn from the medications listed in the preceding paragraph. Because the bed partner's sleep is often disrupted by the PLMs, asking the bed partner about the presence of rhythmic kicking movements of the legs or rhythmic movements of the arms during the night can be quite informative. If PLMs are suspected, the patient should be referred to an accredited sleep disorders center for a nocturnal polysomnogram. Treatment efficacy is varied; medication may reduce the number of limb movements yet produce little or no change in sleep duration or efficiency (Diagnostic Classification Steering Committee, 1990). In other patients, low doses of Sinemet at bedtime greatly improve sleep duration and efficiency.

Insomnia is also associated with the development of many neurologic disorders (sleep disorders associated with neurologic disorders). The effects of degenerative disorders on sleep are varied; sleep fragmentation is common as a result of the involuntary movements associated with many of these diseases; reduced deep sleep (stages 3 and 4) is associated with olivopontocerebellar degeneration, spinocerebellar degeneration, and Huntington's disease, and REM is completely absent with spinocerebellar degeneration (Diagnostic Classification Steering Committee, 1990). Patients with dementia may have difficulties falling asleep, and once asleep may awaken frequently or prematurely (early morning awakening); in addition, sleep efficiency, the amount of deep sleep (stages 3 and 4), and the percentage of REM sleep (a portion of total sleep time) are reduced (Feinberg, Koresko, & Heller, 1967; Prinz et al., 1982). Excessive daytime sleepiness may be present as a result of the disruption of nocturnal sleep. The presence of other sleep disorders such as sleep apnea or periodic limb movements can further exacerbate the sleep disruptions associated with dementia. Sundowning (nocturnal wandering and confusion) rarely appears until the advanced stage of illness, and in the institutionalized elderly it has been shown to be associated with urinary incontinence, increased frequency of bed checks, and better physical health (Evans, 1987). These sleep changes are disturbing to family members and frequently lead to institutionalization (Diagnostic Classification Steering Committee, 1990).

Persons with Parkinson's disease have characteristic changes in their sleep that generally worsen as the disease progresses and the duration of treatment lengthens. Patient complaints of insomnia can be verified by polysomnographic recordings that show a prolonged sleep latency, increased numbers of arousals, increased wake time after sleep onset, and decreased percentage of REM sleep. Tremor usually disappears with sleep onset but may reappear for brief periods during arousals, during sleep stage changes, during stage 2 sleep, and before and after an REM period (Diagnostic Classification Steering Committee, 1990). Stiffness, back pain, difficulty changing position in bed, vivid dreams and nightmares, limb jerks, and visual hallucinations may also disrupt sleep. Daytime sleepiness may also occur as the disease progresses. Drug treatment of Parkinson's disease may have varied effects on sleep, reduce sleep disturbance because of rigidity or bradykinesia, alter or exacerbate existing sleep disorders, or create new sleep disturbances. Up to 80% to 90% of patients who are treated with levodopa or bromocriptine experience medication-induced sleep disruption (Nausieda, Weiner, Kaplin, Weber, & Klawans, 1982; Rabey, Vardi, Glaubman, & Streifler, 1978). Sleep disturbances can be reduced if levodopa administration is restricted to early morning hours or is eliminated. Avoidance of concomitant administration of other antiparkinsonian medications may also help reduce sleep disturbances (Diagnostic Classification Steering Committee, 1990).

• C A S E   S T U D Y   1

Mr. I was a 71-year-old obese man referred to a sleep clinic for evaluation and treatment of his disrupted nocturnal sleep. Included in his rather thick medical chart were the results of tests that his pulmonologist had ordered 6 weeks earlier to rule out the presence of obstructive sleep apnea. No sleep apnea was noted during the nocturnal polysomnogram. However, the patient's nocturnal sleep was moderately to severely disturbed by periodic leg movements. The patient was on oxygen at 2 L/min throughout the study. An MSLT the following day revealed mild to moderate daytime sleepiness.

The patient denied any difficulties with his sleep until an aortic aneurysm repair 2 years earlier. Since that time, Mr. I reported that he was unable to sleep more than 1 hour at a time at night, that he was exhausted, and that he had to take two naps per day (each at least 1 hour in duration). He usually retired between 10 and 10:30 PM but usually awakened 30 minutes later. Instead of staying in bed, he would get a cup of coffee and go to the living room, where he would fall asleep in his recliner for another 1 to 2 hours. When he awakened he would drink more coffee and watch television until he was sleepy again. This pattern was repeated several times throughout the night. A 1-month trial of Sinemet did not improve his sleep. Although he did not attribute his awakenings to difficulties breathing, he did admit to using his albuterol (Proventil) inhaler several times during the night. Mr. I got up between 5:30 and 7 AM, ate breakfast, and then took his first nap of the day. The second nap usually occurred after lunch.

Mr. I consumed approximately four cups of caffeinated beverages during the day and an unknown amount of coffee during the night when he awakened. He reported quitting smoking 2 years earlier and did not use any recreational drugs. However, Mr. I currently consumed hard liquor once per week and, when questioned further, admitted he drank an additional liter of wine per day. His spouse also pointed out that he sipped on wine throughout the day and drank additional wine at night when he awakened.

His history was significant for an aortic aneurysm repair in 1991, two vessel coronary artery diseases, chronic obstructive pulmonary disease (COPD), pancreatitis 5 to 7 years ago, and hospitalization for alcohol treatment 6 or 7 years ago. Current medications included three different inhalers (Proventil t.i.d., Atrovent t.i.d., and AeroBid t.i.d.); Isordil, 40 mg t.i.d.; Lasix, 80 mg t.i.d.; aspirin, one tablet per day; and oxygen at 2 L/min at all times). His physical examination was unremarkable.

The clinical nurse specialist caring for Mr. I concluded that several factors could be disrupting the patient's nighttime sleep. First, difficulties breathing as a result of COPD can fragment sleep. Although the patient denied breathing problems at night, he did spend part of the night sleeping in a recliner and reported using his Proventil inhaler several times during the night. Secondly, Proventil can exacerbate sleep disruptions because of its stimulating effect. Third, Mr. I had a history of alcohol abuse and was currently consuming a substantial amount of alcohol each day. Not only can alcohol itself disrupt sleep, but it can cause or exacerbate PLMs. The fourth possible cause of the patient's disturbed nighttime sleep was the excessive amount of time spent in bed (or in his recliner) sleeping. Between his nocturnal sleep and two daytime naps, the patient was spending approximately 9 to 10 hours in bed. Finally, Mr. I's sleep was disrupted by PLMs.

Nursing diagnoses were inadequate sleep hygiene related to excessive time in bed and ingestion of caffeine and alcohol during the night; potential for impaired respiration during sleep related to the need to sleep in a recliner and to the frequent use of a bronchodilator at night; and noncompliance with recommended medical therapy (use of Proventil inhaler no more than three times per day). Several methods of improving sleep hygiene were discussed with the patient and his wife. First, sleep restriction therapy was explained and a plan decided on for restricting time in bed at night to 7.5 hours with one daytime nap of no more than 1 hour per day. Second, the patient was advised to eliminate all caffeine and to drink decaffeinated coffee. He was also advised to stop drinking all alcohol. When Mr. I remarked that it wouldn't be a problem to stop drinking, the nurse reminded him that it is often very difficult to stop drinking without some additional help and recommended that he participate in Alcoholics Anonymous meetings or obtain counseling. He was also advised to elevate the head of his bed and to talk to his pulmonologist about using his Proventil inhaler during the night. Finally, the clinical nurse specialist emphasized that although PLMs were certainly disrupting Mr. I's sleep, they were not the only cause of his fragmented and nonrestorative sleep and the prescription of medications for PLMs would probably not eliminate his difficulties sleeping. Although Mr. I was instructed to contact the clinical nurse specialist in 1 month to evaluate the effectiveness of these recommendations and to discuss the need for medication to reduce the PLMs, he did not follow through on this recommendation.

Disorders of Excessive Sleepiness

When the presenting complaint is of difficulty maintaining desired wakefulness or of an excessive amount of sleep, the patient should be evaluated carefully. First, it must be ascertained whether the patient is complaining of fatigue or of sleepiness. Physical fatigue with decreased mental alertness, without an increase in sleep behavior, should not be categorized as excessive sleepiness; nor should the normal daily sleepiness occurring during a monotonous activity or following a sleepless night be considered excessive sleepiness. Persons with excessive sleepiness easily fall asleep whenever left alone, and episodes of sleepiness occur daily and often in inappropriate circumstances (e.g., while driving, conversing, waiting for a stoplight to change from red to green). However, patients may not be aware of their excessive sleepiness or may deny that they are abnormally sleepy. It is often helpful to question the patient's spouse or partner about episodes of daytime sleepiness. If assessment reveals that the person is not fatigued and may be excessively sleepy, he or she should be referred to an accredited sleep disorders center for further evaluation, including a nocturnal polysomnogram and an MSLT, which is an objective measure of daytime sleepiness. Referral to an appropriate specialist is a critical nursing intervention, because disorders of excessive sleepiness often profoundly affect the patient's quality of life and can increase morbidity and mortality (obstructive sleep apnea).

Obstructive sleep apnea syndrome is characterized by repetitive episodes of upper airway obstruction that occur during sleep and is usually associated with a reduction in blood oxygen saturation (Diagnostic Classification Steering Committee, 1990). Apnea is defined as the cessation of breathing for more than 10 seconds' duration; shorter respiratory pauses are not counted. Single apneas may last from 10 to 120 seconds (typically 20 to 40 seconds) and end with partial arousal. Although normal adults may have up to five apneic events per hour of sleep, five or more apneic episodes per hour are considered abnormal, particularly if these apneic events are associated with arterial oxygen desaturations, bradytachycardia, and frequent arousals. Mean sleep latencies on the MSLT are often less than 10 minutes (normal sleep latency is 10 to 20 minutes) (Diagnostic Classification Steering Committee, 1990).

Sleep is associated with the relaxation of upper airway muscles, and the airway can become smaller, become partially obstructed (hypopnias are characterized by more than a 50% reduction in airflow), or completely collapse (obstructed). Inspiratory efforts usually continue throughout the apneic episode. Hypoxemia, sometimes with an oxygen saturation of less than 50% (measured by pulse oximetry) during apneic episodes is typical. Once breathing resumes, however, oxygen saturation usually returns to normal. Cardiac arrhythmias are not uncommon and range from sinus arrhythmia to premature ventricular contractions, atrioventricular block, and sinus arrest (Diagnostic Classification Steering Committee, 1990). Bradytachycardia is often associated with apneic episodes: bradycardia occurs during the apneic pause and alternates with tachycardia, which occurs on the resumption of ventilation. Left untreated, obstructive sleep apnea can cause profound functional impairments and life-threatening complications (Diagnostic Classification Steering Committee, 1990; National Commission on Sleep Disorders Research, 1992. Daytime sleepiness may result in job loss, accidents, self-injury, marital and family problems, and poor school performance (Diagnostic Classification Steering Committee, 1990). Impaired memory, secondary depression, personality changes, and loss of both libido and erectile ability may also occur. Hypertension, coronary heart disease, myocardial infarction, and stroke are more common in patients with obstructive sleep apnea. In fact, more than 50% of patients with obstructive sleep apnea also have sustained elevations of blood pressure (National Commission on Sleep Disorders Research, 1992).

Current estimates suggest that more than 18 million adults in the United States have obstructive sleep apnea; this disorder is more common in adulthood than is asthma (National Commission on Sleep Disorders Research, 1992). Persons more at risk of developing obstructive sleep apnea include children with enlarged tonsils and adenoids, middle-aged or older adults, and adults who have cranial-facial abnormalities, who are obese, or who have an endocrine disorder such as hypothyroidism or acromegaly. Sleep apnea in adults is seen predominantly among males and postmenopausal females; the male-to-female ratio for occurrence of sleep apnea is about 15:1 (Ingbar & Gee, 1985). In children, however, this difference does not occur; about equal numbers of boys and girls are affected (National Commission on Sleep Disorders Research, 1992).

Obstructive sleep apnea is a medical diagnosis based on data obtained from a patient's history, a nocturnal polysomnographic evaluation that includes assessment of the patient's sleep, breathing, oxygen saturation, and cardiac status and often an MSLT. This test involves five or six 20-minute–nap trials at specified times during the day. With polysomnographic monitoring, sleep latencies are calculated and the record examined for the appearance of sleep-onset REM periods (SOREMPs). Although sophisticated diagnostic testing is required, knowledgeable laypersons or nurses are often the first to suspect the presence of obstructive sleep apnea. Loud snoring, sometimes loud enough to be heard several rooms away, is quite common. These loud snores often alternate with episodes of silence that usually last 20 to 30 seconds. Gasping, moaning, and snorting sounds may occur when breathing resumes. Nocturnal sleep is often restless and unrefreshing, and some patients—particularly the elderly—are quite disturbed by their fragmented nocturnal sleep and may present with a complaint of insomnia rather than of excessive sleepiness.

The severity of daytime sleepiness may vary and does not seem to be related to the severity of the obstructive sleep apnea (Diagnostic Classification Steering Committee, 1990). Young children may not be excessively sleepy during the day, but developmental delays, learning difficulties, decreased school performance, and behavioral disorders with hyperactivity are common (Guilleminault, 1987). Any patient, particularly if obese or with cranial-facial abnormalities (e.g., micrognathia, retrognathia), with symptoms of loud snoring and excessive daytime sleepiness should be referred immediately to a sleep disorders center for further evaluation. Until a diagnosis is obtained and the disorder is effectively treated, the patient should be advised to limit driving and cautioned not to drive at all if drowsy.

After diagnosis, the treatment plan may include both medical and behavioral approaches. Treatment approaches for patients with mild obstructive sleep apnea may include any or all of the following: avoiding sleep in the supine position, reducing weight if obese, taking low doses of protriptyline at bedtime, avoiding all potentially sedating drugs (including alcohol), and avoiding sleep fragmentation and deprivation. For patients with moderate to severe obstructive sleep apnea, additional treatment approaches are required. Any existing oropharyngeal or mandibular abnormalities may be surgically repaired, and continuous positive airway pressure (nasal CPAP) may be prescribed. Tracheotomy, once the standard treatment for obstructive sleep apnea, is now used only in extremely severe cases.

Nursing interventions after diagnosis are educational and supportive. Patients may need to review and clarify information that they have been given about obstructive sleep apnea and its treatment. Assessing compliance with treatment regimes, particularly weight loss and use of nasal CPAP, is particularly important. Although nasal CPAP therapy is quite effective, compliance rates are somewhat low because of patient discomfort and inconvenience (Krieger, 1992). Sometimes switching to a different type of mask, using nasal pillows instead of a mask, adding a humidifier to the unit, or taking a decongestant at bedtime will improve compliance with nasal CPAP therapy. Patients and their spouses or partners may also benefit from participating in a patient support group (American Sleep Apnea Association, 2700 E Main Street, Suite 206, Columbus, Ohio 43209). Excessive sleepiness is usually significantly reduced by effective treatment; however, if excessive sleepiness continues to be a problem or reappears after several years of effective treatment, further evaluation is needed.

Narcolepsy is a disorder of unknown etiology that is characterized by excessive sleepiness associated with abnormal manifestations of REM sleep. Although it was once thought to be a rare disease, epidemiologic studies suggest that its prevalence is comparable to that of multiple sclerosis or Parkinson's disease (National Commission on Sleep Disorders Research, 1992). The main symptoms of narcolepsy are sleep attacks, cataplexy, sleep paralysis, hypnagogic hallucinations, and disturbed nocturnal sleep. All patients experience sleep attacks, and many have one or more auxiliary symptoms (e.g., cataplexy, sleep paralysis, hypnagogic hallucinations, disturbed nocturnal sleep). In addition to sleep attacks, persons with narcolepsy suffer from high levels of sleepiness throughout the entire day. Some episodes of excessive sleepiness may be combined with automatic behavior and amnesia (Montgomery et al., 1982).

Cataplexy is the brief (seconds or minutes), sudden loss or weakness of skeletal muscle tone without the loss of consciousness. Severity of this symptom can range from a mild sensation of muscle weakness in the neck to a complete postural collapse, with a fall to the ground. Cataplexy is believed to be caused by the intrusion of the muscle atonia associated with REM sleep into waking (Guilleminault, 1976). Frequency may vary; some patients may have only one or two episodes during a lifetime, whereas others may have many episodes of cataplexy each day. Episodes of cataplexy are always precipitated by a sudden emotional stimulus, such as laughter, anger, or surprise. Patients are often reluctant to report these attacks for fear they will be labeled as having psychiatric problems. Although these episodes can be dangerous or embarrassing, many patients consider cataplexy to be less troublesome than excessive daytime sleepiness (Rogers, 1984).

Sleep paralysis occurs in some narcoleptics during the transition between sleep and wakefulness. When falling asleep or waking up, the individual experiences a temporary paralysis of all striated muscles. The person is unable to move any muscles other than the muscles of respiration. The episode usually lasts a few minutes and may be accompanied by intense fear or hypnagogic hallucinations. Sleep paralysis ends spontaneously or terminates immediately when the individual is touched or spoken to by another person. Like cataplexy, the frequency of these episodes is highly individual; sleep paralysis may occur daily, weekly, or once or twice in a lifetime. Nonnarcoleptics may have occasional episodes of sleep paralysis when awakening. Sleep paralysis is attributed to a disturbance in the production and maintenance of wakefulness and in the mechanisms producing the muscle atonia of REM sleep.

Hypnagogic hallucinations are vivid, lifelike sensory experiences that appear as a person is falling asleep but still conscious. The visual, auditory, or tactile hallucinations occur for approximately 1 to 15 minutes. Hypnagogic hallucinations are thought to arise from a SOREMP.

Persons with narcolepsy may also complain of disturbed nocturnal sleep. Nocturnal sleep is often fragmented and shortened. Although fragmented nocturnal sleep is a common symptom of narcolepsy, it is not the cause of excessive daytime sleepiness. Daytime sleepiness is the first symptom of narcolepsy and often develops several years before any difficulties with nighttime sleep are noticed. Moreover, studies have demonstrated that improving the nocturnal sleep of these patients does not lead to any improvements in daytime sleepiness (Thorpy, Snyder, Aloe, Ledereich, & Starz, 1992). One study suggests, however, that daytime sleepiness may contribute to nocturnal sleep disruptions. Patients whose daytime sleepiness was eliminated by stimulant medications had nocturnal sleep patterns that were indistinguishable from those of normal sleepers, whereas subjects whose sleepiness was not controlled by stimulants had fragmented and shortened nocturnal sleep (Rogers, Aldrich, & Caruso, 1994).

A long-standing history of excessive daytime sleepiness (since the teens or early twenties) and the presence of auxiliary symptoms is suggestive of narcolepsy. A history of cataplexy is a characteristic and unique symptom of narcolepsy. In the United States, narcolepsy is differentiated from other disorders of excessive sleepiness by the appearance, on the MSLT, of at least two SOREMPs (Diagnostic Classification Steering Committee, 1990). Although sleep deprivation, withdrawal from a REM-suppressing drug, and endogenous depression can occasionally lead to the appearance of one SOREMP, it is extremely rare to record more than one SOREMP during an MSLT. A nocturnal polysomnogram is also required to rule out excessive sleepiness resulting from obstructive sleep apnea or PLMs. Human leukocyte antigen (HLA) typing of patients with narcolepsy almost always shows the presence of HLA-DR2 and -DQwl regardless of ethnic group (only a small number of African Americans are HLA-DR2 negative) (Diagnostic Classification Steering Committee, 1990). Because this histocompatibility antigen (DR2) is present in about 10% to 35% of the general population, the presence of HLA-DR2 is not diagnostic for narcolepsy. However, if the patient is not positive for HLA-DR2, it is very unlikely that the patient has or will develop narcolepsy. This finding can be quite helpful in distinguishing idiopathic hypersomnia (another disorder of excessive sleepiness) from narcolepsy and is also of use to parents who might be worried about the possibility that their child might develop narcolepsy. Although the exact mode of inheritance (in humans) remains unclear, first-degree relatives of persons with narcolepsy are eight times more likely to develop narcolepsy than are members of the general population (Diagnostic Classification Steering Committee, 1990).

Sleep attacks and daytime sleepiness are treated with stimulant medications such as pemoline (Cylert), methlyphenidate (Ritalin), and dextroamphetamine (Dexedrine). Despite many years' experience with these medications, information about their effectiveness in controlling daytime sleepiness and sleep attacks is limited. Recently, Mitler, Hajdukovic, and Erman (1993) demonstrated that high doses of methamphetamine (40 to 60 mg) can reduce daytime sleepiness and normalize sleep latencies on the MSLT. When Rogers et al. (1994) used 24-hour ambulatory polysomnographic recordings to examine the sleep-wake patterns of treated narcoleptic subjects, they found that stimulant medications eliminated daytime sleep in slightly less than half of the subjects (45.8%). Despite treatment with stimulants, the other narcoleptic subjects remained sleepy, sleeping, on average, 81 minutes during the day (range: 30.0 to 263.0 minutes).

Although some physicians recommend regular drug holidays (e.g., during the weekend), there is no evidence that drug holidays reduce the amount of stimulant needed or are beneficial to the patient (Mitler, Aldrich, Koob, & Zarcone, 1993). Three to six short (15-minute) daytime naps are often prescribed in addition to stimulant medications. However, there is only limited evidence of their efficacy, and further testing is needed (Rogers & Aldrich, 1993). Cataplexy may or may not be treated, depending on the severity of this symptom. If treatment is needed, small doses of tricyclic or serotonergic antidepressants such as protriptyline, imipramine, or fluoxetine (Prozac) usually completely eliminate this symptom.

Narcolepsy is a lifelong disorder that significantly affects an individual's quality of life. Although medical management may provide drug therapy, nursing intervention is also needed to provide accurate information and practical coping strategies for adaptation to the illness. Problems and coping strategies identified by narcoleptics cluster into six areas: driving, education, work, family, social life, and medical care (Rogers, 1984). Driving, household, and smoking accidents and near accidents are significantly higher among narcoleptics (Broughton et al., 1981). Sleep attacks and a drowsy appearance often affect occupational, academic, and social performance. Family and friends may show a lack of understanding or negative reactions to daytime sleepiness, sleep attacks, or cataplexy. Narcoleptics report that their symptoms limit their choice of educational major and occupation, leisure-time activities, social events, close friends, and scheduling of daily activities. Other problems are fear of addiction, medication compliance, social isolation, scheduling of naps, pregnancy, and denial of the illness. Narcoleptic patients benefit from accurate information about their disease and its treatment, assistance in identifying periods of peak alertness or intense drowsiness, assistance in identifying factors that precipitate or aggrevate symptoms, emotional support, and practical strategies for minimizing the effects of the disease on their quality of life (Rogers, 1984).

Nurses should also assess patient compliance with the prescribed medical regimen. Attention should also be paid to monitoring the efficacy of the prescribed treatment; many patients may report that they are able to remain alert, yet polysomnographic studies will indicate that they are very sleepy. Again, important data can be obtained from family members or friends. Sometimes, numerous adjustments in the type and dosage of medications may be needed to significantly reduce or eliminate the symptoms of narcolepsy. Patients should also be referred to an accredited sleep disorder center if their symptoms seem to be getting worse. As patients with narcolepsy get older or gain weight, it is not uncommon for them to develop mild or moderate sleep apnea or PLMs, (Diagnostic Classification Steering Committee, 1990) two other sleep disorders that can further exacerbate their daytime sleepiness.

• C A S E   S T U D Y   2

Ms. C was a 31-year-old sales representative for an industrial supplies company referred to a medical center neurology clinic for evaluation and management of narcolepsy. She had recently moved to the city and experienced difficulty obtaining prescriptions for the stimulants used to treat narcolepsy. She reported the onset of excessive sleepiness at about age 20 years. Inappropriate sleep began occurring during driving, college examinations, and sexual activity. The problem had caused her to switch her career choice from accounting to marketing. She also felt that misunderstandings over her symptoms were the major cause of a divorce. Her strategies for coping with excessive daytime sleepiness and sleep attacks included informing her employer about the illness, scheduling two naps each day of about 20 minutes in duration, scheduling sales calls for after naps, and choosing a nonsedentary, flexible, independent job with productivity measured by output rather than by hours spent in the office. She limited driving to short distances, took extra medication beforehand, rolled the car windows down, and drank cold water to fend off any drowsiness. She stopped driving whenever she became sleepy; walking around or a short nap was used to increase alertness.

At about age 28 years, Ms. C noticed that during laughter or intense emotions, her knees and neck muscles became weak. Her knees would buckle slightly, and her head and jaw dropped downward for 2 to 5 seconds. The examiner observed several of these episodes while taking the history. Ms. C found these cataplectic attacks socially embarrassing and increasingly bothersome at work. She never went to parties ("I can't relax, and I absolutely can't drink alcohol") and had a very limited social life. Thinking about a joke or enjoying a beautiful piece of music would also trigger attacks. She reported viewing "life in a peculiar distanced way" in order to prevent precipitating attacks. On further questioning, she revealed that driving was sometimes accompanied by automatic behaviors (e.g., driving to an unknown place and not remembering how she got there). Near accidents had caused her to rely more on public transportation; her new job required less independent travel. Symptoms of sleep paralysis and hypnagogic hallucinations were not reported.

Other than the observed sudden, brief muscle atonia, Ms. C's physical and neurologic examinations were essentially negative. Tests performed by her previous physician had revealed a mean sleep-onset latency of 2.5 minutes and more than two SOREMPs during an MSLT. After the evaluation, Ms. C's physician renewed prescriptions of methylphenidate, 20 mg twice a day, and imipramine, 25 mg three times a day. Nursing diagnoses were potential for injury related to daytime sleepiness and cataplexy and social isolation related to embarrassment about cataplexy. Regular return to clinic appointments was emphasized and scheduled. Nursing interventions included discussion of driving, safety, social activities, and emotional support, with continued follow-up planning. The clinician and Ms. C maintained telephone contact between clinic visits; numerous adjustments in prescription dosages were made. Over time, Ms. C continued to show resourcefulness in managing the disease-related problems and in developing coping strategies. At present, she is an active member of a peer support group.

ASSESSMENT OF ALTERED SLEEP-WAKE PATTERNS AND NURSING INTERVENTIONS

When a patient complains about his or her sleep or inability to remain awake during the day, the nurse should first find out more about the problem, the person's habits, the family history, and the social history and should obtain information about that person's health (Table 9–3). When assessing a sleep complaint, it is important to remember that no one is accurate in describing his or her own sleep. A patient may present with an initial complaint of difficulties falling asleep but on further questioning reveal that he or she cannot stay awake at work during the day and is a loud snorer. If possible, information should be obtained from both the patient and the bed partner or some other person living with the patient. The assessment should also be guided by the nurse's knowledge of the types of sleep disruptions frequently associated with certain developmental stages, including middle age and aging, and with gender, body build, and presenting complaints.

Depending on the results of the health history, the nurse may decide that more information is needed. Further information may be obtained from a physical assessment or through more objective measurements of sleep. Sleep diaries, such as one described in nursing research (Rogers, Caruso, & Aldrich, 1993), and various questionnaires can be used to obtain data about the patient's usual sleep patterns.

Interventions need to be guided by data obtained when assessing the patient and need not be confined to what is traditionally considered nursing. Referral to a sleep disorder specialist who may be a physician, psychologist,

TABLE 9–3 • ASSESSMENT OF SLEEP-WAKE PATTERNS

1. Presenting complaint
   A. What does the patient think is wrong with his or her sleep?
   B. Why is the patient concerned about this problem?
2. History of current problem (input from bed partner should be obtained whenever possible)
   A. Nature and duration of problem
   B. Severity of sleep problem
      1. Frequency of occurrence
      2. Interference with usual activities
      3. What has the patient done to remedy the problem?
   C. Habits
      1. Usual sleep times; because recall may be inaccurate, ask about specific days (e.g., yesterday, over the weekend)
      2. Use of caffeine, tobacco, alcohol, and recreational drugs; have patient estimate amount used each day and describe time of day when used
   D. Changes in weight and collar size in males; very important if patient is obese or snores loudly
   E. Family history of sleep problems
      1. Insomnia
      2. Obstructive sleep aprea
      3. Narcolepsy
3. Medical history
   A. Review of systems, including psychiatric history
   B. Family history
4. Current and past use of medications
   A. Both prescription and nonprescription drugs
   B. Medications especially for the treatment of sleep problems
5. Social history
   A. Demographic data, including educational level and occupation
   B. Living arrangements (e.g., with spouse or roommates, in a dormitory)
   C. Any unusual stressors or the presence of infants or other family members requiring care during the night

or doctorally prepared nurse may be the most appropriate nursing intervention. If a disorder of excessive sleepiness is suspected, the patient should always be referred to an accredited sleep disorder center. Referral to an accredited sleep disorder center is also needed if sleep disruption has been present longer than 3 to 6 months. An updated list of accredited sleep disorder centers in any area of the United States can be obtained by contacting the Association of Professional Sleep Societies (604 Second Street SW, Rochester, Minnesota 55902). If the nurse suspects that the patient's sleep problem may be caused by a medical or psychiatric disease, then the patient should be referred to an appropriate specialist for management of the underlying problem.

If referral to a specialist is not needed, nurses can be instrumental in providing information about changes in sleep associated with maturation (e.g., infancy and childhood, pregnancy and menopause, normal aging) or in teaching the patient about particular sleep disorders. Nurses can also suggest improvements in sleep hygiene and institute stimulus control, sleep restriction therapies, and relaxation therapies. Finally, nurses can provide support and practical assistance to the patient with a sleep disorder. Examples of this type of intervention include encouraging the patient to try several different types of CPAP masks rather than immediately discontinuing CPAP if the mask is irritating; explaining to family members that stimulants are not a crutch for patients with narcolepsy and that they cannot control their daytime sleepiness with will power or by getting more sleep at night; and helping the patient with narcolepsy obtain new prescriptions for stimulant medications in a timely fashion (schedule II drugs such as amphetamines and methlyphenidate cannot be refilled, cannot be dispensed in quantities of more than 100 tablets, and may require that the prescription be written on a special form).

SUMMARY

Although researchers are gaining knowledge about sleep and waking behaviors, no one really knows why we sleep or exactly which neurotransmitters and structures control sleep and waking states. We do know, however, that certain rhythmic functions are linked to sleep and that sleep is exquisitely sensitive to maturational changes, environmental influences, psychologic stressors, and illness. Appropriate nursing assessment and interventions can assist patients to awaken refreshed in the morning and remain alert throughout the day.

References

Adam, K., & Oswald, I. (1979). One gram of L-tryptophan fails to alter the time taken to fall asleep. *Neuropharmacology, 18*(12), 1025–1027.

Agnew, H. W., Webb, W. B., & Williams, R. L. (1967). Comparison of stage 4 and REM sleep deprivation. *Perceptual and Motor Skills, 24*(3), 851–858.

Ahnve, S., Theorell, T., Akerstedt, T., Frogberg, J., & Halberg, F. (1981). Circadian variations in cardiovascular parameters during sleep deprivation. *European Journal of Applied Physiology, 46*(1), 9–19.

Akerstedt, T., & Torsvall, L. (1985). Napping in shift work. *Sleep, 8*(2), 105–109.

Anders, R. F., Emde, E., & Parmlee, A. (1971). *A manual of standardized terminology, techniques and criteria for scoring states of sleep and wakefulness in newborn infants.* Los Angeles: UCLA Brain Information Service.

Antonioli, M., Solano, L., Torre, A., Volanti, C., Costa, M., & Bertini, M. (1981). Independence of REM density from other REM sleep parameters before and after REM deprivation. *Sleep, 4*(2), 221–225.

Baddeley, A. D., Hatter, I., Scott, D., & Snashall, A. (1970). Memory and time of day. *British Journal of Psychology, 22*, 605–609.

Bates, R. C. (1972). Delirium tremens and sleep deprivation. *Michigan Medicine, 71*(32), 941–944.

Blake, M. J. F. (1967). Time of day effects on performance in a range of tasks. *Psychosomatic Science, 9*, 349–350.

Bliwise, D. L. (1989). Normal aging. In M. H. Kryger, T. Roth, & W. C. Dement (Eds.), *Principles and practice of sleep medicine* (pp. 24–29). Philadelphia: W.B. Saunders.

Bootzin, R. R., & Nicassio, P. N. (1978). Behavioral treatments for insomnia. In M. Hersen, R. Eisler, & P. Miller (Eds.), *Behavioral treatments for insomnia: Progress in behavior modification* (p. 6). Academic Press.

Bootzin, R. R., & Perlis, M. I. (1992). Nonpharmacological treatment of insomnia. *Journal of Clinical Psychiatry, 53* (Suppl.), 37–41.

Bremmer, F. (1977). Cerebral hypnogenic centas. *Annals of Neurology, 2*(1), 1–6.

Broughton, R. J. (1989). Chronobiological aspects and models of sleep and napping. In D. F. Dinges & R. J. Broughton (Eds.), *Sleep and alertness: Chronobiological, behavioral, and medical aspects of napping* (pp. 71–98). Lancaster, CA: Raven Press.

Broughton, R., Ghanem, O., Hishikawa, Y., Sugita, Y., Nevsimalova, S., & Roth, B. (1981). Life effects of narcolepsy in 180 patients from North America, Asia, and Europe compared to matched controls. *Canadian Journal of Neurological Sciences, 8,* 199–204.

Carskadon, M. A., & Dement, W. C. (1987). Sleepiness in the normal adolescent. In C. Guilleminault (Ed.), *Sleep and its disorders in children* (pp. 53–66). Lancaster, CA: Raven Press.

Coble, P. A., Kupfer, D. J., Reynolds, C. F. III, & Houck, P. (1987). EEG sleep of healthy children 6 to 12 years of age. In C. Guilleminault (Ed.), *Sleep and its disorders in children* (pp. 29–41). Lancaster, CA: Raven Press.

Czeisler, C. A., Weitzman, E. D., Moore-Ede, M. C., Zimmerman, J. C., & Knauer, R. S. (1980). Human sleep: Its duration and organization depend on its circadian phase. *Science, 210*(4475), 1264–1267.

Czeisler, C. A., Zimmerman, J. C., Ronda, J., Moore-Ede, M. C., & Weitzman, E. D. (1980). REM sleep is coupled to the circadian rhythm of body temperature in man. *Sleep, 2*(3), 329–346.

Diagnostic Classification Steering Committee. (1990). *International classification of sleep disorders: diagnostic and coding manual.* Rochester, MN: American Sleep Disorders Association.

Dinges, D. (1989). Napping patterns and effects in human adults. In D. Dinges & R. Broughton (Eds.), *Sleep and alertness: Chronobiological, behavioral and medical aspects of napping.* (pp. 171–204). Lancaster, CA: Raven Press.

Drucker-Colin, R., & Espejel, R. M. (1980). Chronic administration of chloramphenicol, a protein synthesis inhibitor, selectively decreases REM sleep. *Behavioral and Neural Biology, 29*(3), 410–413.

Evans, B. A., & Rogers, A. K. (1994). 24 hour sleep/wake patterns in healthy, elderly persons. *Journal of Applied Nursing Research, 7,* 75–83.

Evans, L. K. (1987). Sundown syndrome in institutionalized elderly. *Journal of the American Geriatrics Society, 35,* 101–108.

Feinberg, I., Koresko, R. L., & Heller, N. (1967). EEG sleep patterns as a function of normal and pathological aging. *Journal of Psychiatric Research, 5*(2), 107–144.

Francesconi, R. P., Stokes, J. W., Banderet, L. E., & Kowal, D. M. (1978). Sustained operations and sleep deprivation: Effects on indices of stress. *Aviation, Space, and Environmental Medicine, 49*(1), 1271–1274.

Friedman, L., Bliwise, D. L., Yesavage, J. A., & Salom, S. R. (1991). A preliminary study comparing sleep restriction and relaxation treatment for insomnia in older adults. *Journal of Gerontology, 46*(1), 1–8.

Guilleminault, C. (1976). Cataplexy. In C. Guilleminault, W. C. Dement, & P. Passouant (Eds.), *Narcolepsy: Advances in sleep research* (vol. 3, pp. 125–144). Corte Madera, CA: Spectrum Publishing.

Guilleminault, C. (1987). Obstructive sleep apnea syndrome in children. In *Sleep and its disorders in children* (pp. 213–224). Lancaster, CA: Raven Press.

Haslam, D. R. (1984). Military performance of soldiers in sustained operations. *Aviation, Space, and Environmental Medicine, 55*(3), 216–221.

Hauri, P. J., Hayes, B., Sateia, M., Hellekson, C., Percy, L., & Olmstead, E. (1982). Effectiveness of a sleep disorders center: A 9-month follow-up. *American Journal of Psychiatry, 139*(5), 663–666.

Horne, J. (1978). A review of the biological effects of sleep deprivation in man. *Biological Psychology, 7*(1), 55–102.

Horne, J. A., & Reid, A. J. (1985). Sleep EEG effects of exercise with and without additional body cooling. *Electroencephalography and Clinical Neurophysiology, 60*(1), 33–38.

Horne, J. A., & Wilkinson, S. (1985). Chronic sleep reduction: Daytime vigilance performance and EEG measures of sleepiness with particular reference to "practice effects." *Psychophysiology, 22*(1), 69–78.

Ingbar, D. H., & Gee, J. B. L. (1985). Pathophysiology and treatment of sleep apnea. *Annual Review of Medicine, 36,* 369–395.

Ingvar, D. H. (1979). Cerebral circulation and metabolism in sleep. In R. Priest, A. Pletscher, & J. Ward (Eds.), *Sleep research* (p. 13). Baltimore, MD: University Park Press.

Jones, B. (1979). Elimination of paradoxical sleep by lesions of the pontine gigantocellular segmental field in the cat. *Neuroscience Letters, 13*(3), 285–293.

Jouvet, M. (1969). Biogenic amines and the state of sleep. *Science, 163*(862), 39–41.

Kales, A., & Kales, J. D. (1984). *Evaluation and treatment of insomnia,* New York: Oxford University Press.

Kant, G. J., Genser, S. G., Thorne, D. R., Pfalser, J., & Mougey, E. H. (1984). Effects of 72 hour sleep deprivation on urinary cortisol and indices of metabolism. *Sleep, 7*(2), 142–146.

Karacan, I., Thornby, J. I., Anch, A. M., Williams, R. L., & Perkins, H. M. (1978). Effects of high ambient temperature on sleep in young men. *Aviation, Space, and Environmental Medicine, 49*(7), 855–860.

Karacan, I., Wolff, S. M., Williams, R. L., Hursch, C. J., & Webb, W. B. (1968). The effect of fever on sleep and dream patterns. *Psychosomatics, 9*(6), 331–339.

Kolka, M. A., Martin, B. J., & Elizondo, R. S. (1984). Exercise in a cold environment after sleep deprivation. *European Journal of Applied Physiology, 53*(3), 282–285.

Krieger, J. (1992). Long term compliance with nasal continuous positive airway pressure (CPAP) in obstructive sleep apnea patients and nonapneic snorers. *Sleep, 15,* S42–S46.

Lacks, L. (1987). *Behavioral treatment of persistent insomnia.* Tarrytown, NY: Pergamon Press.

Lazoff, B., Wolf, A., & Davis, N. S. (1985). Sleep problems seen in a pediatric practice. *Pediatrics, 75*(3), 477–483.

Mancia, G., & Zanchetti, A. (1980). Cardiovascular regulation during sleep. In J. Orem & C. D. Barnes (Eds.), *Physiology and sleep* (pp. 2–56). McLean, VA: Academic Press.

McCarley, R. W., & Hobson, J. A. (1975). Neuronal excitability modulation over the sleep cycle: A structural and mathematical model. *Science, 189*(4196), 58–60.

McClusky, H. Y., Milby, J. B., Switzer, P. K., William, V., & Wooten, I. (1991). Efficacy of behavior versus triazolam treatment in persistent sleep onset insomnia. *American Journal of Psychiatry, 148*(1), 121–126.

Metcalf, D. R. (1969). The effects of extrauterine experience on the ontogenesis of EEG sleep spindles. *Psychosomatic Medicine, 31*(5), 393–399.

Mitler, M. M., Aldrich, M. S., Koob, G. F., & Zarcone, V. P. (1993, June 22). The use of stimulants in the treatment of narcolepsy. In *Controversies in the Treatment of Narcolepsy* (pp. 1–27). Paper presented at the Seventh Association of Professional Sleep Societies Meeting, Los Angeles.

Mitler, M. M., Hajdukovic, R., & Erman, M. K. (1993). Treatment of narcolepsy with methamphetamine. *Sleep, 16*(4), 306–317.

Monnier, M. (1983). Sleep dream, and waking as an integral function. In M. Monnier & M. Meulders (Eds.), *Functions of the nervous system* (p. 7). New York: Elsevier.

Monnier, M., & Gaillard, J. (1980). Biochemical regulation of sleep. *Experientia, 36*(1), 21–24.

Monnier, M., Schoenenberger, G., Dudler, L., & Herkert, B. (1975). Production, isolation and further characteristics of the sleep peptide delta. In P. Levin & W. Koella (Eds.), *Sleep* (p. 41). New York: S. Karger.

Montgomery, I., Trinder, J., & Paxton, S. J. (1982). Energy expenditure and total sleep time: Effects of exercise. *Sleep, 5*(2), 159–168.

Morgane, P. J. (1981). Monamine theories of sleep: The role of serotonin—A review. *Psychopharmacology Bulletin, 17*(1), 13–17.

Munroe, R. H., Munroe, R. L., & Whitting, B. (1980). *Handbook of cross-cultural human development.* Columbus, GA: Garland Press.

Muzet, A., Libert, J. P., & Candas, V. (1984). Ambient temperature and human sleep. *Experientia, 40*(5), 425–429.

Naitoh, P., Pasnau, R., & Kollar, E. (1971). Psychophysiological changes after prolonged deprivation of sleep. *Biological Psychiatry, 3*(4), 309–320.

National Commission on Sleep Disorders Research. (1992). *Report of the National Commission on Sleep Disorders research* [DHHS Pub. No. 92-XXXX]. Washington, DC: U.S. Government Printing Office.

Nausieda, P., Weiner, W., Kaplin, L., Weber, S., & Klawans, H. (1982). Sleep disruption in the course of chronic levodopa therapy. An early feature of the levodopa-induced psychosis. *Clinical Neuropharmacology, 5*(2), 183–194.

Nicholson, A. N., Pascoe, P. A., Roehrs, T., Roth, T., Spencer, M. B., Stone, B. M., & Zorick, F. (1985). *Aviation, Space, and Environmental Medicine, 56*(2), 105–114.

Opstad, P. K., Ekanger, R., Nummestad, M., & Raabe, N. (1978). Performance, mood and clinical symptoms in men exposed to prolonged, severe physical work and sleep deprivation. *Aviation, Space, and Environmental Medicine, 49*(9), 1065–1073.

Orem, J., & Keeling, J. (1980). Appendix A: Compendium of physiology in sleep. In J. Orem & C. D. Barnes (Eds.), *Physiology in sleep* (pp. 315–355). McLean, VA: Academic Press.

Pappenheimer, J. R. (1979). "Nature's soft nurse." A sleep-promoting factor isolated from brain. *Johns Hopkins Medical Journal, 145*(2), 49–56.

Parker, D. C., Rossman, L. G., & Van der Laan, E. F. (1973). Relation of sleep-entrained human prolactin release to REM and non-REM cycles. *Journal of Clinical Endocrinology and Metabolism, 38*, 646–651.

Parkes, J. D. (1985). *Sleep and its disorders*. Philadelphia: W.B. Saunders.

Parmeggiani, P. L. (1980). Temperature regulation during sleep: A study in homeostasis. In J. Orem & C. D. Barnes (Eds.), *Physiology in sleep* (pp. 98–145). McLean, VA: Academic Press.

Piro, C., Fraioli, F., Sciarra, F., & Conti, C. (1973). Circadian rhythm of plasma testosterone, cortisol, and gonadotropins in normal male subjects. *Steroid Biochemistry, 4*(3), 321–329.

Pompeiano, O., & Valentinuzzi, M. (1976). A mathematical model for the mechanism of rapid eye movements induced by anticholinesterase in the decerebrate cat. *Archives Italiennes de Biologie, 114*(2), 103–154.

Prinz, P. (1977). Sleep patterns in the healthy elderly: Relationship with intellectual function. *Journal of Gerontology, 32*, 179–186.

Prinz, P. N., Vitaliano, P. P., Vitiello, M. V., Bokan, J., Raskind, M., Peskind, E., & Gerber, C. (1982). Sleep EEG and mental function changes in senile dementia of the Alzheimer's type. *Neurology of Aging, 3*(4), 361–370.

Rabey, J., Vardi, J., Glaubman, H., & Streifler, M. (1978). EEG sleep study in Parkinsonian patients under bromocryptine treatment. *European Neurology, 17*(6), 345–350.

Ramm, P. (1979). The locus coeruleus, catecholamines, and REM sleep: A critical review. *Behavioral and Neural Biology, 25*(4), 415–448.

Rechtschaffen, A., & Kales, A. (1990). *A manual of standardized terminology, techniques, and scoring system for sleep stages of human subjects*. Baltimore, MD: U.S. Department of Health, Education, and Welfare.

Reinberg, A., & Smolensky, M. H. (1983). *Biological rhythms and medicine*. New York: Springer-Verlag.

Richman, N. (1987). Surveys of sleep disorders in children in general population. In C. Guilleminault (Ed.), *Sleep and its disorders in children* (pp. 115–127). Lancaster, CA: Raven Press.

Riley, T. L. (1985). Normal sleep patterns. In T. L. Riley (Ed.), *Clinical aspects of sleep and sleep disturbance* (pp. 61–80). Stoneham, MA: Butterworth Publishers.

Rogers, A. K. (1984). Problems and coping strategies identified by narcoleptic subjects. *Journal of Neurosurgical Nursing, 16*(6), 326–334.

Rogers, A. K., & Aldrich, M. S. (1993). Do regularly scheduled naps reduce sleep attacks and excessive daytime sleepiness associated with narcolepsy? *Nursing Research, 42*(2), 111–117.

Rogers, A. K., Aldrich, M. S., & Caruso, C. C. (1994). Patterns of sleep and wakefulness in treated narcoleptic subjects. *Sleep, 17*, 590–597.

Rogers, A. K., Caruso, C. C., & Aldrich, M. S. (1993). Reliability of sleep diaries for assessment of sleep/wake patterns. *Nursing Research, 42*(6), 368–371.

Rose, R. M., Kreuz, L. E., Holaday, J. W., Sulak, K. J., & Johnson, C. E. (1972). Diurnal variation of plasma testosterone and cortisol. *Journal of Endocrinology, 54*(1), 177–178.

Ross, G., Maira, G., & Vignati, A. (1975). Intracranial pressure during sleep in man. In P. Levin & W. Koella (Eds.), *Sleep* (p. 169). New York: S. Karger.

Sakai, F., Meyer, J., Karacan, I., Derman, S., & Yamamoto, M. (1980). Normal human sleep: Regional cerebral hemodynamics. *Annals of Neurology, 7*(5), 471–478.

Sassin, J., Franz, A., Weitzman, E., & Kapen, S. (1972). Human prolactin: 24-hour patterns with increased release during sleep. *Science, 117*(55), 1205–1207.

Shaver, J. L., Giblin, E., & Paulsen, V. (1991). Sleep quality in midlife women. *Sleep, 14*(1), 18–23.

Small, J. G., Milstein, V., & Golay, S. (1979). L-Tryptophan and other agents for sleep. *Clinical Electroencephalography, 10*(2), 60–68.

Spielman, A. J., Saskin, P., & Thorpy, M. J. (1983). Sleep restriction treatment of insomnia. *Sleep Research, 12*, 286.

Sullivan, C. E. (1980). Breathing in sleep. In J. Orem & C. D. Barnes (Eds.), *Physiology in sleep* (pp. 214–272). McLean, VA: Academic Press.

Thoman, E. B. (1975). Early development of sleeping behaviors in infants. In N. R. Ellis (Ed.), *Aberrant development in infancy: Human and animal studies* (p. 122). New York: John Wiley & Sons.

Thorpy, M. J., Snyder, M., Aloe, F. S., Ledereich, P. S., & Starz, K. E. (1992). Short-term triazolam use improves nocturnal sleep of nacroleptics. *Sleep, 15*(3), 212–216.

Tune, G. S. (1968). Sleep and wakefulness in normal human adults. *British Medical Journal, 2*(600), 269–271.

Vallet, M., & Mouret, J. (1984). Sleep disturbance due to transportation noise: Ear plugs vs oral drugs. *Experientia, 40*(5), 429–437.

Van de Burg, W., & Van den Hoofdakker, R. H. (1975). Total sleep deprivation in endogenous depression. *Archives of General Psychiatry, 32*(6), 1121–1125.

Vogel, G. W. (1975). A review of REM sleep deprivation. *Archives of General Psychiatry, 32*(6), 749.

Webb, W. B., & Dinges, D. F. (1989). Cultural perspectives on napping and the siesta. In D. F. Dinges & R. J. Broughton (Eds.), *Sleep and alertness: Chronobiological, behavioral, and medical aspects of napping* (pp. 247–266). Lancaster, CA: Raven Press.

Williams, R. L., Karacan, I., & Hursch, C. J. (1974). *Electroencephalography of human sleep: Clinical applications.* New York: John Wiley & Sons.

COGNITION PHENOMENA

Cognition: An Overview

BARBARA J. BOSS

COGNITION: AN OVERVIEW

Cognition is a complex concept composed of a number of relevant phenomena including attention, memory, learning, concept formation, abstraction, thinking or thoughts, judgment, reasoning, executive functions, and insight. "Cognition refers to all the processes by which the sensory input is transformed, reduced, elaborated, stored, recovered, and used" (Neisser, 1967). Understanding of cognitive networks has dramatically increased over the past 10-15 years, predominantly because of position emission tomography (PET) and related technology.

No universally accepted definition or concept of attention exists. There are at least three predominant uses of the term in the literature. Attention may be defined as general alertness or arousal. Attention may also be defined as the selection of specific information from available, competing environmental and internal stimuli for further neural processing. This attention network is often referred to as selective attention. The third use of the term attention is to describe executive attentional networks that sustain concentration over time and allow for a delay in response until all pertinent information is known. These executive attentional networks include the vigilance network, the detection network, and the working memory network (Posner, 1994).

Memory is the process by which learned information is stored and retrieved, while learning is the process of acquiring knowledge about the world. Kupfermann and Kandel (1995) argued that the neural basis of learning and memory can be summarized in three principles that relate to the anatomic and physiologic correlates of memory: (1) memory has stages; (2) long-term memory may be represented in different places throughout the nervous system; and (3) implicit and explicit memories may involve different neuronal circuits.

Perception is the brain's construction of an external representation of external physical events (Kandel, 1995a). Perception is an active and creative process involving more than just the intake of sensory information (Kandel, 1995a). A person constructs a perceived world from sensory information.

Complex cognitive (mental, intellectual) operations—that is, operations of the brain requiring analysis and interpretation (including concept formation and abstraction)—are yet to be fully explained neurophysiologically. The cellular mechanisms have not yet been determined, but many facts are known. Even complex cognitive processes are correlated with patterns of firing of individual cells in specific brain regions (Kandel and Kupfermann, 1995). "Each assembly of cells acts as a more or less discrete module and contributes a critical component to the overall mental activity" (Posner and Raichle, 1994). The brain focuses attention on specific types of information. The different qualities of each set of information signals—that is, each sensory experience—are dissected away from the central signal and transmitted to the various areas of cell assembly that are specifically designed for analyzing the quality or qualities of the sensory experience. New information is compared to old information in the memory stores by the brain through determining patterns of stimulation. Previous experiences of the same or similar type are thus recognized and associated. But how the comparisons are made is not known (Guyton, 1992).

Thinking may be defined as the process of logic and reasoning assumed to exist inside the individual and accessible through a study of verbalized associations and actions, whereas a thought may be defined as the act or power of thinking, cogitation, or meditation (Gove, 1986). The neurophysiologic substrate of thought is proposed to most likely involve simultaneous activation (parallel nerve impulse transmissions) in the cerebral cortex, thalamus, limbic system, and reticular formation of the brain stem. "Thinking, such as analyzing the meaning of a word, activates the frontal cortex" (Kandel, 1995a). The activated limbic system, thalamus, and reticular formation areas are believed to determine the general nature of the thought, including its qualities such as pleasant or unpleasant and painful or comfortable, the crude modalities of sensation, the gross localizations to a body area, and other such characteristics. The activated cortical areas are believed to discriminate specific features of the thought such as specific body part, location of sensations, or exact location or objects in the visual field, distinct sensory patterns, and specific characteristics, all of which are reaching awareness at any one time (Guyton, 1992). It is recognized that some primitive thoughts may be mediated entirely by the lower brain centers. A person with destruction of large areas of the cerebral cortex is still able to have thoughts. The degree of awareness of surroundings is reduced after such an injury.

Reasoning is defined as the process of drawing conclusions or inferences from facts or premises, and judgment is defined as the act of deciding or passing decision on something. Insight has been defined as the understanding of oneself or self-understanding (Armstrong, Howe, Smith, Smith, & Snider, 1979; Gove, 1986).

Executive functions may be described as a system of programming, verifying, and correcting. These overseer functions may include motivation; goal formation or selection; planning; initiation, maintenance, and discontinuation of motor acts; self-monitoring; and incorporation of feedback. The executive attentional networks are fundamental to a person's ability to lead an independent and autonomous life.

RELATIONSHIP BETWEEN BRAIN ANATOMY AND COGNITION

There are two major theoretical views regarding cognition: the aggregate field view and the localization view. The aggregate field (holistic) view argues that all brain areas have equal potential in function and that for many cognitive functions, as well as other functions, any part of the brain could substitute for any other part. This viewpoint was dominant throughout the late 19th and first part of the 20th century, and its proponents included British neurologist Henry Head, German neuropsychologist Karl Goldstein, and American psychologist Karl Lashley of Harvard University. Lashley (1929) formulated the "mass action" theory of brain function, which proposed that brain mass is the relevant feature for cognitive function rather than individual neurons and specific neuronal connections. The aggregate field view is closely related to the theory of intelligence first proposed by Spearman that suggested that there is a general factor of intelligence (g factor) that contributes to all human performance (Adams & Victor, 1997). Proponents point to the positive correlation among all tests of cognitive ability as evidence to support this view (Kandel, 1991).

The localization view (cellular connectionism) proposes that the neuronal architecture with its individual neurons and specific neuronal connections is of primary importance to brain function, including cognition (Kandel, 1995a). The areas are not equipotential as to function. The great neuroscientists Broca, Wernicke, and Penfield have been proponents of this view. Again, this view is closely aligned with the psychologic theory of intelligence, which holds intelligence to be the sum total of a number of primary cognitive abilities such as memory, verbal skill, numerical ability, and visuospatial perception, that was first proposed by Thurstone. Proponents do not accept the existence of a general cognitive factor.

Neuropathologic studies have offered little support to the aggregate field theory and to the existence of a general factor of intelligence (Adams & Victor, 1997). These viewpoints, if true, would lead to the assumption that diffuse cortical brain injury would impair cognition (or g factor) proportionally to the brain mass involved. The pathologic studies of damaged brains across all age groups have never demonstrated a universal cognitive deficit associated with injury, nor has this general cognitive ability been demonstrated to decrease consistently with age (Adams & Victor, 1997; Kandel, 1991).

The neuropathologic studies do support the relationship between specific cognitive deficits and injury and dysfunction in particular parts of the cerebral hemispheres (Adams & Victor, 1997). PET and related technology are enabling neuroscientists to localize general reasoning and thinking during certain activities. The findings from clinical and laboratory studies are more consistent with the localization theory. The evidence weighs in favor of localization and even in favor of asymmetrical representation of function in the human cerebral cortex (Kandel, 1995a). Highly complex cognitive functions are associated with operation of specific brain areas (Kandel, 1995a), but most require the integrative actions of neurons in different regions of the brain (Kupfermann, 1995). Hebb first introduced this idea of integration as "cell assemblies," the "Hebbian synapse," and the hierarchical structure of cell assemblies now called networks (Hebb, 1949). Kononki furthered the notion of the complexity of central processes. Cognitive neuroscientists are studying networks of anatomic areas that become active during the performance of mental tasks (Posner & Raichle, 1994).

Left and Right Brain Distinction

Dramatic evidence for the support of asymmetry of hemispheric localization of function to one hemisphere has arisen since the early 1960s, from Geschwind and Levitsky (1968) and from the split-brain research initiated by Sperry, Gazzanga, and Byran. It has been clearly demonstrated that both hemispheres perform sensory analysis, have memory, and are able to learn, form thoughts, and make judgments (Kelly, 1991; Springer & Deutsch, 1989). Much of the analysis, memory, learning, and thoughts, however, appear to be different. The two hemispheres have different interpretative capacities. The right hemisphere is limited related to tasks requiring complex reasoning or analysis (Kelly, 1991; Posner & Raichle, 1994).

The left hemisphere demonstrates a superior ability for tasks requiring an orderly, logical, and systematic assessment of components such as language, mathematical calculations, complex abstraction, and reasoning. The left hemisphere functions in an analytic mode using sequential analysis. Memories are thought to be stored as the component parts and in language format (Kandel, 1991a; Springer & Deutsch, 1989).

The right hemisphere is superior at simultaneous processing such as required for spatial-visual tasks. It is vital for the analysis and interpretation of nonlanguage sounds such as music, of visual experiences, and of spatial relationships. The right hemisphere functions to process whole sensory experiences (input) simultaneously. This hemisphere functions on a holistic level. Memories are apparently stored in a holistic fashion as the auditory, visual, and spatial stimuli are experienced. In addition, the right hemisphere orchestrates holistic performance such as athletic or ballet performance (Kandel, 1991a; Springer & Deutsch, 1989).

Clearly, the right and left hemispheres mediate different types of cognition (intelligence). Thus, overall research findings support the idea that cognition is a gestalt of cognitive functions that have some degree of anatomic localization. Certain regions are more concerned with one cognitive ability than others, although these cognitive abilities are not mediated exclusively by only one area. Cognition, then, is the result of an integrated action of neurons located in different regions (Adams & Victor, 1997; Kupfermann, 1995). More elaborate cognitive capacities are constructed from serial and parallel interconnections of several brain regions (Kupfermann, 1995). Interrelated functions are processed by many neural pathways distributed in parallel (Kupfermann, 1995); thus, the term *network* is the appropriate label for these pathways (Posner & Raichle, 1994).

COGNITION: NORMAL DEVELOPMENT

Nervous system development is characterized by differentiation and cell multiplication during early prenatal life (Table 10–1). Establishment of a mature pattern of neuronal connections occurs in six major stages: (1) a uniform population of neural precursor cells is induced from ectodermal cells, (2) the precursor cells begin to diversify, (3) immature neurons migrate from germinal zones to their final position, (4) neurons extend axons, (5) axons form synapses, and (6) some initial synaptic connections are modified (Jessell, 1995).

During development, especially at times of rapid biomechanical differentiation, the nervous system is sensitive to environmental influences that play a significant role in advancing or hampering normal development. Nutrition, hormones, oxygen levels, and external stimulation have been identified as factors that affect normal development. Protein is necessary to maintain the rates of proliferation of developing neurons and glial cells from the second trimester through the first year of life. Undernourishment during fetal life and early postnatal life probably results in a decreased number of neurons and glial cells and retardation of dendritic growth and synaptic formation (Jacobson, 1991). The normal nervous system maturation sequence requires availability of vitamins, minerals, and calories during fetal development and in the first postnatal year. Exposure to androgens at a critical period is necessary to organize the neural components that mediate male sexual orientation and behavior. Androgens at this critical period effect a permanent change in certain brain tissues (Kelly, 1991). Thyroid hormone is essential during fetal life for increasing cell proliferation, microtubule assembly, axonal and dendritic outgrowth, synapse formation, and myelination (Jacobson, 1991). Glucocorticoids induce glial cell differentiation and enzymes for synthesizing neurotransmitters in cells of the neural crest. Continuous oxygen availability is essential for nervous system development.

Synaptic connections are stabilized by the appropriate environmental conditions in prenatal life. Reinforcement by environmental stimuli is required for complete development of each pathway (Boss, 1998; Jessell, 1995). Environmental agents may impair or prevent normal nervous system development. Such environmental factors include infectious agents (such as rubella and syphilis), excessive radiation, various chemical toxins, and trauma.

Magnetic resonance imaging (MRI) studies have documented that postnatal myelination in the nervous system takes place in three major stages (Hayakawa, Konishi, Kuriyama, Konishi, & Matsuda, 1991). Stage 1 takes place during the first 6 months of life. Stage 2 occurs from 6 months until possibly

TABLE 10–1 • MACROSCOPIC AND MICROSCOPIC DEVELOPMENTAL CHANGES

Time Period	Macroscopic Changes	Microscopic Changes
Approximately 18 days after conception		Ectoderm along what will be the back differentiates and thickens to form neural plate. Ectoderm in head region differentiates and thickens to form placodes (origin of special senses).
Approximately 25 days after conception		Lateral edges of neural plate rise and grow medially until they unite to form the neural tube (the primordial structure that gives rise to the CNS including all neurons and glial cells). Tube detaches from skin and slips beneath surface.
Before 1 month after conception	Cephalic end of neural tube differentiates and enlarges into three dilatations (primary brain vesicles—rhombencephalon [hind-brain], mesencephalon [midbrain], and prosencephalon [forebrain]).	Upper portion of the neural tube proliferates into four concentric zones. Ventricular zone, composed of ventricular cells (pseudostratified columnar epithelium), is for the most part the germinal zone where cell proliferation takes place. Subventricular zone, next to ventricular zone, derives certain classes of neurons and all the macroglia of the CNS. Intermediate (mantle) zone formed from migrating cells of the ventricular and subventricular zones, appears to evolve into gray matter of the CNS. Marginal zone, the outermost zone, has no primary cells of its own, is cell sparse, and eventually forms much of the white matter of the CNS.
Second fetal month	Differentiation into a five-vesicle brain—prosencephalon divides into telencephalon and diencephalon. Telencephalon surrounds diencephalon.	Neurons of the neocortex originate from the ventricular zone as postmitotic cell with an exception. Some cortical cells migrate to subventricular zone and proliferate again. Cortical cells from the ventricular and subventricular zones migrate through the intermediate zone to the cortical plate in an "inside-out" migration. Deeper layers of cortex are formed before more superficial layers are. The initial wave of cells migrates as far as possible between the marginal layer and the white matter. Succeeding waves migrate past these cells and come to lie in the middle third of the mature cortex. Later, cells migrate to the superficial layers of the cortex. Differentiation of cortical neurons progresses in the following sequence: efferent cells (pyramidal cells), primary afferent neurons (thalamic afferent fibers), intrinsic interneurons of the major

TABLE 10–1 • MACROSCOPIC AND MICROSCOPIC DEVELOPMENTAL CHANGES *Continued*

Time Period	Macroscopic Changes	Microscopic Changes
		neuronal pathways (stellate cells), lateral interactions by intrinsic interneurons (horizontal cells and pyramidal axon collaterals), secondary extrinsic afferent neurons (callosal and associational neurons). Glial cells develop after neurons.
Third fetal month	Lateral sulci appear.	Neuronal maturation takes place in four stages: (1) growth and elongation of axons, (2) elaboration of dendritic processes, (3) expression of appropriate biochemical properties, and (4) formation of synaptic connections.
Fifth fetal month	Central sulci, calcarine sulci, and parieto-occipital sulci appear.	
Seventh fetal month	All gyri amd major sulci are present.	
Eighth fetal month	Precentral and postcentral gyri are prominent. Lateral sulci are wide, and the insula is visible. Secondary sulci develop. Occipital lobes override the cerebellum.	Apical dendritic system of cortical pyramidal cells develops in the following progression: apical dendrites, basilar dendrites, axodendritic synapses, axosomatic synapses, axodendritic synapses on spines. Initial formation and orientation of dendrites appears to be determined by intrinsic factors (called developmental programmed maturation). Final shape and morphological specialization appear to be dependent on local interactions with afferent synaptic input (called environmentally arranged learning).
Term	Brain weight is 350 g. Frontal and temporal lobes are short. Insula covered by overlying structures. Few tertiary sulci exist. Subcortical white matter tracts are unmyelinated except for a few somatic afferent tracts (general somatic, auditory, and visual systems).	
First postnatal year	All areas of the neocortex develop synchronously.	Basilar dendritc system of the pyramidal cells develops.
1 year	Brain weighs 1000 g (extremely rapid growth rate).	
Second postnatal year	Slightly slower growth rate occurs. Synchronous neocortical development continues.	
2 years	Relative size and proportions to adult exist. Gray matter is demarcated from myelinated subcortical white matter. Adult myelination pattern exists. Tertiary sulci are predominant.	
Up to third year	Synchronous neocortical development continues. Female brain grows more rapidly, and myelination takes place at a faster rate.	

Table continued on following page

TABLE 10–1 • MACROSCOPIC AND MICROSCOPIC DEVELOPMENTAL CHANGES *Continued*

Time Period	Macroscopic Changes	Microscopic Changes
After third year	Synchronous neocortical development continues. Male brain grows more rapidly.	
6 years	Development of sensory and motor system is predominant.	
7½ years	Frontal executive area development accompanies sensory and motor cortex development.	
At puberty	Female brain weighs approximately 1250 g. Male brain weighs approximately 1375 g. Visuoauditory, visuospatial, and sensory systems peak in development.	
17 to 21 years	Frontal executive system development peaks.	

CNS, central nervous system.

as late as 18 months. Stage 3, where the "adult" myelination pattern is reached, begins after 1 year and is completed by age 2 years.

Electroencephalogram (EEG) analyses have led researchers to conclude that cognitive maturation produces immediate and abrupt changes that occur in five distinct, but uneven, stages of brain maturation postnatally (Hudspeth & Pribram, 1992). During stage 1, all areas of the neocortex—frontal, temporal, parietal, and occipital—that govern executive visuoauditory, somatic, and visuospatial functions appear to develop synchronously until about 6 years. Infants as young as 2 to 3 weeks have been found to carry out tasks that require cross-modal functioning, which is the ability to use two or more systems at once (e.g., imitating an adult by sticking out the tongue) (Kupfermann & Kandel, 1995).

The hippocampus develops quite early and progresses to full development more rapidly than do other areas of the neocortex. By birth, the hippocampus is 40% matured and is 50% matured by 1 month. Full maturity is reached by 15 months, and the child is fully able to transfer memory to permanent storage (Kupfermann, 1991).

Peak development occurs at 2½ years. During stage 2, the child perfects such skills as ability to form images, use words, and place things in serial order. The child also begins to develop tactics for solving problems.

Reinforcement by environmental stimuli postnatally is required for normal nervous system development. But current evidence supports a relatively strict constructionist view related to this requirement. The major connections within the nervous system are established primarily under genetic and developmental control. The initial establishment of connections occurs in the absence of learning. Learning is important for subsequent fine-tuning and maintenance and for regulating the strength of the connections, as in the case of memory.

Initially, stage 2 is marked by only sensory and motor system development involving the parietoccipital and central motor-sensory areas. At about 7½ years (the peak for development in this stage), the frontal executive areas evidence accelerated development. The child begins to perform simple operations such as determining of weights and logical-mathematical reasoning.

The third stage of postnatal brain development is characterized predominantly by further development of visuospatial functions (parietal-occipital areas) but also involves maturation in the visuoauditory regions (temporal lobes). This stage takes place between the ages of 10½ and 13 years, with the peak development at age 12 years. During this stage, the child is able to perform formal operations such as calculations and to perceive new meaning in familiar objects.

Stage 4, called the stage of dialectic ability, occurs between ages 13 and 17 years, with peak development at age 15 years, and involves the development of the visuoauditory, visuospatial, and somatic systems sequentially. The systems successively reach peak development within 1 year of each other. Young teenagers begin to review formal operations, find flaws in them, and create new formal operations. Jernigan, Trauner, Hessehink, and Tallar (1991) reported that "sculpting" (i.e., a decrease in gray matter in the superior anterior and posterior cortical regions) accompanies the hormonal shifts triggered by puberty and viewed this as evidence of the end of plasticity in the younger brain.

The fifth, and final, stage of cerebral maturation occurs between the ages of 17 and 21 years as the frontal executive functions mature to full capacity. Older adolescents begin to question information given to them, reconsider it, and form new hypotheses incorporating ideas of their own. Peak development takes place at 18½ years.

NEUROANATOMY AND NEUROPHYSIOLOGY OF COGNITIVE SYSTEMS

The study of the neural correlates of cognition is best undertaken by examining the neuroanatomy and neurophysiology of the cognitive networks. The cognitive networks include attentional networks, memory networks, and the executive attentional networks. This examination of neuroanatomy and neurophysiology of the cognitive systems will be done by first examining attention and memory networks, including the primary sensory, high-order sensory, and association areas of the cerebral cortex, which participate in the remote memory network and the selective attention network.

Attentional Networks

Attention is fundamental to cognition. The attentional networks provide each person with the ability to be awake and alert. These are anatomically complex networks located in multiple brain stem, diencephalon, and cortical areas mediating complex and highly integrated attention processes.

The arousal network mediates awakeness and sleep and is located throughout the ascending reticular nuclei of the upper brain stem from midpons to thalamic level. When activated, this network produces a person who is obviously awake, with open eyes and ability to respond to his or her internal and external environment. Arousal is further divided into *tonic* and *phasic* arousal.

Tonic arousal refers to "how awake the person is from one time of day to another" (Posner & Rafal, 1987) and therefore accounts for not only sleep-wake cycle differences in arousal but also other diurnal influences of arousal. Phasic arousal refers to "sudden increased attentiveness which immediately follows a warning signal [for] which the person will soon require a quick response" (Posner & Rafal, 1987). The person is "conscious."

The selective attention network provides the person with the ability to orient to selective sensory signals. Authorities believe the selective attention network mediates selective biasing of neural mechanisms to facilitate processing of specific sensory information for special treatment while other available signals are ignored (Posner & Rafal, 1987). The signal may be either exogenous (from the external environment) or endogenous (from within the person). This selective orienting of attention may be either overt or covert. The movement of the head, eyes, and body to the point of interest is overt orienting, whereas the mental shifting of attention to the source of interest is covert orienting. Selective attention has been found to have three components—the disengage component, the move component, and the enhance component—each mediated by different neuroanatomic regions (Posner, 1980; Posner & Rafal, 1987; Posner, Warren, Frederich, & Rafal, 1984; Tsal, 1983). The disengage component is mediated by the right posterior parietal lobe. The move component is controlled by brain stem centers (e.g., the superior colliculi) related to a visual signal. The enhance component is controlled by the pulvinar nuclei of the thalami. Selective attention is viewed as an automatic and unconscious function with simultaneous processing of the elements in a signal by different centers.

Memory Networks

Memory is central to cognition. Two memory networks have been demonstrated that mediate two different kinds of memory.

Implicit memory, also called procedural memory, reflexive memory, unconscious memory, nondeclarative memory, inactive representation, or habit, is memory that can be demonstrated but of which the person is not aware (Diamond, 1990; Kupfermann, 1991b). Change in the rate at which the material is learned provides the evidence that the first exposure is remembered. Implicit memory mediates nonassociative learning (e.g., habituation, sensitization, imitative learning) and associative learning (e.g., classical or operant conditioned behavioral responses) (Kupfermann & Kandel, 1995). Priming is believed to be related to implicit memory (Kupfermann & Kandel, 1995). Implicit memory can be impaired by injury to certain cerebellar nuclei and to the amygdala (Kupfermann & Kandel, 1995). The study of implicit memory in animal models has given scientists and clinicians an understanding of the cellular mechanisms of short-term and long-term memory.

Explicit memory, also called declarative memory, fact memory, conscious memory, or symbolic representation, is memory of which the person is aware (Diamond, 1990; Kupfermann & Kandel, 1995). Explicit memory is described as having two components—episodic memory and semantic memory. Episodic memory is the memory of the persons, objects, and events (episodes) in one's life—one's personal history (autobiographic knowledge) (Kupfermann & Kandel, 1995). Semantic memory is the memory of facts, principles, and information usually obtained in formal learning situations and from reading (factual knowledge) (Kupfermann & Kandel, 1995). The hippocampus, entorhinal cortex, subiculum, and parahippocampal cortices are involved in the process by which explicit memories are stored and retrieved from storage. The hippocampus and its adjacent areas are now thought to play the role of separating important information from nonessential information and coding this information as well as rehearsing the memory store to consolidate it into a long-term memory store (Fig. 10–1). In amnesia, there is a severe impairment of explicit memory, whereas implicit memory is intact. The explicit long-term memory storage areas are located in the somesthetic, visual, and auditory cortices.

SHORT-TERM MEMORY SYSTEM

Short-term memory (immediate memory, working memory, primary memory) is the memory of (1) behavior in the implicit memory network or (2) a few facts, words, numbers, letters, or other bits of information in the explicit memory

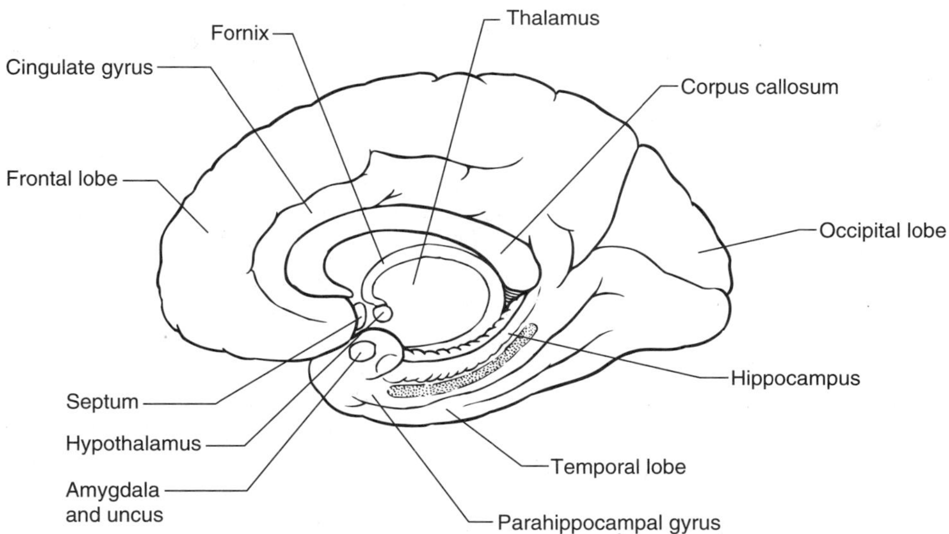

FIGURE 10–1 • The hippocampus and related temporal lobe structures are shaded.

network, for a few seconds to minutes or more at a time (Guyton, 1992). The stored information is referred to clinically as immediate recall. This memory has a very limited survival time. For example, the average individual cannot maintain more than five to nine digits in the short-term memory system. Immediate recall in the explicit memory network seems to be partly dependent on rehearsal of the information and is therefore very distraction labile. If another stimulus interrupts the rehearsal, the information is not held in the short-term memory system.

Short-term memory storage results from changes in neurons that are functional components of the neural pathways (Kandel, 1995b). Several neural mechanisms probably mediate short-term memory. Visual afterimages, called iconic memory, are thought to be due to photochemical processes in the retina (Kupfermann, 1991a). Thus, one very simple form of short-term memory appears to be encoded by a transient physical change in the peripheral receptors. Longer-lasting short-term memory also appears to be encoded by plastic changes in synaptic transmissions, such as posttentanic potentiation and pre-synpatic inhibition, or by ongoing neural transmissions that are maintained by excitatory feedback systems, called reverberating circuits (Guyton, 1992; Kupfermann, 1991a). Short-term habituation involves depression of synaptic transmissions (Kandel, 1995b). Sensitization involves enhancement of synaptic transmission by establishing connections with interneurons that enhance transmitter release in the invertebrate models that have been studied (Kandel, 1995b).

LONG-TERM MEMORY SYSTEM

For a memory to be retained, it must be transferred from short-term to long-term memory. Long-term memory (fixed memory, permanent memory, remote memory) is the storage within the brain of information that may then be recalled at some later time—minutes, hours, days, or years later (Guyton, 1992). The long-term memory system is subdivided into long-term secondary or intermediate memory, which is somewhat equivalent to recent memory and is sensitive to disruption, and truly long-term tertiary memory, which is very insensitive to disruption and which includes most of the remote memory system. Squires (1987) and colleagues have further quantified long-term memory into recent events (1 to 2 years old), old events (3 to 9 years old), and very old events (9 to 16 years old). Squires' (1987) work gives support to the idea that although long-term memory is relatively stable, over time there is gradual loss of the stored information or diminished capacity to retrieve the memory. Thus, memories undergo continuous change.

Neuroanatomically, all parts of the nervous system appear to have the type of plasticity (that is, potential for a persistent functional change) and the neuronal properties required for memory storage (Kupfermann, 1991a). Long-term memory is not mediated in a localized area. Several parallel channels of information are often used in memory storage (Kupfermann, 1991a). Even simple memories appear to consist of patterns of changes in specific connections that are distributed throughout the nervous system network (parallel processing).

Long-term memory is not dependent on continued activity of the brain as in the case of short-term memory. Long-term memory has been demonstrated via electron microscopy to be an anatomic (structural) change in the synapse or cell membrane leading to changes in the effectiveness of synaptic transmission (Kandel, 1995b). The changes probably enhance (facilitate) or suppress signal conduction in specific neuronal circuits. Nerve impulses thus pass through the neuronal circuits with increasing ease, referred to as a facilitated circuit. Long-term facilitation requires gene activation and protein synthesis (Kandel, 1995b).

In invertebrate animals studied using electron microscopy, the development of long-term memory traces involves increase in the vesicular release site in the presynaptic terminal. Likewise, during periods of inactivity, the release site decreases in size and may actually disappear. In addition, growth of the release site depends on activation of specific genetic control mechanisms for the required protein synthesis needed to construct the release structures (Guyton, 1992). Additionally, long-term memory development is associated with an increase in the number of release vesicles in the presynaptic terminal, as well as, in some cases, an increase in the number of presynaptic terminals (Guyton, 1992). The above structural changes probably represent the process of consolidation frequently referred to in the literature.

The brain is thought to rehearse new information so that the important aspects of the sensory experiences become more and more fixed in long-term memory stores. An essential feature of consolidation is codifying of the sensory experiences into different classes of information. Similar patterns are retrieved and recalled from the memory stores to help codify the new information. Information about similarities and differences of the and new information is stored, not the unprocessed information in the original sensory experience. Thus, memory stores are dynamic and changing over time.

Because long-term memory involves structural changes, it is not rehearsal dependent; a person may attend to other stimuli without loss of the previous memory store. Long-term memory is distraction stable. But recent memory stores may be disrupted by extreme stimuli such as head trauma, electroconvulsive shock therapy, extreme psychologic stress, and so on, causing what is labeled *retrograde amnesia.*

Neurophysiologically, long-term memory may be affected by a failure in (1) transferring information from short-term to long-term memory, (2) consolidating the long-term memory store, or (3) retrieving and recalling the memory or by a physical loss of the memory stores. Bilateral failure (destruction) of the hippocampus and associate temporal lobe structures results in a profound explicit recent memory deficit that is irreversible. There is a loss of ability to form new long-term memories, called anterograde amnesia. However, previously acquired long-term memories remain intact. Implicit memory and attention are also unaffected. The transition from short-term to long-term memory appears to be affected for certain types of learning. In Korsakoff's psychosis, the severe explicit recent memory deficit appears to be an inability to suppress interfering memories from previously learned materials. Thus, the primary defect may be in memory retrieval rather than in memory storage in at least some of the recent memory dementias or anterograde amnesias. Consolidation may be impaired by trauma or other stressors.

Physical loss of the memory stores may result from compression, injury, ischemia, surgical resection, or many of the dementing illnesses. Additionally, failure to be able to retrieve and recall memories may account for the retrograde amnesia.

Explicit Remote Memory Network

The explicit remote memory network cannot be adequately understood without also addressing the perceptual networks involved, so the primary sensory areas are discussed in addition to the higher-order and association areas. The primary and higher-order (secondary) sensory areas of the cortex identify, localize, and begin to analyze sensory stimuli (Table 10–2). The higher-order areas of the cerebral cortex perform more in-depth analysis, interpretation, and integration

TABLE 10–2 • LOCATION AND FUNCTION OF THE PRIMARY, HIGHER-ORDER, AND ASSOCIATION CORTICAL AREAS

Area	Function
Primary sensory areas	
Postcentral gyrus (1,2,3—parietal lobe)	Somatic sensory
Calcarine fissure (17—occipital lobe)	Vision
Heschl's gyrus (41, 42—temporal lobe)	Auditory
Higher-order sensory areas	
Dorsal bank of sylvian fissure (operculum portion of 2—parietal lobe)	Somatic sensory
Occipital gyri (18—occipital lobe)	Vision
Occipital gyri and superior temporal sulcus (19 and rostral to 19—occipital and temporal lobes)	Vision
Anterior and inferior temporal cortex (20, 21—temporal lobe)	Vision
Posterior parietal cortex (5 somatic, 7 visual—parietal lobe)	Somatic sensory Vision
Superior temporal gyrus (22—temporal lobe)	Auditory
Association cortex	
Junctions of parietal-temporal-occipital lobes (39, 40, portions of 19, 21, 22, and 37)	Polymodal sensory Language (left side) Prosody (right side)
Rostral portion of dorsal and lateral frontal lobes (area rostral to 6)	Attention over time Goal formation Planning
Cingulate and parahippocampal gyri, temporal pole, and orbital surface of frontal lobe (11, 23, 24, 28, and 38)	Motivation Emotion Recent memory

From Kandel, E.R., Schwartz, J.H., & Jessell, T.M. (1991). *Principles of neural science* (p. 824). New York: Elsevier Publishing.

of sensory data across sensory modalities (Fig. 10–2). By comparing new sensory information with stored memories that are of a similar nature, new sensory experiences are analyzed.

In the analysis process, the individual aspects of the sensory experience are separated and then each aspect is analyzed by comparing it with past sensory experiences. The exact mechanisms by which this is done are not well understood, but in analyzing sensory information, patterns of stimulation seem to be of primary importance. One of the predominant methods of analysis appears to be dissecting information into its component patterns. Sensory information is apparently processed to determine patterns, yet how such patterns of sensation are detected is not known.

The different areas of the cortex reacting to specific types of sensory information include the somesthetic cortical areas, the visual cortical areas, and the auditory cortical areas (see Figure 10–2).

Somesthetic Cortex. The parietal cortex plays a principal role in the processing of somatic sensory information. The primary somesthetic areas, located in the postcentral gyri, receive somatic sensory input from the ventroposterior thalamus areas (Fig. 10–3). These primary somesthetic areas are believed to analyze only the simple aspects of sensation. The somesthetic cortex has a map of the body for each submodality of sensation (Kandel & Kupfermann, 1995); they mediate the analysis of localization of sensations, appreciation of movement and position sense, and identification of cutaneous stimuli. This gives the individual the ability to appreciate weight, texture, and temperature and to form concepts from somesthetic experiences used later to learn new sensory discriminations.

The higher-order somesthetic areas of the parietal cortex, occupying the superior parietal lobes posterior to the postcentral gyri, receive input from the

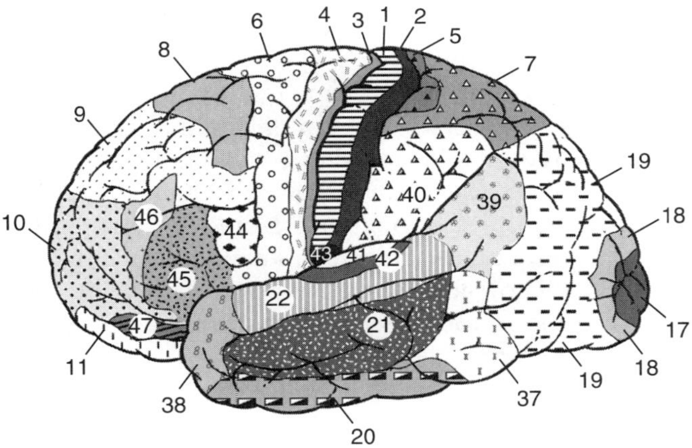

FIGURE 10–2 • This schematic drawing of the lateral surface of the human brain shows the regions of the primary sensory and motor cortices, the higher-order motor and sensory cortices, and the three association cortices.

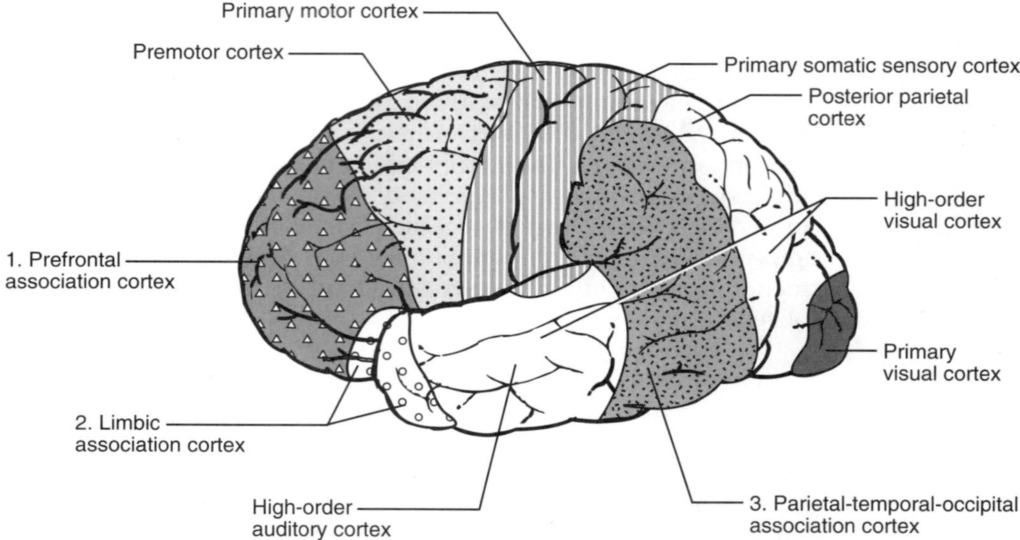

FIGURE 10–3 • Brodmann's division of the cerebral cortex. Each symbol represents a distinct area, numbered as shown.

primary and secondary somesthetic areas and the lateral thalami (see Figs. 10–2 and 10–3). These areas function to interpret somesthetic sensations and store memories of sensory experiences. The discriminative aspects of the primary somesthetic senses are integrated in the high-order somesthetic cortex. The submodality cells converge on common cells, allowing, for example, the recognition of three-dimensional objects (Kandel & Kupfermann, 1995). The somesthetic areas provide an individual with the ability to conceptualize qualities of objects such as shape, form, texture, size, and smoothness. Quantity estimates, such as weight, degree of pressure applied, and temperature change may also be made. Not only may this information be drawn from manual manipulation of an object, but such qualitative and quantitative information may be given by the person even in the absence of direct sensory stimuli. For example, if an individual is asked to give such sensory component information about a pen, a coin, or a leather armchair, that person is able to draw up the sensory images from the long-term stores. Dysfunction of the higher-order somesthetic areas reduces the person's ability to analyze and interpret different characteristics of somatic sensory experiences. Ability to recognize complex objects and forms by touch is impaired, and the person loses the sense of her or his own body form.

Visual Cortex. The primary visual areas, located on the medial portion of each occipital lobe, called the striate area, are the primary receptive areas for visual stimuli (see Figs. 10–2 and 10–3). Here, initial perception of the visual stimulus such as form, brightness, shading, and the like takes place. Color is thought to be partially analyzed by the primary visual cortices, although initial recognition of color is at the subcortical level. Unlike somesthetic sensation, there is no conscious perception of visual stimuli at a subcortical level. An individual is blind without an intact primary visual cortex (Guyton, 1992).

The higher-order visual areas—that is, the secondary visual areas—are located on the lateral surface of the occipital lobes and the medial and inferior temporal lobes; receive input from the striate area; mediate further processing of visual information, responding to more complex patterns than do the primary visual areas; and thus are involved in analysis of complicated visual patterns of stimuli. Dysfunction of the higher-order visual areas does not result in blindness but does diminish the individual's ability to recognize and interpret what is seen—that is, to perceive form, size, and meaning of objects. Loss of function or impaired function of the higher-order visual area in the left (dominant) hemisphere produces an inability to read written language, referred to as dyslexia or word blindness. Loss of reading ability does not occur with dysfunction of the right (nondominant) hemisphere, but performance of tasks requiring visuospatial perception, such as drawing, is impaired.

From the higher-order visual cortices, the processed visual information is projected to the posterior portions of the temporal lobes, where the highest level of visual image integration is thought to take place. Here, tasks that require visual perception are learned, such as using vision to cue eating, to drive, or to read this chapter. Impaired function in this area of the left (dominant) hemisphere begins to impair language comprehension and all cognitive functions that rely heavily on language comprehension. Likewise, impairment of this area within the right (nondominant) hemisphere impairs all visual-perceptual comprehension and all cognitive functions that rely on accurate visuospatial appreciation.

Auditory Cortex. The auditory cortices—that is, primary auditory areas and auditory higher-order (secondary) areas—are located in the medial superior temporal gyri. The primary and higher-order (secondary) auditory areas of the left (dominant) hemisphere mediate language sounds. The primary and higher-order (secondary) auditory areas of the right (nondominant) hemisphere mediate nonlanguage sound analysis and interpretation.

The primary auditory areas, which receive input directly from the medial geniculate body, detect individual elements—that is, pitches and patterns of the auditory stimuli. For example, a simple sound may be identified as being weak or loud (low or high intensity) and low or high frequency. Simple patterns can be interpreted. However, the primary auditory cortex alone cannot provide normal auditory experiences. The meaning of the sound cannot be interpreted. There is no perception of words or intelligible sounds. Dysfunction in the auditory cortex results in hearing loss (Guyton, 1992).

The primary auditory areas working in conjunction with their respective high-ordered (secondary) auditory areas provides for the analysis of complicated sounds. The primary auditory cortex and the thalamic association areas adjacent to the medial geniculate body provide input to the higher-order (secondary) areas. Dysfunction in the higher-order (secondary) auditory areas does not result in loss of hearing but produces difficulty in interpreting sounds—that is, a reduced ability to understand the meaning of the auditory stimuli. If there is dysfunction in the left (dominant) hemisphere's higher-order auditory area, language comprehension is impaired. The individual has a reduced ability to understand spoken language. If the dysfunction is in the right higher-order area, the individual has a reduced ability to appreciate and interpret nonlanguage sounds such as music.

ASSOCIATION CORTICES

Higher cognitive functions are associated with areas of the cerebral cortex that are concerned with the integration of more than one sensory modality and with the planning of movement (see Table 10–2) (Kupfermann, 1995). These true association cortices have proven to be secondary and tertiary processing centers for sensory and motor information (Kupfermann, 1995). They are located in three regions: the parietal-temporal-occipital association cortex, the prefrontal association cortex, and the limbic association cortex (see Figs. 10–2, 10–3, and 10–4).

Parietal-Temporal-Occipital Association Cortex. The parietal-temporal-occipital association cortex functions to integrate sensory functions and language. This cortical region is "thought to link information from several sensory modalities, a step important in the processing of sensory information for perception and language" (Jessell, 1995).

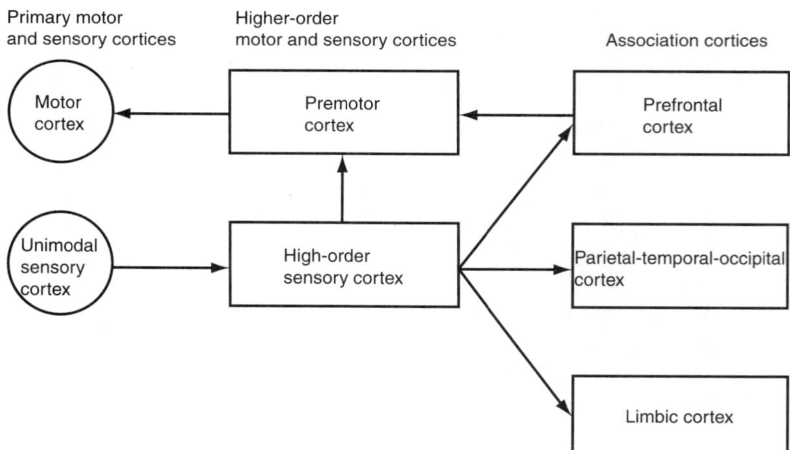

FIGURE 10–4 • The intercortical connections of primary motor and sensory cortices, high-order motor and sensory cortices, and association cortices are shown here in a simplified form. (From Kandel, E.R., Schwartz, J.H., & Jessell, T.M. [Eds.] [1991]. *Principles of neural science* [p. 826]. New York: Elsevier Publishing.)

The parietal lobe functions in attending to the spatial aspects of sensation, to form body image, and to plan movements in extrapersonal space (Kupfermann, 1991b). Damage to the parietal lobes results in alteration in body image, perception of spatial relations, visuomotor integration, and directed attention (Kandel & Kupfermann, 1995).

Dysfunction in the left posterior parietal cortex results in astereognosis, the inability to recognize the form of objects by touch. The individual is unable to appreciate the meaning of the sensory stimuli. For example, when the person with a supramarginal area dysfunction on the right side has a comb placed in the contralateral hand, the person is not able to recognize the object as a comb or visualize it in the imagination through manual examination of the object. The person is able to state isolated qualities about the object but is unable to integrate the bits of information into the concept of a comb.

Dysfunction in the left parietal lobe leaves the person with not only a Wernicke's (sensory, receptive, posterior) dysphasia but also a loss of cognitive functions associated with language or symbolism, such as the ability to perform mathematical calculations and to think through logical problems. Damage to the inferior areas of the left parietal cortex produces Gerstmann's syndrome, which is characterized by right-left confusion, finger agnosia, dysgraphia, and dyscalculia.

The parietal-temporal-occipital area of the left hemisphere is usually very highly developed and, because it mediates complex language, plays the largest single role of any area of the cerebral cortex in the higher levels of brain function that are referred to as cognition. A majority of our sensory experiences are converted into language equivalents and then analyzed, interpreted, and stored in the left parietal-temporal-occipital area.

A person with dysfunction in the parietal-temporal-occipital area on the left is able to hear without difficulty and to read printed words and has no loss of sensation but is unable to recognize the thought conveyed or the meaning of sensory experiences. Such dysfunction in terms of interpretation leaves an individual with a tremendous cognitive deficit.

Bilateral damage to the parietal-temporal-occipital regions produces Balint's syndrome, which is characterized by inability to voluntarily move one's eye to a specific point in space, inability to use visual guidance to grasp an object, and difficulty attending to visual stimuli.

The parietal-temporal-occipital association areas of the right (nondominant) hemisphere mediate understanding and interpretation of prosody (e.g., voice modulation, tone, emotional quality), music, nonverbal visual experiences such as gestures and facial expressions, spatial relationships between the person and the surroundings, and probably somatic experiences related to hand and extremity use. Persons with dysfunction in the right parietal-temporal-occipital area lose cognitive functions associated with nonlanguage sounds (e.g., appreciation of tone and delivery of speech), nonverbal communications such as gestures and facial expression, and visuospatial dimensions (e.g., drawing, art appreciation, athletic performance). Right parietal lobe injuries result in a loss of appreciation of the spatial aspects of all sensory information from the left side of the body as well as external space (Kupfermann, 1991b). The person may exhibit a neglect syndrome varying in severity to include denial of illness and constructional dyspraxia. Persons with an inferior right parietal injury may also be unable to appreciate the nonlanguage components of communication such as tone, loudness, and emotion. They may have difficulty modulating their own language output (Heilman, Schole & Watson, 1975).

PREFRONTAL ASSOCIATION CORTEX

The prefrontal association cortex is anterior to the premotor cortex and is concerned with complex motor activities. This area contributes to the planning of responses (an executive function). The person is able to weigh the consequences of future actions and to plan accordingly. This permits the selection of appropriate motor responses. The area of the principal sulcus is directly concerned with the strategic planning of motor actions including those involved in cognitive tasks (Kupfermann, 1995). This area is needed for execution of complex motor activities in which essential information is not available at the moment of response but has to be temporally held in the working memory network. It is the temporary storing of information to be used shortly to guide a future action, especially spatial actions (delayed spatial response tasks). The inferior prefrontal convexity below the principal sulcus contributes to all types of delayed responses, spatial or otherwise. Delayed response is involved in visual discrimination, planning, and execution of visual motor tasks. Dysfunction in the inferior prefrontal convexity affects ability to delay any response. The person cannot inhibit motor response until an appropriate time. Perseveration and failure to inhibit inappropriate responses are seen. These areas are predominantly dopaminergic. The prefrontal association cortex receives input from various areas of higher-order sensory cortex and the posterior parietal association cortices in particular (Kupfermann, 1995).

This working memory network provides "short-term representational memory" or working memory; that is, it provides a representation of information in its absence and controls the activation of these representations. This working memory provides a temporary area from which the brain can retrieve instructions and other information needed to guide behavior. The person is able to use internal knowledge to guide behavior in the absence of informative external cues (Posner & Raichle, 1994). It permits the reprogramming of mental operations, giving the person control over information processing, which is referred to by Posner and Raichle (1994) as top-down processing. Thus, the person is willfully or consciously able to formulate a plan of action and carry it out. Lateral areas, including areas around the principal sulcus and the anterior cingulate gyrus, contribute to working memory. The left hemisphere areas play a role in word associations, whereas the right hemisphere areas participate in spatial position of visual events held in memory when the original stimulus is removed from view.

Imaging studies have provided data that clarify that the right frontal cortex mediates the attentional network, called *vigilance*. This attentional network, when active, mediates alertness—that is, a sustained state of alertness (sustained attention, attention-over-time, concentration, concentration-over-time) enabling the person to be on guard, scanning and searching the environment (external or internal) for relevant stimuli, noticing anything that should then activate selective attention.

LIMBIC ASSOCIATION CORTEX

The limbic association cortex, located on the medial and ventral surfaces of the frontal lobe, the medial surface of the parietal lobe, and the tip of the temporal lobe (called the temporal pole), includes the orbitofrontal cortex, the cingulate region, and the parahippocampal areas. The limbic association cortex receives input from higher-order sensory areas and sends output to the other cortical areas, including the prefrontal areas. This is one pathway through which emotions influence motor planning.

This detection network contributes to bringing an object into conscious awareness by mediating the selection of a target from among many alternatives and permits the conscious execution of an instruction, including ensuring that the instruction is followed. The detection network has been demonstrated to include the anterior cingulate gyrus for words as well as the basal ganglion areas for colors, motion, and form. Automatic responses are inhibited, and the person can overcome preestablished preferences. An akinetic mute state exemplifies complete failure of the cingulate gyrus area.

The orbitofrontal cortex and the cingulate gyrus are concerned with emotional behavior—that is, the emotional responsiveness of the person. Electrical stimulation of the orbitofrontal cortex results in the appearance of many autonomic responses associated with activation of the sympathetic nervous system. Injury to the orbitofrontal cortex reduces the normal aggressiveness and emotional responsiveness of animals and persons even to intractable pain.

Neuropathophysiologically, a person with dysfunction in the frontal limbic cortex acts impulsively without apparent consideration of the consequences of the behavior or the appropriate degree of response that is called for. In addition, this impulsiveness contributes to the emergence of socially unacceptable behavior.

Stimulation of the superior temporal gyrus results in alterations in the perceptions of sound as well as auditory illusions and hallucinations with a remarkably real quality to them (Penfield, 1958). Also, stimulation of the anterior and medial portions of the temporal lobe causes the person to experience emotional feelings, especially fear (Penfield, 1958). The anterior poles of the temporal lobes have been demonstrated on brain imaging to activate during emotional experiences, including before a panic attack (Reiman, Fusselman, Fox, & Raichle, 1989; Reiman, Raichle, Butler, Herscovitch, & Robins, 1984; Reiman et al., 1989).

The temporal lobe portion of the limbic association cortex is concerned with memory functions. This has been discussed under memory networks.

Persons with left temporal lobe injury have difficulty remembering verbal material (e.g., lists of nouns). Persons with right temporal lobe injury have difficulty remembering patterns of sensory input such as human faces and irregular line drawings.

COGNITION: NORMAL AGE-RELATED CHANGES

Neurons begin to decrease in number after age 30 years, whereas neuroglial cells increase in size and number throughout life. Dendrites and dendritic spines decrease in number (Boss, 1993). Striking changes in the somatodendritic apparatus lead to this loss of dendrites with age. Initially, these changes appear to begin as swelling and distortion of the somatodendrite followed by dendritic loss. However, the dendrites of surviving aged neurons have been shown to have the ability to branch and respond to loss of neurons by developing new synapses (Buell & Coleman, 1979). Axon diameter thins, as does the myelin sheath. In addition, the special and general sensory receptors decrease in number. Likewise, receptors for dopamine, norepinepherine, and acetylcholine have been found to decrease in number in various areas of the nervous system (Gove, 1986). This reduces nerve impulse generation.

Lipofuscin, granulovacuolar organelles, and neurofibrillary tangles may be found in some cells (Adams & Victor, 1997; Goldman & Cote, 1991). Lipofuscin is thought to be composed of large end-stage lysosomes that have accumulated recycled membranes and other cellular debris that cannot be catabolized further by the neuron. Lipofuscin granules have not been demonstrated to impair neuronal function. Different types of neurons appear to accumulate lipofuscin at different rates. Degenerating neurons of the hippocampus and adjacent cortex accumulate granulovacuolar organelles in their cytoplasm and dendrites. These vacuoles are encapsulated by membranes and possess a dense, small granule in the center. Neurofibrillary tangles (Alzheimer's bodies) are large bundles of twisted fibers composed of a pair of filaments. Small numbers of neurofibrillary tangles are found in aging neurons, particularly in the hippocampus and the adjacent temporal lobe areas (Adams & Victor, 1997; Goldman & Cote, 1991).

Neuritic (senile) plaques may be seen extracellularly. The plaque is composed of a central amyloid core that is surrounded by degenerating neuronal processes and an outer covering of glial cells. Plaques are anywhere from 5 to 100 μm in diameter and are found most densely in the hippocampus but are common in the neocortex as well (Goldman & Cote, 1991).

Macroscopic changes include a decrease in brain weight and volume of less than 15% by age 80 years. Atrophy of portions of the cerebral cortex is present, especially in the limbic lobe, insula, and orbital gyri of the frontal lobe. Thus, the gyri narrow in width and the sulci widen. There is an increase in ventricular size and an increased volume of cerebrospinal fluid to fill the space vacated by cortical neurons. The white matter tracts become thinner, and the meninges thicken (Boss, 1993).

Biochemically, total brain protein is reduced by 30% but total brain DNA is increased, presumably as a result of glial cell proliferation. Lipid content of the brain is only minimally changed. Amount of available neurotransmitters is decreased, probably as a result of changes in enzymes and coenzymes. The enzymes and coenzymes required for dopamine and norepinepherine synthesis are drastically reduced. A less severe reduction occurs in the enzymes and coenzymes that catalyze acetylcholine and glutamic acid production. Neuronal activity is decreased, evidenced by a decrease in the frequency and amplitude of brain waves on an EEG. Cerebral blood flow has been shown to remain unchanged (Dastur et al., 1963; Duara et al., 1984). Oxygen and glucose consumption is decreased (Dastur et al., 1963). There is about a 10% decrease in conduction velocity (speed of transmission), thereby increasing response time (Goldman & Cote, 1991; Guyton, 1992).

Neurophysiologic Consequences of Aging Changes

The executive attentional network and working memory are not affected by aging (Prigatano, 1987; Schale & Zelinski, 1978). Explicit memory decreases with normal aging to some degree. More than 25% of persons show memory changes by age 75 years, while 50% of persons show memory changes by the beginning of their eighties (Prigatano, 1987). Twenty-five percent of persons after age 65 years were found to have mild recent memory problems (Jenkyn et al., 1985). Although recall of digits is fairly intact, recall of paragraphs and paired-associate words and recall of geometric designs decrease at age 35 years. Incidental memory decreases after age 35 years. This decrease in recent memory increases learning time to some degree.

Within the explicit remote memory network, visuospatial memory declines between 60 and 80 years to a much greater extent than does verbal recall, which remains fairly stable (Muramoto, 1984). Naming decreases after age 70 years, probably as a result of a retrieval (remote memory) deficit (Penfield, 1958). Language is apparently stable despite aging, except for naming (Prigatano, 1987). With these changes in explicit remote memory, response time increases.

Vocabulary and fund of information (subscales on intelligence tests) are stable across the adult life span, but scores on performance subscales, such as block design picture arrangement and object assembly, decline with age (Adams & Victor, 1997; Ohler & Albert, 1985; Prigatano, 1987). Probably this decline on speeded tests reflects a decreased speed of information processing and an increased response time.

The effects of normal aging on the attentional network of selective attention, implicit memory, and the executive attentional network vigilance were not found in the literature.

SUMMARY

What is the neurophysiologic basis of attention, memory, concept formation, abstraction, thinking, reasoning, forming and carrying out plans, making judgments, or gaining insight? The neuroanatomic structures involved in cognition have not been fully established. It has been demonstrated that different parts of the brain, predominantly in the cerebral cortices, focus on specific aspects of sensory experiences and that other cortical areas mediate integration of various sensory experiences. Data support a localization view proposing that cognition is the result of primary, higher-order, and association processes carried out by specific neural networks. However, often parallel processing takes place so that many cortical areas may be simultaneously activated.

Development of the neuroanatomic structures necessary for cognition starts early in the prenatal period, with the proliferation and generation of classes of neurons and other cells that shortly thereafter migrate to their appropriate location and begin the process of cell maturation with the establishment of specific interneuronal connections. The processes are probably genetically and developmentally determined. The presence of internal environmental influences, such as specific nutrients, oxygen, and hormones, and external environmental influences, such as external stimulation, exerts a definite influence on the developing cortical areas and cognitive neural networks prenatally and postnatally. Final cortical development appears to result from environmentally induced learning, which enables the strengthening and fine-tuning of cognitive networks with the brain.

The attentional and memory networks are fundamental to learning and cognition. The ability to establish, retain, and retrieve long-term memories is the basis of all learning. Within the explicit (declarative) memory, information, knowledge, principles, and facts are retained and retrieved. The hippocampus and related temporal lobe structures play a major role in establishing, retaining, and retrieving the explicit memories. Within the implicit (procedural) memory system, responses such as motor activities, skills, habits, and performances are retained and retrieved. The initial dynamic changes within an activated circuit (short-term) memory are eventually transferred into a permanent anatomic change in synapses within the neural circuit (long-term) memory. Memory is impaired if there is a failure or impairment in the ability to establish, retain, or retrieve memories.

The primary, higher-order, and association areas of the cortex contribute to cognition by mediating the identification, localization, analysis, and interpretation of sensory information. The primary and higher-order areas deal with only one sensory modality, whereas the association cortices integrate information across all the sensory modalities.

The parietal-temporal-occipital association cortex integrates sensory perception. The left parietal-temporal-occipital association areas mediate language and language-dependent cognitive functions. The right parietal-temporal-occipital association areas mediate visuospatial functions, including nonlanguage aspects of communication such as prosody, gesture, facial expression, appreciation of music, spatial perception, and much of nonlanguage visual experiences.

The prefrontal association cortices contribute to cognition by mediating working memory (i.e., the ability to perform delayed response tasks by holding information in a working memory circuit until all required information has been received). Impairment in working memory manifests as an inability to plan or inhibit motor response as well as a failure to self-monitor. Perseveration may be seen.

The limbic association cortices contribute to cognition by mediating emotional responsiveness to environment that serves to motivate the individual to respond. Without such activation, the person lacks motivation, is apathetic and listless, and appears affectless or without emotional responsiveness. The limbic association cortex within the temporal lobe includes the hippocampus and the related memory structures, which are essential to the establishment, retention, and retrieval of explicit memories. Anterograde and retrograde amnesia is the result of impairment of function of this portion of the limbic association cortex.

Neuroanatomically, neurons age by decreasing the number and size of the neuronal bodies and neuronal processes and the thickness of the myelin sheaths. Neuronal metabolic processes decrease, and therefore neuronal functions slow. Neurophysiologically, explicit memory is slightly decreased and visuospatial memory declines somewhat while language-mediated cognitive functions remain relatively intact. Reaction and response time are increased, causing a decline in any speed-testing situations.

References

Adams, R.A., & Victor, M. (1997). *Principles of neurology* (6th ed.). New York: McGraw-Hill.

Armstrong, M.E., Howe, J., Smith, A.P., Smith, M.M., & Snider, M.J. (1979). *McGraw-Hill nursing dictionary*. New York: McGraw-Hill.

Boss, B.J. (1998). Concepts of neurological dysfunction. In K. McCance & S. Huether (Eds.), *Pathophysiology: Biological mechanisms in adults and children* (3rd ed., pp. 460–508). St. Louis: C.V. Mosby.

Buell, S.J., & Coleman, P.D. (1979). Dendritic growth in the aged human brain and failure of growth in senile dementia. *Science, 206,* 854–856.

Dastur, D.K., Lane, M.H., Hansen, D.B., Kety, S.S., Butler, R.N., Perlin, S., & Sokoloff, L. (1963). Effects of aging on cerebral circulation and metabolism in man. In J.E. Birren, R.N. Butler, S.W. Greenhouse, L. Sokoloff, & M.R. Yarrow (Eds.), *Human aging: A biological and behavioral study* (Public Health Pub. No. 986, pp. 59–76). Washington, DC: U.S. Government Printing Office.

Diamond, A. (1990). Introduction. The development and neural bases of higher cognitive functions. *Annals of the New York Academy of Sciences, 608,* xiii–xv.

Duara, R., Grady, C., Haxby, J., Ingvar, D., Sokoloff, L., Margohin, R.A., & Raporport, S.I. (1984). Human brain glucose utilization and cognitive function in relation to age. *Annals of Neurology, 16,* 702–719.

Geschwind, N., & Levitsky, W. (1968). Human brain: Left-right asymmetries in temporal speech region. *Science, 161,* 186–187.

Goldman, J., & Cote, L. (1991). Aging of the brain: Dementia of the Alzheimer's type. In E.R. Kandel, J.H. Schwartz, & T.M. Jessell (Eds.), *Principles of neural science* (pp. 974–982). New York: Elsevier Science Publishing.

Gove, P.B. (1986). *Webster's third new international dictionary of the English language*. Springfield, MA: Merriam-Webster.

Guyton, A.C. (1992). *Basic neuroscience* (2nd ed.). Philadelphia: W.B. Saunders.

Hayakawa, K., Konishi, Y., Kuriyama, M., Konishi, K., & Matsuda, T. (1991). Normal brain maturation in MRI. *European Journal of Radiology, 12*(3), 208–215.

Hebb, D.O. (1949). *Organization of behavior: A neurophysiological theory*. New York: John Wiley & Sons.

Heilman, K.M., Schole, R., & Watson, R.T. (1975). Auditory affective agnosia. Disturbed comprehension of affective speech. *Journal of Neurology, Neurosurgery, and Psychiatry, 38,* 69–72.

Hudspeth, W.J., & Pribram, K.H. (1992). Psychophysiological indices of cerebral maturation. *International Journal of Psychophysiology, 12*(1), 10–29.

Jacobson, M. (1991). *Developmental neurobiology* (3rd ed.). Reading, MA: Plenum Press.

Jenkyn, L.R., Reeves, A.G., Warren, T., Whiting, R.K., Clayton, R.J., Moore, W.W., Rizzo, A., Tuzan, I.M., Bonnett, J.C., & Culpepper, B.W. (1985). Neurologic signs in senescence. *Archives of Neurology, 42,* 1154–1157.

Jernigan, T.L., Trauner, D.A., Hessehink, J.R., & Tallar, P.A. (1991). Maturation of human cerebrum observed in vivo during adolescence. *Brain, 114,* 2037–2049.

Jessell, T.M. (1995). Development of the nervous system. In E.R. Kandel, J.H. Schwartz, & T.M. Jessell (Eds.), *Essentials of neural science and behavior* (pp. 89–110). New York: Appleton and Lange.

Jessell, T.M. (1995). The nervous system. In E.R. Kandel, J.H. Schwartz, T.M. Jessell (Eds.), *Essentials of neural science and behavior* (pp. 71–88). New York: Appleton & Lange.

Kandel, E.R. (1991a). Brain and behavior. In E.R. Kandel, J.H. Schwartz, & T.M. Jessell (Eds.), *Principles of neural science* (pp. 3–16). New York: Elsevier Publishing.

Kandel, E.R. (1991b). Cellular mechanisms of learning and the biological basis of individuality. In E.R. Kandel, J.H. Schwartz, & T.M. Jessell (Eds.), *Principles of neural science* (pp. 1009–1030). New York: Elsevier Publishing.

Kandel, E.R. (1995a). Brain and behavior. In E.R. Kandel, J.H. Schwartz, T.M. Jessell (Eds.), *Essentials of neural science and behavior* (pp. 5–19). New York: Appleton & Lange.

Kandel, E.R. (1995b). Cellular mechanisms of learning and memory. *Essentials of neural science and behavior* (pp. 667–669), E.R. Kandel, J.H. Schwartz, T.M. Jessell (Eds.). Appleton & Lange.

Kandel, E.R. (1995a). Brain and behavior. In E.R. Kandel, J.H. Schwartz, & T.M. Jessell (Eds.), *Essentials of neural science and behavior* (pp. 5–19). Stamford, CT: Appleton & Lange.

Kandel, E.R. (1995b). Construction of the visual image. In E.R. Kandel, J.H. Schwartz, & T.M. Jessell (Eds.), *Essentials of neural science and behavior* (pp. 387–405). Stamford, CT: Appleton & Lange.

Kandel, E.R., Kupfermann, I. (1995). From nerve cells to cognition. In E.R. Kandel, J.H. Schwartz, & T.M. Jessell (Eds.), *Essentials of neural science and behavior* (pp. 321–346). Stamford, CT: Appleton & Lange.

Kelly, D.D. (1991). Sexual differentiation of the nervous system. In E.R. Kandel, J.H. Schwartz, & T.M. Jessell (Eds.), *Principles of neural science* (pp. 959–973). New York: Elsevier Publishing.

Kupfermann, I. (1991a). Learning and memory. In E.R. Kandel, J.H. Schwartz, & T.M. Jessell (Eds.), *Principles of neural science* (pp. 997–1008). New York: Elsevier Publishing.

Kupfermann, I. (1991b). Localization of higher cognitive and affective functions: The association cortices. In E.R. Kandel, J.H. Schwartz, & T.M. Jessell (Eds.), *Principles of neural science* (pp. 823–838). New York: Elsevier Publishing.

Kupfermann, I. (1995). Cognition and the cortex. In E.R. Kandel, J.H. Schwartz, & T.M. Jessell (Eds.), *Essentials of neural science and behavior* (pp. 347–363). Stamford, CT: Appleton & Lange.

Kupfermann, I., Kandel, E.R. (1995). Learning and memory. In E.R. Kandel, J.H. Schwartz, & T.M. Jessell (Eds.), *Essentials of neural science and behavior* (pp. 651–666). Stamford, CT: Appleton & Lange.

Lashley, K.S. (1929). *Brain mechanisms and intelligence: A quantitative study of injuries to the brain.* Chicago: University of Chicago Press.

Malorye, A. (1992, October–November). The effects of neurologic injury on the maturing brain. *Headliners,* 2–10.

Meltzoff, A.N. (1990). Towards a developmental cognitive science. *Annals of the New York Academy of Science, 208,* 1–27.

Muramoto, O. (1984). Selective reminding in normal and demented aged people: Auditory verbal versus visual spatial task. *Cortex, 20,* 461–478.

Neisser, U. (1967). *Cognitive psychology.* Paramus, NJ: Appleton-Century-Crofts.

Ohler, L.K., & Albert, M.L. (1985). Language skills across adulthood. In J.E. Birren & E.W. Schale (Eds.), *Handbook of the psychology of aging* (pp. 463–478). New York: Van Nostrand Reinhold.

Penfield, W. (1958). Functional localization in temporal and deep Sylvian areas. *Research Publication of the Association for Nervous and Mental Disorders, 36,* 210–226.

Poon, D.W. (1985). Differences in human memory with aging: Nature, courses and clinical implications. In J.E. Birren & E.W. Schale (Eds.), *Handbook of the psychology of aging* (pp. 427–462). New York: Van Nostrand Reinhold.

Posner, M.I. (1980). Orienting of attention. The VIIth Sir Frederick Barlett lecture. *Q J Experimental Psych, 32*, 3–5.

Posner, M.I., Raichle, M.E. (1994). *Images of mind.* New York: Science American Library.

Posner, M.I., Rafal, R.D. (1987). Cognitive theories of attention and the rehabilitation of attentional deficits. In M. Meier, A. Benton, & S.L. Diller (Eds.), *Neuropsychological rehabilitation* (pp. 182–201). New York: The Guilford Press.

Posner, M.I., Warren, J., Frederich, F.J., & Rafal, R.D. (1984). Effects of parietal injury on covert orienting of visual attention. *J Neuroscience, 4*, 1863–1874.

Prigatano, G.P. (1987). Neuropsychology of aging: A survey. *BNI Quarterly, 3*(3), 38–44.

Reiman, E.M., Fusselman, M.J., Fox, P.T., & Raichle, M.E. (1989). Neuroanatomical correlates of anticipatory anxiety. *Science, 243*, 1071–1074.

Reiman, E.M., Raichle, M.E., Butler, F.E., Herscovitch, P., & Robins, E. (1984). A total brain abnormality in panic disorder, a severe form of anxiety. *Nature, 310*, 683–685.

Reiman, E.M., Raichle, M.E., Robins, E., Mintun, M.A., Fusselman, M.E., Fox, P.T., Price, J.L., & Hackman, K.A. (1989). Neuroanatomical correlates of a lactate-induced anxiety attack. *Archives of General Psychiatry, 46*, 493–500.

Schale, E.W., & Zelinski, E. (1978). Psychometric assessment of dysfunction in learning and memory. In F. Hoffmeister & C. Mullens (Eds.), *Brain function in old age* (pp. 134–150). New York: Springer-Verlag.

Springer, S.P., & Deutsch, G. (1989). *Left brain, right brain.* New York: W.H. Freeman.

Squires, L.R. (1987). *Memory and brain.* New York: Oxford University Press.

Tsal, Y. (1983). Movements of attention across the visual field. *J Experimental Psych, 9*, 523–530.

Assessment of Cognition

MARGARETHE CAMMERMEYER

ASSESSMENT OF COGNITIVE FUNCTION IN THE CLINICAL SETTING

Assessment of cognitive functioning is an evaluation of brain function that occurs with each verbal and nonverbal interaction. Cognitive assessment may be formal or informal, conscious or unconscious, or part of a professional or social interaction. For example, a family determines, from daily contact, that a member is no longer capable of performing activities of daily living. In contrast, a neuropsychologist uses formal tests to identify impaired cognitive functioning. Both the family and the professional identify impaired cognition, but the methods of assessment differ.

This chapter focuses on methods of assessing cognitive processes such as memory, information processing, and goal-oriented behaviors. It does not focus on assessing primary functions such as hearing (not to be confused with understanding), vision (not to be confused with spatial-perceptual ability), or primary motor functioning (not to be confused with praxis). Such assessment is described in Chapter 23. The presumption in this chapter is that the peripheral organs, such as the eyes and the ears, are working properly.

Nursing assessment of cognition is directed toward discovering dysfunctions that have an impact on daily living. It is, therefore, useful to consider an organizational framework that emphasizes brain functioning.

FUNCTIONAL ORGANIZATION OF THE BRAIN

Luria (1973) organized the brain into three primary functional units. Anatomically, the first functional unit includes the brain stem (with the reticular activating system), the mesial cortex, and the diencephalon. It is the seat of arousal (alertness), memory, and emotion. This first unit is, therefore, the center for "regulating and modifying the body's tone and control over inclinations and emotions of the person. . . . [It is] the center for memory and consciousness" (Luria, 1973, pp. 60, 67).

Anatomically, the second functional unit comprises the posterior cerebral hemispheres and the temporal, parietal, and occipital areas (Luria, 1973). The second functional unit is the seat of reception, analysis, and storage of sensory information. Peripheral sensory organs of hearing, vision, smell, and touch transmit information from the external environment through the sensory system into the second functional unit. The diencephalon must be intact, and the person must be aroused or alert to receive and process the incoming information. The sensory information integrates with information from the first functional unit. For example, memory and emotional processing of information occur in response to the sensory stimulus.

The third functional unit described by Luria (1973) programs, regulates, and verifies input. The anterior portion of the brain, from the premotor cortex, receives information from the first and second functional units and responds to the information, culminating in some motor output or autonomic response. The output may take the form of movement or speech, or it may be limited to cortical integration of information, considered "thought" or "emotion." The limbic system and the deeper cortical structures are presumed to compose the third functional unit.

In contrast to Luria (1973), Plum and Posner (1980) considered cognition to be a part of consciousness. They ascribed cognitive functions to the content of consciousness, as contrasted with the arousal functions of consciousness. As described in Chapter 5, arousal is measured by the observable responsiveness of a person to a variety of stimuli. Cognitive functioning, or the content of consciousness, cannot be tested adequately in people with altered arousal.

Functionally, the content of consciousness, as defined by Plum and Posner (1980), includes higher cortical activities, such as receiving, processing, organizing, and storing information. The content of consciousness can also be measured, in part, through determination of a person's orientation in time and space, reasoning, abstract thinking, and goal-oriented behaviors. These behaviors are comparable to those mediated by Luria's third functional unit—information about what a person can do and how much a person knows. In addition, Lezak (1985) described cognitive executive functions as those abilities that determine whether and how a person cares for herself or himself, whether the person is employable, and whether and how the person maintains normal social relationships (p. 38).

Both structural changes and metabolic processes may alter cognition or information processing. For example, a space-occupying lesion in the left parietal region results in communication difficulties. Metabolic imbalance alters the chemical substrate of brain metabolism and produces changes in cognitive functioning; for example, low blood glucose, hypoxemia, and hyponatremia can all produce confusion and loss of consciousness.

Ascertaining specific cognitive skill levels or deficits is, therefore, an important aspect of ongoing assessment. Objectifying cognitive skills and deficits using predesigned validated instruments is useful for ongoing assessment and to communicate findings between and among health professionals.

TYPES OF COGNITIVE ASSESSMENT

Cognitive functioning is presumed to be measurable. The kinds of higher-level executive functions that have an impact on people's lives include communication, perceptions, visual and manual praxis, memory, orientation, attention, self-regulation, and personality (Lezak, 1985). These functions are evaluated by determining an individual's ability to perform specific actions or responses that are purported to reflect specific cognitive processes. The areas assessed are shown in Table 11–1.

The methods and tools used to assess cortical functioning, however, cannot fully capture the dimensions of cognitive processes or how those processes interact to create the "humanity" of the individual. The methods used to evaluate cognitive functioning are derived from developmental theory and neuropsychology and tend to measure cortical functioning in isolation, that is, not in the context of the activities of daily living.

Nurses can make a useful contribution to the evaluation of cognitive functioning by integrating results from neuropsychologic assessment with the client's functional skills in performing activities of daily living. Information from a neuropsychologic assessment must therefore be clinically appropriate, and

TABLE 11–1 • COGNITIVE FUNCTIONS AND THEIR GENERAL EVALUATION

Function	Evaluation
Orientation	Orientation to time, place, person, and situation; ability to self-regulate; impulse control; and grasp of gestalt of situation
Verbal function	Verbal fluency, repetition of words, fluency of making and understanding spoken and written language
Perceptual function	Visual: Recognition of object from visual cues; picture recognition Auditory: Evaluated by asking patient to repeat a sentence Tactile: Construction with tiles or identifying objects; following sequence of commands using objects
Visuospatial functions and dexterity	Entails creating designs from two-dimensional pictures
Memory function	Broad area requiring evaluation of visual, auditory, immediate, short-term, and long-term memory; evaluated through historical interview, repetition of words, numbers, nonsense words, sentences, or stories at various time intervals after first presentation; pictures drawn from visual memory or stories repeated from auditory recall
General fund of knowledge and gestalt for situations	Assimilation in general areas of evaluation
Construct formation and reasoning ability	Use of judgment and previous life experiences; becomes encompassed in backdrop of memory functioning

results must be available to incorporate into the planning of the total care of the client.

Cognitive functioning can be evaluated by using formal neurobehavioral batteries, screening neuropsychologic tests, or tests that evaluate specific cognitive functions. These tests also need to be specific to the developmental age and culture of the individual.

Life Trajectory and Cognitive Evaluations

Imprecise testing of neuropsychologic functioning has been done since the beginning of time. Parents observe their newborn, noting the first smile, the first word, and the first step. These are the developmental milestones that every human is expected to reach at specific points in time. The milestones are unique to the age of the person and the culture into which she or he is born and reared. It is vital to assimilate cultural norms with the developmental skills of the infant when determining the normal variation for a specific child and skill. For example, in the United States, a 3-year-old who does not walk is considered developmentally delayed, whereas this may be normal in cultures in which toddlers are carried for the first 3 years of life (Williams & Williams, 1987).

Similarly, in aging populations there will be cultural influences that determine the cognitive and psychomotor skill levels of the individual. With aging, the processing of information and the retrieval of memory are normally slowed and delayed; this must not be construed as being pathologic (Kiernan, Mueller, Langston, & Van Dyke, 1987).

Formal Neurobehavioral Batteries

Formal neurobehavioral batteries are useful in that they (1) systematically evaluate numerous areas of cognitive function, (2) provide a complete evaluation, (3) have established interrater reliability among administrations and administrators, (4) have been used repeatedly and show stability, and (5) have been validated against other measures of brain function.

The major disadvantages of such batteries are that they are time consuming and costly to perform, that they require patients be highly attentive and cooperative, and that they have a high level of specificity in dealing with both normal and abnormal areas of cognitive function. Further, they require specialty training to administer and interpret. These tests are also difficult to administer in the acute care setting (Lezak, 1985). Examples of such neurobehavioral batteries include personality inventories, intelligence tests, and neuropsychologic tests.

There are no adequate or specific measures of personality—only measures of behavioral traits. Traits commonly described as components of personality include somatization, obsessive-compulsive behavior, interpersonal sensitivity, depression, anxiety, hostility, phobic anxiety, paranoid ideation, and psychosis. Tests such as the Minnesota Multiphasic Personality Inventory (MMPI) and the Symptom Checklist-90, Revised (SCL-90 R) are used as measures of these behavioral traits (Derogatis, 1977) and have been used to describe personality traits. The MMPI takes several hours to complete and may be offensive to people who feel the test is being administered to see if they are "crazy." The MMPI does not assist in localizing diseases, per se, but it provides a pattern of responses noted in subjects with psychiatric or neurologic disorders. There are 566 questions on the MMPI, with no time limit to complete them. It is scored by computer, which may delay receipt of results. It is, therefore, of limited value in the acute care setting.

The SCL-90 R is a brief, 90-item self-report symptom inventory designed to reflect "psychological symptom patterns." Each item is rated on a five-point response scale from "not at all" depressed to "extremely" depressed. The test takes from 15 to 20 minutes to complete, is not usually found offensive by patients, and provides useful information that assists in identifying personality patterns of behavior. Personality, emotions, social stresses, and hospitalization affect the results of neuropsychologic tests and may alter the interpretation of test results (Derogatis, 1977).

The most commonly used test of general "intellectual ability" is the Wechsler Adult Intelligence Scale (WAIS). Adjusted versions have been developed for children of preschool and primary school age that are similar to the adult version but downgraded and revised as appropriate to developmental age. These three versions of the WAIS evaluate verbal and performance ability. The verbal scale includes testing of general information, comprehension, arithmetic, similarities, digit span, and vocabulary. The performance scale includes digit symbols, picture completion, block design, picture arrangement, and object assembly. The results provide information about verbal comprehension, perceptual organization, and memory. Numerous studies have been performed to standardize the test scores, and they have established reliability and validity of these tests (Buron, 1978). The major limitation of the WAIS is that it takes from 6 to 8 hours to administer. The written report accompanying the WAIS score provides specific information on how the person performed on each subtest, but the final result is expressed in a single number.

Another commonly used formal neuropsychologic test is the Halstead Neuropsychological Battery. The Halstead Battery was composed of six tests: a category test, an actual performance test, a rhythm test, a speech sounds test, a perception test, and a finger-tapping test. To that battery, Reitan added the Trail Making Test, an aphasia screening test, a sensory examination, and a motor strength evaluation. The combined test battery, called the Halstead-Reitan Neuropsychological Battery, takes from 6 to 8 hours to administer. Although the Halstead-Reitan Neuropsychological Battery has limited value in patients with a dense motor or sensory deficit, it is useful as a neuropsychologic test of cognitive deficits (Reitan, 1987; Reitan & Tarshes, 1959).

Neuropsychologic Screening Tests for Adults and Elderly Persons

Administration of formal test batteries is often not practical for acutely ill patients because of their physical disabilities and limited attention spans. There are also times when a clinician will observe abnormal social interaction and want a method of further evaluating the client. Under each of these conditions, an abbreviated screening assessment tool is more useful than the full neuropsychologic battery. Screening tests assess several areas of functioning in a brief time period and can be performed by individuals without formal neuropsychologic training. Nurses, speech therapists, rehabilitation specialists, and others are developing neuropsychologic screening instruments to use in the acute care setting. The objectives are that such an instrument be able to assess multiple areas of cognitive function; be able to identify cognitive dysfunction; and be reliable, reproducible, valid, and clinically relevant for patient care, safety, autonomy, and self-esteem. It must also be practical to administer.

Screening assessment is begun during the admission or intake interview. The assessment includes evaluation of the client's ability to hear, to communicate, to maintain visual contact, and to have an affective and effective interaction. The content of responses allows for additional evaluation of communication skills, coping, orientation, judgment, and emotional and social interaction. The screening neuropsychologic assessment instrument is used to corroborate initial clinical impressions. One such screening tool, adapted from the Reitan-Indiana Aphasia Screen, can be adapted for bedside administration. It is composed of the following six components:

1. Copy these figures: ■ ▲ †
2. Name the figures.
3. Spell the names of the figures.
4. Repeat the sentence, "He shouted the warning."
5. Explain the meaning of the sentence.
6. Write the sentence.

These questions explore the patient's visual-spatial ability and ability to communicate, repeat words, understand, use abstract reasoning, and write. This is an example of a screening assessment of language skills.

The Reitan-Indiana Aphasia Screen itself takes a little longer to administer. The subject is shown a series of pictures, words, and numbers on a small handheld flip chart and is asked specific questions regarding the illustrations. Each question purports to evaluate a specific cognitive skill. The person is asked to draw a square and if unable to do so, in the absence of developmental or motor deficits, is considered to have constructional apraxia. If unable to name the object on the flip chart, the person is considered to have anomia. If the person is unable to respond appropriately to a specific command, the cognitive deficit is as defined on the back of the flip chart. The second half of the Reitan-Indiana Aphasia Screen evaluates sensory and spatial-perceptual function. The subject is asked to identify objects by touch and to identity where he or she is touched when the eyes are closed. The test also evaluates the patient's visual field perception. The Reitan-Indiana Aphasia Screen is used as a screening tool to evaluate cognitive abilities such as communication skills, spatial-perceptual intactness, gestalt of a situation, judgment, and abstract thinking. There are no scores when the screen is completed. Answers are either correct or incorrect. Therefore, serial evaluations will not be sensitive to gradual deterioration or improvement. The test is useful, however, because it can identify specific cognitive deficits that can then be further evaluated (O'Donnell, Romero, & Leicht, 1990). It is also useful because it can be administered with minimal training.

A widely used neuropsychologic screening instrument is the Trail Making Test (Reitan, 1955). Originally, the Trail Making Test was called the Taylor Number Series and was used by the U.S. Army in 1945 to test general ability, because the test requires attention to detail and ability to alternate sequences of events. The Trail Making Test has two sections, A and B. Trail Making A consists of 25 consecutively numbered circles spread out over an 11 by 8.5–inch sheet of paper. The purpose of the test is to draw a line as rapidly as possible from circle to circle in consecutive sequence. Trail Making B consists of 25 circles of numbers and letters. The purpose is to draw a line alternating between the numbers and the letters in alphabetical and numerical sequences. The Trail Making Test has been used to evaluate organic brain damage. A patient with a metabolic disorder may be able to complete both Trail Making A and Trail Making B but will do so very slowly. With structural changes in the brain, the patient may be unable to organize thoughts sufficiently to follow through on the sequencing of the numbers or may be unable to alternate between the numbers and the letters. Translated into real-life situations, the patient may have difficulty with self-care activities. Normative scores and average time to completion have been developed for various age groups from 20 years through 79 years (Brown, Cased, Fisch, & Neuringer, 1958; Conn, 1977; Davies, 1968; Reitan, 1955).

In the early and mid-1970s there was an insurgence of newly developed neuropsychologic screening tests such as the Mini-Mental State (MMS), the Short Portable Mental Status Questionnaire (SPMSQ), the Mental Status Questionnaire, and the Cognitive Capacity Mental Examination. Each of these instruments has been used in clinical practice and clinical research for years. They are particularly useful to corroborate the existence of cognitive deficits identified by the family or identified during the intake interview or through observations of social behaviors. The selection of the instrument to be used should be based on the desired parameter one is interested in evaluating as well as on the sensitivity and specificity of the instrument. A comparison of the functions evaluated by several screening neuropsychologic tests is illustrated in Table 11–2.

The MMS (Anthony, LeResche, Niaz, Von Korff, & Folstein, 1982; Folstein, Folstein, & McHugh, 1975) is a general neuropsychologic screening tool used in such clinical areas as medicine, psychiatry, and geriatrics. The MMS tests orientation, registration, attention, calculations, recall, and language and takes 5 minutes to administer. Subtest scores are added so that there is one single number that represents the client's score. The MMS focuses on communication ability and does not deal with spatial-perceptual skills or other right-brain functions. When using the MMS, the quality of the answers may have a more

TABLE 11–2 • COMPARISON OF MENTAL STATUS EXAMINATIONS WITH FUNCTIONS TESTED

Examination	Ori*	Att	Calc	Lang	Const	Mem	Reas
Mental Status Questionnaire	+						
Short Portable Mental Status Questionnaire	+		+				
Mini-Mental State	+	+	+	+	+	+	
Galveston Orientation and Amnesia Test	+					+	
Cognitive Capacity Mental Examination	+	+	+	+		+	+
Neurobehavioral Cognitive Status Examination	+	+	+	+	+	+	+

* Ori, orientation; Att, attention; Calc, calculation; Lang, language; Const, construction; Mem, memory; Reas, reasoning.

pragmatic value than will the single number score. Difficulty with orientation, attention, recall, and language will interfere with ability for self-care. The MMS shows general agreement with the WAIS test in identifying cognitive impairment in psychiatrically and neurologically impaired populations. Several studies in both the United States and Europe have substantiated that a cutoff point from 23/24 is consistent with a diagnosis of dementia with an 80% to 90% reliability (Hooijer, Dinkgreve, Jonker, & Lindeboom, 1992; Myers, 1987). Dick et al. (1984) noted a false-positive result rate of 39% in older people and in patients with less education. Subjects with a lower intelligence quotient (IQ), as in the developmentally disabled with concurrent psychologic disorders, performed worse on the MMS than did those without psychologic disorders (Myers, 1987). The MMS had a false-negative result rate of 42% when compared with the results of the Neurobehavioral Cognitive Status Examination (NCSE) administered to neurosurgical patients with confirmed abnormal head computed tomography (CT) scans (Kiernan et al., 1987).

Another brief neuropsychologic screening instrument is the SPMSQ (Pfeiffer, 1975). This is a 10-item test of orientation, recent and long-term memory, and serial calculations. The total score is a single number that purports to measure normal intelligence or mild, moderate, or severe impairment. The test employs commonly used questions and quantifies the patient's answers. The test scores have been found to be affected by the education level of the client. In addition, the SPMSQ has a modified normative score for the geriatric population. Hooijer et al. (1992) found no significant difference between the MMS and the SPMSQ in ability to identify cognitive deficits.

The Mental Status Questionnaire (Kahn, Goldfarb, Pollack, & Peck, 1960) is a 10-item questionnaire of orientation to time, place, person, and past and current presidents. The total number of correct responses determines the single number score. Zero to 2 errors is considered normal or "no brain syndrome," 3 to 8 errors is considered moderately severe brain syndrome, and 9 or 10 errors is considered severely impaired.

The Cognitive Capacity Mental Examination (Jacobs, Bernhard, Delgado, & Strain, 1977) is a 30-item questionnaire of time, place, attention, calculations, immediate and short-term memory, and abstracting ability. A total correct score of 30 is possible. A score of less than 20 is considered diminished cognitive capacity, and the patient should be further evaluated with medical and neuropsychologic testing.

Another brief neuropsychologic instrument is the NCSE (Kiernan et al., 1987; Mueller, 1984). The NCSE provides information in 10 cognitive areas: level of consciousness, orientation, attention, communication, memory, constructional ability, calculations, reasoning, abstracting, and similarities. Specific questions are asked for screening purposes. The NCSE takes 20 minutes to administer and requires several props (tiles, pencil, stopwatch, key, coin, flash cards) and a manual. If the screening questions are answered accurately, the next area of cognitive functioning is evaluated. If the person does not pass the screen, a metric portion of the subset of questions is asked. The questions become progressively more difficult until the person is no longer able to answer the metric questions or until the questions reach the same level of complexity as that of the screening questions. The scores are tabulated and recorded on a visual graph. Normative ranges are noted in the shaded portion of the graph. Subjects older than 65 years have an expected decrement in performance in the construction, memory, and similarities portions of the test.

A major advantage of the NCSE is that it evaluates a full range of cognitive abilities, is inexpensive, and can be repeated readily on serial assessment. Little test-retest effect has been noted in patients with neurologic dysfunction. The test can be administered by people with minimal additional training. The major drawbacks are that the instrument relies on communication and language skills for many of the questions. Patients with dysphasia do poorly on the NCSE. The social and cultural bias that is evident in the test can be overcome by rewording some of the judgment questions (depending on the country and population under study). The rating of moderate or severe impairment does not necessarily reflect a patient's ability to function in the real world.

Neuropsychologic Screening Tests for Children

There are numerous neuropsychologic batteries used by neuropsychologists to evaluate children. Many of these are adaptations of the adult versions, such as the Luria-Nebraska Children's Battery and Wechsler's Intelligence Scale for Children. Although there are screening neuropsychologic tests that have been developed and tested, few are easily adaptable to the clinical setting of nurses.

The Denver Developmental Screening Test (DDST) evaluates gross motor, fine motor–adaptive, language, and personal social skills for children up to the age of 6 years (Frankenburg, Dodds, & Fandal, 1970). The test is more a screening evaluation for childhood development, based, in part, on the environment in which the child was raised and the cultural and social status of the family. Cultural differences in childrearing profoundly influence performance on the DDST and must be considered in the evaluation of any child who is not living in Denver, Colorado, where the test was developed (Williams & Williams, 1987). When cultural norms are not available, serial evaluations with the DDST can be used to detect trends of changes in developmental skills, which can then guide the decision as to whether further evaluation is indicated. Poor performance on serial evaluations of the DDST has been used to predict those children who should undergo more complete neuropsychologic evaluation (Greer, Bauchner, & Zuckerman, 1989).

There is a modified Reitan-Indiana Aphasia Screen for young children (ages 6 to 8 years) that can be administered in 10 to 15 minutes. The test consists of 22 performances including naming simple objects, copying simple figures, identifying body parts, reading (to developmental level), counting, performing arithmetic problems, and printing (Reitan, 1987; Reitan & Wolfson, 1992). The main difference between the adult and child versions is in the scoring. The child's response is ranked on a four-point scale (0 = perfectly normal performance; 1 and 2 = intermediate performance; and 3 = seriously defective performance). The sum of the scores represents the child's Reitan-Indiana Aphasia Screen score. This type of evaluation is especially useful with test-retest to identify changes in performance (Reitan & Wolfson, 1992).

Several other neurobehavioral screening tests can be used for children, but the results should be interpreted with caution. As the child develops fine motor–adaptive skills, the combined figures from the Gesell, Standford-Binet, and Bender-Gestalt tests provide examples of the complexity of drawings a child should be able to copy at various ages. This tool can be used to assess for visual deficits and perceptual and motor skills because it is not language bound or culture bound (Weiner, Bresnan, & Levitt, 1981).

The Trail Making Test (A and B) (Reitan, 1955) has been modified so that it can be administered to preschool children who have not developed language skills. Trail Making X and Y are similar to Trail Making A and B in terms of the placement and number of items on the page. The difference is that Trail Making X illustrates a series of clock faces that show 15-minute increments in time. The purpose is to draw a line from one clock to the next clock in sequence to show time progressing. In Trail Making Y there is a series of progressively larger circles that change by 1-mm increments. A line is drawn between the circles as they increase in size. Trail Making X and Y tap into spatial abilities (Stanczak, 1986). The X and Y versions of the Trail Making Test have been useful in identifying learning disabilities. These tests may be particularly useful in children younger than 9 years (Davis, Adams, Gates, & Cheramie, 1989).

Haber et al. (Haber, 1992; Haber & Norris, 1991; Haber & Norris, 1983) have developed a series of infant and child cognitive and developmental screening instruments applicable to clinical practice. The Infant Rapid Screen (IRS) is administered in 1 to 2 minutes on infants from 2 to 15 months. This is a developmental screening instrument for ages 2, 4, 6, 9, 12, and 15 months. The areas of evaluation of the IRS include social adaptive, fine motor, language-visual, and gross motor skills and reflexes. A simple yes or no answer determines the scores. A negative score in two or more areas is sufficient to recommend further evaluation. If one negative response is noted, the clinical evaluation of the person administering the IRS should determine if more in-depth evaluation is warranted. There is a high correlation between results of the IRS and results of the Denver Developmental Screening Test when the results of 380 infants and children with and without known risk factors are compared (Haber & Norris, 1991).

The Toddler Rapid Screen (TRS) is a developmental screening instrument for continuation of child evaluation for ages 18 months, 2 years, 2.5 years, and 3 years (Haber, 1992). The skills evaluated include social adaptive, language, fine motor, and gross motor skills. In a sample of 152 children to whom the TRS was administered, 23 subjects failed the TRS. A subsample of those passing the TRS indicated that 28 of 29 had an IQ greater than 95. Of the 23 children who failed the TRS, all but one had an IQ below 95 and impaired language skills (Haber, 1992). If a child has two or more negative responses on the age-matched screening evaluation, he or she should be tested with the test for the next-younger age group. If the child does not achieve the skills expected for the younger-age screen twice, referral for further evaluation is appropriate.

Using the same basic format as the IRS and the TRS, the Texas Preschool Screening Inventory was developed in the early 1980s (Haber & Norris, 1983) to identify children of ages 4 to 6 years who are at risk for language or learning difficulty. The test evaluates eight aspects of language and attention. It can be administered in 10 minutes without previous training. This test screens for auditory memory, visual memory, and auditory sequencing. If the child fails the visual and auditory portions of the test, she or he has more than a 50% chance of having difficulty in school; further evaluation should be instituted.

Discrete Testing of Cognitive Functioning

A third method of neuropsychologic evaluation involves administering tests that evaluate discrete functions. For example, the patient with Alzheimer's disease may be given only memory tests. Serial administration of these tests can then document incremental changes in memory over time. These specific tests are efficient and less demanding of the patient's and the examiner's time and concentration. However, the integration of the specific cognitive function into the total social functioning of the person will be missed by evaluating specific cognitive skills. The Galveston Orientation and Amnesia Test (GOAT) (Levin, O'Donnel, & Grossman, 1979) is a brief quantitative scale that measures orientation and memory. It is used specifically for evaluation of posttraumatic and retrograde amnesia. Questions address orientation to time, place, person, and present and past events. It is a 10-item scale, with a total sum as the score obtained. Deficits in memory and orientation exist if the score is below 66. A negative score of -100 is possible. (For more details, see Chapter 12).

INTEGRATION OF NURSING AND NEUROPSYCHOLOGIC ASSESSMENT

The most basic, yet essential, aspects of assessing cognitive processing are the interview with the client and the observations made during that interview. The interview helps identify the client's fund of knowledge based on age, culture, and educational background. The history the person and the family describe and observations of their interpersonal interactions provide extensive information for more in-depth evaluation. Subsequent evaluations can be viewed in the following context from the interview:

1. Communications—ability to speak, understand, and respond appropriately

2. Orientation—alertness and awareness of time, place, person, and situation at all times

3. Judgment—decision making governed by insight into self and situation

4. Emoting—ability to express full range of emotions

5. Coping—response to major stressors or presence of anxiety, tension headaches, or irritability

6. Social interaction—presence of family and support; ability to form relationships

If the interview suggests cognitive deficits (Table 11–3), further evaluation is often useful. The briefer neurobehavioral screening tests have pragmatic value in such clinical settings. Some tests are more specific than others; for example, the GOAT is useful when evaluating memory function. If evaluating for dementia, the SPMSQ or the MMS may be more useful. If there is interest in determining if a client can follow a series of complex instructions, as with diabetes management or driving a car after a head injury, or in corroborating inability to perform self-care, the NCSE is useful as a broader test of cognitive functioning in the acute care setting. These tests are easy to administer, inexpensive to score, and take little time to perform. They can be used in the test-retest, before and after treatment, and when observing for changes over time, and the client therefore serves as his or her own control. The information obtained from these tests is communicated easily to other health care providers and therefore is useful in planning and providing patient care. The usefulness of integrating formal testing and everyday observations can best be demonstrated through a case study.

TABLE 11–3 • GUIDELINES OF INDICATIONS TO FORMALIZE NEUROPSYCHOLOGIC ASSESSMENTS

- Patient or family describes changes in mental status or cognition.
- Behavior and responses are aberrant to situation in view of age, education, or culture.
- There is evidence of or concern about learning disabilities.
- There are difficulties with behavioral or psychologic problems or developmental psychosocial difficulties.
- There is evidence of difficulty adapting to change.

• C A S E   S T U D Y

Mr. G was a 53-year-old self-employed furniture upholsterer in good health except for a history of alcohol abuse. Two days before admission, he had complained of a severe headache and confusion. On the day of admission, Mr. G was found obtunded by his wife. After admission, he had a CT scan of the head and an arteriogram, which confirmed a subarachnoid hemorrhage. An aneurysm was located at the most caudal portion of the basilar artery.

On admission, Mr. G was drowsy but would open his eyes, respond appropriately to commands, and move all extremities. He was oriented to time, place, and person. He was aware that he had abnormal bleeding around his brain and that his condition was serious. His reduced attention span necessitated reiteration of his treatment plan and restrictions each time he was awakened. Although he smiled and was superficially socially appropriate, he did not appear unduly concerned about his life-threatening situation and slept most of the time. When questioned, he was able to describe the events leading up to his hospitalization as he drifted in and out of sleep. When he was awake, he recognized his family and would talk with them briefly. Attempts were made to administer the NCSE on three occasions. He was so drowsy that the test could never be completed. He never completed the naming or construction on the NCSE because he fell asleep (Fig. 11–1).

A week after his subarachnoid hemorrhage, Mr. G had a craniotomy with clipping of the basilar artery aneurysm. Postoperatively, his only noticeable neurologic deficit was a third cranial nerve palsy (eyelid ptosis, dilated pupil, and loss of adduction of the right eye). Subsequently, a head CT scan and arteriogram confirmed that the aneurysm had been successfully clipped.

The implications of any behavioral changes that the family may have noted in his behavior were masked by their relief that he had survived surgery. They verbalized that he was a little slower in his thinking and did not talk as spontaneously as before surgery. They thought that these changes would improve after he went home and recuperated. The nursing staff had noticed changes in Mr. G's behavior after surgery also; the preoperative gleam in his eyes had dulled, and his face was not as expressive or affectively spontaneous. He was also less spontaneous and did not initiate conversations as he had done before surgery. He required instruction to complete self-care activities, was passive in planning his own care, and was more dependent than he had been preoperatively.

Postoperatively, he was able to complete the NCSE. Cognitive deficits were identified in construction and memory (see Fig. 11–1). On the Trail Making Test (A and B) he had difficulty with sequencing and set changes. Discharge planning and family teaching centered on incorporating information from the NCSE and the Trail Making Test with potential problems at home. Mr. G was discharged from the hospital neurologically stable and was expected to have full recovery of cognitive deficits.

One month after surgery, Mr. G was evaluated by a physician who concluded that the patient's mental status had returned to normal. However, his family described his persistent difficulty in dressing himself, particularly in tying his shoes. On many days he would not even get out of bed. Mr. G did not acknowledge these difficulties as problems but attributed them to his worsening vision. His wife and mother-in-law had to attend to his upholstery business because he was unable to resume work.

In view of the family history and because Mr. G's cognitive abilities had not improved as expected, the NCSE was repeated. Mr. G's verbal communication and verbal judgment

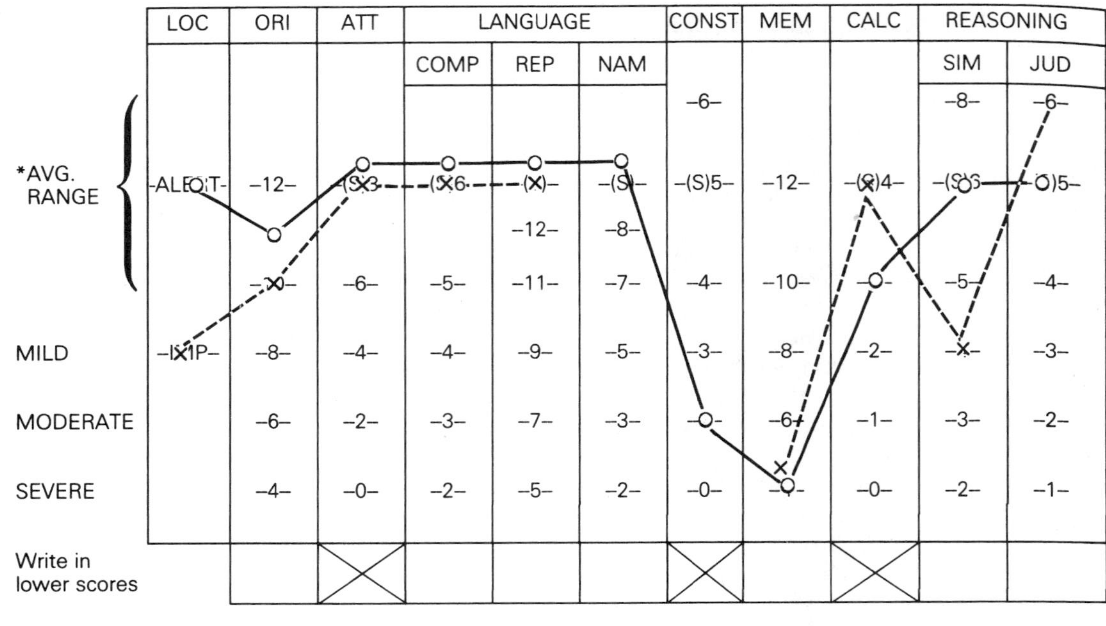

FIGURE 11–1 • The cognitive status profile of a patient diagnosed with an aneurysm. The x–x path indicates the preoperative aneurysm clipping profile; the o–o path indicates the profile 2 weeks after the aneurysm clipping.

were within normal limits, but construction and ability to follow through and complete tasks were markedly impaired (Fig. 11–2). Because the NCSE results indicated persistent cognitive deficits, a repeat head CT scan was performed that demonstrated enlargement of the ventricles and communicating hydrocephalus (a common complication of subarachnoid hemorrhage). He was admitted to the hospital, where he had a lumboperitoneal shunt surgically implanted.

Six weeks after the shunting, Mr. G returned to the clinic with a gleam in his eye and an engaging smile. He was taking care of himself without any assistance from his family and was back at work full-time. The follow-up head CT scan confirmed resolution of the hydrocephalus. His NCSE results were now within the normal range (see Fig. 11–2).

For Mr. G, the neuropsychologic tests initially guided the family discharge planning. When he did not continue to improve as expected, the NCSE confirmed the persistence of cognitive impairment beyond what was expected. The resulting medical evaluation and surgical intervention corrected the underlying medical problem. Subsequently, the NCSE, with repeated testing, confirmed the return of cognitive function, which was substantiated by Mr. G's return to work and ability to function independently.

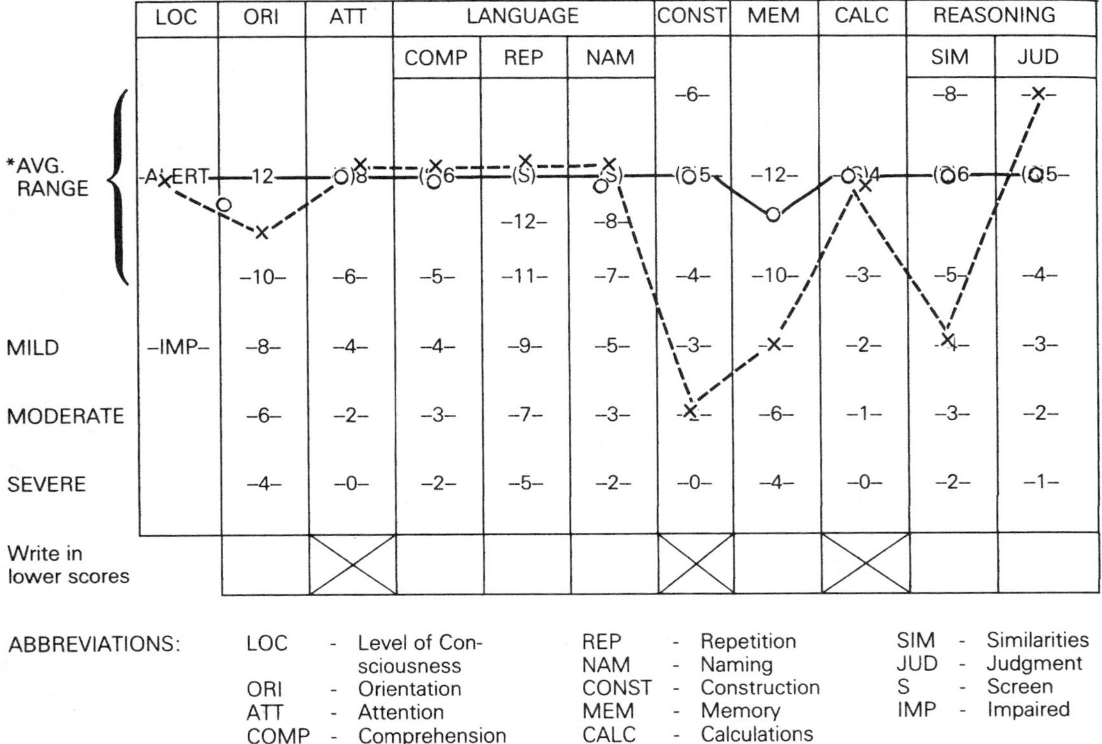

FIGURE 11–2 • The cognitive status profile of a patient diagnosed with hydrocephalus. The x–x path indicates the preoperative shunting profile; the o–o path indicates the profile 10 weeks after shunting.

If the screening evaluation is considered incomplete or if isolated new or progressive changes are identified, then further neuropsychologic testing is warranted. Formal neuropsychologic tests are administered by neuropsychologists to obtain more precise and extensive information about the individual's cognitive ability. Such testing is time consuming and costly and has limited clinical value in the acute care setting because of fluctuations in the client's health status. The tests are useful, however, to obtain specific information on all aspects of cognition not available by cursory evaluation using the less sophisticated neuropsychologic screening tests.

The value of effective, accurate assessment to ensure appropriate client assessment, nursing diagnosis, and interventions cannot be overemphasized. The nurse is in the unique position of spending more time than does any other health professional with the patient and family. The nurse makes the initial interview assessment, may perform brief specific or screening neuropsychologic tests, and observes the moment-to-moment behavior of the patient. After further evaluation, the nurse can integrate the findings of the neuropsychologic assessment into real-life interventions to improve the quality of patient care and patient self-esteem and to develop realistic long-term planning for and with the patient and family.

References

Anthony, J. C., LeResche, L., Niaz, U., Von Korff, M. R., & Folstein, M. F. (1982). Limits of the Mini-Mental State, a screening test for dementia and delirium among hospital patients. *Psychological Medicine, 12,* 397.

Brown, E. C., Cased, A., Fisch, R. I., & Neuringer, C. (1958). Trailmaking test as a screening device for the detection of brain damage. *Journal of Consultinq Psychology, 22*(6), 469.

Buron, O. K. (Ed.) (1978). *The eight mental measurement yearbook.* Minneapolis: Gryphon Press.

Conn, H. O. (1977). Trailmaking and number-connection tests in the assessment of mental state in portal systemic encephalopathy. *Digestive Disease, 22*(6), 541.

Davies, A. (1968). The influence of age on trailmaking test performance. *Journal of Clinical Psychology, 24,* 96.

Davis, R. D., Adams, R. E., Gates, D. O., & Cheramie, G. M. (1989). Screening for learning disabilities: A neuropsychological approach. *Journal of Clinical Psychology, 45*(3), 423.

Derogatis, L. R. (1977). *SCL-90: Manual for the revised version.* Baltimore, MD: Johns Hopkins University Press.

Dick, J. P. R., Gjuiloff, R. J. H., Steward, A., Blackstock, J., Bielawska, C., Paul, E. A., & Marsden, C. D. (1984). Mini-Mental State examination in neurological patients. *Journal of Neurology, Neurosurgery, and Psychiatry, 47,* 496.

Folstein, M. F., Folstein, S. E., & McHugh, P. R. (1975). Mini-Mental State, a practical method for grading the cognitive state of patients for the clinician. *Journal of Psychiatric Research, 12,* 189.

Frankenburg, W. K., Dodds, J., & Fandal, A. (1970). *The Denver Developmental Screening Test manual.* Denver, CO: University of Colorado Press.

Greer, S., Bauchner, H., & Zuckerman, B. (1989). The Denver Developmental Screening Test: How good is its predictive validity? *Developmental Medicine and Child Neurology, 31,* 774.

Haber, J. S. (1992). *Toddler Rapid Screen.* Fort Worth, TX: Department of Communication Sciences and Disorders, Texas Christian University.

Haber, J. S., & Norris, M. L. (1983). *Texas Preschool Screening Inventory manual.* Fort Worth, TX: Department of Communication Sciences and Disorders, Texas Christian University.

Haber, J. S., & Norris, M. L. (1991). *Infant Rapid Screen: IRS.* Fort Worth, TX: Department of Communication Sciences and Disorders, Texas Christian University. Reviewed in *American Family Physician,* January, 1991.

Hooijer, C., Dinkgreve, M., Jonker, C., & Lindeboom, J. (1992). Short screening tests for dementia in the elderly population. I: A comparison between AMTS, MMSE, MSQ and SPMSQ. *International Journal of Geriatric Psychiatry, 7,* 559.

Jacobs, J. W., Bernhard, M. R., Delgado, A., & Strain, J. J. (1977). Screening for organic mental syndromes in the medically ill. *Annals on Internal Medicine, 86*(1), 42.

Kahn, R. L., Goldfarb, A. I., Pollack, M., & Peck, A. (1960). Brief objective measures for the determination of mental status in the aged. *American Journal of Psychiatry, 117,* 326.

Kiernan, R., Mueller, J., Langston, J. W., & Van Dyke, C. (1987). The Neurobehavioral Cognitive Status Examination: A brief but differentiated approach to cognitive assessment. *Annals of Internal Medicine, 107,* 481.

Levin, H. S., O'Donnel, V. M., & Grossman, R. G. (1979). The Galveston Orientation and Amnesia Test. *Journal of Nervous and Mental Diseases, 167*(11), 675.

Lezak, M. (1985). *Neuropsychological assessment* (2nd ed.). New York: Oxford University Press.

Luria, A. R. (1973). *The working brain.* New York: Basic Books.

Mueller, J. (1984). The mental status examination. In H. H. Goldman (Ed.), *A review of general psychiatry* (p. 206). Los Angeles: Lange.

Myers, B. A. (1987). The Mini Mental State in those with developmental disabilities. *Journal of Nervous and Mental Disease, 175*(2), 85.

O'Donnell, J. P., Romero, J. J., & Leicht, D. J. (1990). A comparison of language deficits in learning-disabled, head-injured, and nondisabled young adults: Results from an abbreviated aphasia screening test. *Journal of Clinical Psychology, 46*(3), 310.

Pfeiffer, R. (1975). A Short Portable Mental Status Questionnaire for the assessment of organic deficits in elderly patients. *Journal of the American Geriatrics Society, 23*(10), 433.

Plum, F., & Posner, J. B. (1980). *Diagnosis of stupor and coma* (2nd ed.). Philadelphia: F.A. Davis.

Reitan, R. M. (1955). The relation of the Trail Making Test to organic brain damage. *Journal of Consultinq Psychology, 19*(5), 393.

Reitan, R. M. (1987). *Neuropsychological evaluation of children.* Tucson, AZ: Neuropsychology.

Reitan, R. M., & Tarshes, E. L. (1959). Differential effects of lateralized brain lesions on the Trail Making Test. *Journal of Nervous and Mental Disease, 129,* 257.

Reitan, R. M., & Wolfson, D. (1992). A short screening examination for impaired brain functions in early school-age children. *Clinical Neuropsychologist, 63,* 287.

Stanczak, D. (1986). *Trail Making Test—forms X & Y.* Unpublished tests.

Weiner, H. L., Bresnan, M. J., & Levitt, L. P. (1981). *Pediatric neurology for the house officer* (2nd ed.). Baltimore, MD: Williams & Wilkins.

Williams, P. D., & Williams, A. R. (1987). Denver Developmental Screening Test norms: A cross-cultural comparison. *Journal of Pediatric Psychology, 12*(1), 39.

Alterations in Memory

REBECCA A. SISSON

A frequent sequela of brain disturbances is a change in the ability to remember. Loss of memory for events concurrent with traumatic injury or disease onset is a consistent clinical feature. Alteration in memory is categorized as a cognitive deficit and is a complex phenomenon that encompasses a variety of higher cortical functions. Intact memory is evidence of higher cortical functioning.

The loss of memory occurs as the consequence of many types of neurologic disorders. These disorders affect individuals across the life span and can be developmental, degenerative, traumatic, or a result of exposure to toxic substances. There is increasing evidence that alterations or deficiencies in neurotransmitters have an effect on memory. Loss of memory, or amnesia, is a symptom of either a physiologic or a psychologic disturbance. The impact of memory loss is similar regardless of the age of the person affected and regardless of the cause.

In physiologic disturbances, the symptom indicates a change in usual function and rarely occurs in isolation. The person with amnesia probably also has other symptoms, such as weakness, sensory loss, or mood swings. The nature of these associated problems will vary according to the location of the lesion. Physiologically based memory problems can originate at the storage or the retrieval stage of memory development, with different pathologies producing one or both disturbances in memory processing.

Memory traces are not localized to any one brain structure. Neurons show many kinds of plasticity, and all parts of the nervous system appear to have the plastic properties needed for memory storage. However, the hippocampus and the temporal lobes seem to be the most important in human memory processing (Kupfermann, 1985; Squire, 1987).

In disorders of psychologic function, the symptom of memory loss is frequently associated with other symptoms such as depression and difficulty concentrating (Straub & Black, 1985). Memory loss is very disorganizing whether the cause is physiologic or psychologic, and it is often difficult to differentiate between organic and psychiatric disease.

THEORIES OF MEMORY

Research has shown that there are multiple memory systems. This complex and integrated set of systems allows an individual to remember and learn. Memory has been defined by Squire (1987) as the persistence of learning in a state that can be revealed at a later time. Three stages of memory have been identified; information is (1) received and registered, (2) stored, and (3) retrieved. Once something has been learned, the ability to remember varies depending on the task, the retrieval effectiveness, and the individual's current physiologic state. For learning to occur, the experience must be imprinted. An engram is the set of changes in the nervous system that represents stored memory.

Memory storage occurs in different areas of the brain depending on the type of memory system. Studies using neuroimaging techniques have provided evidence that these memory systems have different mechanisms of operation, process different types of information, and use different brain structures for operation (Squire, 1992). The most widely accepted subsystems of memory are short-term memory and long-term memory. These two subsystems have been further subdivided according to the type of information being processed. Working memory is considered a component of short-term memory, and declarative memory and nondeclarative memory are subsystems of long-term memory.

Short-Term Memory

Also known as primary memory to some researchers, short-term memory is said to be immediate—the information is reproduced rapidly, having never left consciousness. This ability allows an individual to keep several aspects of a problem in mind while trying to reach a solution or to keep temporarily in mind the elements of information being presented so that conclusions can be drawn. Recall is easy for a limited amount of information, and there is a tendency for rapid decay—for example, looking up a telephone number and remembering it just long enough to dial the number. For short-term memory storage, attention is necessary.

The theory of a working memory was initially proposed by Baddeley and Hitch and suggested that working memory had two components, an attentional loop and an articulatory loop (Baddeley, 1984). These components allowed for temporary storage of a limited amount of information. Further research reported by Baddeley (1992) elaborated on the theory and proposed that there are three components. This model includes a central executive or attentional controller and two slave systems, the articulatory loop or phonologic loop and the visuospatial sketchpad. The central executive has several functions, which include controlling attention and coordinating information from separate subsystems. The phonologic loop is responsible for maintaining and processing speech-based information and assists in verbal learning. The visuospatial sketchpad is responsible for registering visuospatial information such as pictures, patterns, or patches of color. Because working memory has been more extensively studied, the components of this theory are more widely accepted.

Long-Term Memory

Frequently called secondary or remote memory, this memory store has been shown to effect actual structural, synaptic change in the brain. This physical change is what allows memories from the past to be retained. The imprinting or engram occurs when the information or experience has specific meaning for the individual. Long-term memory is divided into two subsystems: the declarative or fact memory and the nondeclarative or procedural memory.

Declarative memory allows the recollection of facts and events—for example, knowing the name of the current president or the dates of parents' birthdays. Declarative memory is described as explicit and has two components: episodic memory, which stores information about facts and events that are personal or autobiographic, and semantic memory, which stores general knowledge, world facts, and concepts.

Nondeclarative memory is known as procedural or implicit. This memory system functions to help us learn skills, develop habits, or acquire conditioned responses. Because of implicit memory, we are influenced by previous experience, and this affects how we react to similar situations. According to Squire (1992), this is called priming and facilitates performance because recent experience improves the ability to process a perceptual object.

Patients with amnesia seem to retain an intact implicit or nondeclarative memory but have severe impairment of explicit or declarative memory. Research indicates that this is because declarative memory is fast and accessible to conscious recollection whereas nondeclarative memory is unconscious (Squire, 1992). This helps explain why amnesic patients have memory deficits for new knowledge but can easily recall past experiences or retain old habits.

Sensory Memory

This type of memory is of interest to some researchers who study memory systems, but it is generally believed to be a part of both short-term and long-term memory. Information from a range of sensory input channels influences memory storage. Visual, tactile, auditory, and gustatory stimuli may enhance memory. Most sensory information is believed to be stored only temporarily; however, certain sensory stimuli can evoke past memories. Patients have related that pleasant odors, music, or the taste of a favorite food has brought past experiences to mind. Sensory stimulation is a current therapeutic mechanism being used in the treatment of comatose patients to promote increased cognitive functioning (Baddeley, Bressi, Della, Logie, & Spinnler, 1991).

The research on memory and memory systems is rapidly producing knowledge about how memories are stored, where they are stored, and what can be done to enhance memory function. Multiple forms of memory exist, and different areas of the brain store memories; thus this complex system with many different characteristics offers a challenge to those who study and diagnose memory disorders.

PATHOPHYSIOLOGY OF MEMORY LOSS

An alteration in memory can result from a variety of central nervous system pathologies, including infection, tumors, seizure disorders, strokes, toxicity, metabolic response, or trauma. Across the life span, the pathology of memory problems can usually be categorized into age groups. In children and adolescents, memory problems are associated with developmental disorders, trauma, seizure disorders, and toxic substances or drugs. The young to middle-aged adult can have memory difficulties resulting from metabolic disturbances, infection, trauma, tumors, or progressive neurologic diseases. The older adult and elderly person have memory disorders primarily from neurologic disease, degenerative brain disorders, and trauma.

The mechanisms producing changes in the structure of nervous tissue that result in memory loss are multiple. The following general categories will be used to describe the types of pathology that produce memory problems: developmental, metabolic, degenerative, and traumatic. The specific mechanisms for each category will be described as well as research related to the diagnostic categories.

Developmental

Difficulties with memory are poorly addressed during the developmental years. Cognitive deficits, including those of memory, are seen in learning-disabled children, speech-disordered children, children with seizure disorders, and children receiving cancer therapy. Very little research has been done related to memory problems in children. One study by Rodgers, Britton, Morris, Kemahan, and Craft (1992) reported on memory impairment in children following treatment for acute lymphoblastic leukemia. This study found that these children had significant memory deficits in tasks that required planning. Short-term memory impairment was found in a pilot study of adolescents with heavy marijuana use (Schartz, Gruenewald, Klitzner, & Fedio, 1989). These were 14- to 16-year-olds in a drug treatment program, and after 6 drug-free weeks there was still significant impairment of short-term auditory and visual memory. It was also noted by the authors that children with learning disabilities are at risk for marijuana addiction. Because there is so little research describing memory deficits in children with developmental difficulties, it is hard to know the extent of the problem.

Possibly included in the developmental category is the loss of memory during pregnancy. Two studies by the same group of researchers found significant impairment of recall memory in women with normal pregnancies (Brindle, Brown, Brown, Griffith, & Turner, 1991; Sharp, Brindle, Brown, & Turner, 1993).

The cause of this impairment does not appear to be physiologic and is present in all trimesters. This is obviously an area that needs further study and could have implications for the health care education of pregnant women.

A newly defined memory disorder is termed age-associated memory impairment (AAMI) and is found in nondemented persons age 50 years and older (Baddeley et al., 1991). This is believed to be a normal decline in memory and is associated with normal developmental processes (aging). The criteria for the diagnosis of AAMI are age of at least 50 years; difficulty with rapid recall and with remembering names, items to be purchased, and telephone numbers, as well as misplacement of objects; impairment on memory test performance; adequate intellectual function; and absence of dementia. This decline in memory is gradual, but it causes problems for middle-aged and older adults who are still engaged in intellectually demanding jobs or other activities.

Metabolic

Not only can memory be affected by direct injury or degeneration of the brain, but it can also be affected by metabolic and endocrine disorders. There is increasing evidence in the literature that metabolic imbalance or disturbances can have permanent effects on cognitive function.

A study by Sachon et al. (1992) examined the effects of severe hypoglycemic episodes on the cognitive function of insulin-dependent diabetics. Their results support other studies that demonstrated permanent memory impairment in insulin-dependent diabetics who had experienced several severe hypoglycemic episodes producing coma.

Another endocrine disorder that seems to affect memory is Cushing's disease. Patients with Cushing's disease as well as persons treated with large doses of corticosteroids have been shown to develop cognitive disturbances. A study to evaluate memory impairment in patients with Cushing's disease showed a moderate degree of impairment, and this impairment increased with age (Mauri et al., 1993).

Since the 1980s, there has been more evidence to show a relationship between cardiovascular disease and cognitive dysfunction. Decreased cardiac output and dysrhythmias as a result of myocardial infarction, cardiac surgery, and cardiac arrest have been shown to produce impaired intellectual function and cognitive dysfunction. A study assessed memory and cognitive abilities of patients undergoing permanent pacemaker implantation (Rockwood, Dobbs, Rule, Howlett, & Black, 1992). The results indicated a high prevalence of cognitive impairment in patients with complete heart block (Cerny & McNeny, 1983). These data lend support to the idea of a relationship between hypoperfusion and impaired cognitive ability. Short-term memory seemed to be most affected, and pacemaker implantation produced only minimal improvement in some of the patients.

Degenerative

Certain neurologic diseases have associated cognitive deficits, including memory loss. In Parkinson's disease, there are a number of neuropsychologic disturbances, one of these being memory function. Episodic memory, auditory verbal learning, spontaneous recall, and procedural memory have all been found to be impaired (Levin, Tomer, & Rey, 1992). Although patients with Parkinson's disease seem to have minimal difficulty in memory storage, they do have a problem with retrieval and high-order processing.

Memory difficulty is one of the most common complaints of patients with multiple sclerosis (MS). A review article by Mahler (1992) describes the types of memory disturbances seen in MS. Immediate and delayed recall, remote memory, and anterograde memory have all been found to be affected. This indicates that the primary area of difficulty is retrieval. Of interest is the fact that chronic progressive MS seems to produce greater memory problems than does the relapsing-remitting type.

The incidence of memory problems in patients with epilepsy has been frequently reported. Often the source of the problem is the underlying pathology of brain tumor, trauma, or cerebrovascular disease. Most research on seizure disorders has shown that temporal lobe origin of seizures puts an individual at more risk for memory problems. Another risk factor for persons with epilepsy is age of onset. Onset of epilepsy during adolescence places one at risk for learning and memory difficulties (Thompson, 1991). The most commonly reported problems are difficulty learning new material and impaired recent memory (e.g., patients forgetting what they were told the day before).

One of the most frequently occurring degenerative disorders is dementia. This term applies to chronic encephalopathy, which results in such severe deterioration of intellectual function that there is interference with personal and social activities (American Psychiatric Association, 1980). The most classic symptom of dementia is memory impairment, particularly recall of recent information. As the degeneration progresses, recent and remote recall are impaired.

Alzheimer's disease (AD) is a type of dementia that has impaired memory as its earliest symptom. The memory deficit in AD is the inability to learn new material, indicating that imprinting does not occur. Baddeley et al. (1991) suggest that the central executive function of working memory is impaired in AD. This function is to coordinate information from several different sources and requires the ability to sustain attention. Patients with AD have difficulty in this area.

Korsakoff's syndrome is a degenerative brain disease with predominantly frontal lobe atrophy; it is attributed to alcoholism. This syndrome includes impaired recent memory, defective retrieval of retrograde memory, and confabulation.

Traumatic

The most common cause of memory loss is trauma. Included as trauma are closed head injury, skull fracture, stroke, and missile injury. Trauma causes a disruption in blood flow, in neuroconduction, and in neurotransmission. Also, with trauma there may be actual tissue loss. Posttraumatic amnesia (PTA) is the period following trauma when the person lacks the ability to acquire and retrieve new information. The duration of PTA is thought to be predictive of outcome—the longer the duration of PTA, the poorer the outcome.

Anterograde amnesia and retrograde amnesia are memory deficits usually attributed to trauma. Anterograde amnesia is the loss of memory of events after the trauma and is also the inability to learn new material. During this period, the person may be aware of his or her surroundings but unable to store memory of the events. Disorientation may be present during the period of anterograde amnesia.

Retrograde amnesia refers to loss of memory of events before the brain injury. This memory rarely returns, and it is believed that the events are not stored as a result of the physiologic disruption associated with trauma. Although retrograde amnesia tends to be relatively short, there are cases in which the amnesia extends back several months. As PTA resolves, the retrograde amnesia shrinks. Resolution of the amnesia generally occurs to the point that the immediate events related to the injury are the only missing pieces.

There is increasing evidence of memory problems following minimal or mild traumatic brain injury (MTBI). A review article by Szymanski and Linn (1992) described the neuropsychologic changes following MTBI. Memory problems were reported in all the studies on MTBI. The definition of MTBI is loss of consciousness of less than 30 minutes and a Glasgow Coma Score of 12 to 15. In the past, it was believed that these patients would experience no significant signs or symptoms of neurologic dysfunction. A study by Strugar, Sass, Buchanan, Spencer, & Lowe (1993) reported that patients with minimal brain injury, some without loss of consciousness, continue to have memory problems for up to 2 years after trauma. Thus, even minor traumatic brain injury has the potential to cause persistent memory impairment.

DIAGNOSES OF SPECIFIC PATHOPHYSIOLOGY

The diagnosis and treatment of memory disorders is complex and challenging. When local brain lesions can be identified, it appears that memory disturbances are specific to regions of the brain. Luria (1976) was the first to describe specific areas of the brain where certain memory functions are located. Memories are known to be stored in multiple regions of the brain. Memory storage can be localized, but complex memory requires several brain areas. It is difficult to localize the region of injury in many cases of brain trauma, however, especially in the severely injured patient with coma lasting longer than a week. Frequently, it is not possible to assess memory function accurately after brain injury because of associated depression, distractibility, and poor concentration. It is best to assess each patient individually, because no true pattern of memory disturbance can be identified according to location of lesion.

Three categories of neuropathology are used in this chapter to organize and illustrate the appropriate nursing management when alteration in memory occurs. These categories are (1) stroke, (2) head injury, and (3) brain lesion. Although other pathologies produce memory loss, these are the most common. (The principles used to intervene when these conditions exist can be applied to other neuropathologic disturbances.)

Impaired Long-Term Memory and Recall Ability

• C A S E   S T U D Y   1

Stroke

Mrs. L, a 78-year-old woman, was admitted with the diagnosis of stroke, right hemiparesis. She was stuporous and appeared dehydrated. She responded to pain, moved her left side spontaneously, and opened her eyes when she heard her name. The pupils were equal and reactive, and the cranial nerves were normal. Mrs. L became aware, in several days, that she was in the hospital. She was confused by her surroundings and did not remember coming to the hospital. She did not know what day it was or how much time had passed. When the nurse came into her room, Mrs. L tried to ask what had happened. The words would not come, and the sounds that she heard herself making were strange. The nurse, in a loud voice, told Mrs. L that she had had a stroke and was going to be all right. Mrs. L was very upset; she could not remember anything.

Gradually, in the course of a week, Mrs. L began to make herself understood, and some words were becoming easier to remember. She was still confused about many things. A general physical assessment and neurologic examination revealed a well-nourished but slightly dehydrated woman. All findings were essentially normal except for right upper extremity weakness and decreased sensation to light touch. The right lower extremity could perform gross motor movement; sensation was intact.

To assess memory, orientation, and other cognitive abilities, the Galveston Orientation and Amnesia Test (GOAT) and the Neurobehavioral Rating Scale (NRS) were used. The GOAT score was 54, indicating impairment (a score of 65 or less indicates impairment). The NRS score showed a moderately severe rating on conceptional disorganization, memory deficit, and decreased initiative; a moderate rating on expressive deficit and poor planning; and a mild rating on anxiety, agitation, depressed mood, and inaccurate insight and self-appraisal.

Observations and direct questions revealed that Mrs. L could not remember her address and did not know where she was, except that she was in a hospital. (She did not know the hospital's name.) Mrs. L stated that she remembered nothing before awakening in the hospital room. She was able to name three articles correctly after 5 minutes and to describe her sister's visit the previous evening. She could not describe the exercise taught to her by the physical therapist. The appropriate nursing diagnosis was altered thought processes related to loss of memory as evidenced by impaired recall ability.

At this stage of recovery, the most important nursing intervention is to provide reality orientation and memory cues. Mrs. L's sister, her only relative, should be included in the planning, teaching, and reorienting. A calendar and clock should be used to reinforce time and date orientation. The large printed name of the hospital and Mrs. L's room number near the bedside will orient her to place. Personal belongings and reminders of home will provide the stimuli to remind her of where she lives. A daily schedule should be posted to remind Mrs. L of mealtimes and of times for physical therapy, speech therapy, and occupational therapy.

Most important is a consistent approach. All staff and the patient's sister should use the same cues. Short, simple phrases are best for giving instructions, and positive reinforcement will provide encouragement. The outcome criteria for this patient are that she will remember the day, time, and place; recall her home and address; and relate her daily routine schedule.

Impaired Long-Term Memory and Retention Ability

• C A S E   S T U D Y   2

Head Injury

Mike was recovering from a closed head injury. He also had abdominal injuries, requiring a splenectomy, and a lumbar fracture that was fused. The critical period was past, and he was in a rehabilitation program. The physical weakness in his right arm and leg had greatly improved, and he was able to walk without a cane. There was still a slight problem with fine motor movement and coordination in his right hand.

It had been 3 months since the automobile accident that resulted in Mike's head injury, and he had been in a coma for 6 days. Since regaining consciousness, he had made remarkable recovery, and his prognosis was favorable. In talking with Mike, it became evident that there were areas of memory difficulty. He had no memory of the events just before the accident; his last memory was of a friend's wedding 1 month before the accident.

The physical and neurologic examination assessments were essentially normal except for right-side weakness of the face, arm, and leg. The computed tomographic (CT) scan done after the injury revealed a left cerebral contusion with temporal lobe hemorrhage. A mental status evaluation revealed good short-term memory but retrograde amnesia for 1 month before the injury and PTA of approximately 1 month. The GOAT score was 75, which is in the borderline range.

Mike described his memory as "not good" and said he had trouble concentrating, especially when reading. He denied experiencing headaches or dizziness. He stated that his right arm and leg were weak and that he had decreased vision in his right eye. The rating on the NRS indicated a moderate expressive deficit, memory deficit, and inaccurate insight and self-appraisal. Mike was a dentist and said he planned to go back to work soon after returning home. The nursing diagnosis was altered thought processes related to loss of memory as evidenced by impaired remote memory and impaired retention.

Family involvement is critical in the planning and use of selected techniques in intervention. Mike will require many memory cues from his family and friends. Reminders of home, such as pictures, letters, and personal items, will help resolve the PTA. Practicing activities of daily living in a realistic setting will be beneficial in reminding Mike of his previous routines. Gaining skill in reading and in following instructions will mean practice in short sessions to decrease tiring and loss of concentration. A notebook may be helpful for taking notes that will aid memory.

Mike's lack of insight into his deficiency is a difficult problem. Reviewing books of dental procedures and practice may help Mike; however, his alteration in memory may not become evident to him until he actually tries to go back to work. The family should be prepared to cope with this situation. The outcome criteria for this client are that he will recall home and describe the setting, describe the acute care hospital before the rehabilitation unit, demonstrate the ability to recall events and retain information, and discuss decisions related to his future plans.

Impaired Short-Term Memory and Retention Ability

• C A S E   S T U D Y   3

Brain Lesion

Mr. S was a 71-year-old man admitted with a diagnosis of left frontoparietotemporal mass, possibly a cyst. Over the past several months, he had progressively developed temporal area headache, personality change, loss of short-term memory, and dementia. The CT scan localized a large, fluid-filled cyst, and surgery was performed to remove it.

In the postoperative assessment, Mr. S had essentially normal physical and neurologic findings. Some right homonymous hemianopia persisted, and he remained disoriented and confused.

Mental status examination revealed a GOAT score of 50, which is in the impaired range. Mr. S was not oriented to time and place and could not remember events before surgery. When questioned about his memory, he stated that it wasn't "too good." He could not remember what he had for breakfast or if the doctor had visited.

When the family was interviewed, they were very concerned about Mr. S's memory. He constantly repeated himself and did not seem able to retain anything he was told. He would get lost as soon as he left his hospital room. The family expressed apprehension about Mr. S's return home. The nursing diagnosis was altered thought processes related to loss of memory as evidenced by impaired short-term memory.

Initially, Mr. S will need constant reality orientation. Nursing intervention includes reminding him of the time, date, and place whenever possible. A large calendar near the bed and a clock can be used as aids. Mr. S will also need aids to remind him of personal hygiene routines and daily schedules. It often is helpful to label drawers, cabinets, and closets with their contents; for example, the bathroom cabinet could have a label that says "razor." Another helpful aid is a list of activities or instructions in the appropriate room at home. The family could be instructed to post lists in the bathroom (e.g., instructions to wash face and hands, brush teeth, and shave) and in the kitchen (e.g., instructions for making coffee). Mr. S can be helped to learn to write everything in a notebook, especially messages, appointments, and names. Important telephone numbers should be posted by the phone along with the names.

The family should be involved from the beginning in suggesting interventions and in learning about techniques to aid memory. The family must understand the importance of allowing Mr. S to be as independent as possible; he should be encouraged to do as much as he is able and gradually to increase the complexity of his activities. The outcome criteria are that Mr. S will be able to state the day and time, relate information about activities of the day, and carry out personal hygiene.

MANIFESTATIONS OF MEMORY DEFICIT

In the past, there has not been an emphasis on assessment of mental status, including memory, by nurses. One reason for this has been the lack of instruments or assessment guides. Mental assessment is an area that nurses have generally left to physicians and psychologists because there has been little in the nursing literature to provide guidance. However, with increased knowledge and advanced training, the neuroscience nurse has begun to develop tools for assessing cognitive function, communication skills, and memory.

There are several reports in the literature of tools developed and used by nurses to assess cognitive function after head trauma (Brooks, 1983; Crosby & Parsons, 1989; Dowling, 1985; Turner, Kreutzer, Lent, & Brockett, 1984; Warren, Goethe, & Peck, 1984). Such general assessment of cognitive function is described in Chapter 11. Specific memory assessment aids are discussed in this chapter.

Initial Assessment

The neuroscience nurse has the knowledge and skill to assess patients' neurologic function accurately. Physical and mental assessment are required to plan appropriate nursing care. An important part of the assessment is obtaining a pertinent history. Because patients with memory problems frequently deny difficulty or confabulate information, patient answers should be verified so that accuracy of responses can be determined. The chart, the physician, other health care providers, and the family are all resources to verify data. Accurate assessment is often difficult in patients with memory disturbances because of associated problems such as attention disorders, poor concentration, lack of insight, and confusion.

The initial assessment includes the nursing history, which contains the following information: (1) individual's description of present problem; (2) past illnesses and injuries; (3) coping mechanisms; (4) education level; (5) occupation; (6) family, interpersonal, and social information; and (7) usual daily activities—sleeping, waking, eating, and activity patterns. This information is essential to plan care and establish realistic outcome goals.

A thorough physical assessment is also important, and special attention should be given to motor and sensory evaluation. Sensory deficits can affect performance in activities of daily living and in therapeutic regimens. Visual problems, hearing loss, and decreased sensation can cause difficulty for the patient and can interfere with memory-training techniques.

Any missing information or additional data should be obtained from family members. It is especially important to have the family's perspective on the patient's personality and previous coping mechanisms. Alteration in memory is very frustrating, and it is helpful to have family input and involvement from the beginning. The more comprehensive the assessment, the more likely it is that the neuroscience nurse will arrive at an accurate diagnosis and treatment plan. Many creative and individualized aids could be developed by the nurse to identify problems in remembering daily routines.

Behavioral Observations

In the day-to-day interaction with a patient, the neuroscience nurse can make many observations that provide evidence of a memory problem. The most obvious manifestation is forgetting—names, dates, events, activities, current news, appointments, or visitors. Casual conversation with some specific questions interjected can disclose gaps in memory. It is important to determine whether new (recent) or old (remote) memory is affected. Such questions as "When were you born?" "What time did you wake up today?" "Where did you go on vacation last year?" "Who were the visitors here yesterday?" "When is your physical therapy appointment?" and "What year did you graduate from school?" are helpful in determining which type of memory loss is present. Another manifestation of memory alteration is losing items or getting lost. Not remembering where items are placed, where personal articles are stored, which door is to the bathroom, what direction to take to physical therapy, or how to find one's room are all common occurrences for a person who suffers from memory deficits.

Determining whether a patient can follow through on a series of activities of self-care identifies areas of memory loss. Does the person remember when to get up, bathe, dress appropriately, and eat breakfast, or does he or she forget some items in the sequence? It is particularly important when discharge is anticipated to determine if the deficit affects activities of daily living. An ongoing assessment and observation of memory function will provide the nurse with valuable data for making a nursing diagnosis and planning interventions.

Formal Assessment Tools

Another method for assessing memory is the use of tools developed by nurses and other health professionals for this purpose. Objective data can be obtained that may help pinpoint specific problem areas of memory function. Several such tools are listed in Table 12–1. The author, in collaboration with Levin et al. (1987), developed the NRS, which is designed to assess 27 areas of cognitive and behavioral sequelae of head trauma. It was first tested on 108 head-injured patients, and high interrater reliability was obtained. This author used the NRS to evaluate cognitive and emotional outcomes of stroke and found a significant correlation between cognitive dysfunction and functional ability in activities of daily living (Sisson, 1992). Memory loss is one item for which the NRS is

TABLE 12–1 • TOOLS TO ASSESS MEMORY AND COGNITIVE DEFICITS

Tool	Author
Wechsler Memory Scale	Wechsler (1945)
Galveston Orientation and Amnesia Test	Levin et al. (1979)
Disability Rating Scale	Rappaport et al. (1982)
Neurobehavioral Rating Scale	Levin et al. (1987)
Brief Neuropsychological Mental Status Exam	Turner et al. (1984)
Mini-Mental State	Folstein et al. (1975)
Neurobehavioral Cognitive Status Examination	Kiernan et al. (1987)
Crook's battery	Crook et al. (1990)

very sensitive. A brief, structured interview is used by the clinician to obtain data, followed by the rating, which is done without the patient present. The interview and rating take less than 30 minutes. This rating scale requires minimal training and is useful in evaluating neurobehavioral status over time. A nurse specialist can easily use this tool to assess outcomes after various types of head trauma and stroke.

Another tool, the GOAT, is useful during the early stages after head trauma to document the resolution of PTA (Fig. 12–1) (Levin, O'Donnell, & Grossman, 1979). The author has used it to assess recovering stroke victims; however, a brief orientation test has proven to be more useful in assessing stroke victims (Fig. 12–2).

Mental status examinations are another source of data for the nurse in making a comprehensive assessment. These tests identify which aspects of memory are affected and which are intact. Usually such testing is done by a

Name ____   Date of Test ⌊__⌊__⌊__⌋
Age _________ Sex   M   F   mo day yr
Date of Birth ⌊__⌊__⌊__⌋   Day of the week s m t w th f s
              mo day yr   Time   AM   PM
Diagnosis ____________________________________   Date of injury ⌊__⌊__⌊__⌋
                                                                     mo day yr

GALVESTON ORIENTATION & AMNESIA TEST (GOAT)

Error Points

1. What is your name? (2) ________________ When were you born? (4) _________   ⌊__⌊__⌋
   Where do you live? (4) _______________
2. Where are you now? (5) city ____________ (5) hospital _______________   ⌊__⌊__⌋
   (unnecessary to state name of hospital)
3. On what date were you admitted to this hospital? (5) __________________   ⌊__⌊__⌋
   How did you get here? (5) ____   ⌊__⌊__⌋
4. What is the first event you can remember *after* the injury? (5) ___________   ⌊__⌊__⌋
   Can you describe in detail (e.g., date, time, companions) the first event you can recall after injury? (5) _______________________________________

5. Can you describe the last event you recall *before* the accident? (5) _______   ⌊__⌊__⌋.
   ________________________ Can you describe in detail (e.g., date, time, companions)
   the first event you can recall *before* the injury? (5) _______________
6. What time is it now? ______ (1 for each ½ hour removed from correct time to maximum of 5)   ⌊__⌊__⌋
7. What day of the week is it? ______ (1 for each day removed from correct one)   ⌊__⌊__⌋
8. What day of the month is it? ______ (1 for each day removed from correct date to maximum   ⌊__⌊__⌋
   of 5)
9. What is the month? ______ (5 for each month removed from correct one to maximum of 15)   ⌊__⌊__⌋
10. What is the year? ______ (10 for each year removed from correct one to maximum of 30)   ⌊__⌊__⌋

                                              Total Error Points   ⌊__⌊__⌋
                          Total Goat Score (100-total error points)   ⌊__⌊__⌋

FIGURE 12–1 • Galveston Orientation and Amnesia Test. (From Levin, H. S., O'Donnell, V. M., & Grossman, R. G. [1979]. The Galveston Orientation and Amnesia Test. *Journal of Nervous and Mental Disease, 167*[11], 675–684. Copyright by Williams & Wilkins.)

1. Person

What is your name? _______________________________

How old are you? _________________________________

When is your birthday? ____________________________

2. Place

Where are we right now? ___________________________

What is the name of this place? _____________________

What kind of place is this? _________________________

How did you get here? _____________________________

What city are we in now? ___________________________

What is your home address? ________________________

3. Time

What is today's date (year, month, day)? ______________

What day of the week is it? _________________________

What time is it right now? __________________________

What is the season? _______________________________

How long have you been in the hospital? ______________

On what date were you admitted? ____________________

FIGURE 12–2 • Orientation test. (Adapted from Straub, R. L., & Black, F. W. [1985]. *The mental status examination in neurology* [p. 81]. Philadelphia: F.A. Davis.)

neuropsychologist, but others, including nurses, can be trained to administer these tests. One such test that has been used by nurses is the Neurobehavioral Cognitive Status Examination; it is discussed in detail in Chapter 11 (Kiernan, Mueller, Langston, & Van Dyke, 1987).

The widely used Wechsler Memory Scale has seven subtests used to provide a summary score (memory quotient). This scale is not particularly sensitive to impairment of memory for visual material; thus, another test should be used to assess this component. The test batteries chosen for use should contain verbal and visual memory assessment (Brooks, 1983).

The Mini-Mental State is a very reliable and brief test that has been used extensively in research and in practice (Folstein, Folstein, & McHugh, 1975). Although developed to evaluate psychiatric patients, it has been found to be reliable in evaluating the cognitive state of many types of neurologic disorders.

A postconcussion screening tool was developed to follow up with patients after minor head injuries (Bader & Thompson, 1993). This tool can be administered by the nurse specialist and has been found to be helpful in identifying symptoms of postconcussion syndrome (Fig. 12–3).

Some neuropsychologists prefer to use a collection of specific tests rather than one battery. This allows the clinician to assess particular aspects of memory. Such a collection should include the following:

1. Logical recall—a story is read to the patient, who is asked to explain it.

2. Word pairs association learning—a word pair is read, then one word is given to the patient and he or she is asked to name the other.

Name: ____

Age: ______________ Trauma # ____________________ MR # ________________________

GCS at scene: ________________ GCS on arrival in ER ________________________

Loss of consciousness: Yes/No   Amnesic to event: Yes/No   ETOH: ________________

CT scan: Yes/No   Results of CT scan: ________________________________

GOAT (Galveston Orientation and Amnesia Test): ________________________________

1. Introduce self

2. How are you feeling? ____

Are you back to work/school? ____

If no—Why? ____________________________________ When will you go back?____________

If yes—Are you having any problems at work/school? ________________________

What are the problems? ____

3. Occasionally certain symptoms occur after a minor head injury. I'm going to describe some symptoms—answer yes or no if you are experiencing any of these:

Somatic		Cognitive		Affective	
Headache	Y/N	Memory	Y/N	Anxiety	Y/N
Dizziness	Y/N	Difficulty concentrating	Y/N	Depression	Y/N
Decreased energy	Y/N	Difficulty completing tasks	Y/N	Sleep disturbance	Y/N
Vision problem	Y/N	Visuospatial problems	Y/N	Fatigue	Y/N
Weakness	Y/N	Problems with reasoning	Y/N	Easily irritated	Y/N
Nausea	Y/N	Problems with judgment	Y/N	Anger	Y/N
Ringing ears	Y/N	Slowed thinking	Y/N	Problems with initiating activities	Y/N

4. Grade your recovery period from what you were like before the accident to the present (scale 0–10) 0 = poor 10 = complete recovery

0   1   2   3   4   5   6   7   8   9   10

Follow-up. Send a note with card informing the patient another follow-up call will occur in eight weeks.

FIGURE 12–3 • Postconcussion screening tool. (From Bader, M. K. & Thompson, D. [1993]. *Journal of Neuroscience Nursing, 25*[4], 249–253.)

3. Visual memory tests—the patient is shown geometric shapes and then asked to reproduce them from memory.

4. Delayed recall (verbal or visual)—the patient is told a story or shown pictures and, after a time lapse (usually 30 minutes), is asked to tell the story or draw the picture.

One technological advance in memory assessment was developed by Crook and uses a computer program to evaluate memory function (Crook, Larrabee, & Youngjohn, 1990). There are 10 tests in the computerized test battery, and patients respond to the stimuli on the screen. Examples of test content are grocery list recall, name-face association, a first names–last names test, and facial recognition. This test battery has been used in the United States and in several other countries and has been found to be very beneficial in detecting memory disorders, especially in patients with progressive dementias and AAMI (Crook et al., 1990).

The major disadvantage to most tests of mental status is that they do not relate to everyday problems or difficulties encountered in daily life. Crook's battery is the first memory test to use relevant material from daily life to assess memory function.

NURSING DIAGNOSES FOR THE INDIVIDUAL AND THE FAMILY

After the in-depth assessment, the neuroscience nurse will be able to arrive at the specific problem or nursing diagnosis. The identified problem areas reflect the patient's deficits in carrying out functional activities of daily living. Because of the patient's deficits, the family also faces problems in how to help the family member adapt. There is evidence that the cognitive and memory disturbances of the person with brain damage have the greatest effect on the caregiver (Bishop & Evans, 1990; Grant & Bean, 1992). The following are possible nursing diagnoses for the individual when there is alteration in memory:

- Altered thought processes related to loss of memory as evidenced by impaired short-term memory with problems recalling or recognizing events that occurred in the immediate past; impaired remote memory with problems recalling or recognizing events of the remote past; impaired recall ability with problems recalling material or procedures learned in practice sessions, such as an exercise procedure, making coffee, or how to use public transportation; impaired retention with problems remembering short instructions, basic routines of daily life, assignments or appointments, and personal decisions.

- Self-care deficit related to impaired memory retention as evidenced by impaired recall ability and impaired retention

The following outcomes would be the goal of nursing intervention: to gain ability to use memory aids to improve independence and to carry out self-care activities with minimal assistance.

The following nursing diagnoses apply to the family:

- Altered family processes related to change in family roles, as evidenced by caregiving activities

- Ineffective family coping: compromised, related to the chronic health problem as evidenced by irritability and impatience with the affected family member

Nursing intervention for these diagnoses should focus on the following outcomes: family will relinquish some caregiving activities, family will encourage self-care activities and techniques, and family will use respite care and other community resources.

There are many concurrent and related problems that the brain-injured person might experience. These frequently influence and compound the diagnoses for the patient and the family. Problems with attention, concentration, language, and judgment affect the person's ability to cope with memory deficits and compound the coping skills required by the family. Because these other deficits frequently occur in conjunction with impaired memory function, these related problems may serve as etiologies for the nursing diagnoses.

NURSING INTERVENTIONS

The neuroscience nurse has the knowledge and skill to develop or adapt intervention techniques to meet the needs of specific patient populations. This is particularly important in planning care for patients with memory disturbances. It requires creativity and good patient assessment to arrive at treatment strategies that are appropriate for each individual. Using variations of the techniques tested in laboratory settings, the nurse can design individualized ways to improve memory function in the real-life setting.

The nurse specialist can use the research literature and other resources to develop innovative intervention techniques to assist patients with memory loss. Modification of reported therapeutic strategies and application of intervention techniques from other disciplines are ways the nurse specialist can assist in planning memory-retraining activities.

The goals of nursing are to improve the patient's ability to function more independently and for the family to participate in helping the patient attain increased independence. The focus of nursing intervention for the family is to include them in problem identification, treatment approaches, and teaching.

Initially, the focus is on in-hospital activities. The neuroscience nurse can design activities and provide memory aids that promote memory retraining. Of course, this is not done in isolation. The nurse should incorporate in her or his interventions the goals and activities of the other health team members—for example, encouraging the patient to practice exercises learned in physical therapy or skills learned in occupational therapy.

The following three principles should be remembered when planning activities to improve memory function (Kupfermann, 1985):

1. Make tasks simple and measurable so that progress is easily evaluated.

2. Space out the learning sessions and make them brief.

3. Provide positive reinforcement of appropriate behaviors.

The literature on memory retraining is sparse, and most of it has not been updated in recent years. The methods described are often useful in the clinical setting but not appropriate for preparing the patient for the real world. The nurse has a great challenge in trying to design memory aids that will help the patient deal with everyday activities. When there is permanent brain damage, the return of function is slow and often minimal. More recent research indicates promise with the plasticity theory, and there is evidence that transfer of function to other areas of the brain occurs or that certain areas of the brain assume new functions. For the present, the nurse must use creativity to work with the patient with a memory deficit.

Several researchers have described external memory aids as the most useful (Harris, 1992; Moffat, 1984). These include notebooks, calendars, charts, lists, alarms, timers, and prompt cards. These aids can be used by patients and families to remind them of schedules, appointments, and activities of daily life.

Internal memory aids described in the literature include visual imagery and verbal strategies (Glasgow, Zeiss, Barrera, & Lewinsohn, 1977; Lewinsohn, Danaher, & Kikel, 1977; Moffat, 1984; Zarit, Zarit, & Reever, 1982). Most of these have been tested only in laboratory settings and offer little for rehabilitation of the patient with memory loss as a result of brain damage.

Several useful memory aids have been developed. One that can easily be individualized is the memory wallet. This is a collection of sentence and picture stimuli that are designed to prompt the recall of factual information—for example, a picture of a family member with the identifying statement underneath, "This is my sister, Mary." One study of the use of memory wallets with dementia patients found that just the preparation of the wallets and the orientation to their use improved the patients' and their families' interaction and conversation (Bourgeois, 1993). There are also commercially prepared memory aids or wallets called passports that are most useful in community reorientation, such as eating in restaurants, grocery shopping, purchasing personal items and prescription drugs, or shopping in malls.

A therapy that was developed for use with psychiatric and geriatric patients has been found to be useful for the head-injured patient. Reality orientation aims to retrain a person's awareness of time, place, and current events. It is a process of continuous stimulation and repetition of basic orientation information (Cerny & McNeny, 1983). To be effective, reality orientation must be used on a 24-hour basis by all members of the staff. The program should begin as soon as the patient arouses from coma. The two basic components of the therapy are consistency and repetition. Whenever any staff member interacts with the patient, he or she should provide some orientation information. The family must be involved and can provide valuable information as well as bring personal and familiar objects from home. Photographs, posters, clothing, clocks, calendars, radios, and other favorite personal possessions can be used in reality orientation. A daily schedule board should be posted in full view to remind the patient of activities and therapies. This also helps the family and staff to reinforce the schedule and encourage the patient to follow it. Family involvement is crucial because this therapy should be continued throughout rehabilitation and when at home.

Another therapy that has been tried in some rehabilitation settings is memory groups. These groups share various memory aid strategies, discuss the difficulties related to having a memory problem, and play games that are designed to improve memory function. These groups may not work for all types of memory disorders, but for short-term memory loss they seem to have some benefit.

SUMMARY

The challenge to neuroscience nurses is to assess the patient accurately and to plan interventions that assist in adjustment to the disabilities that accompany neurologic disorders. Mental alterations present a particularly difficult task. Memory loss is distressing to the patient and the family and is the problem dealt with least by nurses. Often, the inability to remember is viewed as the result of hospitalization and, therefore, is expected to improve when the person returns to familiar surroundings. Unfortunately, this is usually not the case when there has been an intracranial insult.

With the development and use of specific assessment tools, the neuroscience nurse can better determine the extent of neurologic deficit. Once a memory loss has been determined, the nurse can begin a realistic plan to help the patient and family adjust.

References

American Psychiatric Association. (1980). *Diagnostic and statistical manual of mental disorders* (3rd ed.). Washington, DC: Author.

Baddeley, A. D. (1984). Memory theory and memory therapy. In B. Wilson & N. Moffat (Eds.), *Clinical management of memory problems* (pp. 5–27). Gaithersburg, MD: Aspen.

Baddeley, A. D. (1992). Working memory: The interface between memory and cognition. *Journal of Cognitive Neuroscience, 4*(3), 281–288.

Baddeley, A. D., Bressi, S., Della, S. S., Logie, R., & Spinnler, H. (1991). The decline of working memory in Alzheimer's disease: A longitudinal study. *Brain, 114*(Pt. 6), 2521–2542.

Bader, M. K., & Thompson, D. (1993). The year after: Post-concussion syndrome. *Journal Neuroscience Nursing, 25*(4), 249–253.

Bishop, D. S., & Evans, R. L. (1990). Family functioning assessment techniques in stroke. *Stroke, 21*(Suppl. 2), 50–51.

Bourgeois, M. S. (1993). Evaluating memory wallets in conversations with persons with dementia. *Journal of Speech and Hearing Research, 35*(6), 1344–1357.

Brindle, P. M., Brown, M. W., Brown, J., Griffith, H. B., & Turner, C. M. (1991). Objective and subjective memory impairment in normal human pregnancy. *Psychological Medicine, 21,* 647–653.

Brooks, D. N. (1983). *Outcome of severe head injury.* New York: Oxford University Press.

Cerny, J., & McNeny, R. (1983). Reality orientation therapy. In M. Rosenenthal, E. R. Griffith, M. Bond, & J. D. Miller (Eds.), *Rehabilitation of the head-injured adult* (pp. 345–353). Philadelphia: F.A. Davis.

Crook, T. H., & Larrabee, G. J. (1991). Diagnosis, assessment and treatment of age associated memory impairment. *Journal of Neural Transmission, 33*(Suppl.), 1–6.

Crook, T. H., Larrabee, G. J., & Youngjohn, J. R. (1990). Diagnosis and assessment of age associated memory impairment. *Clinical Neuropharmacology, 13*(Suppl. 3), S81.

Crosby, L., & Parsons, L. C. (1989). Clinical neurologic assessment tool: Development and testing of an instrument to index neurologic status. *Heart and Lung, 18*(2), 121–125.

Dowling, G. A. (1985). Levels of cognitive functioning: Evaluation of interrater reliability. *Journal of Neurosurgical Nursing, 17*(2), 129.

Folstein, M. F., Folstein, S. E., & McHugh, P. R. (1975). "Mini-mental state": A practical method for grading the cognitive state of patients for the clinician. *Journal Psychiatric Research, 12,* 189–198.

Glasgow, R. E., Zeiss, R. A., Barrera, M., & Lewinsohn, P. M. (1977). Case studies on remediating memory deficits in brain-damaged individuals. *Journal of Clinical Psychology, 33*(4), 1049.

Grant, J. S., & Bean, C. A. (1992). Self-identified needs of informal caregiver of head injured adults. *Family and Community Health, 15*(2), 49–58.

Harris, J. (1992). Methods of improving memory. In B. Wilson & N. Moffat (Eds.), *Clinical management of memory problems* (pp. 59–85). Gaithersburg, MD: Aspen.

Kiernan, R. J., Mueller, J., Langston, J. W., & Van Dyke, C. (1987). The neurobehavioral cognitive status examination: A brief but differentiated approach to cognitive assessment. *Annals of Internal Medicine, 107,* 481.

Kupfermann, I. (1985). Learning. In E. Kandel, & J. Schwartz (Eds.), *Principles of neural science* (2nd ed., pp. 570–579). New York: Elsevier North-Holland.

Levin, B. E., Tomer, R., & Rey, G. J. (1992). Cognitive impairments in Parkinson's disease. *Neurologic Clinics, 10*(2), 471–485.

Levin, H. S., High, W. M., Goethe, K. E., Sisson, R. A., Overall, J. E., Rhoades, H. M., Eisenberg, H. M., Kahsky, Z., & Gary, H. E. (1987). The neurobehavioral rating scale: Assessment of the behavioral sequelae of head injury by the clinician. *Journal of Neurology, Neurosurgery, and Psychiatry, 50,* 183–193.

Levin, H. S., O'Donnell, V. M., & Grossman, R. G. (1979). The Galveston Orientation and Amnesia Test: A practical scale to assess cognition after head injury. *Journal of Nervous and Mental Disease, 167,* 675.

Lewinsohn, P. M., Danaher, B. G., & Kikel, S. (1977). Visual imagery as a mnemonic aid for brain-injured persons. *Journal of Consulting and Clinical Psychology, 45*(5), 717.

Luria, A. R. (1976). *The neuropsychology of memory.* New York: Halsted Press.

Mahler, M. E. (1992). Behavioral manifestations associated with multiple sclerosis. *Psychiatric Clinics of North America, 15*(2), 427–438.

Mauri, M., Sinforiani, E., Bono, G., Vignati, F., Berselli, M. E., Attanasio, R., & Nappi, G. (1993). Memory impairment in Cushing's disease. *Acta Neurologica Scandinavica, 87*(1), 52–55.

Moffat, N. (1984). Strategies of memory therapy. In B. Wilson & N. Moffatt (Eds.), *Clinical management of memory problems* (pp. 63–88). Gaithersburg, MD: Aspen.

Rappaport, M., Hall, K. M., Hopkins, K., Bellexa, T., & Cope, D. N. (1982). Disability rating scale for severe head trauma: Coma to community. *Archives of Physical Medicine and Rehabilitation, 63,* 118.

Rockwood, K., Dobbs, A. R., Rule, B. G., Howlett, S. E., & Black, W. R. (1992). The impact of pacemaker implantation on cognitive functioning in elderly patients. *Journal of the American Geriatrics Society, 40*(2), 142–146.

Rodgers, J., Britton, P. G., Morris, R. G., Kemahan, J., & Craft, A. W. (1992). Memory after treatment for acute lymphoblastic leukaemia. *Archives of Disease in Childhood, 67*(3), 266–268.

Sachon, C., Grimaldi, A., Digy, J. P., Pillon, B., Dubois, B., & Thervet, F. (1992). Cognitive function, insulin-dependent diabetes and hypoglycemia. *Journal of Internal Medicine, 231*(5), 471–475.

Schartz, R. H., Gruenewald, P. J., Klitzner, M., & Fedio, P. (1989). Short-term memory impairment in cannabis-dependent adolescents. *American Journal of Diseases of Children, 143*(10), 1214–1219.

Sharp, K., Brindle, P. M., Brown, M. W., & Turner G. M. (1993). Memory loss during pregnancy. *British Journal of Obstetrics and Gynecology, 100*(3), 209–215.

Sisson, R. A. (1992). Cognitive and emotional function of stroke patients. In S. G. Funk, E. M. Tornquist, M. T. Champagne, & R. A. Wiese (Eds.), *Key aspects of elder care: Managing falls. Incontinence and cognitive impairment* (pp. 300–308). New York: Springer.

Squire, L. R. (1987). *Memory and brain.* New York: Oxford University Press.

Squire, L. R. (1992). Declarative and nondeclarative memory: Multiple brain systems supporting learning and memory. *Journal of Cognitive Neuroscience, 4*(3), 232–242.

Straub, R. L., & Black, F. W. (1985). *The mental status examination in neurology.* Philadelphia: F.A. Davis.

Strugar, J., Sass, K. J., Buchanan, C. P., Spencer, D. D., & Lowe, D. K. (1993). Long-term consequences of minimal brain injury: Loss of consciousness does not predict memory impairment. *Journal of Trauma, 34*(4), 555–558.

Szymanski, H. V., & Linn, R. (1992). A review of the postconcussion syndrome. *International Journal of Psychiatry in Medicine, 22*(4), 357–375.

Thompson, P. J. (1991). Memory function in patients with epilepsy. *Advances in Neurology, 55,* 369–382.

Turner, H. B., Kreutzer, J. S., Lent, B., & Brockett, C. A. (1984). Developing a brief neuropsychological mental status exam: A pilot study. *Journal of Neurosurgical Nursing, 16,* 257.

Warren, J. B., Goethe, K. E., & Peck, E. A. (1984). Neuropsychological abnormalities associated with severe head injury. *Journal of Neurosurgical Nursing, 16*(1), 30.

Wechsler, D. (1945). A standard memory scale for clinical use. *Journal of Psychology, 19,* 87.

Zarit, S. H., Zarit, J. M., & Reever, K. E. (1982). Memory training for severe memory loss: Effects on senile dementia patients and their families. *Gerontologist, 22*(4), 373.

Alterations in Cognitive Processing

SR. CALLISTA ROY

Cognitive processing is a significant and distinctive human life process. Cognitive abilities are used to take in and interact with the physical and social environments. These special competencies empower a person to adapt and to reach higher levels of integration within the self and with society. Health potential is closely related to the use of cognitive and emotional capabilities to enhance integration. One consequence of this generally held assumption is that cognitive deficits are crucial concerns for all patients and particularly so for patients encountered in neuroscience nursing practice.

Cognition is a broad term encompassing the human abilities to think, feel, and act. It has been a subject of philosophical and scientific study through the ages. Aristotle divided mental functions into cognitive functions, or thought processes, and emotional and moral aspects. From the middle of the 19th century, psychologists postulated several basic mechanisms behind mental processes. Principles of association were thought to be the essence of human mental life. Later, complex mental phenomena such as active perceptions and symbolic forms were studied. In the early decades of the 20th century, the socialist transformation of Soviet society provided the natural laboratory to suggest that the very structure of human cognitive processes differs according to the ways that social groups live out their various realities (Luria, 1976). Today, neuroscience nurses, neurobiologists, neuropsychologists, cognitive scientists, cultural anthropologists, linguists, philosophers, and others chart the relationships among brain organization, mental activities, human life processes, and social environments.

The societies of developed countries have opened wide the information highway. The incomparable social changes of this era will significantly affect the cognitive processing of each person. Every human cognitive ability will be influenced and potentially enhanced in the information-processing society. As a major profession within society, nursing focuses on understanding all human life processes. Understanding cognitive processing and cognitive deficits from an information-processing approach is key to all nursing activity today and in the future. Clinical practice in neuroscience nursing both provides for and calls for developing this specific knowledge.

MODELS OF COGNITIVE PROCESSING

Cognitive science is the study of intelligence and intelligent systems, and particularly of human behavior as information processing. Since about 1950, a branch of computer science called artificial intelligence has been studying the intelligence exhibited by machines. Developments in this field have greatly influenced the study of human thinking processes; however, the human processes are the focus of this chapter. Early models of human intelligence focused on memory, thinking, and behavior. Models later evolved to study the underlying mechanisms of processing information.

The study of information-processing models can be approached on the basis of three aspects of the information-processing continuum. On the input side of the continuum, models deal with perception, such as visual or auditory stimulation held in memory and then recoded. Second, literature has focused extensively on memory-related information-processing models and their empirical consequences. These investigations denote stages such as rehearsal, recognition, and acoustic representation for linguistic material. In addition, the processes that underlie forgetting, or memory loss, and retrieval and responding, as distinct from storage, are studied. The resulting models pay little attention to input variables, recognizing only that stimulation precedes storage. The third emphasis noted in cognitive information-processing models is on problem-solving behavior and verbal associative learning. In this emphasis as well, less attention is paid to perceptual processes as such. This focus is most apparent in the study of artificial intelligence, in which deep thinking has proved easier to understand and simulate than eye-hand coordination. The problem lies in delicate issues of adaptive design presented in the interface between intelligent systems and their external environments—that is, sensory and motor organs. Hence the design of white-collar expert systems, including diagnostic systems, is carried out with far more assurance than is the design of robots (Simon & Kaplan, 1989).

Das (1984) argued cogently that if we want to understand how information is processed by human beings, we must comprehend how processing occurs in the brain rather than in the computer. Following Hunt's (1980) three components of intelligence, he proposed an information integration model in which the structure is the brain, the processes are neuropsychologic, and the knowledge base is provided by the experience and education of the person. Das' work was based on Luria's clinical studies. In addition to his work on sociocultural issues of cognitive development, Luria worked for more than 40 years in the mid-20th century to describe disturbances of the higher cortical functions in the presence of local brain lesions (Luria, 1973, 1980). Detailed and insightful observations of victims of World War II resulted in systematic treatment to restore brain functions deranged by head injuries.

Luria conceptualized three main functional divisions of the brain, one for controlling arousal, one for coding, and one for planning and decision making. The theory was distinct in that it emphasized functional units of the brain. The functional units, according to Luria, have depth, cortically and subcortically, as well as spread across hemispheres. Processing of information in simultaneous quasispatial arrays, for example, is spread over a large area comprising the occipital and parietal lobes. Successive information processing—that is, ordering information temporally—is also located widely, mainly in the temporal and frontotemporal areas of the brain. Planning and decision making seem to involve the whole of the frontal lobes. At the same time, depth is involved, in that coding, such as coding of visual information, passes through hierarchical levels of the brain consistent with its topography.

Luria's theory of the holistic function of the cerebral hemispheres rejected traditional views of localization. If there are not discrete centers for aspects of language, of calculation, or of writing, then there must be a reanalysis of conditions such as agnosia and apraxia. Luria's more holistic view is supported in the burgeoning multidisciplinary scientific literature. One example is the astute clinical studies of Anderson et al. (1992) in which they showed that three severely aphasic hearing patients were able to acquire competency in aspects of the American Sign Language (ASL) lexicon and finger spelling. The investigators suggested that conceptual knowledge is represented independently of auditory-vocal records, and that left anterior temporal cortices outside traditional language areas are part of the neural network that supports the linkage between conceptual knowledge and linguistic signs.

A combination of approaches has been used to obtain functional maps of the brain and to understand better the activity of information-processing networks. These approaches involve topographic studies of the effects of brain damage, stimulation of the exposed cortex during surgery, microelectrode recordings of cortical activity evoked by behavior or sensory stimuli, radioactive isotope techniques, and monoclonal antibodies to measure the enhanced blood supply to cortical areas that are activated by the performance of specific sensory, motor, and mental tasks. Active neurons have the ability to change their own local blood supply. Such changes can be measured by an injection of a small amount of radionuclide known as a tracer. The activity of the tracer is detected by a positron emission tomography (PET) scanner. Similarly functional magnetic resonance imaging (fMRI) can detect changes in metabolism or blood flow in the brain during cognitive tasks. A consistent finding from imaging studies is that any given task activates a network of areas, including both frontal and posterior cortical areas as well as subcortical areas.

Willis and Grossman (1981) acknowledged the great advances of the 1970s in neuroanatomy and neurophysiology. Still, they cautioned that it must be recognized that the neural substrates related to cognition are poorly known. The authors provided a very generalized summary of current knowledge at that time. Willis and Grossman (1981) noted that participation and interaction of many brain areas appear to be involved in most of these processes, that cortical and subcortical areas are involved, and that processes of consciousness, attention, and perception are intimately interrelated. Less than a decade later, Sejnowski and Churchland (1989) listed 12 neurobiologic developments that provide organizational parameters for the cognitive neuroscientist in developing functional brain-mind hypotheses. They noted a new, if cautious, optimism for achieving some measure of integration and explanatory unification of the various levels of organization in nervous systems. The decade of the brain in the 1990s provided prospects that "favor genuine progress in generating theories that honor neurobiological and psychological constraints to explain how networks of neurons achieve high-level effects" (Sejnowski & Churchland, 1989, p. 344).

Two classical review articles were done by Mountcastle (1979 and 1997) that draw conclusions from a century of brain-mapping work. Initially Mountcastle (1979) concluded that each neocortical area has a distinctive cytoarchitecture and a distinctive function; however, it also possesses in its own unique set of extrinsic connections. The columnar organization of the neocortex is further described in the later work. Mountcastle (1997) notes that the modular organization of the nervous system is a widely documented principle for human and animal brains of which the columnar organization of the neocortex is an example. The well-known areas of the neocortex are composed of smaller units, and the local neural circuits are repeated within each area. Areas located at some distance from one another have some common properties and may be linked by long-range intracortical connections. Mountcastle (1997) notes that the remarkable success of neuroanatomical studies of brain connectivity during the last decades has revealed the vast number and diversity of connections that link brain structures to each other. When these findings are considered together with the results of neurophysiological studies, a new concept of brain function emerges. The author notes, in support of Luria's earlier insights, that the brain operations and particularly those of the higher functions are distributed in nature. Further, there are some hierarchical and quasi-serial linking operations to the afferent and efferent systems of the brain.

Nursing assessments and interventions related to patient cognitive processes are influenced greatly by these developments and by the plasticity of cerebral function they reflect. On the basis of this developing knowledge and of the author's career work in nursing theory, Figure 13–1 proposes a model for nursing's view of cognitive processing. The inner circle lists basic internal processes of arousal and attention, sensation and perception, coding and concept formation, memory and language, and planning and motor response. These functions are dependent on the brain structure, neurologically and neurochemically, and they occur within the field of consciousness (Willis & Grossman, 1981). The next circle represents the situation immediately confronting the person, which he or she is processing. Roy refers to this as the focal stimulus (Roy, 1984; Roy & Andrews, 1999). The outer circle represents the education and experience of the person within which the current processing situation is embedded. In terms taken from the Roy Adaptation Model of Nursing, these are considered contextual and residual stimuli. The broken lines in the figure indicate the permeability between the stimulus fields.

The circles of the model highlight contemporary views in both nursing and cognitive science that the individual is a participant and partner in the developmental process. Cognitive processing abilities throughout the life span are subject to interactional factors that have bidirectional and multidirectional influences. Development involves biologic aspects, or maturation, and environ-

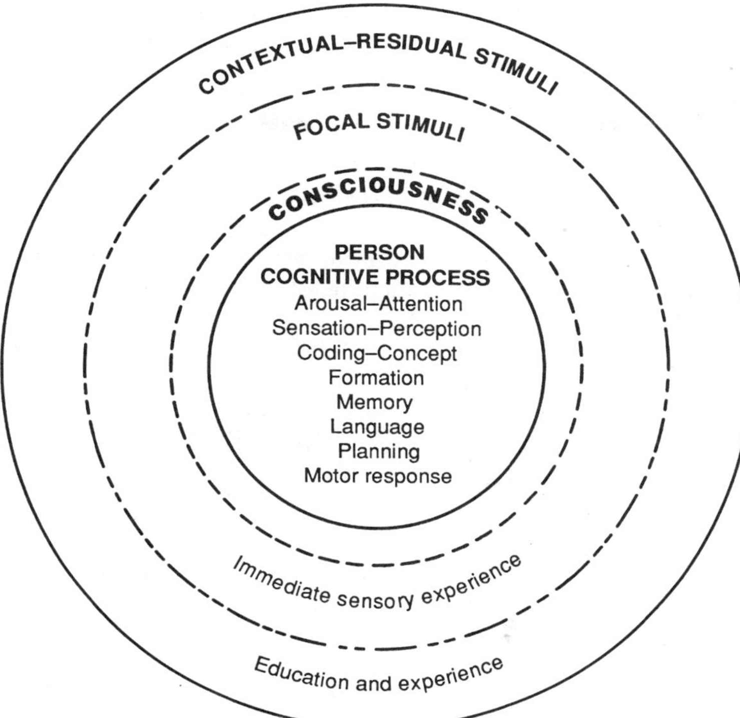

FIGURE 13–1 • Nursing models for cognitive processing.

mental factors, such as learning opportunities. Rather than naming a single factor (e.g., age affecting development at a steady pace), this interactive model includes individual participation and historical, social, biologic, and environmental influences. Children and the elderly have a much greater degree of variability in expression of abilities and have less well-studied and inherently more difficult to understand cerebral organizations (Horton & Puente, 1990). Children are subject to poorly understood growth spurts, developmental stages, and developmental lags. Changes associated with aging can be either primary, nonpathologic changes, such as alterations in sensory functioning, or secondary, pathologic processes, such as the changes associated with Alzheimer's disease.

The clinical discussion that follows is based on the growing knowledge of integrated brain function presented here and the nursing model derived from that knowledge. The model is inclusive of increasing awareness of life-span issues related to cognitive processing.

DOMAINS OF COGNITIVE PROCESSING

Brain and behavior literature is both impressive and bewildering. Markowitsch (1988) recognized the common agreement that information processing is the principal function of the nervous system. Still, he pointed out that these actual mechanisms are poorly understood. Thus we rely on the use of metaphors in the study of brain-behavior relationships. For example, diagrams are used metaphorically to present hypotheses. They are not pictures of the brain but sketches of interpretations of observations (Heilman & Valenstein, 1993). It is useful, then, for the purposes of this chapter to organize a person's cognitive processing according to functions within each stage of the information-processing system (Fig. 13–2). The input stage of processing involves the functions of arousal and attention as well as sensation and perception. Central processing includes the functions of coding and concept formation, memory, and language. Functions that can be examined at the output stage are planning and motor response.

HUMAN RESPONSES TO ALTERED COGNITIVE PROCESSING

In various conditions affecting the central nervous system, there are changes in all or some of these domains of cognitive processing. The section that follows discusses these deficits, which are considered in making nursing diagnoses; their clinical manifestations; and the nursing interventions that are based on an understanding of the specific deficit (Table 13–1).

Impaired Cognitive Input Function

Deficits related to the person's ability to take in information occur within the domains of arousal and attention and sensation and perception.

AROUSAL AND ATTENTION

In the domain of arousal and attention, deficits occur in relation to selective attention, speed of processing, and alertness (van Zomeren, Brouwer, & Deelman, 1984). Arousal and attention direct perceptual mechanisms to stimuli in the field of consciousness. Behaviorally, the occurrence of arousal and attention is defined by orienting of sensory receptors to a stimulus. This orienting

INPUT ⟶	CENTRAL PROCESSING ⟶	OUTPUT
Arousal–Attention	Coding–Concept Formation	Planning
Sensation–Perception	Memory Language	Motor Response

FIGURE 13–2 • Information-processing system.

TABLE 13–1 • DEFICITS OF COGNITIVE INPUT PROCESSES

Deficits by Function	Behavioral Manifestations	Interventions
A. Arousal and Attention		
1. Selective attention		
a. Focused attention deficit (FAD)	Automatic response to stimulus and inability to modify response Perseveration Inability to establish a new focus of attention	• Remove the stimulus that is eliciting the automatic response. • Change the stimulus-response bond through behavioral modification. • Include the automatic response in a desired behavior pattern.
b. Divided attention deficit (DAD)	Inability to maintain a focus of attention to the immediate situation in context of ordinary background stimuli Decreased number of pieces of information consciously held in mind Slowness in following instructions or learning a new task Frustration with the environment	• Use verbal cues to maintain focus. • Minimize distractions. • Give information in small amounts and of minimal complexity. • Wait patiently for series of cognitive operations to be made. • Encourage efforts in spite of frustration. • Teach safety awareness.
c. Unilateral neglect	Impaired ability to attend to both left and right hemispaces, shown by hemi-inattention, hemi-intention, and hemineglect	• Teach compensation techniques to the individual, family, significant others, and health care providers. • Use computer programs.
2. Speed of processing	Manifestations as in DAD	• Use interventions used for DAD.
3. Alertness		
a. Receptivity deficit	Decreased general receptivity to stimulation or hyperkinesis	• Use verbal, tactile, and pain stimulation to rouse, or protect from stimulation.
b. Phasic alertness deficit	Decreased expectancy response shown in facial expression, posture, or electroencephalogram	• Provide verbal cues to increase readiness to respond.
c. Tonic alertness deficit	Impaired ability to sustain a specific focus of attention over an extended period	• Recognize limits of extended alertness and divide tasks into time frames matching patient pattern. • Challenge attention in games such as making matches of objects. • Perform self-instructional training, involving self-verbalizations. • Use selected computer programs paired with one-to-one interaction. • Use reality orientation programs.
B. Sensation and Perception		
1. Primary sense processing		
a. Partial or complete blindness	Inability to detect or difficulty detecting things in the visual environment	• Maintain safety and integrity of body parts without sensation. • Preserve optimal sensory function.

Table continued on following page

TABLE 13–1 • DEFICITS OF COGNITIVE INPUT PROCESSES *Continued*

Deficits by Function	Behavioral Manifestations	Interventions
b. Hearing disorders	Impaired reception of sound	• Develop and use a systematic method to compensate for loss of sensation.
c. Olfactory or gustatory disorder	Impaired sense of smell or taste	
d. Somatic sensory disorder	Impaired sense of touch, temperature, vibration, pain, position, and discrimination	• Adapt lifestyle and need for independence within the context of deficit.
e. Integrative multimodal sensory disorder	Impaired coordination of sensory inputs from two or more systems	
2. Pattern recognition		
a. Visual, auditory, and somatosensory agnosias	Loss of ability for identification, recognition, discrimination, or classification of stimuli that is out of proportion to the loss of perception of the existence of the stimuli	• Structure the environment with simplicity, order, and routine. • Encourage patient to use alternative senses and cues for identifying objects.
b. Alexia	Severe impairment of ability to read words and sentences	• Use exercises to reactivate patient's comprehension of words.
c. Dyslexia	Reading difficulties, especially seen in school-aged children	• Provide aids for reading (e.g., ruler, large print, supervised practice).
d. Topographic disorientation	Acquired inability to locate places	• Accompany patient to any new location and provide written instruction even in familiar places.
3. Naming and association		
a. Naming and association deficits	Inability to name and associate correctly	• Teach patient to recognize deficits and to compensate for them.
b. Disorders of color naming	Inability to name colors in spite of ability to experience sensation of color	• Simplify the environment. • Use exercises that construct visual images and practice charades.
c. Spatial analysis deficits	Inability to grasp the whole visual field Unstable useful visual field Difficulty perceiving moving objects Misjudgments of depth or direction of sound	• Simplify the environment. • Maintain safety. • Develop and use a systematic method to compensate for deficit.

is triggered by (1) a change in stimulus level—for example, in attempting to arouse a moribund elderly patient, the nurse raises his or her voice above the level of the background noise in the emergency department; (2) presentation of a novel stimulus—for example, in assessing an infant's visual capacity, a striped stuffed zebra is moved into the visual field; and (3) presentation of a stimulus that has been learned as a signal for reward or punishment—for example, the public address system announcement of a fire drill orients all personnel at a long-term care facility to that stimulus. For research purposes, electrophysiologic signs of the process of paying attention can be observed by recording sensory evoked potentials from the cerebral cortex.

A continuous stream of stimuli reaches the senses, and a vast amount of information is present in the memory system. Yet actual behavior, of an acutely ill patient, of a worker in a health promotion program, or of a nurse in any health care setting, is determined by only a fraction of this information. A number of theories of selective attention have been developed to explain the process of attending to one stimulus and stopping all others below the level of awareness. Early theories assumed that information could be filtered by the person according to how meaningful or pertinent it was. A later theory (Schneider & Shiffrin, 1977) proposed that selectivity was not structurally connected to any fixed level of abstraction, that is, not connected to the process of giving meaning to the stimulus. Rather, if one views processing as both automatic and controlled by the individual, then there are different kinds of attentional deficits. Allport (1989) cited the general agreement that attention is limited or selective. However, he noted that data point to a multiplicity of attentional functions. His work on visual capacity suggests a significant interdependence between the orienting of spatial attention and the preparation for action. In doing concurrent quasi-independent tasks, such as running over uneven ground to catch a baseball, it is necessary to keep the streams of information appropriately segregated to avoid unwanted crosstalk between them that interferes with effective processing. Allport (1989) acknowledged the significance of the shift away from the earlier focus on informational limitations in the message system to the emphasis on issues of task preparation and attentional control. He credited the groundbreaking work of Schneider and Shiffrin and others for this progress but still maintained that further theoretical development would recognize that attentional control is what is to be explained, rather than an explanation itself (Shiffrin & Schneider, 1977).

In a review article on the neurobiology of selective attention, Posner and Carr (1992) noted the substantial progress in the field of selective visual attention. In particular, neuroimaging and electrical recording results indicate that selective attention amplifies neural activity in the prestriate areas concerned with basic visual processing. Networks of anatomic areas that serve as the source of attentional modulation are being delineated with the suggestion that these networks are anatomically distinct from the sites of the resulting amplifications. Unresolved issues suggest that the conceptualization of attentional functions—their purposes and constraints—deserves more thorough reapprasial. Identifying further explanatory theory will provide the basis for describing additional clinical implications.

Empirical generalizations made by Shiffrin and Schneider (1977) are particularly useful in describing problems of neuroscience patients. In their theoretical formulations, these authors described two forms of processing. Automatic processing does not demand conscious effort but rather is the result of learning and practice—for example, the skill of driving a car regularly. Controlled processing, on the other hand, is the temporary activation of a sequence of elements that can be set up quickly and easily but require attention, like driving an unfamiliar car. The capacity for controlled processing is limited; it usually occurs in serial steps and typically in new situations. All information entering the system is processed automatically up to the highest level possible without conscious control. Processing is initiated by the appropriate input, based on activation of a learned sequence of long-term memory elements, and then proceeds automatically to the response. This framework specifies two kinds of limitations of selective attention: focused attention deficits (FADs) and divided attention deficits (DADs).

FADs result from automatic response tendencies conflicting with responses required by the task at hand. There is a conflicting stimulus-response bond. Thus the nurse who has always used emergency equipment from a certain cupboard will reach in that direction when an emergency occurs, even though she or he has been transferred to another unit where emergency equipment is stored in a different place. If the person cannot interrupt a learned automatic process, then a FAD occurs.

DADs, however, result from speed limitations of consciously controlled processing. Controlled processing makes use of results of automatic processing and operates on this information by means of a strategy formed on the basis of instruction, prior learning, and context. Transformations of the input information are carried out, and responses have to be selected from the behavioral repertoire. Because this processing is speed limited, the available processing capacity must be divided over several cognitive operations required for the task. For example, if an elderly patient who is being discharged from the hospital receives a detailed list of instructions about home care, he or she is likely to politely answer, "Thank you." The patient may or may not have processed the entire list of instructions. Limitations of rate of processing will be discussed further below.

Unilateral neglect has been described as a specific type of selective attention deficit (Mesulam, 1985). This composite phenomenon can be analyzed from the perspective of complex perceptual, motor, and motivational aspects. Yet it appears that this phenomenon represents a fundamental disturbance in a vector aspect of attention—namely, the spatial distribution of directed sensory attention. Mesulam (1985) noted that the possibility of unilateral neglect merely reflecting a combination of elementary sensory motor deficits can be dismissed. Repeated studies have shown that the extent of sensory loss does not correlate with the severity of neglect. Some patients with intact visual fields may still show neglect, whereas patients with hemianopia do not necessarily neglect the blind field, but rather move the head and eyes to take in the field on the visually impaired side.

Mesulam (1985, pp. 156–158) developed a hypothetical model of a neural network for the distribution of attention based on observations of the three regions of the entire cortex that consistently lead to unilateral neglect when damaged (Fig. 13–3). In this model, the distribution of directed attention is coordinated by a neural network that contains three independent but interacting representations of the extrapersonal world. The posterior parietal cortex may contain a sensory template of the extrapersonal world. The frontal eye fields and the related cortex may contain a motor map for the distribution of orienting and exploratory movements in the extrapersonal space. Mesulam's model shows a third representation to contain a map for the distribution of expectancy and relevance, perhaps centered on the cingulate cortex. Arousal tone may

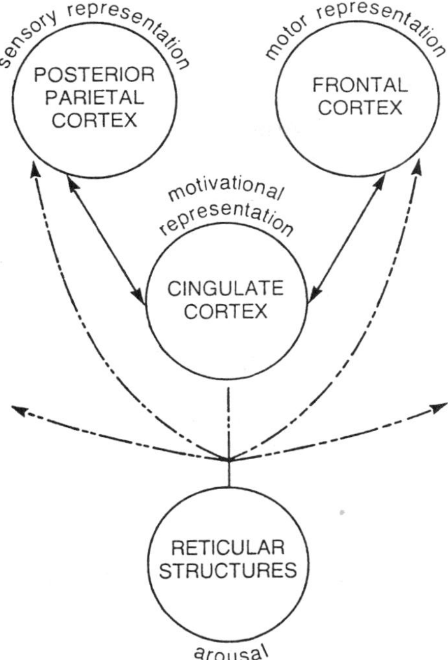

FIGURE 13–3 • The components of a neural network involved in modulating directed attention. (From Mesulam, M. M. [1981]. A cortical network for directed attention and unilateral neglect. *Journal of Annals of Neurology,* *10*[4], 309.)

be provided by reticular structures that provide input for each of the three representations. Finally, each representation has specific connections with the striatum and thalamus. Assuming this mechanism, the effective distribution of attention within the extrapersonal space requires a flexible interaction among the three representations. This model, based on empirical and clinical data, is consistent with Luria's notion of functional systems of the brain that have both depth and spread. In discussing unilateral neglect, the integrity of the entire network, or, as Mountcastle (1979 and 1997) called it, the complex of reciprocally interconnected systems, is more relevant than theories of cortical localization.

A second major category of deficits in the cognitive functions of arousal and attention relates to speed of processing. The speed with which the person can process information will partly determine what will be noticed and how much will go unnoticed. As described earlier in Schneider and Shiffrin's notion of controlled processing, the number of operations possible in a certain time unit is finite. Whenever controlled processing fails to deal with all information that should be processed for optimal task performance, a DAD occurs. A dramatic example of this type of deficit seemed apparent in the decision to launch the space shuttle Challenger in January 1986. In the months of investigation that followed the fatal explosion of the spacecraft, details of information were laid out that were not processed adequately during the much shorter time span of the launch decision. Unfortunately, a speed of processing deficit can have catastrophic effects, as well as account for the most ordinary errors.

In head-injured patients, several studies provide convincing evidence that there is a slowing down of controlled processing of information. The person must expend even greater energy paying attention, because he or she has less attention to pay. Because of this speed of processing deficit, these patients are greatly influenced by the number of stimulus alternatives. With more things to pay attention to and less attention to pay, they are easily distracted and then feel frustrated when their efforts to take in their environment prove unsuccessful. Using the Paced Auditory Serial Addition Task, Gronwall and Sampson (1974) compared a hospital control group with head-injured patients classified in two degrees of severity. The nature of errors did not discriminate patients from those in the control group, and without time pressure both patients and controls could do the task almost perfectly. Gronwall and Sampson concluded that the poor performance of head-injured patients in the usual testing condition is probably the result of a slow but qualitatively normal processing strategy.

The third type of arousal and attention deficit to be discussed is related to alertness. Posner (1975) used the term alertness to refer to a hypothetical state of the central nervous system that affects general receptivity to stimulation—for example, variations in wakefulness and sleep. The half-asleep patient may not readily take in and and respond appropriately to all questions asked at 6 AM during neurosurgery rounds. This highlights the significance of the nurses' recorded observations over the 24-hour period. Human performance is not constant over time, and researchers describe fluctuations in efficiency that have both phasic and tonic shifts.

Phasic changes occur rapidly and depend on the person's interests and intentions. Such changes have been described by what is called the expectancy wave (EW) on the electroencephalogram (EEG). It is as if the brain of a person driving a car and waiting for a traffic light to change is idling like the car engine is idling. When cues are noted that the light is about to change, such as the cross traffic stopping, the EW would occur. Tonic changes of alertness, on the other hand, occur slowly and involuntarily. Because tonic changes cover minutes or hours, they are studied by vigilance tasks that measure the person's efficiency at detecting a signal. Lapses of attention are measured by changes in the EEG wave patterns. Research on alertness such as this is used to guide decisions related to safety standards in certain occupations—for example, the number of consecutive hours an airline pilot may fly.

It often is assumed that patients with various neurologic or neurosurgical conditions have deficits of "sustained attention." Decreased EWs were found in some early studies of alertness in head-injured patients. It was then suggested that the basic deficit after head injury is the inability to sustain attention of a level required for normal performance on some tests. However, in studies using more precise measures, this hypothesis is not supported. A research group in Holland (Brooks, 1984, p. 94) reported studies of control subjects and head-injured patients who performed auditory vigilance tasks lasting 30 minutes.

Every 4 seconds, a click was presented by means of headphones, with one out of five clicks being 4 decibels weaker than the standard clicks. Normal subjects showed clear performance decrements during the second half of the session. Their EEGs indicated signs of drowsiness. In the severely head-injured patients tested, the relationship between EEG and performance was not found. In fact, these patients showed persistently alert EEGs during the task, while their heart rates were higher. Their signal detection performance was decidedly poorer but was quite steady over time. The investigators found some evidence that phasic alertness may be nonoptimal after head injury but also noted that these patients may have higher tonic levels of alertness.

Attentional problems in children are manifested as hyperactivity and impulsivity. These behaviors may be part of a broader syndrome called minimal brain dysfunction (MBD). Given differing views on this disorder, a national task force (Clements, 1966) stated that the term MBD should be used only to describe those children with at least near-average intelligence whose learning and behavioral disabilities are the consequence of certain perceptual, cognitive, and attentive dysfunctions. The list of 99 signs and symptoms associated with MBD diagnosis was reduced to 10 major characteristics. Symptoms tend to occur in clusters. Satz and Ross (1973) noted that a child assigned this label has one or more of the following symptoms: short attention span, motor impulsivity, hyperactivity, emotional lability, poor eye-hand coordination, motor clumsiness, and defective use of language. Hyperkinesis (HK) is a particular syndrome that has been the subject of wide concern to families and of intensive study by neuroscience investigators. Diagnosis is most frequently made during the child's primary school years because symptoms are manifested in the classroom setting. Conservative estimates of occurrence of HK are as much as 4% to 10% among elementary-school–aged children, with boys affected four times as often as girls. Although phamacologic intervention has been controversial, Stamm and Kreder (1979) reviewed a wide range of scientific studies and noted strong evidence for the beneficial effects of methylphenidate amphetamine in HK children. Reportedly, the drugs result in improvement of selective and sustained attention, impulse control, and restless behavior.

Clinical Applications Related to Arousal and Attention Deficits. Clinically, patients in neuroscience nursing show signs of attention and arousal deficits. On the basis of an understanding of the processes described above, clinical manifestations of deficits related to selective attention, speed of processing, and alertness are discussed. The theoretical understanding also provides direction for specific interventions (see Table 13–1, Part A).

As noted earlier, FADs involve automatic response tendencies based on already-established stimulus-response bonds. This is recognized in the patient who automatically responds to stimuli and is unable to modify the response. Behaviorally, perseverations may occur, such as always repeating the name of a certain person regardless of the specific question asked about persons the patient has known. The persistence of overlearned behaviors inhibits the person's ability to establish a new focus of attention. Thus the stroke patient whose bathroom at home was to the left of his or her bed may continue to go in that direction when he or she has the urge to void in spite of efforts to teach the patient to go in the correct direction (i.e., to the right).

In general, the nurse deals with this type of attention deficit by removing the stimuli that are eliciting the automatic response; changing the stimulus-response bond through behavioral modification techniques; or including the automatic response in a desired behavioral pattern. In the example of the stroke patient, the first approach is not appropriate, while the second approach might take a great deal of time and effort for both the patient and the nurse. Thus the third approach might be most useful. In the above example, the patient's bed may be turned to face in the other direction so that turning left becomes the desired response.

DADs are manifested by an inability to maintain a focus of attention on the immediate situation in the context of ordinary background stimuli. The patient shows a decrease in the number of pieces of information that can be consciously held in mind and a slowness in following instructions or learning new tasks. The patient's awareness of this deficit, or the reactions of others to the person's being slow, often result in great feelings of frustration for the patient. Similar frustrations are felt when the crosstalk interference of processing occurs.

Nurses can help patients with this attention deficit by managing the environment and their own input to the patient. When the patient must attend to a given task, the nurse uses verbal cues to maintain focus (e.g., in the dayroom of a long-term care facility, the nurse may tell the elderly patient, "It's lunchtime now, and you are to be eating."). At the same time, background distractions can be minimized by arrangements such as having the television off and limiting interaction with other patients in the room during mealtime. Any information given to the patient will be provided in simple terms and in small amounts at a time.

Recognizing that the patient is going through a series of cognitive operations to complete processing of the information, the nurse will wait patiently for the process to be completed. She or he will watch for cues that the patient has successfully processed the input or has not done so. Her or his response will be encouraging of the patient's efforts in either case. She or he continues to modify the amount of information to match the patient's speed of processing ability and prevents interfering crosstalk. The nurse can help family determine how much time is needed for processing and thereby increase successful task performance.

We noted Mesulam's (1985) description of unilateral neglect as a disturbance in the spatial distribution of directed attention. Given that the patient does not have the necessary intact neural network, he or she will show an impaired ability to attend to both left and right hemispaces as shown by hemi-inattention, hemi-intention, or hemineglect. Interventions for this condition involve teaching safety awareness, teaching compensation techniques, and using computer programs to relearn the extent of the sensory field. The individual and the family and significant others, as well as the health care staff, will also learn these techniques. Their knowledgeable input to the patient's program of rehabilitation is key for recovery and for their own sense of satisfaction in contributing to that recovery. Too often, nurses do not have the most recent knowledge available to plan the care of patients throughout the continuum of care from acute illness or injury through long-term recovery and living with remaining cognitive deficits.

Speed of processing has been discussed as a dimension of attention and arousal separate from selective attention. Deficits in this area are reflected in DADs because a limitation in the speed of processing results in attention having to be divided over the total amount of input. Thus the clinical problems with speed of processing and the appropriate interventions are the same as those discussed for DADs. Again, the nurse is aware of the great amount of energy the patient must expend to accomplish a series of cognitive operations slowly. In a busy neurologic unit, it is not always easy to wait for the patient's response, but the nurse's use of this knowledge can provide the patient with the opportunity to be a thinking person who can interact meaningfully with the environment.

The last category of deficits listed in Table 13–1 relates to alertness. These deficits may be manifested by a decreased general receptivity to stimulation or by HK. When a patient seems not to be responding to stimulation, the nurse uses verbal, tactile, and, if necessary, pain stimulation to arouse the person. This category of deficit overlaps somewhat with discussions of consciousness in the text but refers to the person who is conscious but has a decreased level of alertness.

With phasic alertness deficits, there is a decreased expectancy response, as shown in a nonalert or vacant facial expression. Posture may be slumped, the patient may look unready for a response, and it may be possible to identify an alertness deficit on an EEG by use of averaged evoked potentials. If there is a tonic alertness deficit, the patient will also show an impaired ability to sustain a specific focus of attention over an extended period. In providing care, the nurse uses verbal cues to increase readiness to respond. For example, he or she may address the patient by name on entering the room and tell the patient that he or she is there to help the patient get ready for a family visit. The patient may still look quizzical, but with the patient aroused, the nurse may proceed with the task. In doing this, the nurse uses another basic intervention for alertness deficits. The nurse recognizes limitations and divides the task into time frames that match the patient's tonic alertness. For example, helping the patient dress may take 10 minutes. Because this is the limit of the patient's alertness ability, the nurse will come back to help the patient ambulate to the sunroom during another short period of alertness.

Readily available interventions for children with a variety of attention deficits include make-a-match games. Pairs of objects, pictures, or playing cards may be used. These can be purchased in educational supply or toy departments, or they may be adapted from household items, such as two cups, two spoons, two forks, two socks, two gloves, and so forth. Sets of cards with animal pairs are commercially made or can be cut out from magazines. Children readily become involved in finding the matches, especially when the exercises are structured for competition with an adult opponent or with a digital stopwatch that counts down in seconds. Care must be taken that the task is age appropriate and ability appropriate so that attention is the one skill being challenged.

Self-instructional training (SIT) has been described as an intervention for attentional problems, including hyperactivity, in children. This approach involves the child's use of self-verbalizations. A five-step fading procedure, pioneered by Meichenbaum and Goodman (1971), is used in an SIT program. A model—for example, the nurse—begins the process by verbal demonstration of self-instruction statements, followed by a behavioral display of the statements. Second, the model verbally provides self-instruction statements while the child rehearses these statements and performs the behaviors included in the statements. The third step involves the model prompting the child with the first word of each self-instruction statement and the appropriate behaviors. Next, the model whispers the prompt, followed by the child's whispering of the entire statement and demonstration of the motor behaviors. Finally, the model silently thinks the statement and instructs the child to do the same, as he or she displays the motor behaviors of the statement. Research evidence for maintenance of SIT treatment of hyperactive children is inconclusive (Braswell & Kendall, 1988). Still, there is a broad and rapidly developing literature based on the clinical applications of SIT and related research topics that merits investigation by neurosciences nurses. When SIT was used with head-injured individuals to improve attention and help alleviate memory difficulties as a result of attentional deficits, follow-up testing showed a normal range of immediate recall and a significant decrease in errors on verbal memory tests (Webster & Scott, 1983).

Computer programs have provided sophisticated interventions for attention and concentration. Although some of these packaged sets of programs for cognitive rehabilitation are in their fifth or sixth generation, empirical research documenting their effectiveness lags behind the production of new programs. One difficulty with these modules is that they have no unifying theoretical framework for cognitive processing or for remediation (Brown, Gouvier, & Blanchard-Fields, 1990). In addition, it is the experience of clinicians that although such programs are useful, they cannot replace the costly one-to-one work of the health care provider with the patient.

For the elderly, attentional impairments are often the initial focus of assessment and intervention owing to the importance of sustaining attention for any learning and for responding appropriately to the environment. Three key features of any reality orientation (RO) program have been identified: 24-hour RO, environmental RO, and classroom RO. Many of these approaches are familiar to nurses but can be more purposefully used as they are understood within the information-processing approach to cognitive deficits. In the hospital setting, 24-hour RO involves staff, volunteers, and visitors. Each person communicates information such as person, place, time, activities, and expectations at all times when the patient is awake. Environmental RO is used to assist 24-hour RO in both hospital and long-term care settings. It includes using reminders to orient the patient such as RO boards, color-coded doors and hallways, personal identifying symbols and labels, holiday decorations, and so forth. The principle of making the stimulus stand out from the ongoing backgound is particularly applicable in designing and changing environmental RO. Lastly, what is called classroom RO uses orientation tasks for a group of four to six patients in a small setting that maximizes attentional cues. Such classes may be at the basic or the advanced level and offer practice of person, place, time, and current events orientation. Again, the research literature is mixed in reporting the success of such programs. Measurement and design issues make evidence of improvement in attention difficult to demonstrate.

SENSATION AND PERCEPTION

The second domain of cognitive functions related to the person's ability to take in information is that of sensation and perception. The model of integrated brain function implies that all cognitive processes are interrelated. The processes of sensation and perception presuppose arousal and attention, and they provide the initial step for central processing by coding, memory, and language. However, for the purpose of describing cognitive deficits and their clinical implications, these functions can be considered separately.

Kolb and Whishaw (1985) made the simple distinction that sensation is the result of activity of receptors and their associated afferent pathways to the corresponding neocortical sensory areas, whereas perception is the result of activity of cells in the cortex beyond the first synapse in the sensory cortex. From the nursing model of information processing proposed in this chapter (see Fig. 13–1), we might consider that immediate sensory experience is transformed into a percept in the neocortex by such factors as education and experience. That is, the focal stimulus is processed in light of contextual and residual stimuli. Here, the mind as a symbolic system comes into human action.

During the 1980s, there was an enormous growth in studies of mental models. Versions of the mental-model hypothesis, based on the early contention of Craik (1943), are used to explain such different and complex processes as visual perception, comprehension of communication, reasoning, and representation of knowledge and expertise. Perception is considered the primary source of mental representations (Johnson-Laird, 1989). In the simple single-cell paramecium, the creature merely reacts physically to the immediate environment; for instance, if it bumps into an obstacle, the resulting chemical changes cause the cilia of the paramecium to beat in the opposite direction. However, more complicated creatures use the information impinging on the sensorium to compute an internal representation that in turn is used to control action. Human mental models need to integrate information from all the senses and from general knowledge, that is, the sights, sounds, smells, and possibilities of the world (Johnson-Laird, 1989). For example, if smoke covers the last two letters of an exit sign during a fire, the sign will still be perceived as "EXIT" even though the sense perception is only "EX." Sensation is a more passive process (e.g., light on the retina creates the visual sensation of the outline of two letters), but perception is the active process of encoding the impulses transmitted by the aroused retina into a pattern of letters that makes a word that has meaning in the current situation. That is, the person perceives the exit sign as a way to leave the burning building.

Researchers have described the relationship between the sensory experience during development and the forming of perceptual mechanisms. Deprivation of visual experience has been shown to result in malformation of a proportion of the dendritic spines of visual cortex neurons in the mouse, although some spines develop normally in the absence of vision. Visual deprivation also produces changes in the shapes of the receptive fields of feline visual cortex neurons (Willis & Grossman, 1981). Studies of perception look at the way in which the physical characteristics of stimuli, such as intensity, quality, and position in space, are encoded by neural activity. Transformations in the neural activity at each relay station in the sensory pathway are studied throughout the somatosensory system. Laws are described that relate the physical property of the intensity of the stimulus to the psychologic property of the intensity of the percept. For example, a power function best describes the transformation of stimulus energy to the intensity of the percept. The intensity of a series of stimuli, then, must increase exponentially to produce equally spaced increments of sensation and thus the person's report of the perception of the sensation.

Several important properties of normal sensation and perception help in understanding deficits of these cognitive functions. For example, intact visual perception is characterized by the constancy of the percepts. An example of this phenomenon is size constancy. A bed observed from a distance of 5 feet does not look twice as large as a bed observed from a distance of 10 feet, even though its retinal image is twice as large as the one seen from 5 feet. Learning plays a role in developing such constancies. In this way, there is a sensation of stability of the external world that is important in being able to manipulate the environment. Another significant aspect of perception is the recognition of objects. This aspect of perception is related to the philosophical notion of the knowledge of universals. Thus we can recognize (classify) a particular object, such as a bed, that we have never seen before as an example of a class of objects (beds) even when the object is presented to us in a different spatial orientation, such as upside down. By perceptual mechanisms, we tend to group objects into patterns. Human phenomenologic experience of the world is a triumph of natural selection, according to Johnson-Laird (1989). People seem to perceive the world directly, not a representation of it. However, this phenomenology is an illusion because what is perceived depends on both what is in the world and what is in a person's head. Perception is based both on what evolution has wired into the human nervous system and on what the person knows as a result of experience. To what extent organizational tendencies in perception are innate and to what extent they are learned remains a fruitful area of study.

Willis and Grossman (1981) indicated that there may be a considerable degree of inherent, or "prewired," organization of responses to particular types of stimuli built into the nervous system. They cited work of recordings from single neurons at various levels of the visual system in amphibia and in mammals that revealed the presence of neurons that act as detectors for certain properties of the stimulus, such as motion detectors, edge detectors, or contour detectors. Mesulam (1985) likewise drew heavily on relevant evidence in nonhuman primates to describe neural connectivity in the cortex that includes primary sensory and motor areas, modality-specific (unimodal) association areas, and high-order (heteromodal) association areas. This description of cortical zones of the human brain is consistent with Luria's concept of functional divisions described earlier in this chapter. Within and across these zones and their depth projections into the paralimbic and limbic areas, sensory signals are transformed into complex percepts. For example, facial recognition is a complex nonverbal perceptual task performed by the whole right hemisphere. The extensive cortical distribution and complexity of perceptual activities make them highly vulnerable to brain injury, yet also perhaps more available for recovery processes.

Clinical Applications Related to Sensation and Perception. The distinction between sensation and perception and the descriptions of peripheral and central neural networks are useful because they allow understanding of the effects of lesions on lower (sensory) and upper (perceptual) components of the somatosensory system. Clinically, nurses in neuroscience practice will encounter patients with deficits in at least four categories: primary sensory deficits such as blindness and deafness, disorders of pattern recognition, acquired disorders of naming and association, and disorders of spatial analysis.

Primary sensory deficits and their nursing interventions are discussed in Chapters 23 to 25. Alterations in abilities of primary sensation are noted here only in relation to clarity of input for cognition. Deficits in this area, together with relevant behavioral manifestations and nursing interventions, are summarized in Table 13–1, Part B. Techniques for assessing these deficits are described in greater detail by Bickley (1999, pp. 586–589). In visual processing, the major deficit is partial or complete blindness. Hearing disorders involve impaired reception of sound by reason of distortions or loss of acuity. Patients with hearing impairments may complain that people speak too softly for them to hear or that the words are loud enough but run together and are incomprehensible. For some patients, tinnitus, or noise heard inside the head, interferes with sensory input from the environment. These internal noises are described as ringing, hissing, buzzing, thumping, whistling, or roaring. Disorders of the olfactory and gustatory senses result in an impaired sense of smell or of taste. Whereas vision and hearing are highly significant for a person's safety, taste and smell are more pleasing and satisfying than essential for well-being. Still, disturbances of smell and taste are annoying and can be very distressing. Generally, the person has not experienced the adaptive and protective mechanisms of these senses, so they are not keenly developed or used. However, some persons rely on these senses more than others do, and therefore find deficits of taste and smell more distressing. For example, a wine connoisseur is temporarily disabled in relation to his or her job when he or she has a cold. Likewise, a blind person may have learned to use the sense of smell to identify whether or not it is a familiar person who is heard entering the room and will feel the loss of this sense disproportionately when he or she has a cold. Somatic sensation involves touch, temperature, vibration, pain, position, and discriminatory sense, any of which may be impaired. Finally, primary sense processing involves integrative multimodal sensation. A disorder of this function is observed as an impairment of the coordination of sensory input from two or more different sensory systems, for example, impairment of the ability to coordinate vestibular and visual input, as in reaching for an object while adjusting body position with respect to it.

Any decrease or distortion in receiving input of sensory data affects the person's ability to interact effectively with the environment, to learn, and to grow. Even minor alterations of sensory function can affect normal living. In considering the context for such changes, the meaning of the deficit and the effect that it has on one's chosen lifestyle will be key factors in nursing management. For example, the loss of sensation in one or two fingers would be an annoyance to a teacher, but it would be a major physical and emotional burden for the person who plays classical guitar. Nursing intervention for deficits of primary sense processing will be specific to the particular deficit. The common goals are to maintain safety and the integrity of body parts without sensation, to preserve optimal sensory function, to develop and use a systematic method to compensate for lost sensation, and to adapt lifestyle and need for independence within the context of the deficit.

The presence of normal primary sensation in itself does not mean that the person can use the information obtained by the senses. The discriminative functions involve pattern recognition and look at the ability of the sensory cortex to correlate, analyze, and interpret sensations. The term agnosia is used to describe, in Teuber's words, "a normal percept stripped of its meanings" (cited by Damasio, 1985, p. 259). Damasio (1985) provided an operational definition of visual agnosia that further clarified the distinction between primary sensory deficits and pattern recognition deficits. Visual agnosia is defined as

> *a disorder of higher behavior confined to the visual realm, in which an alert, attentive, intelligent, and nonaphasic patient with normal visual perception gives evidence of not knowing the meaning of those stimuli—that is of not recognizing them (Damasio, 1985, p. 259).*

Damasio maintained that although perception and recognition are part of a continuum, it is possible to identify, both behaviorally and neurophysiologically, some components of the process that are mainly related to perception and some that are mainly related to recognition. The painstaking search for supporting evidence of effective perception precedes the identification of an agnosia. Furthermore, the correct identification of a deficit as one of sense processing or of pattern recognition affects the design of appropriate nursing interventions.

Agnosias occur in the visual, auditory, and somatosensory realms. It is difficult to isolate a disturbance to a given realm, just as it is difficult to distinguish agnosias from sensory deficits. Still, the types of major agnosias and the functions that may be affected are listed below based on classification and discussion by Kolb and Whishaw (1985, pp. 205–233):

Type of Altered Function

Visual Agnosias

Object agnosia	Naming, using, or recognizing objects
Agnosia for drawings	Recognition of drawn stimuli
Prosopagnosia	Recognition of faces
Color agnosia	Association of colors with objects
Color anomia	Naming colors
Achromatopsia	Distinguishing hues
Visual-spatial agnosia	Stereoscopic vision, topographic concepts

Auditory Agnosias

Amusia	Tone deafness; melody deafness; disorders of rhythm, measure, or tempo
Agnosia for sounds	Identifying meaning of nonverbal sounds

Somatosensory Agnosias

Astereognosia	Recognition of objects by touch
Anosognosia	Awareness of illness
Anosodiaphoria	Response to illness
Autotopagnosia	Localization and naming of body parts
Asymbolia for pain	Reaction to pain

Alexia is a particular disorder of visual pattern recognition and in pure form is called alexia without agraphia or "word blindness." This deficit is manifested by severe impairment of ability to read most words and sentences, and in many patients even the reading of single letters is defective. The patient can see sentences, words, and letters and can copy them but cannot read them. Mechanisms of this deficit are thought to lie in parallel distributed processing (PDP) models rather than in more traditional serial processing models. The processing capacity is thought to be divided among several units linked in parallel. In neural-type PDP networks, for example, neurons in a given anatomic area may be richly interconnected into an ensemble with certain computational properties (Friedman, Ween, & Albert, 1993). Several such ensembles, often in widely disparate areas of the brain, may be interconnected, via white matter fiber tracts, into highly complex neural networks. Hierarchical interconnections also exist, as noted in brain architectural schemas. The combined activity of this widely distributed, multiply interconnected system brings about a behavioral function, such as visuospatial orientation or word recognition. Information is represented in patterns of activity within these networks. Cross-mapping of information between ensembles, or networks, is observed and interpreted as processing.

Dyslexia is a common developmental deficit in pattern recognition that often has a strong familial history. This disorder can lead to reading difficulties, especially in school-age children, because the identification of words is a major component of the reading process. Visual word identification has been the subject of intensive study since the 1970s. Two related issues often addressed are the relationship between the identification of words and letters and the role of recoding to sound in word identification. Research methods focused on the process of reading use on-line measures such as reaction times or the pattern of eye movements. These methods are more direct in the assessment of pattern recognition than are the more traditional research methods that examine the products of reading using measures such as recall and comprehension.

Summarizing some of this work, Pollatsek and Rayner (1989) noted that data are quite clear that words are accessed through a level best termed "abstract letter identities" and that the letters (for short words, at least) are processed in parallel. Sound coding is involved in the process of getting to the meaning of a word, but the details of this involvement are not clear. From a review of 95 references related to visual word recognition, Posner and Carr (1992) concluded that a combined cognitive and anatomic analysis may be of considerable benefit in developing more adequate models of human information processing. This work provides significant implications for understanding better ways of studying other deficits of pattern recognition.

A variety of disorders involving spatial orientation are included in the designation of topographic disorientation. The acquired inability to locate a public building in a city, to find one's bedroom at home, or to describe either verbally or by means of a map how to get to a specific room or place are all behavioral manifestations of this deficit. The cause of this deficit is based on the mechanisms of agnosia and is differentiated from similar behaviors on the basis of unilateral hemispatial neglect or on a global amnestic syndrome.

In the four types of pattern recognition deficits discussed—agnosia, alexia, dyslexia, and topographic disorientation—the behavioral manifestations generally involve a loss of ability or an impaired ability to identify, recognize, discriminate, or classify stimuli that is out of proportion to the loss of perception of the stimuli. Interventions related to these deficits focus first on simplifying the environment. Because the person has difficulty making sense of the perceptual world, the task of taking it in will be simplified by having fewer stimuli and by ensuring that the stimuli present are meaningful. For example, at mealtimes only one dish is placed in front of the person at a time and another is added only when the first is eaten. Taylor and Ballenger (1980) recommended a structured environment with the key elements of simplicity, order, and routine for brain-damaged patients, and these suggestions are relevant particularly for persons with pattern recognition deficits.

Second, the patient can be encouraged to establish awareness of the deficit and then to use alternate senses or cues for identifying and recognizing a stimulus. For example, the patient with prosopagnosia may be taught to touch his or her eye and then his or her face, saying, "I don't see faces." Then the patient practices relying on voices, mannerisms, uniforms, and so forth to identify health care personnel. Specific learning exercises may help reactivate a person's comprehension of words. These exercises are often included in handbooks for families of stroke patients or head-injured patients. One example (Pi Lambda Theta, 1983) is to use fairly large, colorful pictures and a list of words related to the pictures as well as words unrelated to the pictures. The person is shown a group of words and a picture and is asked to point to the word or words that go with the picture. The task may be reversed so that the person is shown a group of pictures and a word and then asked to point to the pictures that go with the word. Another variation is to show the person a group of words, all but one of which belong in the same category (e.g., animals), and then to ask the patient to pick out the word that doesn't belong (e.g., tree).

Aids to reading such as a ruler to follow the line and large-print publications may help some patients improve pattern recognition. Lastly, the person with topographic disorientation must be accompanied to any new location and will need written instruction even in familiar places. It is clear that an infinite amount of patience is required of the person with a pattern recognition deficit, as well as of the family and of all health care providers, in adapting lifestyle and need for independence in the context of the remaining abilities.

Luria (1973) discussed the fact that perceptual ability is not confined to the processes of perception. Rather, as noted in the discussion of dyslexia related to reading, visual perceptual activity necessarily includes the active formation of visual images corresponding to a single word meaning. This active perceptual process includes search for the most important elements of information, their comparison with each other, the creation of a hypothesis concerning the meaning for the information as a whole, and the verification of this hypothesis by comparing it with the original features of the object perceived. A person may have an intact ability to create a visual synthesis of an object or a picture yet be unable to relate it to past experience or—in other words—be unable to associate it in memory. The mechanisms underlying naming and association deficits are not entirely clear. Geschwind suggested a disturbance that effectively separates a primary sensory or sensory association area from the dominant hemisphere language area (Benson & Geschwind, 1985; Geschwind, 1965).

Luria (1973, p. 239) provided clinical observations showing the behavioral characteristics of such deficits. These patients can still see clearly an object or a picture of it. However, either they cannot relate it to their personal experience (for example, when looking at a picture of a group of soldiers on a tank, one patient said, "This is my family, my father, sisters, and children") or they will assess the meaning of a picture on the basis of irrelevant associations (for example, another patient interpreted a picture of a boy who had broken a window and been caught by the owner of the house as follows: "Someone from Buryat Republic has won a competition, and they are presenting him with a cup").

Disorders of color naming and color association are particular types of this perceptual deficit. Damasio (1985) differentiates disorders of color naming from achromatopsia, or loss of color vision. This deficit occurs when otherwise nonaphasic patients can experience the sensation of color and can match colors according to hue but are unable to name those colors that they apparently perceive without difficulty. Damasio's discussion of efforts to analyze the lesion that leads to this deficit provides further insight into the complexities of the neurophysiology of human sensory and perceptual processing.

Studying an extensive series of patients, Damasio concluded that the lesion necessary for color-naming defects is located in the left hemisphere, mesially, in the transition between the occipital and temporal lobes in a subsplenial position. The right homonymous hemianopia that is also present in these patients is caused by an additional lesion in the geniculate body, in the visual cortex, or in the optic radiations. Damasio notes that, regardless of the lesion that causes it, the net effect of a right field cut is to circumscribe visual information to the right visual cortex. The effect of the occipitotemporal lesion is to interfere with the ability of language areas in the left hemisphere to receive visual information related to color. This lesion may simply disconnect color information conveyed by the corpus callosum, or another possibility is that some crucial step in the processing of that information takes place in the occipitotemporal transition cortex.

Other types of visual information still reach the remainder of the left visual association cortices, thus explaining the preservation of other aspects of visual naming.

In his discussion of disorders of color association, Damasio further noted that the cognitive basis of the concept of color is fragile, being principally dependent on (1) the association of a verbal tag with a given color and (2) the association of a given color with objects that commonly carry it (an association that must be, at least in part, verbally mediated). The author suggested that a functional dissociation between visual and verbal processes is likely to prevent the concomitant arousal of verbal and visual memory traces on which the attribution of meaning to a normal color perception must depend.

Deficits of naming and association as described here, and all the variations of those reported in the literature, have the common behavioral manifestation of inability to name and to associate correctly. Interventions for such deficits are similar to those listed for primary sensory and pattern recognition deficits. Simplification of the enviornment is key, as is developing an awareness of the deficit and assisting the person to use remaining abilities. Exercises that have the person construct visual images may be useful. For example, ask the patient to describe a house he or she has been in, then a house the patient has never been in; a familiar bird, then a strange bird; a person he or she knows well, then someone the patient has never met. The nurse or family member can use magazine pictures, naming words for various things seen. The patient repeats each word to help build association of words and pictures. Charades may be used to recall and name words.

The fourth type of deficit of sensation and perception is that of spatial analysis. Damasio (1985) described one of the most striking of these disorders, Balint's syndrome, an acquired disturbance of the ability to perceive the visual field as a whole, resulting in the unpredictable perception and recognition of only parts of it (simultanagnosia), which is accompanied by an impairment of target pointing under visual guidance (optic ataxia) and an inability to shift gaze at will toward new visual stimuli (ocular apraxia).

Essentially, these patients become unable to grasp the whole field of vision in its entirety and will report seeing clearly in only a small fraction of the panorama, with vision outside that spot described as hazy. The subjective problem becomes more difficult because this fragment of useful field is not stable and moves erratically from quadrant to quadrant. Such patients commonly fail to detect and orient to new stimuli that may appear in the periphery of the visual field. Also, an object that is clearly seen at a given moment may suddenly disappear from view as the center of vision shifts. Patients will complain about objects vanishing from the scene they are inspecting and of an inability to report more than one or two components of the visual field at any one time. They may find that moving objects are especially difficult to perceive. With optic ataxia, these patients can point with accuracy to targets on their own body or clothing, using somatosensory information, and also to a source of sound. Depending on vision, however, there is marked difficulty in reaching toward small targets and in finger pointing. These patients are unable to direct the gaze voluntarily toward a new stimulus appearing in the periphery of the visual field. Even if told that the stimulus has entered the field, they will not orient to it, or, if they do, the gaze will be inaccurate.

Related visual disturbances are the inability to discriminate depth on the basis of binocular visual information and the inability to judge directional orientation of lines. Disorders of auditory-spatial analysis are considered inconsequential in relation to visual disorders, although these can also be distressing to a person and can present threats to saftey. For example, a woman suffering recent one-sided hearing loss after acoustic neuroma surgery reported spending an inordinate amount of time trying to locate visually the source of an annoying whirling sound in her office. In desperation, she called a colleague in the office next door to ask if the noise was outside the window. The colleague responded that there was not an unusual noise coming from outside the window but that she would come and investigate the sound. Entering the office, the colleague pointed directly to a copier in the corner and said, "That machine is on."

The main behavioral feature of this disorder is inaccurate and distorted perception. Clinically, then, interventions are designed as they are for persons with primary sensory losses, particularly partial or complete blindness. The nurse focuses on maintaining safety and developing a systematic method to compensate for the deficit. In addition, the patient and family must learn to adapt their lifestyle and the patient's need for independence within the constraints of the deficit.

The person's ability to use arousal, attention, sensation, and perception to take in the environment is a preparation for central processing. This aspect of cognitive processing and the deficits of central processing are described in the next section.

Impaired Function of Central Cognitive Processing

The person's relationship to the environment has been described in terms of arousal and attention acting to direct perceptual mechanisms that take in immediate sensory experience. At this point in human information processing, the central processes become primary. Input stimuli are further processed by way of coding and concept formation, memory, and language. Because memory and language are such significant areas of deficit for neuroscience patients, they have been covered more extensively in Chapters 10, 12, 14 and 15.

CODING

The brain's unique power is due mainly to its ability to store information—that is, to code a representation of experience for future use. In Luria's (1973, p. 67) description of functional units of the brain, the second of these complex working systems is for the reception, coding, and storage of information. Some years ago Lashley (described by Pribram, 1969) reviewed the experimental evidence related to how the brain goes about storage and retrieval. He then stated, somewhat wryly, that on the basis of the available evidence, learning and remembering were obviously impossible. Pribram (1969) noted that what appears to happen is that the nervous system is so constructed that it analyzes from the complexities of the receptive mechanisms some sort of alphabet that can be used as a code to represent the input. He used the notion of the neural hologram analogously to photographic holograms. In the photographic process, a record of wave patterns emitted or reflected from an object is frozen until it is read out by a process called wave-front reconstruction. Scientists continue to pursue the answer to the intractable question of how information is stored.

The next generation of understanding central cognitive processes—that is, how the brain functions to code, store, and use information—was summarized by Willis and Grossman (1981). They noted that central higher functions are thought of as producing a structural or electrophysiologic change in the brain. This change was called the memory trace even though no particular type of localization or mechanisms of storage were yet identified. Various models were used to study the processes that produce the memory trace and the processes for gaining access to the trace, for recalling it to consciousness, and for producing motor activity. The general principles that these authors provided for the foundation of clinical neuroscience include the following:

1. Storage of information is a function of the brain as a whole.

2. The hippocampus may be involved in processes of sorting, assembling, and supplying information—for example, with sensory information that is emotionally significant.

3. Such processes, in the broadest sense, can be thought of as plasticity or modifiability of synaptic function.

4. Short-term changes in synaptic function have been identified in work on habituation and conditioning, but how such short-term changes might be converted into long-term learning or memory lasting for years is not known.

5. Such changes in synaptic function imply either growth of new synaptic connections or change in the functional effectiveness of synapses.

6. Metabolic activity or protein synthesis might be important in the processes under consideration.

Woody (1982) discussed the chemical forms theoretically available for controlling engram or code formation—that is, subionic particles, ions and molecules, macromolecules, and complex molecular aggregates. The six classical principles have been useful in directing two decades of further research on central cognitive processing.

In a review of 46 papers, Damasio, Tranel, and Damasio (1990) noted that evidence suggests that knowledge storage systems are specialized with respect to their capacity for supporting acquisition and retrieval of different domains and levels of knowledge. A demonstration of networks for conceptual knowledge was given from the tradition of skillful clinical observations (Anderson et al., 1992). Three severely aphasic hearing patients were able to acquire competency in signs from ASL, in contrast to their near complete inability to speak the English counterparts of the signs. On the basis of the comparison of task performance with specific brain lesions, the authors suggested that conceptual knowledge is represented independent of the auditory-vocal records for the corresponding lexical entries and that left anterior temporal cortices outside identified language areas are part of the neural network that supports the linkage between conceptual knowledge and linguistic signs, especially as they are used for production or comprehension of meaningful sentences.

Formulations that have been suggested in neuropsychologic investigations are supported by current experimental work in animals. Furthermore, refinements of neuroimaging techniques—-computed tomography (CT), positron emission tomography, single photon emission tomography, nuclear magnetic resonance imaging (MRI), and magnetoencephalography—permit elaborate clinical and experimental work related to the processing of complex information in the human brain. Used with powerful computers, these techniques can capture in real time images of the physiology associated with central cognitive processes. Such powerful tools of brain imaging produce data for "visualizing the mind," with research centers across the world investigating mental activities such as attention, creation of images, memory, perception, motor control, and emotion (Raichle, 1994). Neuroscience databases can be organized and quickly disseminate the resulting repository of information to aid the understanding and care of people who have problems ranging from developmental learning disorders to language disabilities arising from stroke or head injury.

Given these advances, it is timely to approach cognition with the aim of relating a given function to its corresponding neural organization and activity state. A model of learning temporal sequences by selection (Dehaene, Changeux, & Nadal, 1987) illustrated how neurons coding for relationships between mental objects may differentiate as a consequence of experience. Using complex learning situations in monkeys with reversible cryogenic brain lesions, Horel (1988) looked at the question of whether there are discrete centers for information storage. He concluded that memories for objects could normally be in the temporal cortex but that the lesion conditions force them to be stored elsewhere or cause the animals to use information that is normally in an alternative area and is not normally used with this particular behavior task.

Clinical and empirical investigations provide evidence for the principle that cognitive central processing is a function of the brain as a whole. It is reasonable to note that this function is most sensitive to the effects of changes in the brain regardless of site. Thus, for example, significant changes in memory storage following anesthesia have been noted, as have persistent disorders of learning and memory as long as 10 to 20 years after head injury (Brooks, 1984; White & Wolf-Wilets, 1977). At the same time, these findings also provide evidence for brain plasticity, that is, for predicating recovery of function by the use of different or retrained pathways.

Clinicians use various ways of classifying deficits of processing so that they may plan care for patients with these deficits. The extensive disorders specifically noted in the central processing functions of memory and language are discussed in other chapters. Coding and concept formation, however, are viewed as additional functions of central processing that are requisite for memory and language functions. The deficits observed in these domains, along with their behavioral manifestations and relevant nursing interventions, are listed in Table 13–2.

To simplify current theoretical and empirical studies of brain function, the viewpoint being presented describes coding as involved in the registration of incoming stimuli, the consolidation of it into a form for storage, and the synthesis of consolidated elements with previous brain codings or engrams. Lezak (1994) described registration as the holding of large amounts of incoming information briefly (for 1 or 2 seconds at most) in sensory store. It is neither strictly a memory function nor a perceptual function but rather a selecting and recording process by which perceptions enter the memory system. It has been called the valve to determine which memories are stored. Acquired sensory response patterns, perceptual and response predispositions, and attention-focusing components of perception play an integral role in the registration process. The important clinical concept related to this process is consciousness.

Key Deficits of Coding. As indicated in the nursing model for cognitive processing (see Fig. 13–1), immediate sensory experience takes place within a field of consciousness, with the permeable boundaries of the contextual and residual stimuli (i.e., education and experience) also available to the processing person. The key deficit in this domain might be called altered level of consciousness. Consciousness has been defined as an awareness of the internal and external environments. Crigger and Strickland (1985) provided the distinction that theoretically, consciousness includes two components: arousal, the awakeness of the person, and content, the interpretation of internal and external environment. If a person is having difficulty registering immediate sensory experience, the difficulty may be in either the arousal or the content component. That is, the person may not be alert enough to register experience, or the individual's content storage may be disrupted in such a way that new information cannot enter. Behaviorally, the deficit is manifested by minimal, no, or nonproportionate responses to stimuli. Confusion, delirium, and agitation are further manifes-

TABLE 13–2 • DEFICITS OF COGNITIVE CENTRAL PROCESSES

Deficits by Function	Behavioral Manifestations	Interventions
A. Coding		
1. Registration		
a. Altered level of consciousness	Minimal, no, or disproportionate response to stimuli	Use verbal, tactile, or pain stimulation to rouse to desired level of response. Provide for safety and meeting basic needs. Simplify the environment. Converse as if patient can register information.
	Confusion, delirium, agitation	Develop a sense of trust and confidence. Help family to understand patient's behavior. Use calm, matter-of-fact, nonpunitive approach to reassure patient of protection. Use firm, consistent, personal restraint temporarily with reassurance.
2. Consolidation		
a. Defective information storage	Impaired ability to use prior experience to benefit future actions Defective spontaneous recall	Help patient and family recognize the deficit. Provide continuous flow of useful, orienting information. Develop and use routine for daily living care. Structure the environment for simplicity and safety. Encourage and support patient and family. Be patient with problems inherent in limitations.
3. Synthesis		
a. Lack of perspective	Impaired ability to differentiate and identify common elements in past, present, and future sets of information; to identify differences and relationships among these elements; and to integrate such information into a whole as a basis for a modulated response	Provide protective and supportive supervision. Structure the environment for safety and psychologic comfort. Provide for relief of caregivers. Assist family with issues related to long-term institutional care. Safeguard personal integrity.
B. Concept formation		
1. Integrated recognition		
a. Fractionated recognition	Lack of subjective familiarity with stimulus Absence of responses adequate to the stimulus Loss of ability to identify stimuli	Provide structured, controlled environment. Help patient deal with feelings of perplexity and fear of the unfamiliar.

Table continued on following page

TABLE 13–2 • DEFICITS OF COGNITIVE CENTRAL PROCESSES *Continued*

Deficits by Function	Behavioral Manifestations	Interventions
2. Abstraction and flexibility		
a. Conceptual concreteness	Inability to form concepts and use categories Inability to generalize from a single instance Inability to apply procedural rules and general principles Preference for obvious, superficial solutions Inability to make distinctions related to relevancy, essences, and appropriateness	Limit the need to abstract or symbolize. Maintain the same environment. Show rather than explain. Avoid confusing the patient with details beyond the immediate. Avoid joking and teasing.
b. Conceptual inflexibility	Inability to shift a course of thought or action according to the demands of the situation	Focus on patient concerns. Use simple, direct humor.
3. Calculation		
a. Acquired disorders of calculation	Impaired ability to identify values of digits in a counting system Impaired ability to identify or use symbols or elements of mathematical operations	Teach patient to recognize the deficit and make plans for meeting needs that require calculation. Reasure patient that this is an understood phenomenon, but that it is still being studied further. Encourage patient about likelihood of recovery.
C. Memory 1. Recall of new information 2. Recall from remote memory 3. Sequential skills, abilities, and routines 4. Ongoing planning and awareness of self	Discussed in Chapters 10–12	
D. Language 1. Expressive transmission 2. Receptive transmission 3. Integrated language modalities	Discussed in Chapters 14–15	

tations of changes in levels of consciousness. Assessment and interventions related to altered consciousness are discussed in Chapters 5 to 9.

The nurse is aware that a central processing deficit differs from one of primary sense processing in that the patient cannot use another mode to compensate. The environment is made as simple as possible with the hope that the remaining capacity for registering input can be used effectively. Likewise, the nurse is aware of how much is unknown about central cognitive processing and particularly about the deficit of a given patient. If it is true that sense experiences occurring at a time when the patient is not responding to the environment are stored for later interpretation, the nurse might use greater care with both the content and the tone of her or his conversations at the bedside or to an apparently comatose patient.

For patients with confusion, delirium, and agitation, the nurse aims to develop a sense of trust for and confidence in the caregivers and to help the family understand the reasons for the patient's behavior and respond appropriately. The patient's perceptions are disorganized and distorted; there may be frightening hallucinations (Taylor & Ballenger, 1980). The sights and sounds of the hospital, which the nurse easily processes, take on strangeness for both the patient and the family. What the nurse considers a mildly uncomfortable procedure may appear threatening or exaggerated when the patient is unable to code the input appropriately. Patients are often frightened by their own mental condition, struggling to protect themselves and make sense out of their environment. Even ordinary discomforts such as a distended bladder or bowel or sensations of hunger or thirst cannot be registered at the appropriate level of stimulation and may increase the patient's restlessness and feelings of panic. Such disturbed states may alternate with periods of relative lucidity or with lethargy and stupor. The family may be frightened or embarrassed by the patient's confused, agitated, and combative behavior. A calm, matter-of-fact, nonpunitive approach toward the patient is used to let these patients know that the nurse will protect them from their own uncontrollable behavior. Adequate staff is needed to control the behavior temporarily until the patient can be calmed. Several nurses can hold the combative patient without inflicting injury or sustaining injury themselves. Limbs are held fully extended proximal to the joint for best control (e.g., the legs on the bed with the nurse's arm across the knees and the arms extended while being held above the elbow and at the wrist). One nurse continues talking quietly and reassuringly to the patient, saying, for example, ''You're okay, Mr. Jones. I know you are scared, but you're okay. We'll stay here; you'll be okay.'' A firm, consistent approach over time helps the patient feel more secure and thus more calm.

Lezak's (1994) description of memory and learning processes indicated that registration, short-term storage, primary memory, and rehearsal all depend basically on electrochemical activation at the synapses. However, in keeping with current evidence and theory construction, consolidation and the processes that follow involve semipermanent changes in cell structure or chemistry. Consolidation begins as soon as 1 half-second after information enters short-term storage and may continue as long as information remains there. A likely sequence of events includes biochemical processes of protein synthesis in the nerve cells that bring about transformations, possibly in conjunction with the budding of new cell contact points, and that create transmission patterns between cells to constitute the long-term memory traces. Much of the information being stored at this point appears to be organized on the basis of meaning (such as grandmother's likeness) and according to the principles of association. This differs from earlier stages of short-term storage that use contiguity or sensory properties such as similar sounds, shapes, or colors.

A deficit in the function of consolidation is referred to as defective information storage. Behavioral manifestations include the inability to use prior experience to benefit future actions. The patient may even consciously remember that he or she has practiced a certain task but may find that the experience was not coded for storage in such a way that the practice makes the patient better able to do the task. A further sign of this coding deficit is difficulty with spontaneous recall. Nursing interventions are aimed at recognizing such deficits and helping the patient and family deal with the problems inherent in limitations of information storage. These patients may be able to carry out activities of daily living independently if reminded to do so. They can repond to what they see, hear, and feel in the immediate environment but cannot properly code this information for storage. Therefore, they need a continuous flow of useful, orienting information. The nurse will introduce herself or himself each time she or he enters the patient's room and will let the patient know what will be happening at that moment. A structured environment with attention to safety is needed, as is much patience. Encouragement and support of both the patient and the family are important.

The evidence of the meaningful storage of consolidated elements points to a stage of coding that may be called synthesis. The organized elements consolidated for central processing enter an already highly organized system of stored information. In other words, prior experience and education shape further processing so that what is coded is a synthesis of new and previously stored information. This function involves relating, organizing, differentiating, and integrating. A speculative, general theory of how the brain works in registering, coding, and synthesizing is explained by Poggio (1990). The theory predicts a specific type of population coding that represents an extension of schemes such as look-up tables—that is, it provides a more specific version of the classic theme of information processing in the brain, leading to "grandmother" neurons responding selectively to the precise combination of visual features that are associated with one's grandmother. The main points of this theory are (1) the brain uses modules for multivariate function approximation as basic components of several of its information-processing subsystems, (2) these modules are realized as HyperBF networks, and (3) HyperBF networks can be implemented in terms of biologically plausible mechanisms and circuitry. A HyperBF network is the most general and powerful version of the regularization networks that represent a general framework for learning smooth mappings and that rigorously connect approximation theory, generalized splines, and regularization with feedforward multilayer networks. Specific biophysical mechanisms are suggested as part of a basic type of neural circuitry to approximate multidimensional input and output mappings from sets of examples. These circuits are replicated in different regions of the brain and across modalities.

A deficit in synthesis of coding can be called lack of perspective. Behaviorally, this deficit is manifested by impaired ability to differentiate and identify common elements in past, present, and future sets of information; to identify differences and relationships among these elements; and to integrate such information into a whole as a basis for a modulated response. This basic problem in handling the coding of one's environment calls for aware and sensitive nursing care.

Patients who are not able to integrate the coding of sensory experience in an ongoing way need protective and supportive supervision. A structured and controlled environment can contribute to safety and psychologic comfort. Remaining in a familiar environment as long as is feasible is helpful. Relief for caregivers is often indicated because it takes much energy and patience to help the person synthesize experience on a minute-to-minute basis. Issues related to long-term institutional care may be faced, and the nurse can provide guidance and support in this time of transition. Safeguarding of personal integrity is as significant as protection from physical hazards for these patients. As Taylor and Ballenger (1980) noted, even the most befuddled patient will be acutely aware of the attitudes and behaviors of the caregivers.

CONCEPT FORMATION

The process of concept formation is key to the person's ability to process and deal effectively with the world. Concept formation adds qualitatively different functions to the coding process. Specifically, these functions include integrated recognition, abstraction and flexibility, and calculation.

Pattern recognition has been discussed as the ability of the sensory cortex to correlate, analyze, and interpret sensations. Just as Damasio (1985) regarded perception and recognition as part of a continuum, so here it is maintained that integrated recognition is a further point along that continuum. Powerful recognition capabilities are a major component of expert systems. Therefore, within the domain of concept formation lies the potential for differentiating human abilities and performance.

Some critics claim that agnosic failures, or pattern recognition deficits, can be understood as the combined result of primary sensory processing disturbance and generalized mental deterioration or as a complex mixture of disturbed perception and faulty sensory-motor exploration. Early on, Geschwind (1965) stated that recognition is not a unitary process and suggested that agnosic errors result from disconnection of intact cortical sensory regions from an intact speech area. The term, according to Geschwind, covers the totality of all the associations aroused by any object. Recognition at the central processing end of the continuum encompasses a broad range of behaviors including attention, feature extraction, exploratory behavior, pattern and form perception, temporal resolution, and memory. Damasio, Damasio, & van Hoesen (1982) expanded this thesis by adding that recognition is a combined evocation of pertinent multimodal memories that permit the experience of familiarity. With advances in studying sensory systems, recognition of sensorially presented stimuli is understood as a complex outcome of parallel processing occurring simultaneously at the cortical and subcortical levels.

Bauer (1993) reviewed these advances and noted that much of the problem of agnosia can be reduced to the problem of fractionated recognition abilities. This identification of a problem is consistent with the underlying theory of

HyperBF networks proposed by Poggio (1990). Thus, in dealing with the central cognitive processes, we refer to one deficit of concept formation as fractionated recognition. Behaviorally, this deficit is manifested by a lack of subjective familiarity with the stimulus and by an absence of responses adequate to the stimulus, as well as by a simple loss of ability to identify stimuli. A structured and controlled environment is important for these patients, as it is for patients with other cognitive processing deficits. Because familiarity with the environment is lacking, the nurse will help the person deal with the resulting feelings of perplexity and fear.

Another stage of concept formation involves abstraction and flexibility. Woody (1982) noted that perception involves primary image construction and arises from uncomplicated processing of sensory-coded information. Conceptualization and language, on the other hand, appear to involve extended secondary image construction. An extended image implies some inference drawn from perception. It is an image of an image and may not correspond to physical reality. Such abstracted conceptualizations seem to depend on similarities being detected between primary images.

Woody (1982) defined a primary image as an aggregate of sensory-coded information distributed among a set of neurons. Extended imagery is the process whereby the central nervous system, with all its stored information, orders the matter of primary images in space and time and supplies the concepts whereby we understand experience. Consider the proposal of HyperBF networks. Woody (1982) provided the example of a fish swimming under water going through the following sequence: (1) sensation—"I see something," (2) primary image—"It's worm shaped," and (3) extended image—"Is it food or bait?" Although the use of language is closely related to abstract conceptualization, this does not mean that words are necessary for abstract thinking, as noted earlier in the example of aphasic patients who could use ASL but not English vocabulary. Furthermore, the example is often given of Helen Keller, who was blind and deaf but after learning language could explain, "Ideas derived from material objects appear to me first in ideas similar to those of touch. Instantly, they pass into intellectual meanings. Afterwards, the meaning finds expression in what is called inner speech" (Keller, 1954).

A deficit of the functions of abstraction and flexibility is called conceptual concreteness and mental inflexibility. Behaviorally, the person who is having difficulty thinking abstractly will show an inability to form concepts, use categories, generalize from a single instance, or apply procedural rules and general principles such as grammar or conduct. There will be a preference for obvious, superficial solutions. The person cannot comprehend subtle underlying or intrinsic aspects of a situation and therefore is unable to distinguish what is relevant from what is irrelevant, what is essential from what is inessential, and what is appropriate from what is inappropriate. With this deficit, the person cannot generalize and therefore deals with each event as if it were novel, an isolated experience with its own set of rules. Conceptual inflexibility often occurs with concrete thinking, and the effects of each are mutually reinforcing. However, in some persons, particularly when there is frontal lobe involvement, conceptual inflexibility can be present to a significant degree without much impairment of the ability to form and apply abstract concepts. The key feature of this deficit is the inability to shift a course of thought or action according to the demands of the situation.

Interventions for persons showing concrete thinking or conceptual inflexibility focus on limiting the need to abstract or symbolize and on maintaining sameness in the environment. For these patients, it is better to show them than to try to explain (e.g., to show them a picture of the rehabilitation hospital). Procedures are explained as they are occurring rather than in advance, using simple and concrete language—for example, "You are going to have a spinal tap. I'll help you. First, turn on your side like this. Now the doctor will clean your back. It will feel cold." Conversations generally focus on the patient and on present concerns. Trying to broaden the focus of attention may confuse the patient. Family members can limit their talk to simple, familiar things happening at home or in the person's neighborhood. In particular, Taylor and Ballenger (1980) noted that the patient who cannot deal with abstractions takes everything literally, including teasing or joking statements. Humor and sarcasm are readily misunderstood and should be avoided until the patient can handle them. Showing appreciation for a humorous remark may be an early sign of recovering central processing functions.

Calculation is a specialized function of abstraction. It involves operations of ordering and compounding using numbers. As with other central processes, observations of persons with deficits of calculation show that this is not a unitary function that can be specifically lateralized and localized. The process of calculation is understood as similar to language. There is no unitary aphasia or lesion localization that produces a generalized language disturbance. Rather, language is differentially disrupted by compromise in its various neural substrates. These different lesions produce different patterns of language errors. Contributions to the classification of acalculia (disturbances in calculation) show a trend toward more detailed analysis of errors, just as in the analysis of aphasia.

Levin, Goldstein, and Spiers (1993) noted that this type of analysis can be combined with improved methods of lesion localization by CT and with new techniques to measure regional cerebral blood flow and metabolism to better understand the cerebral organization of calculation. They pointed to Warrington's study of a physician whose language fully recovered within 1 month of a left posterior parieto-occipital intracerebral hematoma. Even though the patient's acute aphasia subsided, he exhibited a residual decline in efficiency and accuracy of calculation for all oral and written arithmetic operations; however, his capacity to follow procedural rules (e.g., borrowing) in solutions to mathematical problems, to provide numerical cognitive estimates (e.g., estimating the height of the average English woman), and to select the larger of two numbers was relatively well preserved. The case analysis demonstrates several points about calculation as a central process. First, it is possible to identify a dissociation between arithmetic processing in general and accurate retrieval of specific computational values. Second, calculation represents a major category of semantic knowledge within which it is possible to identify various subcategories that may become disrupted. Finally, there is further evidence that the left hemisphere is preferentially involved in mediating the fundamental calculation process.

On the basis of current understanding of this central function, acquired disorders of calculation are divided into three categories: acalculia secondary to alexia and agraphia for numbers, acalculia resulting from spatial disorganization of numbers, and anarithmetria or impaired calculation in the strict sense. The major behavioral manifestations of these deficits that the nurse will be aware of are (1) the impaired ability to identify values of digits in a counting system and (2) the impaired ability to identify or use symbols or elements of mathematical operations. Interventions are aimed at having the person recognize the deficit so that alternative plans can be made for meeting needs that require calculation. (The management of a checkbook is a common example.) An understanding of the problem can be comforting to the patient. He or she may be told the nature of the disturbance and reassured that it is a phenomenon that is understood but still being studied. Most especially, the person can be encouraged that abilities in certain areas are likely to improve as the disease condition improves.

The registration, coding, and storage of conceptual information constitute only a phase of human cognitive processes. This central processing acts in preparation for the phase in which conscious activity is organized and carried out.

Impaired Cognitive Functions of Output Processing

The thinking person is also an acting person. For cognitions to be communicated, they must be physically enacted. To help a patient understand human information processing, then, one explains how the person transmits information to the environment, as well as how the person takes information in and codes and conceptualizes it for retrieval. Action is characterized at all levels by a degrees-of-freedom problem—that is, a surplus of options, choices, and potential control variables (Jordan & Rosenbaum, 1989). Human beings even have a capacity for motor equivalence; for example, they can achieve the same physical objective in more than one way. One can get another person's attention by speaking his or her name or by a gentle tap on the shoulder. Theoretically, the problem is to understand how the system discovers effective patterns of action among a plethora of possibilities.

Luria (1973, p. 79) described the third functional system of the brain as the one responsible for programming, regulating, and verifying activity. Lezak (1994) discussed such processes in terms of executive functions and motor performance. The executive functions include four components: goal formulation, planning, carrying out of goal-directed plans, and effective performance. Each of these components, the author noted, is necessary for appropriate social responsibility and for effective adult conduct.

Insight into the significance of human output is provided by Sacks' (1983) descriptions of postencephalitic patients emerging from parkinsonian inactivity when treated with the drug levodopa. Observing patients who were suddenly mobile after years of virtually total immobility led the neurologist to reflect on the truth of Leibniz's dictum *Quod non agit non existit*—what does not act does not exist. Sacks commented, "We are critically dependent on a continual flow of impulses and information to and from all the sensory and motor organs of the body. We must be active or we cease to exist: activity and actuality are one and the same" (1983, p. 302). Sacks called the experiences he was witnessing in his patients "awakenings."

Executive functioning is affected by intactness of the frontal lobes and subcortical areas, particularly the limbic structures, including the thalamic nuclei. Frontal lobe damage affects basic aspects of cognition and of neurologic function. Still, the notion of a unitary frontal lobe syndrome has been refuted by anatomic, clinical, and neuropsychologic evidence. The system of executive functions can break down at any stage in the behavioral sequence that makes up planned or intentional activity. Furthermore, when a person's capacity for these functions is defective, it typically involves a cluster of deficiencies, with one or two components especially prominent. The outlet channel for executive functions is the motor cortex, but as Luria (1980) noted, the motor projection cortex cannot work in isolation; all a person's movements require, to some extent, a tonic background. This background is provided by the basal motor ganglia and the fibers of the extrapyramidal system. Finally, the prefrontal cortex plays an essential role in regulating the state of activity. Activity changes in accordance with the person's complex intentions and with plans formulated with the aid of language. This sequence is key in the organization of human behavior. Luria (1980) further cited investigations that identify a feedback mechanism as an essential component of any organized action. He concluded that the frontal lobes perform not only the functions of synthesis of external stimuli, preparation for action, and formation of programs, but also the function of allowing for the effect of the action carried out and the verification that it has taken the proper course. The deficits involved in the output functions of cognitive processing are described in relation to three major functions: planning, motor response, and self-regulation, including affect.

PLANNING

Planning involves formulating a goal and determining the steps needed to achieve the goal. Goal formulation is a complex process of determining what one needs or wants and conceptualizing some kind of future realization of that need or want. Lezak (1994) pointed out that the capacity to formulate a goal relates to one's motivations and psychologic awareness of self. This is true even at the less well-conceptualized level of forming an intention.

Persons who lack the capacity to formulate goals simply do not think of things to do. They may be capable of performing complex activities, such as swatting away an annoying fly or responding to internal stimuli such as a full bladder. However, they cannot initiate such activity unless instructed to do so. Even simple activities such as eating can be done only with continuing explicit instructions. If deficits are less severe, the person may be able to eat what is set before him or her without the verbal direction to eat but will not seek out food spontaneously, even when hungry. With mild impairment of planning functions, patients can do their usual chores and engage in familiar activities and hobbies without prompting. These persons, however, are typically unable to assume responsibilities that require long-term or abstract goals. Therefore, they do not enter new activities independently.

Lezak (1994) noted that to plan, a person must be able to conceptualize change from present circumstances, deal objectively with the self in relation to the environment, and view the environment objectively. This ability relates to the functions of abstraction and flexibility discussed as a part of the central cognitive processing. The person must be able to conceive of alternatives, to weigh and make choices, and to evolve a conceptual framework or structure that will give direction to carrying out the plan conceptualized. Judgment is the particular weighing of one type of behavior against another. It involves the use of foresight and anticipation of the outcome of one's actions. Some areas to observe in assessing a person's planning abilities are abstract versus concrete reasoning patterns, thought flexibility, egocentrism, and inhibition and disinhibition. The nurse will note the effective strategies the patient has maintained, the strategies that are proving ineffective for the person, and the interplay of the integration of the various processes.

Specific deficits of the planning function include impairment of problem solving, means-end analysis, and judgment. Impaired problem solving is manifested behaviorally by the person's inability to order systematically an internally generated, temporally distributed sequence of activity. Sometimes the patient may be able to perform structured activities within normal limits. However, in unstructured verbalizations and in writing, many patients, including those with mild head injuries, reveal marked difficulty organizing their thoughts.

Impaired means-end analysis refers to failures in identification of a group of subgoals and in organization of those goals into a set of acts leading to the attainment of the larger goal. For verbally related means-end analysis, the critical point is the temporal ordering of the subgoals. Thus what the person does first, second, and so forth is significant. Nonverbal deficits in this processing may appear as difficulty solving a visually presented maze. It is characteristic that persons with such deficits do not make the expected improvement after feedback on their errors. Thus they may make the same wrong turn again.

Impaired judgment is looked at behaviorally as inability to act appropriately in an ambiguous situation. A commonly used assessment of judgment is to ask patients what they would do if they found a sealed, stamped, addressed envelope on the street. Weintraub and Mesulam (1985), however, cautioned that, taking into account studies of moral development, there are distinctions among knowing what to do, knowing why to do it, and actually acting in a real situation. Thus a person may be able to respond appropriately to the examiner's question but might act in an entirely different way that is clearly inappropriate. Weintraub and Mesulam (1985) suggested that a more reliable way to assess judgment is by direct observation of behavior or by interviewing family members carefully about the patient's behavior in situations requiring judgment.

Although much knowledge of frontal lobe function remains elusive, patients with selective frontal lobe damage usually show two features. First, functions attributed to the other three lobes of the brain, such as motor dexterity, perceptual abilities, memory, and language, are relatively preserved. Second, there are deficits in judgment, insight, mental flexibility, reasoning, abstraction, planning, sequencing, and testing of attentional tone—especially in those tests that depend on response inhibition and on the ability to sustain behavioral output.

Patients with more subtle deficits of planning can be assessed in the workplace and in the home. They will report that they can no longer function well because they cannot concentrate or cannot follow complex instructions. Penfield (cited in Mesulam, 1985) reported that at the end of the acute postoperative period, his sister, on whom he had performed a right-sided prefrontal lobectomy, had quite preserved abilities of judgment, insight, social graces, and cognitive abilites. However, when he visited her home as a dinner guest, he noticed a diminished capacity for the planned preparation and administration of the meal and a slowing of thinking. Mesulam (1985) noted that although such subtle changes are rather characteristic of unilateral prefrontal lesions, bilateral involvement leads to the more dramatic disturbances of motivation, insight, judgment, and comportment, seen as highly inappropriate behavior. Because persons with planning deficits cannot generate and carry out a plan for their own daily activities, they need guidance to avoid aimless wandering once they have finished their routine activities. Again, as with other cognitive deficits, interventions are directed toward identifying the nature and extent of the deficit and providing the supervision and supportive care needed for safety and for leading as productive and satisfying a life as possible.

Activities suggested for head-injured patients to overcome difficulties with inferential reasoning can be useful in many other situations of planning deficits. According to Tomlin and Liberto (1993), activities for different levels of reasoning include the following:

Lower level—interpretation of idiom, slang, and expressions in one's language; interpretation of concrete-level jokes; paraphrasing of idioms in sentences; and making basic inferences about pictures (e.g., "I know it is daytime because the sun is shining.")

Middle level—proverb interpretation; matching punchlines to jokes; putting the frames of comic strips in order; interpreting how voice tones and word accents change sentence meaning; stating opinions and explaining other people's opinions; labeling emotions conveyed in situations and pictures; and determining consequences from specific actions and situations

Higher level—interpreting cartoons and comic strips; reading and interpreting metaphoric stories; interpreting poetry; interpreting pictures and captions; analyzing other people's opinions and viewpoints; using humor and abstract language in structured situations and in conversation; and analyzing how different actions will result from various approaches

There are, of course, virtually no human actions that involve only one executive thinking function. Rather, cognitive abilities of interacting with the environment manifest themselves in an integrated manner. In helping patients with this integration, the nurse structures multifaceted tasks that have varied executive thinking skills layered into them. For example, the patient in a busy clinic can be asked to focus on reading a page of the newspaper, then picking out two major stories and interpreting the meaning of each, and finally deciding on two possible future outcomes for each story. There are endless possibilities for using creativity in meeting each patient's needs. In particular, the nurse shares his or her understanding of the deficits with both the patient and the family so that they also can learn to use strategies for strengthening cognitive processing abilities and for compensating for areas of deficit.

MOTOR RESPONSE

The stage of human information processing that translates cognitive activity into overt behavior has been implied in earlier discussion. Lezak (1994) noted that this stage requires a response modality sufficiently integrated with central cortical activity to transform conceptual experience into manifest behavior. As described by Poggio (1990), the cerebellum is a part of the brain that is important in the coordination of complex muscle movements. It provides a set of approximation modules for learning to perform motor skills, both movements and posture. Golgi's cells receive input, and Purkinje's cells are the outputs of the network. Still, the distinguishing features of complex movement have not been described adequately, and thus it is more difficult to discuss motor response as a basic process and to outline the deficits of functioning.

Willis and Grossman (1981) discussed willed movement and noted that it appears to be characterized by the act of initiating the movement. Once the movement is started, it is possible that it may be carried on by centrally programmed or reflex mechanisms. Willed movements have the second characteristic that their purpose is to reach some goal. This may be a goal in the person's sensory field or one that is represented in the person's memory store of information. The motivational aspect of voluntary movement suggests that the descending motor systems are being driven from a core of the person that is related to consciousness, emotion, and memory (see the following discussion of consciousness). Structures with projections to large portions of the cortex are important in the initiation of movement, and therefore Willis and Grossman (1981) suggested that the nonspecific thalamic system might function in voluntary movement. Limbic structures and their thalamic and frontal lobe projections that are apparently involved in emotion, motivation, and memory may also be important.

As listed in Table 13–3, the major functions of motor response include motor planning, initiating action, and regulating action. With motor planning, major deficits are sequencing disorders and dyspraxia. A sequencing disorder is recognized behaviorally as an impaired ability to put together coherent sets of movements and progress from one component to the next. Dyspraxia refers

TABLE 13–3 • DEFICITS OF COGNITIVE OUTPUT PROCESSES

Deficits by Function	Behavioral Manifestations	Interventions
A. Planning		
1. Impaired problem solving	Inability to order systematically an internally generated, temporally distributed sequence of activity	Identify nature and extent of deficit and provide for safety.
2. Impaired means-end analysis	Failure to identify a group of subgoals and to organize those goals into a set of acts leading to attainment of larger goal Poor functioning because of problems with concentration and following instructions	Provide supervision and support for routine activities. Guide toward productive and satisfying activity after routines are completed.
3. Impaired judgment	Inability to act appropriately in an ambiguous situation	Use exercises related to interpreting idioms, jokes, and proverbs. Have patient label emotions in pictures and determine consequences from specific actions and situations. Practice interpreting cartoons and comic strips, and analyzing how different actions will result from various approaches. Teach patient and family about the deficit and how to strengthen abilities and to compensate for areas of deficit.
B. Motor response		
1. Motor planning		
a. Sequencing disorder	Impaired ability to put together coherent sets of movements and to progress from one component to the next	Plan to meet needs of activities of daily living. Provide supervision and support.
b. Dyspraxia	Impaired ability to generate individual, goal-oriented skilled movements	Maintain sensitivity to thinking and feeling person.
2. Initiating action		
a. Deficit of intentional movement	Impaired initiation of planned action	
3. Regulating action		
a. Deficit of monitoring, modulating, and regulating behavior	Unawareness of behavioral errors such as those of intensity and timing or perception of errors that does not lead to correction	Identify nature and extent of the deficit and help family plan for meeting daily needs. Teach the concept of feedback systems and help plan alternative systems for checking behavior.
b. Deficits of social planning	Abnormal social conduct leading to negative consequences (e.g., choosing untrustworthy friends), inability to handle money	Try to activate, by cognitive learning, the link between given situation and eventual somatic state; some computer games are thus programmed.
c. Impaired self-consciousness	Inability to identify one's own feelings	Teach sensory discriminatory skills and use driver metaphor.
d. Impaired intentionality	Irresponsible behavior	Teach and practice discriminatory skills or feelings. Teach basics of human behavior. Build conceptual frameworks that include cultural values.

to an impairment of the ability to generate individual, goal-oriented, skilled movements. Apraxia can be defined as the inability to carry out a motor act despite intact motor and sensory systems, good comprehension, and full cooperation. Deficits of motor planning are not a result of impaired comprehension, motivation, or other such factors. Posture and movement are normal, but skill is lost. Rather than a disorder of movement per se, it is a disorder of the systems that command movement, or, in other words, a failure in output transmission. With such disorders, automatic or habitual movements are frequently preserved.

Initiating action is a specific function of motor response. Difficulties with this function can be termed deficits of intentional movement. Brooks (1984) discussed models of intended movement and provided details of the neural basis of motor control. He described a learned task, such as hitting a baseball, as an action sequence produced by overall plans that create smooth, fast, skillful action. Such motor programs are a set of muscle commands that are structured before the motor action begins, and, in the neurologically intact person, they can be sent to the muscles with the correct timing so that the entire sequence can be performed. Behaviorally, deficits in this function are seen as impaired intiation of planned action.

Impairments related to motor planning and initiating action greatly disrupt the integrated functioning needed for carrying out activities of daily living. Interventions focus on identifying the nature and extent of the deficit and providing for safety, supervision, and support as needed. At the same time, the nurse will be aware that it may be only the output of cognitive functioning that is a difficulty for the patient. Except that these persons cannot execute what they intend, they are normally thinking and feeling people.

Regulating action is the final aspect of motor response discussed. In describing the function of regulating action, Lezak (1994) noted that an activity is as effective as the performer's ability to monitor, self-correct, and regulate the intensity, tempo, and other qualitative aspects of the performance. Similarly, Luria's (1987) emphasis on self-regulation addressed the person's need for a well-functioning response feedback system to continuously monitor and modulate output. Abilities for self-correction and self-monitoring are vulnerable to many different kinds of brain damage. Some patients cannot correct their mistakes because they do not perceive them. Other patients may perceive their errors and even identify them and yet, because of other output deficits, not be able to initiate action to correct them. Behaviorally, this deficit shows up in many ways—for example, in a missed line in an account book or in shoelaces broken because of too much pressure. Cramped writing may leave little or no space between words; responses on paper-and-pencil tests or questionnaires may be skipped.

Clinical studies of a 33-year-old woman described striking deficits in higher cognition, most notably in self-regulation of emotion and affect and in social behavior (Eslinger, Grattan, Damasio, & Damasio, 1992). Of particular note is the evidence of delayed consequences of damage to the frontal lobe sustained 26 years earlier. Analysis of the patient's behavioral development failed to show a pattern of abrupt onset of deficits immediately after the injury. Rather, there was a delayed onset, followed by a period of seeming progression and finally by an arrest of development in adolescence. The neurologic examination was normal, but MRI revealed a lesion in the left prefrontal cortex and the deep white matter. Cerebral blood flow studies showed an abnormal pattern in both the left and the right frontal regions. The investigators suggested that this unusual pattern of symptom development was the natural consequence of the varied changes that occur in brain development and social cognition during formative years.

The pathophysiology of developed deficits revealed in abnormal social behavior has been an enigma. Following damage to ventromedian frontal cortices, adults with previously normal personalities develop defects in decision making and planning. These defects result in abnormal social conduct that repeatedly leads to negative personal consequences. Damasio et al. (1990) proposed that the defect is due to an inability to activate somatic states linked to reward and punishment. These states were previously experienced in association with specific social situations, and they must be reactivated in connection with anticipated outcomes of response options. Failure to reactivate pertinent somatic markers would deprive the individual of an automatic device to signal the eventual harmful consequences of responses that might initially bring immediate reward or, alternatively, to signal ultimately beneficial outcomes of responses that might initially bring immediate pain. Activation of somatic markers would (1) force attention to future negative consequences, permitting conscious suppression of the responses leading to them and deliberate selection of personally beneficial responses and (2) trigger unconscious inhibition of response states by engagement of subcortical neurotransmitter systems linked to appetitive behaviors. Investigation of this theory in patients with frontal damage reveals that their autonomic responses to socially meaningful stimuli are indeed abnormal, suggesting that such stimuli fail to activate somatic states at the most basic level. Still, elementary unconditioned stimuli such as loud noises produce normal autonomic responses.

Consciousness is a significant concept to include when discussing the regulation of action, also known as self-regulation. Consciousness was described in relation to the realm of sensory input and also as a prerequisite for the central process of registering information. However, when dealing with locomotion, reaching and prehension, oculomotor control, and intentional actions, human activity is much more than outputs of a highly complex physical system, ultimately to be understood in terms of musculature and neurocircuitry. Activity, and what is termed intentionality, stem from frameworks including such things as needs, motives, values, and beliefs that are built up in human consciousness. Human consciousness has been termed one of the last surviving mysteries of science. Still, what began as philosophical debate has been joined by psychology, artificial intelligence, neuroscience, ethology, and evolutionary theory to make encouraging progress in understanding the importance of consciousness of self, values, and action. Eccles and Robinson (1985) noted that there is strong support for the hypothesis that the supplementary motor area is the sole recipient area of the brain for mental intentions that lead to voluntary movements. Still, Dennett (1991) insisted that consciousness is a mode of action of the brain rather than a subsystem of the brain and that it is therefore possible for such mode shifts to be timed by outside observers.

The philosopher Immanuel Kant described a person as a subject who is responsible for one's own actions. Self-consciousness is necessary to monitor and regulate one's behavior. To be self-conscious is to have, at a minimum, knowledge of oneself. Self-consciousness involves not just knowledge of one's physical states but knowledge of one's mental states specifically. Also, one's consciousness involves the same kind of continuous apprehension of an inner reality, the reality of one's mental states and activities. Differentiating one mental state from another depends on apprehending them within a conceptual framework that catalogs the various different types of mental states. One can make the recognitional judgment that one is angry, is elated, or believes or hopes in something. Churchland (1988) pointed out that this suggests that there are different degrees of self-consciousness, because presumably one's ability to discriminate subtly different types of mental states improves with practice and increasing experience. Further, the conceptual framework within which explicit recognition is expressed grows in sophistication and comprehensiveness as one learns more about the intricacies of human nature.

The expansion of introspective consciousness is generally viewed as a good thing both for the individual and for the society. Nurse authors such as Newman (1999) viewed health as expanding consciousness. Roy (Roy & Andrews, 1999) views conscious awareness as a basic human ability used to promote adaptation. Churchland (1988) discussed how one might improve or enhance introspective access. Surgical or genetic modification may be possible but is not realistic in the short term. He suggested that we can learn to make more refined and penetrating use of the discriminatory mechanisms we already possess. Illustrating this ability using an external sense modality, he considered the enormous increase in discriminatory skill and theoretical insight that spans the gap between an untrained child's auditory apprehension of Beethoven's Fifth Symphony and the same person's auditory apprehension of the same symphony 40 years later, heard in his or her capacity as conductor of the orchestra performing it. What was before a dimly apprehended tune is now a rationally structured sequence of distinguishable chords supporting an appropriately related melody line. Churchland (1988) gave similar examples in chemistry and astronomy and then noted that in each of these cases, what is finally mastered is a conceptual framework—musical, chemical, or astronomic—a framework that embodies far more wisdom about the relevant sensory domain than is immediately apparent to undeveloped discrimination. Such frameworks result from a cultural heritage that is pieced together over many generations. Their mastery supplies a richness and penetration to our sensory lives that would be impossible without such input. Churchland (1988) then suggested that it is the conceptual framework of a completed neuroscience that will embody the essential wisdom about our inner nature and the dawning in which its marvelous intricacies are finally revealed in self-conscious introspection.

The two-way flow of consciousness was noted in Eccles and Robinson's (1985) discussion of voluntary movement, freedom of the will, and moral responsibility. Arguing against pure materialism, Eccles and Robinson cited the transcendent importance of recognizing that by taking thought we can influence the operation of the neural mechanisms of the brain. In that way we can bring about changes in the world for good or ill. They used the simple metaphor that our conscious self is in the driver's seat. Life can be regarded as made up of successive patterns of choices that could lead to the feeling of fulfillment with the attendant happiness that comes from a life centered on meaning and purpose. The ideal that each human person is to have the maximum freedom to realize his or her potentialities derives from the belief that life has a transcendental meaning and that each life is precious. This value has been stated in many ways in philosophies of nursing (for example, by Roy in 1988 and 1997), but its full impact relative to neuroscience progress has not yet been fully explicated. Herein lies a rich science of intentional health as the pinnacle of human existence.

Deficits of regulating action are important to the patient and to society at large. Legal systems often respond to the person's ability to regulate his or her own actions when those actions have been outside the societal norms specified in law. Again, the nurse can help identify the nature and extent of deficits in the area of regulating action. On the basis of the particular needs of the patient, the nurse can help the family plan for meeting needs of daily living. On the basis of the current understanding of these deficits, as discussed here, other, more specific interventions may be tried. The patient may be taught the concept of a feedback system, learn the deficits that he or she has, and plan to consciously develop alternative systems (for example, manually and visually checking intensity, tempo, and bookwork).

Nurses have long worked with patients who have defects in social planning, under the label of sociopathic personalities. Explaining this defect and its place among the deficits of cognitive output processing may offer new insights for intervention. For example, on the basis of the patient's remaining cognitive skills, the nurse may make efforts to activate learning of the link between given situations and eventual somatic states. Certain computer games can be programmed to include making responses and withholding responses. One teenager who had a head injury was trained with such a computer game. She returned to the clinic saying, "Every time my mother yells, that's a yellow light." The teenager had learned to withhold her response and not perpetuate fights with her mother. The interventions for impaired self-consciousness and impaired intentionality are based on a similar understanding of the deficits. The nurse can begin by teaching sensory discriminatory skills that provide the delight of discovery. Then the patient can begin to identify the feelings of self and others. Newspaper pictures can be used for practice. The nurse will also include lessons in the basics of human behavior. Combinations of material prepared for kindergarten lessons in social skills and adult self-improvement books are used. The careful task of building conceptual frameworks that include cultural values is demanding but can be most rewarding. Using simple picture sequences of social mishaps, the patient can identify what is happening, what feelings are involved, and, finally, what is wrong with the situation. The patient may be given choices of solutions to make what is happening come out right. The metaphor of being in the driver's seat is useful throughout such training.

The nurse can help family and friends understand the deficits and the interventions that have the potential to help.

SUMMARY

This chapter has highlighted cognitive functioning from an information-processing approach. On the basis of a nursing conceptual framework and knowledge from the neural and behavioral sciences, a nursing model of information processing has been described. Clinical applications of the model outlined the cognitive functions of each stage of the model. Deficits of these functions were described, and interventions useful in working with people with deficits were identified. Knowledge in the area of cognitive processing and its neural basis is burgeoning in the laboratories and clinics around the world. Brooks (1986) made the analogy that we need a simple map to board a fast-moving train so that we may recognize the landscape as it flies by the windows. Today, the field may be compared to boarding a shuttle mission to outer space. All the more necessary is a navigational guide that lets us see in broader expanse and greater detail the universe outside the cockpit window. This chapter is an attempt to point out some dazzling changes in the field of neuroscience and to offer planetary marks that can keep us oriented in the universe of knowledge that is richly being charted before us. Most especially, the chapter offers a way to see scientific developments translated into neuroscience clinical practice.

References

Allport, A. (1989). Visual attention. In M. I. Posner (Ed.), *Foundations of cognitive science* (pp. 631–682). Cambridge, MA: MIT Press.

Anderson, S. W., Damasio, H., Damasio, A. R., Klima, E., Bellugi, U., & Brandt, J. P. (1992). Acquisition of signs from American Sign Language in hearing individuals following left hemisphere damage and aphasia. *Neuropsychologia, 30*(4), 329–340.

Bauer, R. M. (1993). Agnosia. In K. M. Heilman & E. Valenstein (Eds.), *Clinical neuropsychology* (3rd ed., pp. 215–278). New York: Oxford University Press.

Benson, D. F., & Geschwind, N. (1985). Aphasia and related disorders: A clinical approach. In M. M. Mesulam (Ed.), *Principles of behavorial neurology* (pp. 193–238). Philadelphia: F.A. Davis.

Bickley, L. S. (1999). *Bates' Guide to Physical Examination & History Taking.* Philadelphia: J. B. Lippincott.

Braswell, L., & Kendall, P. C. (1988). Cognitive-behavioral methods with children. In K. S. Dobson (Ed.), *Handbook of cognitive-behavioral therapies* (pp. 167–213). New York: Guilford Press.

Brooks, N. (1984). Cognitive deficits after head injury. In N. Brooks (Ed.), *Closed head injury: Psychological, social and family consequences* (pp. 44–73). New York: Oxford University Press.

Brooks, V. (1986). *The neural basis of motor control.* New York: Oxford University Press.

Brown, L. M., Gouvier, W. D., & Blanchard-Fields, F. (1990). Cognitive interventions across the life-span. In A. M. Horton, Jr. (Ed.), *Neuropsychology across the life-span* (pp. 133–153). New York: Springer.

Churchland, P. M. (1988). *Matter and consciousness: A contemporary introduction to the philosophy of mind.* Cambridge, MA: MIT Press.

Clements, S. D. (1966). *Task force one: Minimal brain dysfunction in children* (National Institute of Neurological Diseases and Blindness Monograph No. 3). Washington, DC: U.S. Department of Health, Education, and Welfare.

Craik, K. (1943). *The nature of explanation.* New York: Cambridge University Press.

Crigger, N. J., & Strickland, C. C. (1985). Selecting a nursing diagnosis for changes in consciousness. *Dimensions of Critical Care Nursing, 4*(3), 156.

Damasio, A. R. (1985). Disorders of complex visual processing: Agnosias, achromatopsia, Balint's syndrome, and related difficulties of orientation and construction. In M. M. Mesulam, Jr. (Ed.), *Principles of behavorial neurology* (pp. 259–288). Philadelphia: F.A. Davis.

Damasio, A. R., Damasio, H., & van Hoesen, G. W. (1982). Prosopagnosia: Anatomic basis and behavioral mechanisms. *Neurology, 32*(4), 331–341.

Damasio, A. R., & Tranel, D. (1992). Knowledge systems. *Current Opinions in Neurobiology, 2*(2), 186–190.

Damasio, A. R., Tranel, D., & Damasio, H. (1990). Individuals with sociopathic behavior caused by frontal damage fail to respond autonomically to social stimuli. *Behavioral Brain Research, 41*(2), 81–94.

Das, J. P. (1984). Intelligence and information integration. In J. Kirby (Ed.), *Cognitive strategies and educational performance.* McLean, VA: Academic Press.

Dehaene, S., Changeux, J. P., & Nadal, J. P. (1987). Neural networks that learn temporal sequences by selection. *Proceedings of the National Academy of Science, 84*(9), 2727–2731.

Dennett, D. C. (1991). *Consciousness explained.* Boston: Little, Brown.

Eccles, J., & Robinson, D. N. (1985). *The wonder of being human: Our brain and our mind.* Greenwich, CT: New Science Library.

Eslinger, P. J., Grattan, L. M., Damasio, H., & Damasio, A. R. (1992). Developmental consequences of childhood frontal lobe damage. *Archives of Neurology, 49*(7), 764–769.

Friedman, R. F., Ween, J. E., & Albert, M. L. (1993). Alexia. In K. M. Heilman & E. Valenstein (Eds.), *Clinical neuropsychology* (pp. 37–62). New York: Oxford University Press.

Geschwind, N. (1965). Disconnection syndromes in animals and man. *Brain, 88,* 237, 585.

Gronwall, D. M. A., & Sampson, H. (1974). *The psychological effects of concussion.* New Zealand: Auckland University Press.

Heilman, K. M., & Valenstein, E. (1993). *Clinical neuropsychology.* New York: Oxford University Press.

Horel, J. A. (1988). Cortical systems of storage and retrieval. In H. J. Markowitsch (Ed.), *Information processing by the brain: Views and hypotheses from a physiological-cognitive perspective* (pp. 65–78). Toronto, ON: Hans Huber Publishers.

Horton, A. M., Jr., & Puente, A. K. (1990). Life-span neuropsychology: An overview. In A. M. Horton, Jr. (Ed.), *Neuropsychology across the life-span* (pp. 1–15). New York: Springer.

Hunt, E. (1980). Intelligence as an information-processing concept. *British Journal of Psychology, 71,* 449.

Johnson-Laird, P. N. (1989). Mental models. In M. I. Posner (Ed.), *Foundations of cognitive science* (pp. 469–499). Cambridge, MA: MIT Press.

Jordan, M. I., & Rosenbaum, D. A. (1989). Action. In M. I. Posner (Ed.), *Foundations of cognitive science* (pp. 727–767). Cambridge, MA: MIT Press.

Keller, H. (1954). *Story of my life.* New York: Doubleday.

Kolb, B., & Whishaw, I. Q. (1985). *Fundamentals of human neuropsychology.* New York: W.H. Freeman.

Levin, H. S., Goldstein, F. C., & Spiers, P. A. (1993). Acalculia. In K. M. Heilman & E. Valenstein (Eds.), *Clinical neuropsychology* (pp. 91–122). New York: Oxford University Press.

Lezak, M. D. (1994). Domains of behavior from a neuropsychological perspective. *Nebraska Symposium on Motivation, 47,* 23–55.

Lezak, M. D. (1994). *Neuropsychological assessment.* New York: Oxford University Press.

Luria, A. R. (1973). *The working brain: An introduction to neuropsychology.* New York: Basic Books.

Luria, A. R. (1976). *Cognitive development: Its cultural and social foundations.* Cambridge, MA: Harvard University Press.

Luria, A. R. (1980). *Higher cortical functions in man.* New York: Basic Books.

Markowitsch, H. J. (1988). Introducing information processing by the brain. In H. J. Markowitsch (Ed.), *Information processing by the brain: Views and hypotheses from a physiological-cognitive perspective* (pp. 1–4). Toronto, Ontario, Canada: Hans Huber Publishers.

Meichenbaum, D., & Goodman, J. (1971). Training impulsive children to talk to themselves. *Journal of Abnormal Psychology, 77,* 115–126.

Mesulam, M. M. (1985). Attention, confusional states, and neglect. In M. M. Mesulam (Ed.), *Principles of behavioral neurology* (pp. 125–168). Philadelphia: F.A. Davis.

Mountcastle, V. B. (1979). An organizing principle for cerebral function: The unit module and the distributed system. In F. O. Schmitt & F. G. Worden (Eds.), *The neurosciences.* Cambridge, MA: MIT Press.

Mountcastle, V. B. (1997). The columnar organization of the neocortex. *Brain, 120,* 701–722.

Newman, M. A. (1999). *Health as expanding consciousness.* Sudbury, MA: Jones & Bartlett Publishers.

Pi Lambda Theta, San Jose Area Chapter (1983). *Helping head injury and stroke patients home: A handbook for families.* San Jose, CA: Author.

Poggio, T. (1990). A theory of how the brain might work. In *Cold Spring Harbor Symposia on Quantitative Biology* (Vol. LV, pp. 899–910). Plainview, NY: Cold Spring Harbor Laboratory.

Pollatsek, A., & Rayner, K. (1989). Reading. In M. I. Posner (Ed.), *Foundations of cognitive science* (pp. 401–436). Cambridge, MA: MIT Press.

Posner, M. I. (1975). The psychobiology of attention. In M. S. Gazzaniga & C. Blakemore (Eds.), *Handbook of psychobiology* (pp. 441–480). McLean, VA: Academic Press.

Posner, M. I., & Carr, T. H. (1992). Lexical access and the brain: Anatomical constraints on cognitive models of word recognition. *American Journal of Psychology, 105*(1), 1–26.

Pribram, K. H. (1969). *Brain and behavior 3: Memory mechanisms.* New York: Penguin.

Raichle, M. E. (1994, April). Visualizing the mind: Strategies of cognitive science and techniques of modern brain imaging open a window to the neural systems responsible for thought. *Scientific American, (270)*4, 58–64.

Roy, C. (1984). *Introduction to nursing: An adaptation model.* Paramus, NJ: Prentice-Hall.

Roy, C. (1988). An explication of the philosophical assumptions of the Roy adaptation model. *Nursing Science Quarterly, 1*(1), 26–34.

Roy, C. (1997). Future of the Roy adaptation model: Challenge to redefine adaptation. *Nursing Science Quarterly, 10,* 42–48.

Roy, C., & Andrews, H. (1999). *The Roy adaptation model.* Stamford, CT: Appleton & Lange.

Sacks, O. (1983). *Awakenings.* New York: Dutton.

Satz, P., & Ross, J. J. (Eds.) (1973). *The disabled learner.* Holland: Rotterdam University Press.

Schneider, W., & Shiffrin, R. M. (1977). Controlled and automatic human information processing: I. Detection, search and attention. *Psychology Review, 84,* 1.

Sejnowski, T. J., & Churchland, P. S. (1989). Brain and cognition. In M. I. Posner (Ed.), *Foundations of cognitive science* (pp. 301–356). Cambridge, MA: MIT Press.

Shiffrin, R. M., & Schneider, W. (1977). Controlled and automatic human information processing: II. Perceptual learning, automatic attending and a general theory. *Psychology Review, 84,* 127.

Simon, H. A., & Kaplan, C. A. (1989). Foundations of cognitive science. In M. I. Posner (Ed.), *Foundations of cognitive science* (pp. 1–47). Cambridge, MA: MIT Press.

Squire, L. R. (1987). *Memory and brain.* New York: Oxford University Press.

Stamm, J. S., & Kreder, S. V. (1979). Minimal brain dysfunction: Psychological and neurophysiological disorders in hyperkinetic children. In M. S. Gazzaniga (Ed.), *Handbook of behavioral neurobiology* (pp. 119–150). Reading, MA: Plenum Press.

Taylor, J. W., & Ballenger, S. (1980). *Neurological dysfunctions and nursing intervention.* New York: McGraw-Hill.

Teuber, H. L. (1968). Alteration of perception and memory in man. In L. Weiskrantz (Ed.), *Analysis of behavioral change* (pp. 274–328). New York: Harper & Row.

Tomlin, K., & Liberto, L. (1993). Identification and remediation of cognitive-communication impairments following mild head trauma. In S. Mandel, R. T. Sataloff, & S. Schapiro (Eds.), *Minor head trauma: Assessment, management and rehabilitation* (pp. 272–289). New York: Springer-Verlag.

Tourtellotte, W. G., van Hoesen, G. W., Hyman, B. T., Tikoo, R. K., & Damasio, A. R. (1990). Alz-50 immunoreactivity in the thalamic reticular nucleus in Alzheimer's disease. *Brain Research, 515*(1–2), 227–234.

van Zomeren, A. M., Brouwer, W. H., & Deelman, B. G. (1984). Attentional deficits: The riddles of selectivity, speed and alertness. In N. Brooks (Ed.), *Closed head injury: Psychological, social and family consequences* (pp. 74–107). New York: Oxford University Press.

Webster, J., & Scott, R. (1983). The effects of self-instructional training on attention deficits following head injury. *Clinical Neuropsychology, 5,* 69–74.

Weintraub, S., & Mesulam, M. M. (1985). Mental state assessment of young and elderly adults in behavioral neurology. In M. M. Mesulam (Ed.), *Principles of behavioral neurology* (pp. 71–123). Philadelphia: F.A. Davis.

White, M. J., & Wolf-Wilets, V. (1977). Memory loss following halothane anesthesia. *AORN Journal, 26,* 1053.

Willis, W. D., & Grossman, R. G. (1981). *Medical neurobiology.* St. Louis: Mosby–Year Book.

Woody, C. D. (1982). *Memory, learning and higher function.* New York: Springer-Verlag.

COMMUNICATION PHENOMENA

Communication Disorders: An Overview

ROBERTA SCHWARTZ-COWLEY
• ANDREW K. GRUEN

Human communication is often taken for granted despite the fact that it is a tremendously complex process. It represents a sophisticated interplay of language, memory, and reasoning that permits the exchange of ideas, emotions, and desires within one person or among many people. The very foundations of present society, the means of maintaining information from the past, and the projection of plans and aspirations for the future are direct results of this ability to communicate interpersonally and intrapersonally. Impairment or loss of this ability can be catastrophic for an individual and also has implications for the impaired person's family and community.

Communication is a learned system of symbols and codes used to represent thoughts and ideas. When the same group of symbols and codes is learned by more than one individual (a shared system), each can understand what the other expresses. This system is most often called language.

LANGUAGE: DEFINITION AND ACQUISITION

According to Bloom and Leahy (1978), "a language is a code whereby ideas about the world are represented through a conventional system of arbitrary signals for communications" (p. 10).

Definition

Language is a code in the sense that strict rules govern how its signals are formed and used. These signals (symbols) are arbitrary rather than innate.

Symbols, such as speech sounds, spoken and written words, and gestures, were originally invented, maintained, or changed over time by choice. Language is also arbitrary by nature of the cultural variations around the world. For example, the English language varies significantly from the Chinese language, but the English language also varies within itself (Bollinger, 1975).

Language is informative, directive, and expressive: it allows for the exchange of information intrapersonally, interpersonally, and over time (informative); it can be used to cause a person to perform or not perform a specific action (directive); and it conveys feelings and emotions and serves to provide reinforcement and encouragement or their opposite (expressive) (Liles, 1975).

Linguist Noam Chomsky (1968) referred to the fact that, despite a relatively small number of sounds, letters, and gestures, humans have an infinite number of ways to express themselves. This is because the rules for language that govern the content, form, and use of the expressions also allow for creativity and innovation (Perkins, 1971).

Acquisition

Language and its rules are acquired through exposure. A child will learn his or her native language given sufficient exposure to it unless the child is restricted by sensory impairment or learning disabilities (Devilliers & Devilliers, 1978).

Various scales have been compiled to evaluate the emergence of major cognitive, language, and motor milestones. Finding a reasonable balance between the comprehensiveness of such a tool and the time needed to administer it can prove difficult; tests that are sensitive enough to detect mild to moderate problems can be very time-consuming (Wetherby, 1985). A succinct developmental and criterion-referenced scale has been devised by Miller (1983) (Table 14–1). A child who fails to develop a particular language behavior by the age specified should be referred to a speech-language pathologist certified by the American Speech-Language-Hearing Association (ASHA) for further evaluation.

Initially, a child learns how to put sounds together to form words. By 1 to 1.5 years of age, a child will normally have absorbed and begun to use a vocabulary of as many as 50 to 100 words and will have begun to understand sentences spoken by others. Learning and using sounds for verbal expression generally continue until age 7 or 8 years. During that time, the child will learn to combine words to convey more meaning than would be possible with simple word utterances. The child will learn rules that control how these words are used and sentences for appropriate and efficient communication. This overall learning occurs as a gradual acquisition, overgeneralization, and refinement of the symbols of language (Devilliers & Devilliers, 1978; Leonard, 1982; Moskowitz, 1981). Language acquisition at this time is largely passive, reflecting assimilation, modification, and trial and error.

Learning a written language is an active process of associating printed symbols with meaning and verbal correspondents. This learning is achieved through active assistance from others. Gestural communication tends to be

TABLE 14–1 • DEVELOPMENTAL SCALE FOR IDENTIFICATION OF COMMUNICATION DEFICITS IN THE FIRST 2 YEARS OF LIFE

Behaviors that should be present at 6 mo
  Comprehension
    Consistent orienting to sound
  Production
    Syllable repetition (*ba ba ba*)
    Duration of cooing, singing, and babbling, 203 sec
    Variable intonation, both during crying and cooing
    Voiced-voiceless contrast: /p/ vs /b/
    Discrete tongue movements: /d/, /n/
Behaviors that should be present at 12 mo
  Comprehension
    Understands own name or name of present familiar person
  Production
    Ma-ma or da-da, pet name referentially, low frequency and intelligibility
    Imitates speech sounds
  Language use
    Turn-taking vocalizations in communication games, peek-a-boo, pat-a-cake
Behaviors that should be present at 18 mo
  Comprehension
    Understands single words, names for objects within visual field
  Production
    Few intelligible words
    Words frequently note familiar people and objects
    Frequency of vocalization increasing
  Language use
    Requests, comments
    Rejects with motor and vocal or vocal behavior
    Hi and bye with gesture or vocal behavior
Behaviors that should be present at 24 mo
  Comprehension
    Understands at least two words in utterance, such as *throw ball* indicating action object relation
  Production
    Expresses single words, including action verbs and reference to absent objects
    Vocabulary increases to 20 words minimum
    Two-word utterances
    At least two intelligible utterances
  Language use
    Request names, locations: "What's that," "Where's that"
    Uses words for multiple function

From Miller, J. F. (1983). Identifying children with language disorders and describing their language performance. In J. Miller, D. Yoder, & R. Schiefelbusch (Eds.), *Contemporary issues in language intervention* (ASHA Report No. 12, pp. 61–74). Rockville, MD: American Speech-Language-Hearing Association.

learned both passively and actively through recognition, association, assimilation, and inquiry (Hughes, 1962; Knapp, 1981).

Language acquisition, however, is not merely a matter of learning symbols. According to Devilliers and Devilliers (1978), "some changes in child's speech and understanding reflect the growth of linguistic knowledge: others reflect the development of memory capacity, attention span, or reasoning ability" (p. 5).

This fact is important to consider because a person learns the basic rules of word formation and grammar in childhood, but language learning continues throughout life. This continued learning is a result of growth of concept development; better understanding of context, setting, and interpersonal relationships; and increased use of abstraction and problem-solving abilities. This learning is expected to continue passively but may be accelerated or expanded when an individual actively attempts to develop and refine personal language skills as certain needs are encountered.

As people age and mature, they display a high degree of variability in their development of both intrapersonal and interpersonal communication skills. The acquisition and improved use of language seem to slow down the aging process; this decline can be related to a concomitant decline in older people's physiology and auditory capability. Obler and Albert (1981), for example, believed that deterioration of language comprehension and expression with age is likely a manifestation of reduced hearing acuity, attenuation of attending and memory skills, and changes in neuroanatomy and neurophysiology. Expressive language may be further compromised by anatomic and physiologic changes associated with speech, writing, and gestural mechanisms (Kahane, 1981).

Reductions in communication ability during the normal aging process are not predestined, however, and when they do occur, they tend to be individual, like the learning process itself. Obler and Albert (1981) also noted that, for many older people, communication skills (and, thus, language) do not deteriorate. Language efficiency and growth may continue because of improved narrative skills, increased ability to encode thought into language and communicate effectively, and better understanding of what others intend. Furthermore, perceived changes in cognitive skills and memory may not reflect neurophysiologic decline but rather adaptation to the different circumstances and requirements encountered by the geriatric population (Denny, 1981; Smith & Fullerton, 1981).

The likelihood of disrupted language acquisition therefore appears to occur on a highly individualized basis and is not related directly to age considerations. Disorders in language acquisition and use are more readily related to abnormalities that disrupt a person's ability to express and understand. These abnormalities involve anatomic or physiologic changes secondary to vascular, degenerative, and metabolic disorders or to trauma, tumors, infections, or other disorders.

ANATOMY: SPEECH, HEARING, LANGUAGE, AND MOTOR-SPEECH MECHANISMS

A brief review of the structure and physiology of the speech, hearing, language, and motor-speech mechanisms will enhance the discussion of specific communication disorders.

Speech Mechanism

The speech act is a highly complex process involving the coordination of respiratory, laryngeal, palatopharyngeal, lingual, labial, and mandibular musculature. The channel through or adjacent to these structures is the vocal tract, essentially a tube with valves and filters to modify the outgoing airstream (Zemlin, 1968). Principal valving or constriction of the tract occurs at the level of the vocal folds, at the palatopharyngeal sphincter, at various positions of the tongue as it approximates areas within the oral cavity, and at the lips. The quality of sound is related to the sound frequencies generated by the airstream. These frequencies are filtered or modified within the vocal tract by resonance, the characteristic of sound in which existing sound frequencies are magnified or diminished as they pass through the vocal tract (Frey, 1980) (Fig. 14–1).

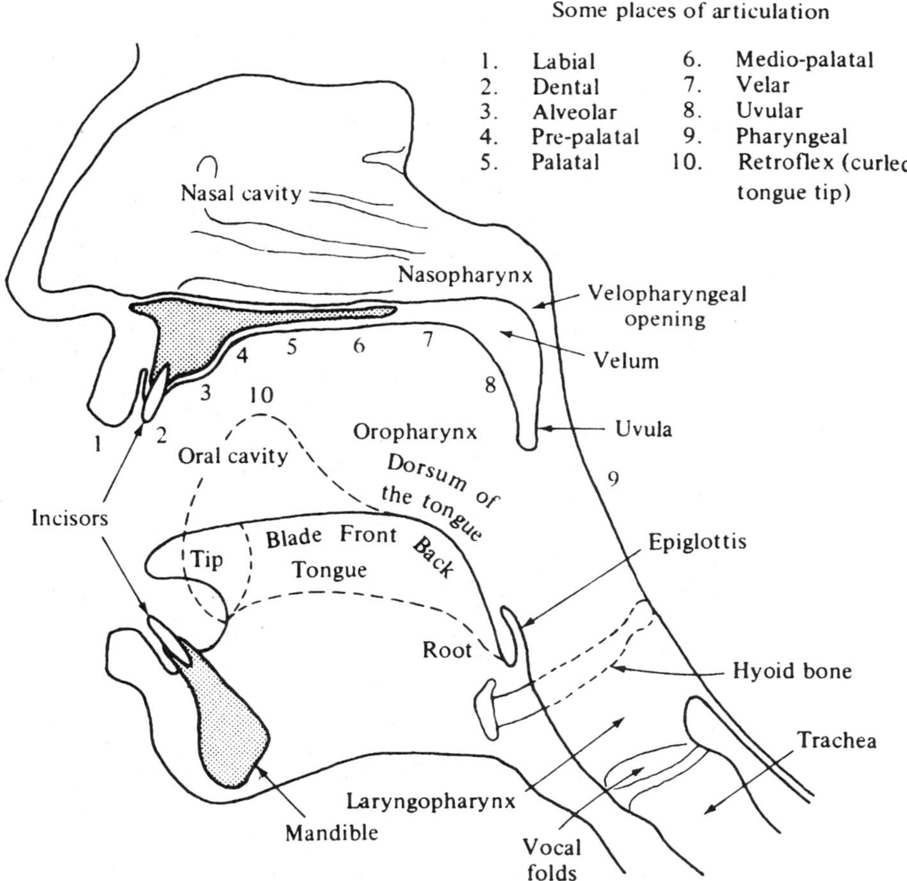

FIGURE 14–1 • The vocal tract and points of articulation: (1) labial, (2) dental, (3) alveolar, (4) prepalatal, (5) palatal, (6) mediopalatal, (7) velar, (8) uvular, (9) pharyngeal, and (10) retroflex (curled tongue tip).

Respiration is the force for speech production. Cooperative interaction of the thoracic and abdominal musculature produces inhalation and exhalation. The exhaled airstream is directed through the bronchial tree and trachea to the larynx. The airstream has no purposeful sound quality until it reaches the larynx. Speech breathing involves quick inhalation and prolonged or extended exhalation; thus, respiration for speech is anticipatory and linguistically conditioned (Perkins, 1971; Zemlin, 1968).

The larynx, a collection of muscles and cartilaginous structures that serves as the first valve in the vocal tract, is suspended between the hyoid bone and the trachea by the exterior or extrinsic laryngeal muscles. The principal cartilages of the larynx for speech purposes are the thyroid, the cricoid, and the paired arytenoids. The interior or intrinsic laryngeal muscles are innervated by the 10th cranial nerve (vagus) and are responsible for phonation or the voicing of speech sounds.

Phonation, an aerodynamic process, occurs through vibration of the vocal folds as air passes through the opening between them (the glottis). The vocal folds are adducted or approximated by contractions of the lateral cricoarytenoid muscles, resulting in increased subglottic pressure as the exhaled airstream gathers below the closed folds. The pressure overcomes the resistance of the elastic vocal folds and forces the folds apart, releasing the airstream and vibrating the vocal folds, which produces phonation or voicing. (The airstream will ascend without voicing if the exhaled air passes through the glottis when the vocal folds are abducted or opened away from each other. Both voiced and unvoiced air are directed upward to the oropharynx for further modification.) The pitch or frequency of the vibrations is relative to the length, mass, and tension of the individual's vocal folds and how these are varied (Frey, 1980; Zemlin, 1968). Finally, air pressure changes and elastic recoil draw the folds back together again.

The second vocal tract valve is the palatopharyngeal sphincter. Most speech sounds are produced in or directed through the oral cavity because the nasopharynx has been sealed off, directing the exhaled airstream through the oropharynx to the oral cavity. The nasopharyngeal port is sealed off by sphincteric closing of the palatopharyngeal isthmus by elevation and tension of the soft palate and approximation of the soft palate by the posterior and lateral pharyngeal walls of the superior constrictor muscles. (The nasopharyngeal port is open for only three speech sounds: the nasal sounds of "M," "N," and "NG.") This palatopharyngeal action is due to innervation by the 10th cranial nerve, with the contribution of motor fibers from the fifth cranial nerve (trigeminal) (Bateman, 1977; Perkins, 1971; Zemlin, 1968).

The airstream receives most of its modification within and as it leaves the oral cavity. The shape of the oral cavity, which is due to the size of the mouth and the amount of space the tongue takes up as it is positioned in different ways, will cause some frequencies to be amplified, some frequencies to be diminished, and some new frequencies to be created secondary to resonance. In addition, specific vowel sounds and consonants will be formed by (1) positioning the tongue, (2) positioning the lips, and (3) moving the lips and jaw. These oral modifications constitute the final valves of the vocal tract.

The complex movements of the tongue are based on interplay of both extrinsic and intrinsic musculature. These movements are principally caused by innervation from the 12th cranial nerve (hypoglossal). Labial or lip movements are variations on sphincteric action owing to the seventh cranial nerve's (facial) innervation. Mouth opening adjustments are related to mandibular or jaw movements secondary to innervation from the motor branch of the fifth cranial nerve. Damage to these structures or disruption of cranial nerve innervation could be catastrophic to speech production.

Hearing Mechanism

Speech and other sounds are heard by way of acoustic, mechanical, and electrical energy that is transmitted through the outer, middle, and inner portions of the ear and through the ascending neural pathways to the cortical association areas (Newby, 1979). The anatomy of hearing is reviewed in Chapter 23.

Language Mechanism

Reception and comprehension of linguistic symbols, association and integration of these symbols, and formulation and programming of expression are associated with activity in the cerebral cortex. Typically, these functions are attributed to the left hemisphere of the cerebrum, although exceptions have been reported. For purposes of this discussion, the left hemisphere is considered the dominant hemisphere for language. Language is a cooperative process that involves many areas of the dominant hemisphere. It also relies on intact input from the nondominant (right) hemisphere and subcortical areas for maximal function and efficiency (Bayles, 1979).

The areas of the brain most often associated with language are located in the temporal and frontal lobes (see Fig. 10–2). The primary auditory cortex (Heschl's gyrus) and Wernicke's area, located in the superior temporal gyrus, are of primary importance for the reception and comprehension of spoken language. The primary speech cortex (Broca's area) is responsible for motor programming of the intended speech message and is also associated with adherence to rules for word and sentence construction. Located in the inferior portion of the third frontal gyrus, Broca's area is adjacent to the precentral gyrus of the frontal lobe, often called the motor strip or motor cortex. The lower portion of the motor cortex, which is responsible for actions of the larynx, tongue, jaw, lips, and face, is situated closest to Broca's area. Transmission between Wernicke's area and Broca's area is accomplished by a tract of nerve fibers called the arcuate fasciculus. Transmission of information from the primary visual cortex to Wernicke's area is accomplished by the angular gyrus of the parietal lobe. This fact is particularly relevant because comprehension of the written word depends on auditory association; that is, auditory symbols are associated with written symbols to allow accurate interpretation and comprehension through reading (Benson, 1979; Benson & Geschwind, 1983).

From a neuroanatomic and neurophysiologic viewpoint, a language model involves a highly complex, cooperative process. It is important to consider the brain's language activities as a diffuse, integrative process involving not isolated, specialized areas but interrelated areas that complement each other for maximal communication.

Motor-Speech Mechanism

Once programmed, the motor-speech act must be transmitted to the appropriate speech musculature to achieve the intended speech production. The speech program is delivered to the motor cortex. The direct pathway of motor activity involves upper motor neurons and is referred to as the pyramidal system. Messages are transmitted to the final common motor pathway (lower motor neurons), comprising the motor nuclei of the cranial nerves, the myoneural junctions, and the muscles themselves. These direct or voluntary processes are regulated by three other more indirect processes: (1) the extrapyramidal system, which consists of neural pathways descending from the basal ganglia and other subcortical bodies to effect involuntary subconscious and automatic monitoring and regulation of the direct processes; (2) the cerebellum, which also influences the coordination and accuracy of control functions; and (3) vestibular-reticular centers in the brain stem, which give rise to pathways projecting to the lower motor neurons for the purpose of regulating reflex activity at the level of the lower motor neurons (Darley, Aronson, & Brown, 1975).

COMMUNICATION DISORDERS

A detailed discussion of communication disorders is best begun with a framework or categorization for accurate description and differentiation. Communication can be oversimplified, but presented correctly, as the transmission and integration of language. Transmission entails both the expressive characteristics of language and the means by which the linguistic symbols are received. Integration includes the process of association, interpretation, and formulation for the purpose of decoding and encoding language.

Disorders may occur at the periphery of receptive or expressive transmission, or they may affect specific structures that reduce transmission. For example, trauma or a disease process could impair hearing at the level of the outer or middle ear, yet sensory and neural components of hearing would remain intact. Likewise, dysarthria secondary to stroke could impair verbal expression markedly, yet the language centers of the brain would remain unimpaired.

Disorders of Transmission

Disorders of transmission should be viewed with regard to (1) the structure (muscle, bone, cartilage); (2) the means of innervating these structures (motor-speech mechanism); and (3) the central system required for both recognition before comprehension and programming of the motor acts after linguistic formulation for expressive purposes.

The patient with communication impairment as a result of a neurogenic disorder may have one or more of the following expressive or receptive transmission disorders: the dysarthrias, dyspraxia, dysgraphia, dyslexia, agnosia, or hearing impairment secondary to conduction, sensorineural, or retrocochlear disorders (Tables 14–2 and 14–3).

EXPRESSIVE DISORDERS OF TRANSMISSION

Expressive disorders of transmission include the dysarthrias, dyspraxia of speech, and dysgraphia.

TABLE 14–2 • DISORDERS OF TRANSMISSION

Disorder	Anatomic Area Affected	Etiology
Receptive		
Hearing impairment	Outer, middle, or inner ear; auditory nerve; subcortical tracts to cortex	Trauma, disease, stroke, tumors, presbycusis
Auditory verbal agnosia	Auditory association area of cortex in superior temporal gyrus	Stroke, trauma, disease, diffuse encephalopathy, degenerative disorder
Dyslexia	Angular gyrus, left occipital lobe with concomitant lesion to splenium of corpus callosum	Stroke, trauma, disease, diffuse degenerative disorders
Expressive		
Dysarthrias		
Flaccid	Lower motor neuron and motor unit	Stroke, trauma, bulbar palsy, myasthenia gravis, trauma
Spastic	Upper motor neurons (pyramidal tracts)	Stroke, trauma, pseudobulbar palsy
Ataxia	Cerebellum	Stroke, trauma, tumors, intoxication, degeneration or demyelinating processes
Hypokinetic	Basal ganglia, substantia nigra, subthalamic nuclei (extrapyramidal tracts)	Reductions in dopamine production secondary to Parkinson's disease
Hyperkinetic	Basal ganglia, substantia nigra, subthalamic nuclei (extrapyramidal tracts)	Reductions in acetylcholine production secondary to stroke, tumors, trauma, dystonia, chorea, torticollis, tardive dyskinesia, infection
Mixed	Combinations of above lesion sites	Variable (e.g., amyotrophic lateral sclerosis, multiple sclerosis, Wilson's disease)
Dyspraxia of speech	Area of third frontal gyrus of left hemisphere adjacent to motor cortex	Stroke, trauma, tumors
Dysgraphia	Frontal lobe, parietal-temporal lobes of left hemisphere, posterior areas of right hemisphere	Stroke, trauma, diffuse cortical lesions

TABLE 14–3 • CHARACTERISTICS OF DISORDERS OF TRANSMISSION

Disorder	Characteristics
Hearing disorder	Reduced ability to receive sounds resulting in impaired reception of speech
	Reduced ability to recognize speech despite intact transmission from ear to cortex
Reading disorder	Reduced ability to recognize letters and words in written or printed form
Speech disorders	Breathy voice and audible inspiration, hypernasality, imprecise consonants, relatively flat pitch and loudness
	Markedly imprecise speech articulation; slow rate of speech; voice reductions owing to strained phonation, low pitch, and harsh quality
	Markedly reduced speech articulation of consonants and vowels, stress changes, prolongations and inappropriate pauses, irregular rhythms and coordination
	Imprecise consonants; reductions and equalizations of pitch, stress, and loudness; short rushes of speech; inappropriate pauses; rate of speech inappropriately varied
	• Slow hyperkinesias resulting in speech disorder characterized by distorted speech movements, inappropriate prolongations, reduced articulation, strained voice, irregular breakdowns
	• Quick hyperkinesias resulting in speech disorder characterized by imprecise speech articulation, prolonged pauses in speech, variable rate and loudness, flat pitch, and harsh voice
	• Combinations of the above characteristics relative to site of lesion and types of dysarthria presented
	Impairment in programming speech movements for intended speech act, highly consistent errors of production at any level of the vocal tract, disorder also characterized by faulty compensation attempts
Writing disorder	Mechanical difficulties secondary to reduced motor control; such symbol errors as reversals, omissions, distortions, and misspellings or visual-spatial difficulties

Dysarthrias. Dysarthria comprises a group of speech disorders resulting from disturbances in muscular control. Because there has been damage to the central or peripheral nervous system, some degree of weakness, slowness, incoordination, or altered muscle tone characterizes the activity of the speech mechanism. The term encompasses coexisting motor disorders of respiration, phonation, articulation, resonance, and prosody (Darley et al., 1975).

In the past, dysarthrias have been classified with regard to neuroanatomy or neurophysiology (Froeschels, 1943; Grewel, 1957). A more recent classification relates a described muscular dysfunction to a specific form of dysarthria (Darley, Aronson, & Brown, 1969; Darley et al., 1975). The dysarthrias are differentiated as flaccid, spastic, ataxic, hypokinetic, hyperkinetic, and mixed.

Flaccid dysarthria results from damage to any portion of a lower motor unit. This unit is composed of the lower motor neuron's body and axon, the myoneural junction, and the muscle itself. Damage may be a result of widespread injury, specific nerve impairment of the myoneural junction, or damage to the muscle fibers themselves. The speech quality of the person with flaccid dysarthria varies, depending on the specific area of disruption, but is typically characterized by breathy voice, audible inspiration, and hypernasality (Darley et al., 1975; Wertz, 1978).

Spastic dysarthria results from suprasegmental (upper motor neuron) damage. These pathways are closely approximated through their courses, and lesions to the pyramidal tracts are more often than not accompanied by lesions to the extrapyramidal tracts. Unilateral lesions to upper motor neurons produce remarkable, but typically mild, impairment of speech. Spastic dysarthria involving bilateral upper motor neuron damage is usually associated with widespread damage to the central nervous system. Spastic dysarthria owing to bilateral involvement causes marked speech deficits, chiefly characterized by markedly imprecise articulation of speech and a harsh voice quality (Darley et al., 1975; Rosenbeck & LaPointe, 1978).

A familiar manifestation of bilateral upper motor neuron impairment is pseudobulbar palsy, which results in spastic dysarthria with characteristic symptomatology similar to that of bulbar palsy. Differentiating between the two involves identifying the areas affected and remembering that spastic dysarthria affects overall movement patterns, whereas flaccid dysarthria secondary to bulbar palsy affects individual motor units (Darley et al., 1969). Increased incidence of emotional lability is also associated with pseudobulbar palsy (Darley et al., 1975).

Ataxic dysarthria is associated with bilateral or widespread damage to the cerebellum (Darley et al., 1975). The predominant role of the cerebellum appears to involve regulating and attenuating the descending cortical speech program (Brown, Darley, & Aronson, 1970). Ataxic dysarthria is related, like other central nervous system disorders, to a variety of injuries. Friedreich's ataxia is a disease process commonly associated with ataxic dysarthria. Speech characteristics include marked speech misarticulations, stress changes, and prolongations. These manifestations are thought to be symptoms of overall reduced coordination and inhibition of the motor-speech program (Darley et al., 1975). The characteristics of ataxic dysarthria are commonly associated with, and at times mistakenly attributed to, alcohol intoxication ("drunk speech").

Hypokinetic dysarthria is a manifestation of damage to portions of the extrapyramidal level of the motor-speech program. Disorders of inhibition with regard to the extrapyramidal system, usually associated with reduced production of dopamine, result in hypokinesis and hypokinetic dysarthria (Bateman, 1977; Darley et al., 1975). The most common form of hypokinesia is parkinsonism (Darley et al., 1975; Rosenbeck & LaPointe, 1978; Wertz, 1978). It is important for the neuroscience nursing clinician to remember that parkinsonianlike symptoms have been known to develop in patients using drugs containing reserpine or one of the phenothiazines (Darley et al., 1975).

Marked limitation of range of movement is the characteristic most often associated with speech impairment secondary to hypokinesia (Darley et al., 1975). Speech characteristics tend to encompass flat or reduced aspects, and occasionally short rushes of words are noted (Darley et al., 1975; Wertz, 1978).

Hyperkinesia (as well as hyperkinetic dysarthria) is related to extrapyramidal dysfunction specific to reduced facilitory function and is often attributed to reductions in the production of acetylcholine. The symptomatology involves quick and slow abnormal involuntary movements. These movement disorders should be thought of on a continuum of quickest to slowest, with occasional overlapping (Fig. 14–2).

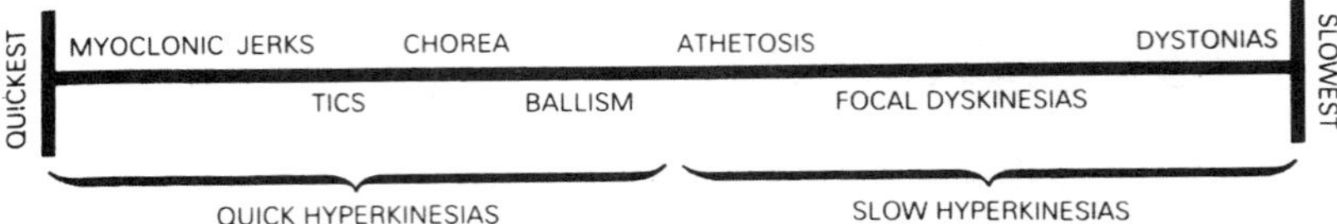

FIGURE 14–2 • Diagrammatic representation of movement disorders associated with hyperkinetic dysarthria.

The quick hyperkinesias are characterized by random, nonpurposeful movements typically accompanying purposeful movement, causing disruption in the normal sequence of motor-speech activity at all levels (respiration, phonation, resonance, articulation, prosody) (Darley et al., 1975).

Characteristics of slow hyperkinesias include twisting and prolonged movement patterns and gradual increases and subsequent decreases in muscle tone (Darley et al., 1975; Rosenbeck & LaPointe, 1978; Wertz, 1978). Slow hyperkinesias are associated with extrapyramidal lesions, but more cortical involvement may be present than that noted in other extrapyramidal disorders (Darley et al., 1975).

The dysarthrias discussed have been viewed as pure and mutually exclusive disorders. The widespread neuropathology associated with stroke, head trauma, toxins, and other causes suggests, however, that combinations of disorders, or mixed dysarthrias, exist. In fact, they do. Although the potential variety of combinations is limitless, three outstanding disorders traditionally have illustrated the symptomatology of mixed dysarthria.

Amyotrophic lateral sclerosis is a disease characterized by progressive degeneration of both upper and lower motor neurons. Speech gradually deteriorates secondary to increasing combinations of spastic and flaccid dysarthrias. In addition, compromise of the bulbar musculature can lead to difficulties with respirations and swallowing.

Multiple sclerosis, although not completely understood, is a demyelinating condition of the central nervous system. Speech is not always affected, but when it is, variable involvement of spastic, ataxic, and flaccid dysarthrias is noted. The severity of dysarthria is directly related to the severity of the overall neurologic involvement.

Wilson's disease, a genetic and metabolic disorder, affects the body's ability to process mineral intake, specifically copper, in the diet, which eventually leads to neuromotor degeneration. A marked symptom of Wilson's disease is dysarthria, with variable combinations of spastic, ataxic, and hypokinetic involvement. Concomitant disorders involve ataxia, dysphagia, intention tremor, rigidity, and drooling.

Other mixed dysarthrias might result secondary to diffuse head injury, multiple strokes, disseminated tumors, Creutzfeldt-Jakob disease, Shy-Drager syndrome, hydrocephalus, and other diffuse encephalopathies.

Dyspraxia of Speech. Motor-speech programming is an almost incomprehensibly complex process that is beyond conscious, voluntary control. Critical to this process is the frontal lobe of the brain's left hemisphere; it provides accurate and efficient programming of the motor-speech process after formulation of linguistic content and grammatical form.

Dyspraxia (sometimes called apraxia) of speech occurs when this motor-speech programmer is impaired by brain damage. It is seen largely as a motor-speech disorder manifested by errors in articulation and the patient's attempts to compensate for these errors (Darley, 1982; Darley et al., 1975; Rosenbeck, 1978; Wertz, 1978).

The speaker has a reduced ability to position the different parts of the speech mechanism for speech sound production and a reduced ability to sequence sounds to produce spoken words. Speech is highly variable, and errors are inconsistent, characterized by groping and frustration of the speaker, who knows what he or she wants to say but cannot produce the words as planned. Substitutions are more common than other types of errors (e.g., "dake a cake" for "bake a cake") (Rosenbeck, 1978).

Dyspraxic speech is believed to occur secondary to a lesion in the third frontal convolution of the left hemisphere. The lesion is usually secondary to stroke or head trauma (Wertz, 1978). The lesion thus occurs within (or close to) Broca's area, which is considered the principal center for verbal expression of language. Not surprisingly, dyspraxia of speech more often than not occurs along with aphasic involvement.

It is important to remember that dyspraxia of speech is clearly distinguished from dysarthria, aphasia, and oral apraxia. Apraxia of speech is a speech disorder secondary to programming impairment; errors are highly inconsistent. Dysarthrias, on the other hand, are speech disorders related to impaired muscle movement; errors are consistent. Aphasia deficits involve word choice and linguistic rules, not the actual motor-speech performance. Oral apraxia involves reduced programming of all volitional acts of the oral musculature, whereas dyspraxia of speech is noticed only during speech production (Benson & Geschwind, 1983; Darley, 1982; Darley et al., 1975; Wertz, 1978).

Dysgraphia. Dysgraphia, a transmission disorder that also impairs expression, is defined as loss or impairment of the ability to produce written language secondary to brain damage (Benson, 1979). It is an expressive disorder that occurs after language formulation.

Abnormalities of writing are complex and difficult to attribute to specific areas of the brain. The most frequently mentioned areas with regard to dysgraphia are (1) the frontal lobe of the dominant hemisphere (impaired motor control), (2) the parietal-temporal area of the dominant hemisphere (symbol errors), and (3) the posterior areas of the right hemisphere (visual-spatial difficulties) (Benson, 1979; Benson & Geschwind, 1983; Darley, 1982).

RECEPTIVE DISORDERS OF TRANSMISSION

Receptive disorders of transmission include hearing impairment, auditory verbal agnosia, and dyslexia.

Hearing Impairment. The diversity of hearing impairments is enormous. Briefly, impairments are typically associated with middle-ear dysfunction (conductive hearing loss), inner-ear dysfunction (sensorineural hearing loss), and dysfunction of the neural pathways beyond the cochlea (retrocochlear hearing loss). These impairments can occur in combination and are discussed in Chapters 23 and 24. Also see the texts by Newby (1979) and Zemlin (1968).

Auditory Verbal Agnosia. Auditory verbal agnosia is a disorder in which the sensations of speech reach the cortex and are experienced, but without recognition or meaning (Darley, 1982; Perkins, 1971; Sies, 1974). It is often associated with reductions in auditory comprehension secondary to aphasia (Sies, 1974) but is considered a sensory deficit rather than an impairment in symbolic language (Darley, 1982).

Dyslexia. Dyslexia, a reading disorder, has both acquired and congenital origins. Simply, it is the loss or impairment of the ability to read (Benson, 1979). Rather than a language disorder of one modality, it is a reduced ability to recognize and interpret written symbols. Dyslexia is often accompanied by dysgraphia, when the lesion is in the parietal-temporal juncture and, more specifically, the angular gyrus.

DISORDERS OF LANGUAGE INTEGRATION

Language integration disorders include aphasia, cognitive-linguistic impairment, and generalized intellectual impairment (Table 14–4).

Aphasia

Aphasia is an integrative language disorder that affects all language modalities. It is secondary to brain damage and is not attributable to dementia or confusion or sensory or motor dysfunction. It is characterized chiefly by reductions in available vocabulary, reduced verbal retention span, and reductions in the ability to use learned linguistic rules (Benson, 1979; Brookshire, 1978; Darley, 1982; Perkins, 1971; Schuell, Jenkins, & Jimenez-Pabon, 1964).

Aphasia is typically associated with lesions to the primary linguistic centers (Wernicke's area, Broca's area), but aphasia is also noted in areas adjacent to these in the cortex (Benson & Geschwind, 1983; Wertz, 1978). New information suggests possible subcortical correlations for aphasia (Benson, 1979; Goodglass & Kaplan, 1983).

Aphasia has been described and categorized based on lesion location and linguistic deficit (Darley, 1982; Goodglass & Kaplan, 1972; Schuell et al., 1964). Because the variety of existing adjectives and labels can be confusing, one framework based on lesion location and derived from research at the Boston Veterans Administration Hospital (Goodglass & Kaplan, 1972) is used here.

Disorder	Anatomic Area Affected	Etiology	Characteristics
Aphasia			
Broca's	Third gyrus of left frontal lobe (Broca's area)	Stroke, trauma, tumors	Halting nonfluent speech, restrictions in vocabulary and grammar, reductions in language modalities of comprehension and expression, reduced verbal retention
Wernicke's	Posterior portion of superior temporal gyrus of left hemisphere (Wernicke's area)	Stroke, trauma, tumors	Fluent speech, reduced meaningful content, paraphasia, reduced auditory comprehension, poor error awareness, circumlocutions, word-finding difficulty, reduced reading and writing ability
Anomic	Parietal-temporal juncture of left hemisphere, angular gyrus	Stroke, trauma, tumors	Fluent speech relatively devoid of substantive words, word-finding difficulty, circumlocutions, less auditory comprehension impairment and less paraphasia
Conduction	Arcuate fasciculus	Stroke, trauma, tumors	Word-finding difficulty, marked paraphasic errors, fluent speech occasionally disrupted for word retrieval, relatively intact error awareness, grammatically intact
Transcortical sensory	Periphery of Wernicke's and Broca's areas, isolating intact language areas	Stroke, trauma, tumors, anoxia	Adequate speech articulation, marked paraphasia and neologisms, often irrelevant and echolalic, intact repetition, severely reduced reading and writing ability
Transcortical motor	Anterior and superior to Broca's area, deep to Broca's area	Stroke, trauma, tumors	Reduced initiation of speech, variably nonfluent and then fluent, word-finding difficulty, relatively intact articulation, repetition and comprehension, rare paraphasias
Cognitive-linguistic impairment	Diffuse cortical and subcortical lesions	Trauma, multiple strokes, diffuse cerebral metastases or infection	Reduced cognitive functioning, including reductions in arousal and alertness, selective attention and concentration, discrimination and categorization, memory, abstraction and associational abilities, and analysis and reasoning; these reductions subsequently impair language usage
Generalized intellectual impairment	Diffuse cortical and subcortical lesions	Dementia secondary to disease, other diffuse degenerative processes	Language impairment relative to severity of intellectual impairment (dementia), characterized by reductions in concentration, memory, generalization, and abstraction

Broca's Aphasia. Broca's aphasia has been called verbal, motor, or expressive aphasia. It occurs as a result of a lesion in the third frontal convolution of the left hemisphere. Its characteristics include restricted vocabulary; sparse, poorly articulated words; and restrictions of grammar to the simplest, most automatically used forms (Goodglass & Kaplan, 1983). Written language follows the pattern of speech impairment and is often found to be more impaired than speech. Numerous efforts at self-correction of expression are attempted but are often unsuccessful (Darley, 1982). Productions are essentially halting or nonfluent, and considerable frustration is shown by the speaker, who is typically aware of the difficulties. The individual with Broca's aphasia comprehends spoken and written language better than he or she can speak or write, but comprehension is still impaired. Productions of more than one or two words tend to be telegraphic (e.g., "Want . . . water . . . drink").

Wernicke's Aphasia. Wernicke's aphasia has been called sensory, acoustic, or receptive aphasia. This language disorder is typically associated with lesions in the posterior portion of the first temporal gyrus of the left hemisphere. Essential characteristics of Wernicke's aphasia include impaired auditory comprehension and speech that is fluently produced but relatively bereft of content. Productions are often circumlocutory or tangential and are frequently interspersed with paraphasic errors or jargon. For example, a person with Wernicke's aphasia might refer to "fire" as "the thing that burns" (circumlocution), "fear" (paraphasia), or "grop" (jargon). The person will make these types of errors because of difficulty comprehending and monitoring his or her own productions as well as difficulty comprehending and monitoring the speech of others (Schuell et al., 1964). Such a person has little frustration with his or her own productions, however, because error awareness is markedly reduced (Benson & Geschwind, 1983).

Word-finding difficulty or naming impairment, an important consideration, is usually associated with this type of aphasia. A person with Wernicke's aphasia may have such severe word-finding difficulty that the person may appear to have an expressive deficit and may be misdiagnosed as an expressive aphasic.

Reading skills are reduced at least as much as are listening skills, primarily because Wernicke's area is believed to be within the area where visual and auditory linguistic symbols are associated and integrated for language use (Goodglass & Kaplan, 1983). Writing, as a reflection of speech, is also reduced in meaningful content and exhibits circumlocutory and tangential characteristics, although the mechanics and legibility should be relatively intact. Paraphasic errors are known to intrude into written expression as well (Benson, 1979; Darley, 1982; Goodglass & Kaplan, 1983).

Anomic Aphasia. Anomic aphasia has been called amnesic aphasia. Like Wernicke's aphasia, anomic aphasia is fluent, with intact grammatical structure. The major difference is that the anomic aphasic has more severe word-finding difficulty, but without paraphasic errors and with relatively little auditory comprehension difficulty. The listener begins to notice that the content of the aphasic's speech is relatively devoid of substantive words: Instead of "I went to the store to buy some bread," one might hear "I went over there [points] to get those things, you know what I mean" (Darley, 1982; Goodglass & Kaplan, 1983).

This aphasia is usually associated with parietal-temporal lesions, and the lesion's proximity to the angular gyrus is noteworthy (Goodglass & Kaplan, 1983).

Conduction Aphasia. Conduction aphasia, sometimes referred to as central aphasia, is an aphasic syndrome most notably associated with increased paraphasic errors and the reduced ability to repeat words (Benson & Geschwind, 1983; Goodglass & Kaplan, 1983). It is often attributed to a lesion in the arcuate fasciculus, the fiber pathway that is believed to be the means of linguistic transfer from Wernicke's area to Broca's area and vice versa (Benson, 1979; Geschwind, 1979; Goodglass & Kaplan, 1983). The fluent conduction aphasic has an anomic component but will usually retrieve paraphasic words in a struggle to recall the correct word. Relatively unimpaired error awareness is manifested by struggle behavior and can be attributed erroneously to the nonfluency of Broca's aphasia. The most language difficulty and the highest incidence of paraphasic intrusion occur primarily in repetition.

Transcortical Sensory Aphasia. Transcortical sensory aphasia is a rare aphasic syndrome that is believed to occur under exceptional circumstances. "Watershed lesions" secondary to stroke or anoxia cause damage about the periphery of the intact Wernicke-Broca language complex (Benson & Geschwind, 1983; Goodglass & Kaplan, 1983). The result is that the language areas function unimpaired, but they are isolated from the higher-level ideation areas of the rest of the brain and from the motor-speech mechanism.

Characteristics include adequate speech articulation but with marked paraphasia and neologisms (new words). Responses are often irrelevant and occasionally echolalic. Confrontation naming of objects is reduced, but repetition is intact. Reading and writing are severely impaired.

Transcortical Motor Aphasia. Transcortical motor aphasia is another uncommon aphasia syndrome that is associated with lesions located either on the anterior-superior periphery of Broca's area or deep within that area (Goodglass & Kaplan, 1983). The person with this type of aphasia has difficulty initiating communication, and his or her responses are typically disorganized and display word-finding difficulty. Such a person tends to be considered more nonfluent than fluent but is capable of sporadic fluent speech with intact grammar (Benson & Geschwind, 1983; Goodglass & Kaplan, 1983).

Aphasia is a language disorder that manifests varying degrees of impairment in all language modalities (auditory comprehension, verbal expression, reading, and writing). The classifications given cannot be considered mutually exclusive, but they tend to highlight the language functions that are most impaired or preserved when lesions to the brain affect certain areas. The etiology of the lesion may involve different destructive or degenerative processes, but aphasia typically results from stroke or traumatic head injury. Aphasia is a disorder of the brain's ability to integrate and associate language and linguistic symbols, not a disorder of transmission.

Cognitive-Linguistic Disorders

Cognitive-linguistic disorders are impaired language skills owing not to disruption of the previously mentioned language areas but to diffuse cortical or subcortical injuries that affect the person's ability to be alert, to concentrate, to remember, and to reason, which, in turn, reduces the efficiency of the person's language. This debility has traditionally been referred to as the language of confusion (Halpern, Darley, & Brown, 1973), but this label refers to only one feature of a vast continuum of cognitive impairment. The disorders may result from space-occupying lesions (e.g., contusions, shearing of axon tracts, open head wounds). A preliminary study at the Shock Trauma Center of the Maryland Institute for Emergency Medical Services Systems suggested that cognitive-linguistic deficits, ranging from mild to severe, occur secondarily to closed head injury despite negative computed tomographic scan results.

The area of cognitive-linguistic disorders has received increasing attention as efforts to rehabilitate head-injured patients have grown nationally (Levin, Benton, & Grossman, 1982; Rosenthal, Griffith, Bond, & Miller, 1983). Work during the 1970s at Rancho Los Amigos Hospital in Downey, CA gave rise to classification systems of cognitive functioning that are beneficial for better understanding of cognitive-linguistic impairment and for prediction of recovery (Hagen, Malkmus, & Durham, 1977).

According to Hagen (1983), "the majority of language impairment characteristics, while similar to aphasia disorders, are symptoms of an underlying impairment, release, suppression, and/or disorganization of the cognitive processes which support language processing" (p. 4). Specifically, it is believed that a hierarchy of cognitive processes is affected relative to (1) the areas of the brain that are injured and (2) the severity of the injuries. The hierarchy begins with the most severe impairment associated with reduced or absent ability to be aroused and alert, followed by deficits in selective attention and concentration. The hierarchy proceeds to consider disruptions of discrimination, separation, and categorization skills. At this point, disorders of memory and association are observed more commonly. Analysis, synthesis, and reasoning are the highest level of cognitive functioning to be impaired. At any level, these deficits would impair the person's ability to use his or her language mechanism maximally, accurately, or efficiently.

Typical language disturbances include varying degrees of impairment for comprehension and expression; the likelihood of confabulation, jargon, or circumlocution; and irrelevant, disinhibited, and tangential expressions. Word-finding difficulty and grammatical disruptions have been reported (Hagen, 1983).

In 1987, the ASHA published a report, developed by its subcommittee on language and cognition, that addressed the role of the speech-language pathologist in the treatment of cognitive impairment (ASHA, 1987). As stated in that document, because the relationship between cognition and language is the basis for effective communication, cognitive impairment can result in communication breakdown. Specific "cognitive communication impairments" that might affect language include the following: impaired attention, perception, and memory; inflexibility, impulsivity, and disorganized thinking or acting; inefficient processing of information; difficulty processing abstract information; difficulty learning new information; inefficient retrieval of information; ineffective problem solving and judgment; inappropriate social behavior; and impaired "executive" functions such as goal-setting, planning, initiating, and self-monitoring.

The term *cognitive-language disorder* more accurately reflects the cause of deficits (both cognitive and language processes) resulting from traumatic brain injury (Kennedy & DeRuyter, 1991). The term *language* is more precise than communicative, because communication disorders may encompass a variety of conditions, such as vocalization problems, dyspraxia, dysarthria, and impaired hearing.

The diffuse nature of the injuries associated with cognitive-linguistic impairment is likely to give rise to other speech and language deficits, such as dysarthria, apraxia, and aphasia. Considerable effort is needed to diagnose these overlapping disorders correctly and differentially.

One means of differentiation is to observe the appropriateness and relevance of the patient's behavior. For example, if the patient displays marked auditory comprehension difficulty after head injury and has difficulties with concentrating, attending, acting appropriately, or reasoning and orientation, the comprehension difficulty is probably a diffuse cognitive-linguistic disorder, not aphasia.

Head-injured patients at the R. Adams Cowley Shock Trauma Center, Maryland's specialty referral center for neurotrauma, typically have cognitive-linguistic deficits secondary to their traumatic brain injury. Reports of the incidence of aphasia secondary to brain injury vary and depend on when the patients are evaluated (Schwartz-Cowley & Stepanik, 1989). Heilman, Safran, and Geschwind (1971) reported a 2% incidence of aphasia in closed head injury patients during the acute hospital admission period. Sarno, Buonaguro, and Levita (1987) investigated closed head injury patients in a rehabilitation center (mean time after injury, 45 weeks) and reported a 28% incidence of aphasia.

According to Luria's theoretical model of functional systems (Luria, 1966, 1973), the brain is organized into three integrated units that are essential to the execution of cognitive tasks. The first unit regulates arousal and wakefulness (brain stem and other subcortical areas). The second functional unit receives, analyzes, and stores tactile, auditory, and kinesthetic sensory information (surface of the brain, primarily the temporal and posterior areas). The third functional unit programs actions and regulates behavior (frontal areas). Any impairment of the basic processes within the functional systems disrupts the system and changes behavior. Thus, function can be recovered by reorganizing functional systems (cognitive retraining).

Bracy (1986) expanded Luria's concept of functional areas into four major areas: the first determines level of arousal, alertness, and responsivity; the second involves sensation and initial processing of sensory information; the third includes the brain areas and functional processes that integrate sensory information, perception, conception, and memory; and the fourth relates to response planning, cognitive organization, and execution of motor programs. In this model, the executive area has a role in every aspect of behavior. Like Luria, Bracy advocated that treatment be directed toward the basic processes that are impaired.

In the process-specific approach to cognitive rehabilitation, Sohlberg and Mateer (1989) oriented treatment toward specific cognitive areas. This model assumes that the cognitive process areas (e.g., language, attention, memory, visual processing, executive function, reasoning) can be treated individually and directly retrained and remediated.

Other theorists stress the relationships of systems and processes. Hagen (1981, 1984) suggested that the treatment goal for communication disorders be the reorganization of the underlying cognitive processes instead of the linguistic consequences of cognitive disorganization. He also reported that, as cognitive processes become more organized, one will automatically see an improvement in the phonologic, semantic, syntactic, and verbal reasoning ability aspects of language.

The relationships between cognitive processes and systems were stressed by Szekeres, Ylvisaker, and Holland (1985) and Smith and Jacobson (1988). They proposed three general aspects of cognition, based on information-processing theories: component processes (operations that take in, interpret, and retrieve information and formulate output); component systems (basic and acquired processes and knowledge); and functional-integrative performances (real-life activities, that is, the interaction of the entire cognitive mechanism with the environment). Rehabilitation of patients with cognitive-linguistic disorders includes retraining specific component processes, teaching personal and environmental compensations, and training for functional daily activities. Because the executive system plays a crucial role in rehabilitation, metacognition instruction is also important to help the patient understand the deficits (Ylvisaker & Szekeres, 1989).

Adamovich, Henderson, and Auerbach (1985) suggested that the appropriate approach to treatment depends on the stage of recovery. Stimulation or arousal and alerting are followed by structured, goal-oriented programs or operative retraining. Subsequently, home and community-oriented programs focused on independent functioning are recommended.

Human Immunodeficiency Virus Infection

Increasing numbers of children are being born with, and living with, developmental disabilities caused by the human immunodeficiency virus (HIV). By 1990, the number of cases of acquired immunodeficiency syndrome among children younger than 13 years totaled 2786. It is estimated that 1500 to 2000 children were born with HIV between 1989 and 1991 (Gwinn et al., 1991).

Neurologic dysfunction is evident in as many as 90% of children with advanced HIV infection. Manifestations include the following: loss of previously acquired milestones or failure to attain milestones at the expected age, intellectual deficits, impaired brain growth, spasticity-rigidity, weakness, ataxia, and seizures.

The rehabilitative strategies used for other populations apply to this new population of children with neurologic and developmental deficits associated with HIV infection (Harris, 1992). In addition to physicians, nurses, and laboratory technicians, the rehabilitation team should include physical therapists, speech-language pathologists, occupational therapists, social workers, psychologists, nutritionists, and developmental specialists. These team members work in concert to accurately assess each child and design comprehensive interventions.

The goals of the speech-language program (Pressman, 1992) that treats children with HIV infection are to establish baselines for comparison during the course of the illness, to provide treatment as indicated, and to help families cope with the illness. Tests for evaluation of neurologic status among HIV-infected children are listed in Table 14–5 (Bangs & Dodson, 1979; Children's Hospital of San Francisco, 1979; Dunn, 1959; Furuno et al., 1984; Glover, Preminger, & Sanford, 1978; Levenson & Kairam, 1991; Zimmerman & Dodson, 1979).

Generalized Intellectual Impairment

The language of generalized intellectual impairment represents a complex of disorders that compose dementia (Wertz, 1978). Like the cognitive-linguistic disorders described previously, the language deficits secondary to generalized intellectual impairment represent impairment of diffuse areas of the brain. Darley (1982) noted that problems cross all language modalities and that the severity of language impairment reflects the severity of intellectual impairment. Differential diagnosis must include an exacting and detailed premorbid history

TABLE 14–5 • NEUROLOGIC FUNCTION TESTS FOR CHILDREN WITH HUMAN IMMUNODEFICIENCY VIRUS
Birth to Three Developmental Scale (Bangs & Dodson, 1979)
Early Learning Accomplishment Profile (Glover, Preminger, & Sanford, 1978)
Hawaii Early Learning Profile (Furuno et al., 1984)
Preschool Language Scale (Zimmerman & Dodson, 1979)
Peabody Picture Vocabulary Test (Dunn, 1959; Levenson & Kairam, 1991)
Expressive One Word Picture Vocabulary Test (Children's Hospital of San Francisco, 1979)

Modified from Pressman, H. (1992). *Communication disorders and dysphagia in pediatric AIDS.* Rockville, MD: American Speech-Language-Hearing Association.

with a variety of formal and informal evaluations of intellect and language facility.

The location of the lesions responsible for dementia is not as relevant as it is for other communication disorders. Typically, large portions of the cortex or the entire brain are involved (Wertz, 1978).

Dementia is associated primarily with disease processes, such as Alzheimer's disease, Pick's disease, Creutzfeldt-Jakob disease, and Huntington's chorea. The severity of the language disorders and the prognosis for recovery are as variable as the wide variety of possible etiologies.

Alzheimer's Disease. The demographic parameter of age structure is changing in the United States (Griffiths, 1992). In 1990, 12.6% of the population was 65 years of age or older; between 2010 and 2030, that age group is projected to increase to 30% (Statistical Abstracts of the United States, 1992). There is a general correlation between advancing years and increasing disability, including dementia (Smith & Jacobson, 1988). The most common degenerative dementia affecting the elderly is Alzheimer's disease (Fraser, 1987).

Alzheimer's disease is primarily a cortical dementia, which induces notable deficits in language abilities. Clinical features include memory disturbance, personality changes, and alterations in intellectual and cognitive processes (French, 1986; Gravell, 1988). The diagnosis of Alzheimer's disease is based on behavioral criteria. Speech-language pathologists assess language abilities using standard batteries such as the Western Aphasia Battery and the Boston Test for Aphasia. In the early phases of the disease, deficits manifest as word-retrieval problems, deficiencies in confrontational naming skills, and circumlocution ("talking around" the unretrieved word). As the disease progresses, patients remain fluent, but speech becomes "empty" and increasingly circumlocutory (Orsini, Van Gorp, & Boone, 1988). Cummings, Darkins, Mendez, Hill, and Benson (1988) observed that test results indicate transcortical or Wernicke's aphasia.

The treatment approach focuses on compensation and on learning how to cope with the changes being experienced by the patient. Therapies are best directed toward those requiring little cognitive flexibility or learning and those that maximize the individual's ability to function effectively by reducing the need for lost functions, where possible, by relying on remaining skills. Treatment should enhance the skills necessary for daily life (Dobson, 1989; Golper & Rau, 1983).

ACUTE AND LONG-TERM IMPLICATIONS

Acquired communication disorders often accompany a variety of debilitating vascular disorders, traumatic injuries, and diseases. These disorders create an enormous potential for crisis and catastrophe in the lives of everyone they affect, be it directly (the patient) or indirectly (the family, the caregiver, and the community).

Effects of Communication Disorders

Communication disorders can cause speech, language, and hearing deficits, which can lead to high frustration and anxiety levels as well as diminished self-image, lack of personal fulfillment, and feelings of pessimism and isolation. In addition, a patient with such a disorder will project his or her deficits and fears beyond the immediate situation: "How will these deficits affect me and my family? My friends? My job?" These reactions may increase the effects of the deficits, laying the groundwork for a downward spiral in terms of adjustment and rehabilitation.

In a similar manner, the patient's family members also experience these feelings. The family and significant others need to adjust to a change in their lives. The family can be expected to go through a period of denial, anger, and depression. It is not unusual for other marked sequelae of brain injury (e.g., hemiplegia, visual-spatial disturbances, incapacitation) to demoralize and affect the family further. Periods of overreaction and underreaction with unrealistic hopes and doubts are often manifested. The family will need considerable counseling and education to assist in their adjustment. The neuroscience nurse can be of direct assistance in this regard and may serve as the coordinator for other assistance from specialists in the areas of medicine and rehabilitation.

In the community, the patient with an acquired communication disorder may have considerable difficulty returning to his or her place of employment or to school, work, or home responsibilities. Job efficiency in fields that require regular verbal interaction (e.g., sales, management) may be drastically altered. Communication deficits in concentration, memory, or accurate reasoning could be catastrophic for employees or students who must work complex and sophisticated tasks with pressures to succeed and meet deadlines. In addition, such disorders can adversely affect personal interests with friends and social or religious organizations and can exert an adverse impact on the management of home duties and economic responsibilities.

The trend in rehabilitation emphasizes the role of the family and community in effecting and sustaining treatment outcomes throughout the recovery process and beyond. This approach is exemplified by the 1992 standards manual of the Commission on Accreditation of Rehabilitation Facilities and by the Americans with Disabilities Act (Kneipp & Paul-Cohen, 1993). Despite this focus on community reentry, many state governments have imposed limitations on funding for rehabilitation. Thus, rehabilitation specialists are increasingly challenged to provide or arrange community-based services.

In the provision of community-based services (i.e., rehabilitative interventions that take place in the home or community), cognitive-communicative impairment can impede the individual's ability to obtain and advance in employment and can contribute to shortened job tenure and termination of employment. These deficits can also influence the likelihood of divorce, dysfunctional family systems, substance abuse, and diminished quality of life (Kneipp & Paul-Cohen, 1993). However, the community offers many contexts that can stimulate functional gains. Those resources include adult education classes, pottery classes, tennis instruction, bowling leagues, spas, and social groups affiliated with churches and synagogues. Community reentry treatment plans should incorporate high-interest, age-appropriate activities in the individual's own community (Kneipp, 1991).

ROLE OF THE NEUROSCIENCE NURSE

It is particularly important for the neuroscience nurse to consult with the speech-language pathologist in the diagnostic and planning stages of treatment. The speech-language pathologist is a trained and accredited specialist in the field of communication disorders, with at least a master's degree in education and at least 9 months of supervised clinical practice. The pathologist is then nationally accredited by the ASHA and holds a certificate of clinical competence that reflects completion of academic and practical experiences and denotes expertise in the field of communication disorders. Collaboration between the neuroscience nurse and the speech-language pathologist will provide comprehensive information during the evaluation, planning, and treatment phases.

The neuroscience nurse cares for the patient not only in the acute and chronic stages but also in the rehabilitation areas. The patient and the patient's family will often approach the nurse for information, assistance, and counseling. The neuroscience nurse must draw on personal expertise and on information about the patient from the patient and family, as well as from the physicians and rehabilitation specialists.

The neuroscience nurse, in collaboration with the speech-language pathologist, will be able to assist the patient in adapting to the environment and minimizing the effects of communication disorders. The nurse augments and implements on the unit the treatment recommendations from the speech-language pathologist.

Family members will need extensive instruction regarding the type of communication disorder as well as counseling to help them adjust to the changes that they will see in the patient and the effect on their relationship to the patient. The neuroscience nurse should intervene early in the patient's care by providing information about the patient's communication disorder as well as by communicating recommendations of the speech-language pathologist. The family can be instrumental along with the staff in continuing the recommendations from the speech-language pathologist.

Arrangements for placement in the community are made in either the acute or the chronic phase, depending on the patient's progress. Extensive planning may be required, depending on the severity and prognosis of the language disorder, that may include contact with the patient's employer, school, friends, and so on. Continued outpatient therapies may be required, and arrangements should be set up before discharge.

SUMMARY

Language and communication are highly sophisticated processes in human relationships. Communication has become more critical in daily life as society places more and more emphasis on the informative, directive, and expressive elements of language and communication. Disorders in communication can markedly disrupt the quality of life for the individual affected as well as for his or her family and community.

Communication disorders are described in this chapter with regard to transmission and integration impairments. Transmission refers to the sensorimotor activities that permit reception and expression of linguistic symbols, such as speech, written symbols, or gesture. Receptive transmission disorders discussed are (1) acquired hearing impairment, which affects transmission and transmutation of sound through the ear to the auditory nerve portion of the eighth cranial nerve; (2) auditory verbal agnosia, which refers to impaired ability to recognize speech; and (3) acquired dyslexia, which refers to impaired ability to recognize written or printed letters or words. Expressive transmission disorders discussed are (1) the dysarthrias, which relate to speech disturbances resulting from paresis or incoordination of speech movements; (2) dyspraxia of speech, which refers to impairment of the cortical programmer for the complex organization of the motor-speech act; and (3) dysgraphia, which refers to various disorders of the ability to write.

Integration disorders are those language impairments that disrupt the brain's ability to associate and process the symbols of language. They are not disorders of transmission to or from people but reductions in comprehension, assimilation, and formulation of symbolic language. The disorders discussed are (1) aphasia, which refers to sudden disruption of language secondary to disorders of specific areas of the brain thought to be primarily responsible for language processes; (2) cognitive-linguistic impairment, which refers to diffuse cortical and subcortical lesions (usually secondary to head injury) that reduce cognitive functioning and, consequently, interfere with language adequacy and efficiency; and (3) generalized intellectual impairment, which is also a diffuse impairment of cognitive and language function but which is usually presented as a gradual onset secondary to disease and age-related considerations.

This chapter and Chapter 15 are directed toward a better understanding of communication and communication disorders and the management of these disorders. The neuroscience nurse specialist is highly involved in direct care of the communicatively impaired patient and serves as coordinator of medical and rehabilitation specialists for the family. The understanding the neuroscience nurse carries into this role will assist in improving interdisciplinary cooperation and will help provide maximum benefit for the patient, the family, and the community to which the patient returns.

References

Adamovich, B. B., Henderson, J. A., & Auerbach, S. (1985). *Cognitive rehabilitation of closed head injured patients: A dynamic approach.* San Diego: College-Hill Press.

American Speech-Language-Hearing Association. (1987). *Role of speech-language pathologists in the habilitative and rehabilitative care of cognitively impaired individuals: A report of subcommittees on language and cognition* (pp. 53–55). Rockville, MD: Author.

Bangs, T. E., & Dodson, S. (1979). *Birth to three developmental scale*. Allen, TX: DLM Teaching Resources.

Bateman, H. (1977). *A clinical approach to speech anatomy and physiology*. Springfield, IL: Thomas.

Bayles, K. (1979). Language and the brain. In A. Akajian, R. A. Demers, & R. Harnish, *Linguistics: An introduction to language and communication* (pp. 306–327). Cambridge, MA: MIT Press.

Benson, D. F. (1979). *Aphasia, alexia, and agraphia*. New York: Churchill-Livingstone.

Benson, D. F., & Geschwind, N. (1985). The aphasias and related disturbances. In A. B. Baker & L. H. Baker (Eds.), *Clinical neurology* (Vol. 1, pp. 1–34). Philadelphia: J.B. Lippincott.

Bloom, L., & Leahy, M. (1978). *Language development and language disorders*. New York: John Wiley & Sons.

Bollinger, D. (1975). The origin of language. In D. Bollinger (Ed.), *The origin of language* (2nd ed., pp. 5–23). New York: Harcourt, Brace, & Jovanovich.

Bracy, O. L. (1986). Cognitive rehabilitation: A process approach. *Cognitive Rehabilitation, 4*, 10–17.

Brookshire, R. H. (1978). Auditory comprehension and the aphasias. In D. F. Johns (Ed.), *Clinical management of neurogenic communicative disorders* (pp. 103–128). Boston: Little, Brown.

Brown, L. R., Darley, F. L., & Aronson, A. K. (1970). Ataxic dysarthria. *International Journal of Neurology, 7*, 302–318.

Children's Hospital of San Francisco. (1979). *Expressive one word picture vocabulary test*. Novato, CA: Academy Therapy Publications.

Chomsky, N. (1968). *Language and mind*. New York: Harcourt, Brace, & Jovanovich.

Cummings, J., Darkins, A., Mendez, M., Hill, M. A., & Benson, D. (1988). Alzheimer's disease and Parkinson's disease: Comparison of speech and language alterations. *Neurology, 38*(5), 680–684.

Darley, F. (1982). *Aphasia*. Philadelphia: W.B. Saunders.

Darley, F. L., Aronson, A. K., & Brown, J. R. (1969). Differential diagnostic patterns of dysarthria. *Journal of Speech and Hearing Research, 122*, 246–249.

Darley, F. L., Aronson, A., & Brown, J. (1975). *Motor speech disorders*. Philadelphia: W.B. Saunders.

Denny, N. W. (1981). Adult cognitive development. In D. Beasley & G. A. Davis (Eds.), *Aging: Communication processes and disorders*. New York: Grune & Stratton.

Devilliers, J. G., & Devilliers, P. A. (1978). *Language acquisition*. Cambridge, MA: Harvard University Press.

Dobson, S. (1989). New skills are needed in adult mental handicap. *Speech Therapy in Practice, 4*, 19.

Dunn, L. M. (1959). *Peabody picture vocabulary test*. Circle Pines, MN: American Guidance Service.

Fraser, M. (1987). *Dementia: Its nature and management*. New York: John Wiley & Sons.

French, A. (1986). A response: Some thoughts on "functional communication" [Bulletin 411]. London: College of Speech Therapists.

Frey, D. B. (1980). *The physics of speech*. Cambridge, MA: Cambridge University Press.

Froeschels, E. (1943). A contribution to the pathology and therapy of dysarthria due to certain cerebral lesions. *Journal of Speech and Hearing Disorders, 8*, 301.

Furuno, S., Inatsuka, T., O'Reilly, K., Hosaka, C., Zeisloft, B., & Allman, T. (1984). *Hawaii early learning profile (HELP)*. Palo Alto, CA: VORT.

Geschwind, N. (1979). Specializations of the human brain. *Scientific American, 241*(3), 180.

Glover, M. E., Preminger, J. L., & Sanford, A. R. (1978). *Early learning accomplishment profile (ELAPJ)*. Winston Salem, NC: Kaplan.

Golper, L. C., & Rau, M. T. (1983). Treatment of communication disorders associated with generalized intellectual deficits in adults. In W. H. Perkins (Ed.), *Current therapy of communication disorders: Language handicaps in adults* (pp. 119–129). New York: Thieme-Stratton.

Goodglass, H., & Kaplan, E. (1972). *The assessment of aphasia and related disorders*. Philadelphia: Lea & Febiger.

Goodglass, H., & Kaplan, E. (1983). *The assessment of aphasia and related disorders* (2nd ed.). Philadelphia: Lea & Febiger.

Gravell, R. (1988). *Communicative problems in elderly people: Practical approaches to management*. London: Croom Helm.

Grewel, F. (1957). Classification of dysarthrias. *Acta Psychiatrica Scandinavia, 32*, 325.

Griffiths, H. L. (1992). The psychiatry of old age. In R. Gravell & J. France (Eds.), *Speech and communication problems in psychiatry* (pp. 194–219). San Diego, CA: Singular Publishing Group.

Gwinn, M., Pappaioanou, M., George, J. R., Hannon, W. H., Wasser, S. C., Redus, M. A., Hoff, R., Grady, G. F., Willoughby, A., & Novello, A. C. (1991). Prevalence of HIV infection in child-bearing women in the United States. *JAMA, 265,* 1704–1708.

Hagen, C. (1981). Language disorders secondary to closed head injury: Diagnosis and treatment. *Topics in Language Disorders, 1,* 73–87.

Hagen, C. (1983). *Diagnosis and treatment of language disorders secondary to closed head injury.* Paper presented at the Rehabilitation of the Brain Injured Young Adult Conference, Leesburg, VA.

Hagen, C. (1984). Language disorders in head trauma. In A. Holland (Ed.), *Language disorders in adults* (pp. 247–281). San Diego, CA: College-Hill Press.

Hagen, C., Malkmus, D., & Durham, P. (1977). *Levels of cognitive functioning.* Downey, CA: Professional Staff Association of the Rancho Los Amigos Hospital.

Halpern, H., Darley, F. L., & Brown, J. R. (1973). Differential language and neurologic characteristics in cerebral involvement. *Journal of Speech and Hearing Disorders, 38*(2), 162–173.

Harris, M. H. (1992). Habilitative and rehabilitative needs of children with HIV infection. In A. C. Crocker, H. J. Cohen, & T. A. Kastner (Eds.), *HIV infection and developmental disabilities: A resource for service providers* (pp. 85–94). Baltimore, MD: Paul H. Brookes.

Heilman, K. M., Safran, A., & Geschwind, N. (1971). Closed head trauma and aphasia. *Journal of Neurology, Neurosurgery, and Psychiatry, 34,* 265–269.

Hughes, J. P. (1962). *The science of language: An introduction to linguistics.* New York: Random House.

Kahane, J. C. (1981). Anatomic and physiologic changes in the aging peripheral speech mechanism. In D. Beasley & G. A. Davis (Eds.), *Aging: Communication processes and disorders* (pp. 21–45). New York: Grune & Stratton.

Kennedy, M. R. T., & DeRuyter, F. (1991). Cognitive and language bases for communication disorders. In D. R. Buekelman & R. M. Yorkston (Eds.), *Communication disorders following traumatic brain injury: Management of cognitive, language, and motor impairments* (pp. 123–190). Austin, TX: Pro-Ed.

Knapp, M. (1981). A structure for the analysis of nonverbal communication. In V. P. Ciark, P. Escholz, & A. Rosa (Eds.), *Language: Introductory readings* (3rd ed., pp. 611–623). New York: St. Martin's Press.

Kneipp, S. (1991). Cognitive remediation within the context of a community re-entry program. In J. S. Kreutzer & P. H. Wehman (Eds.), *Cognitive rehabilitation for persons with traumatic brain injury: A functional approach* (pp. 239–250). Baltimore, MD: Paul H. Brookes.

Kneipp, S., & Paul-Cohen, R. (1993). Community-based services and support for individuals with traumatic brain injury. *Seminars in Speech and Language, 14*(1), 32–43.

Leonard, L. B. (1982). Early language development and language diseases. In G. H. Shames & E. H. Wiig (Eds.), *Human communication disorders: An introduction* (pp. 221–257). Columbus, OH: Merrill.

Levenson, R. L., Jr., & Kairam, R. (1991). Equivalence of Peabody picture vocabulary test—revised, forms L and for children with acquired immune deficiency syndrome (AIDS). *Perceptual and Motor Skills, 72,* 99–102.

Levin, H. S., Benton, A. L., & Grossman, R. G. (1982). *Neurobehavioral consequences of closed head injury.* New York: Oxford University Press.

Liles, B. L. (1975). *An introduction to linguistics.* Englewood Cliffs, NJ: Prentice-Hall.

Luria, A. R. (1966). *Higher cortical functions in man.* New York: Basic Books.

Luria, A. R. (1973). *The working brain: An introduction to neuropsychology.* New York: Basic Books.

Miller, J. F. (1983). Identifying children with language disorders and describing their language performance. In J. Miller, D. Yoder, & R. Schiefelbusch (Eds.), *Contemporary issues in language intervention* (ASHA Report No. 12, pp. 61–74). Rockville, MD: American Speech-Language-Hearing Association.

Moskowitz, B. A. (1981). The acquisition of language. In V. P. Ciark, P. Escholz, & A. Rosa (Eds.), *Language: Introductory readings* (3rd ed. pp. 77–107). New York: St. Martin's Press.

Newby, H. (1979). *Audiology* (4th ed.). Englewood Cliffs, NJ: Prentice-Hall.

Obler, L. K., & Albert, M. L. (1981). Language and aging: A neurobehavioral analysis. In D. Beasley & G. A. Davis (Eds.), *Aging: Communication processes and disorders* (pp. 107–121). New York: Grune & Stratton, 1981.

Orsini, D. L., Van Gorp, W. G., & Boone, K. B. (1988). Dementia. In *The neuropsychology casebook. New York: Springer-Verlag.*

Perkins, W. H. (1971). *Speech pathology: An applied behavioral science.* St. Louis: Mosby.

Pressman, H. (1992, January). *Communication disorders and dysphagia in pediatric AIDS.* Rockville, MD: American Speech-Language-Hearing Association.

Rosenbeck, J. C. (1978). Treating apraxia of speech. In D. F. Johns (Ed.), *Clinical management of neurogenic communicative disorders* (pp. 191–241). Boston: Little, Brown.

Rosenbeck, J. C., & LaPointe, L. L. (1978). The dysarthrias: Description, diagnosis, and treatment. In D. F. John (Ed.), *Clinical management of neurogenic communicative disorders* (pp. 251–310). Boston: Little, Brown.

Rosenthal, M., Griffith, E., Bond, M., & Miller, J. D. (Eds.) (1983). *Rehabilitation of the head-injured adult.* Philadelphia: F.A. Davis.

Sarno, M. T., Buonaguro, A., & Levita, E. (1987). Characteristics of verbal impairment in closed head injured patients. *Archives of Physical Medicine and Rehabilitation, 67,* 400–405.

Schuell, H., Jenkins, J., & Jimenez-Pabon, E. (1964). *Aphasia in adults.* New York: Harper & Row.

Schwartz-Cowley, R., & Stepanik, M. J. (1989). Communication disorders and treatment in the acute trauma center setting. *Topics in Language Disorders, 9*(2), 1–14.

Sies, L. F. (Ed.) (1974). *Aphasia theory and therapy: Selected lectures and papers of Hildred Schuell.* Baltimore, MD: University Park Press.

Smith, A., & Jacobson, B. (Eds.) (1988). *The nation's health: A strategy for the 1990's: A report from an independent multidisciplinary committee.* London: Ring Edward's Hospital Fund for London.

Smith, A. D., & Fullerton, A. M. (1981). Age differences in episodic and semantic memory: Implications for language and cognition. In D. Beasley & G. A. Davis (Eds.), *Aging: Communication processes and disorders* (pp. 139–155). New York: Grune & Stratton.

Sohlberg, M. M., & Mateer, C. (1989). *Introduction to cognitive rehabilitation.* New York: Guilford Press.

Statistical Abstracts of the United States (1992).

Szekeres, S. F., Ylvisaker, M., & Cohen, S. B. (1987). A framework for cognitive rehabilitation therapy. In M. Ylvisaker & E. M. R. Gobble (Eds.), *Community re-entry for head injured adults* (pp. 87–136). Boston: College-Hill Press.

Szekeres, S. F., Ylvisaker, M., & Holland, A. L. (1985). Cognitive rehabilitative therapy: A framework for intervention. In N. Ylvisaker (Ed.), *Head injury rehabilitation for children and adults* (pp. 219–246). Boston: College-Hill Press.

Wertz, R. (1978). Neuropathologies of speech and language: An introduction to patient management. In D. F. Johns (Ed.), *Clinical management of neurogenic communicative disorders* (pp. 1–101). Boston: Little, Brown.

Wetherby, A. M. (1985). Speech and language disorders in children: An overview. In J. K. Darby (Ed.), *Speech and language evaluation in neurology: Childhood disorders* (p. 20). Orlando, FL: Grune & Stratton.

Ylvisaker, M., & Szekeres, S. (1989). Metacognitive and executive impairments in head-injured children and adults. *Topics in Language Disorders, 9,* 34–49.

Zemlin, W. R. (1968). *Speech and hearing science: Anatomy and physiology.* Englewood Cliffs, NJ: Prentice-Hall.

Zimmerman, I. L., & Dodson, S. (1979). *Preschool language scale.* Columbus, OH: Charles E. Merrill.

15 Alterations and Management of Cognitive-Language Disorders

ROBERTA SCHWARTZ-COWLEY
• ANDREW K. GRUEN

The health care community has long recognized that the management of cognitive and communicative disorders secondary to neurologic events must be an interdisciplinary team effort. Each discipline brings expertise from an eclectic background and melds with other disciplines to manage and facilitate communication in the hospital through home care arenas. It is not uncommon for many patients who are admitted to intensive care and step-down units in a neuroscience facility to present with a number of multifaceted and often complex communication issues. Tables 15–1, 15–2, and 15–3 outline multiple factors associated with potential communication disorders in hospitalized patients. Without properly identifying basic causes and implementing effective communication strategies, the patient is left vulnerable and the best care cannot be provided. This lack of efficient, relevant, and cohesive communicative interplay often leads to increased frustration for all parties concerned, decreased tolerance, and increased potential for compromised care of the patient. Nurses are often the primary communicators with patients in the intensive care unit and thus become the patient's primary advocate. Effective communication is an essential component of even the most basic care provided.

In ancient times, wine, berries, roots, herbs, and nuts (particularly cashews) were used for medicinal purposes with the hope of improving functional recovery (Helm-Estabrooks & Albert, 1991). This "salad bar" approach has yielded to modern-day use of caffeine, aspirin, amobarbital sodium, and various other agents. Demonstrative results are still lacking. Hence, traditional evaluative and therapeutic approaches remain the most promising method for functional recovery of cognitive-linguistic and communicative deficits.

Diagnostic measures and treatment strategies vary greatly depending on the basic nature of the disability presented by the patient. This distinction is also crucial in later stages of medical and community care. It is essential in the fast-paced environment of the medical or neuroscience intensive care unit to make quick and accurate determinations regarding the communicative and cognitive skills of each patient. Early specific interventions must translate into

TABLE 15–1 • SELECTED PRIMARY FACTORS RELATED TO COMMUNICATION DEFICITS

- Decreased level of consciousness
- Comprehension difficulties
- Visual-spatial problems
- Decreased hearing
- Decreased understanding or receptive language skills
- Impaired expression capabilities
- Inability to complete automatic speech tasks
- Poor articulation skills
- Decreased intelligibility of speech
- Decreased ability to read
- Impaired writing skills in the absence of motor deficits
- Perseveration
- Word-finding difficulties
- Inability to express basic thoughts
- Difficulty initiating communication

long-term meaningful strategies for effective communication. By increasing patient performance and decreasing overall frustration levels and potential maladaptive behaviors, the neuroscience nurse can effect significant improvement in the patient's ability to communicate basic needs and desires.

To this end, the neuroscience nurse must exert a major effort even in the critical beginnings of the rehabilitative process. This is important in cases of traumatic brain injury. The nurse interested in coma stimulation from a critical

TABLE 15–2 • SELECTED SECONDARY FACTORS RELATED TO COMMUNICATION DEFICITS

- Impulsivity
- Poor judgment or safety awareness
- Increased confusion
- Perceived unacceptable sexual behaviors
- Poor insight or awareness
- Decreased attention
- Disorientation
- Learning difficulties
- Decreased problem-solving skills
- Difficulties in retention of information
- Lack of initiation of communicative events
- Poor language organization skills
- Decreased ability to generalize information
- Disordered sequencing of events
- Decreased mental flexibility
- Inability to correctly determine inferences
- Decreased social pragmatics
- Decreased self-monitoring abilities

TABLE 15–3 • SELECTED TERTIARY FACTORS RELATED TO COMMUNICATION DEFICITS
• Tendency toward verbal or physical abuse
• Anxiety or agitation
• Depression
• Ineffective coping skills
• Mood swings
• Disordered thinking
• Decrease in academic performance

review standpoint is encouraged to review the work of Zasler, Kreutzer, and Taylor (1991).

Many practitioners report that children either recover quickly with minimal deficits or remain severely and often permanently disabled. Although acquired childhood language disorders present more infrequently than their adult counterparts, recovery in children may be as inconsistent and variable as in older individuals. Murdoch (1990) stated that language deficits tend to be less severe in children and adolescents. This positive prognosis for recovery is primarily a result of brain plasticity. Plasticity refers to the ability of certain sections of the developing brain to assume functions not ordinarily associated with that specific anatomic location. Murdoch's (1990) experience relates more positively to children younger than 10 years, the generally recognized period for cerebral plasticity.

The importance of appropriate and timely interventions with children and adolescents cannot be overstated. The entire interdisciplinary team must carefully determine where the child is in developmental terms, understand the nature of basic neurologically based communication disorders in children, and develop effective treatment modalities to enhance recovery and continued progression of developmental milestones. To that end, the nurse must be aware of and empathetic to the overall communicative and cognitive status of the child. This is commonly required when determining effective medication and health-teaching strategies that will facilitate carryover into the home setting.

The goal of rehabilitation is to enable the patient to achieve the highest degree of independence through guidance and instruction by trained specialists in an interdisciplinary team approach to patient care. The team as a whole seeks to maximize the recovery process and to channel reemerging behavior into purposeful activity through progressive stimulation and modification of observed patient behaviors. Specific discipline or specialty boundaries become less apparent and threatening in this type of team interaction, increasing not only the smooth functioning of the team but also the overall level of care given. However, it is equally apparent that the nursing staff interacts the most with patients in the medical setting. Other team members, including the speech-language pathologist, often gain only a glimpse of the patient's overall communicative efficiency and effectiveness. Thus, nursing personnel can often make judgments and report "typical communicative status" to a greater extent than can the rest of the team, which, in turn, can make additional or modified recommendations concerning the most effective communication strategies.

To maximize nursing interventions for the patient who has cognitive or communicative deficits, the neuroscience nurse needs to develop physical and cognitive assessment skills; determine realistic goals; and delineate proper, effective therapeutic procedures. In subacute care centers, for example, the nurse is the overseer of the interdisciplinary care plan, because most, if not all, therapeutic interventions delineated by other rehabilitative personnel have direct implications for the nursing management of the patient. Many centers employ the Minimum Data Set, a federally mandated data collection system in many centers, which evaluates the patient's overall functional abilities in a variety of areas. Current status and changes are tracked over time in a variety of medical, communicative, and social arenas, each of which has direct implications for overall progress or change in status. If the interdisciplinary team, including nurses, can appropriately determine the management strategies necessary for quality patient care relative to communication, the patient's self-esteem will be maintained because the patient will become an active and interactive member of the team. In addition, overall effectiveness of the health care organization and satisfaction of the patient and family will be enhanced.

It is imperative, therefore, for the neuroscience nurse to become adept at (1) observing and documenting cognitive and communicative strengths and deficits, (2) assessing various physical and cognitive capabilities through informal means, and (3) using functional treatment strategies to help the patient overcome the frustrations and difficulties evidenced in the medical or neurologic care units. The strategies so employed require only minor modification for maximal patient benefit regardless of whether the behavior occurs in the critical care, acute, subacute, rehabilitative, or extended care facility.

DISORDERS OF COMPREHENSION AND COGNITION

Communicative endeavors compose an intimate relationship of organizing cognitive information, understanding spoken or written language, and responding by producing verbal or written language. Individuals who have sustained significant neurologic insults or have experienced a gradual decline in cognitive functions as the result of dementia can be left vulnerable in the overall communication process (Cummings & Read, 1988). Children who have sustained traumatic injuries to the brain or have congenital problems related to the central nervous system can also be vulnerable. The neuroscience nurse must take a comprehensive view of such patients to understand where breakdowns occur in the system.

It is often noted that patients are not able to participate in meaningful activities of daily living owing to decreased ability to communicate or express their needs and desires. In many cases, underlying receptive or understanding problems coexist and prevent the patient from responding in an efficient and organized manner. Therefore, all team members must be keenly aware of receptive disorders. Because comprehension cannot be assessed accurately without judging the patient's response to commands, it can be difficult to determine objectively whether an understanding deficit exists and how significant a problem it poses for the patient.

Assessment for possible receptive communicative or cognitive disorders includes both behavioral observations and informal screenings from nursing personnel. Table 15–4 outlines common behaviors that alert the nurse to the potential for cognitive linguistic or receptive language deficits. Health care professionals and family members are often concerned about relative inconsistencies noted in the patient's performance. Questions may arise regarding the overall motivation of the patient and the quality of care that is provided by nursing staff and other members of the interdisciplinary team. Frustration on the part of all parties concerned escalates, and a detrimental cycle occurs that leads to increased additional miscommunication. All caregivers must avoid questioning motivation and quality of care until a true assessment of receptive or understanding skills can be accomplished. In addition, the effect of memory loss, especially noted in patients with traumatic brain injuries (Brockway, 1991) and progressive dementia (Cummings & Read, 1988) cannot be overlooked. Luterman (1991) offered excellent suggestions for effective counseling of family members regarding realistic and fact-based judgments relative to a patient's ability to communicate.

Informal assessment of the patient's ability to understand speech and written material can help identify many of the problem etiologies. Systematic evaluation, careful decision making, and proper referral procedures can expedite effective treatment. The goal of assessment is to provide objective documen-

---

TABLE 15–4 • BEHAVIORAL OBSERVATIONS SUGGESTING POTENTIAL COGNITIVE-LINGUISTIC OR RECEPTIVE LANGUAGE DEFICITS

- Patient appears not to hear what is said and asks for frequent repetition of directions, such as transferring procedures or menu choices.
- Patient appears unable to follow commands consistently, especially commands that entail complex, lengthy, or abstract directions.
- Patient appears to understand commands of varying lengths for short periods, followed by intermittent periods of confusion.
- Patient appears capable of following certain instructions during various times of the day or for certain people but not for other people or at different times of the day, such as when fatigued.
- Patient appears to forget commands or instructions and requires repetition of even simple routine activities.
- Patient demonstrates significant reduction in attention or memory skills.
- Patient appears not to understand written material, such as the menu, even after reading the words aloud.
- Patient contradicts himself or herself by responding in an appropriate manner to questions requiring a yes-or-no response; for example, "Are you cold?" "No." "Do you want a blanket?" "Yes."

tation of strengths and weaknesses of the patient's ability to deal effectively with incoming messages.

Receptive communication screenings initiated by nursing staff should include a variety of specific language categories (Table 15–5). First, the nurse should verbally give the patient simple concrete commands. Care should be taken to minimize accompanying gestures, because they tend to invalidate the assessment. Commands start with simple one-step directives such as "Make a fist," or "Point to the floor." Identification by pointing—whether to body parts, room objects, or specific people in the room—is appropriate. The nurse must take into account the effects of motor weakness and poor motor initiation or control when providing commands to patients with muscle or nerve deficits.

Next, two-step commands consisting of combinations of previous commands should be given. Difficulties following sequential commands in an organized manner or problems dealing with complex thoughts may be presenting hallmark behaviors of either dementia or traumatic brain injury.

As a third step, yes-or-no questions are asked of the patient. Clinical research suggests that a patient whose comprehension is not consistently intact will respond more often in the affirmative (Gruen, 1982). Ascertainment of a reliable "yes" or "no" response is imperative. The nurse should have correct answers available for comparison or validation of patient responses. Questions can incorporate information from the patient's care plan or medical record, such as biographic information or family names. The patient's response can be verbal, written, or gestural, depending on expressive capabilities. If the accuracy of the patient's yes-or-no response is questionable, the nurse can provide similar content questions that require both a positive and a negative response; for example, one might ask the patient if he or she is at home (no) and then ask if he or she is in the hospital (yes). Conflicting answers so obtained can help establish that the patient's comprehension or understanding of verbal messages is not adequate. Should the patient demonstrate difficulty in understanding verbal input, the nurse can present similar information either in writing or by gestures but must be certain to document the modification employed.

Next on the continuum for understanding is determining the patient's baseline literacy and comprehension of the written word. The nurse may supply short paragraph information, such as newspaper articles or a home instruction packet, for the patient to read and then may question the patient's understand-

---

TABLE 15–5 • RECEPTIVE LANGUAGE SCREENING CATEGORIES

- One-step commands
  "Point to the floor."
- Two-step commands
  "Touch your stomach and look at the window."
- Yes-or-no questions
  "Is your name Jane?" (no) "Is your name [insert correct name]?" (yes)
- Reading of words, sentences, and short paragraphs
  Provide newspaper headlines and short articles.

ing of what she or he has read. Simpler forms of reading assessment include matching written words to objects found in the room.

Other informal assessment considerations include observing the duration of selective attention, determining the possibility of hearing loss (noted especially in geriatric and traumatized populations), and assessing the ability to understand English.

Although it is important for the neuroscience nurse to assess the patient's receptive abilities, a certified speech-language pathologist should be consulted for a comprehensive and formalized assessment of communicative behaviors. Objective, standardized evaluative tools such as the Boston Diagnostic Aphasia Examination, the Western Aphasia Battery, and the Minnesota Test for Differential Diagnosis of Aphasia are particularly useful in quantifying and qualifying patient behaviors. Routine readministration of such tools ensures documentation of progress over time.

An otolaryngologist and certified audiologist can provide documentation of a formalized evaluation of the patient's hearing status. The otolaryngologist will physically examine the hearing mechanism and evaluate the outer, middle, and inner ear functions. Recommendations for medical or surgical interventions may be provided. On the basis of audiologic evaluation (which may include air conduction, bone conduction, and impedance testing), the audiologist may recommend environmental or behavioral modifications, such as hearing aids or sign-language instruction, that would serve to maximize the patient's ability to hear and understand verbal communication.

A neuropsychologist is consulted when input regarding the cognitive-linguistic status of the patient is important. Comprehensive standardized evaluations, such as the Halstead-Reitan Neuropsychological Test Battery and the Luria Nebraska Neuropsychological Battery, are commonly used to help delineate specific deficits arising from a cognitive, perceptual, and motor interaction system. It should be noted, however, that the patient must be able to tolerate lengthy assessment sessions and must have basic cognitive and communicative skills in place for the testing to be accurate and appropriate. In cases where patient tolerance or ability to participate is questioned, the neuropsychologist may resort to brief assessment tools or informal screenings.

Bijur, Haslum, and Golding (1990) reported a variety of cognitive issues frequently missed or overlooked when evaluating children with mild brain injuries. Their research focused on review of more than 13,000 children and found that significant sequelae can result from even minor blows to the head. These sequelae may persist for years, affecting normal development of cognitive and language skills.

Consolidation of the cognitive-linguistic evaluation provided by the speech-language pathologist and the results of the cognitive-motor-perceptual examination provided by the neuropsychologist results in an overall comprehensive interpretation from which functional therapeutic guidelines can be established. Schwartz-Cowley and Gruen (1986) outlined a variety of areas that typically are evaluated in this manner.

Gruen and Gruen (1994) reviewed differential diagnosis factors related to symbolic language disorders and cognitive-linguistic deficits. An understanding of these differences will assist the clinician and other team members in developing a reasonable and appropriate treatment program for the patient. Once a diagnosis of a receptive-communicative or cognitive disorder has been established and documented, an appropriate intervention plan is needed. It is important for the neuroscience nurse to realize that many aspects of daily patient care can be transformed into meaningful, functional rehabilitative stimuli appropriate for therapy procedures. This is especially valid when working with children and adolescents. Daily routines can often provide the therapeutic milieu for generalization and carryover. Modifying the communicative environment, the speaker's utterances, or the patient's behaviors will have a positive effect on comprehension. It is widely held that family members should be encouraged to interact and talk with the patient as much as is feasible to stimulate natural conversation in a way that is meaningful and predictable for the patient. With promotion of this type of spontaneous interaction at an informal level, the patient can be assisted to communicate with minimal restrictions and maximal acceptance from family members. Family members, by nature, are an integral part of the interdisciplinary team and can shed considerable light regarding particularities observed by nursing or other therapy staff.

The communicative environment should be as quiet and distraction free as possible. This allows the patient the greatest opportunity to focus on communication attempts and maximizes concentration and sustained attention capabilities. It is well-recognized that a calm, conducive setting will allow for increased understanding abilities from physical (hearing), symbolic (language), and cognitive perspectives (Boss, 1984). If receptive problems are recognized by nursing personnel, it is best to remove any potentially distracting items when attempting to communicate with the patient. Televisions and radios should be turned off and privacy curtains pulled to remove auditory and visual distractions.

The patient is best nurtured in an atmosphere that is caring and encouraging. The communicatively impaired patient can easily perceive a threatening atmosphere through the speaker's tone of voice, facial expressions, or gestures. The patient's own lack of total and complete understanding of verbal messages can result in negative impressions, which, when coupled with harsh tone of voice or condescending facial expressions, can exacerbate the problem. A one-on-one communication situation uses effective environmental control with only one person speaking at a time (Norman & Baratz, 1979). Above all, the patient should be exposed to calm, controlled discourse from others providing ample opportunities to hear speech, because this may aid increased comprehension (Boss, 1984).

When a speaker addresses a listener who has receptive difficulty, it is imperative that the speaker carefully monitor all language and modify characteristics of the message as needed. This goal can be accomplished in several ways. Some nursing personnel and other caregivers will get the patient's attention by calling his or her name and gesturing that a message is forthcoming. Establishing direct eye contact is also productive. Employing these strategies with children and adolescents as well as with patients who have sustained traumatic brain injuries assists in providing a "communication set" and expectancy for communication exchange.

Unless a hearing loss has been identified, using a significantly louder voice or exaggerated mouth movement tends not to enhance comprehension of verbal messages (Norman & Baratz, 1979). On the contrary, the use of such tactics presents increased distractions and loss of natural rhythm and melody of speech, a paralinguistic quality that often enhances comprehension. Serbin and Sommers (1984) suggest that use of normal voice loudness and intonation patterns will facilitate comprehension because of familiarity.

Boss (1984) and Weinhouse (1984) indicate that the addition of gestures, pantomime, and facial expressions supplements auditory comprehension. Multimodal presentation using various input modalities such as written cues, pictures, and drawings can also help (Ryan, 1982). Consistently maintaining topics of conversation, speaking in short precise statements, and using words familiar to the patient also produce beneficial effects. Excessive slowing of the speech signal may actually hinder comprehension because of the loss of natural intonation patterns and the effect of short-term recall difficulties (Hooper & Dunkle, 1984). Inserting pauses between phrases has been found to enhance overall comprehension of verbal messages in clinical trials (Louis & Poyse, 1980). This supports the premise, maintained by Beukelman and Yorkston (1991) and others, that neurologic injuries decrease the speed of understanding verbal messages.

Maintaining adult topics of conversation and establishing a daily nursing routine while encouraging the patient to perform or cooperate with medical treatments also have beneficial results (Ozuna, 1984). Likewise, children who rehearse activities of daily living and are assisted by nursing personnel who are aware of their developmental limitations often comprehend more and retain information better if it is repeated or completed in a routine scheduled fashion.

A common inclination is to believe that if a patient has a verbal communication deficit, a comprehension deficit of equal severity exists. In reality, patients (especially young children) can often understand much more than they can communicate expressively. For this reason, medical personnel working with patients should monitor all bedside conversations. Nothing should be said within a patient's hearing range that the patient should not hear, even if it appears that he or she does not understand. Many potentially embarrassing and often depressing situations can thus be avoided.

Special attention needs to be exercised when dealing with children and adults who show evidence of significant hearing loss. Many communication exchanges can be enhanced by simply facing the speaker and maintaining good eye contact. Often, a hearing-impaired individual will rely on visual cues such as gestures or lip movements to facilitate improved communication. Therefore, a well-lit room is paramount to increasing the amount of information that the patient will understand. It should be noted that hearing loss is an issue of acuity and not usually of content or semantic language skills impairment. Therefore, interactions are best received when they focus on improving the acuity of the listener by eliminating distractors such as television and radio or medical monitoring equipment with a routine auditory signal such as a feeding pump. If environmental factors are controlled as much as possible but the patient continues to be confused, alteration in the length of the verbal message or restating of the message in different words might be helpful.

Sometimes a patient can tell the nurse clearly and concisely what he or she can or cannot hear and can provide suggestions for increasing communicative efficiency. These suggestions should be diligently attended to. The speaker should avoid signs of personal frustration or impatience, because impatience tends to discourage active continued interaction on the part of the hearing-impaired patient.

In general terms, the understanding of a patient with a symbolic language or cognitive disorder (or, to a lesser degree, a hearing impairment) can be increased by decreasing the length of utterances, limiting distractions in the environment, decreasing the complexity and abstract quality of the conversation, increasing the specificity of commands presented, increasing multimodal cues (gestures, pictures, words), and decreasing the number of possible alternatives available to the patient. Although rate of presentation has been suggested as a significant variable in auditory comprehension, clinical research data support insertion of pauses rather than lengthening of the actual time of presentation.

Of paramount importance is the need for the speaker to maintain a positive communicative atmosphere with the patient, routinely checking for comprehension in nonthreatening ways. To achieve this goal, the neuroscience nurse may have to modify her or his own speech in terms of length, complexity, and extraneous information. Consider the following command given to a patient who demonstrates decreased understanding abilities: "Turn over part way on your left side so that I can change the 4-by-4 dressing pad that is soaked with blood and could result in an infection if not changed promptly and carefully." If the patient appears confused or indicates that he does not understand, the following modifications are encouraged. "Mr. Smith [tap patient on his shoulder to get his attention]. I need to change [pause] your dressing [point to dressing site]. Roll this way [gesture to the left and help the patient initiate movement]. Thank you."

DISORDERS OF EXPRESSIVE COMMUNICATION

Expressive capabilities involve an individual's ability to communicate through speech, writing, or gesture. In the medical field, concern is raised when the patient is unable to communicate basic needs effectively and fluently to the nursing staff. Although it is generally accepted that many patients who have sustained neurologic events demonstrate some degree of difficulty with comprehension or understanding, expressive disorders are frequently easier to observe and report, thus providing a more obvious framework for documentation and assessment. Treatment of expressive disorders relies heavily on the processes involved and the general characteristics displayed by the patient.

Expressive communicative or cognitive-linguistic disorders occur in many variations and may reflect significant differences in functional communication difficulties. Table 15–6 displays typical observations commonly found in patients who are referred to speech-language pathologists for communication work-ups.

Some patients appear able to repeat words but cannot communicate personal needs verbally. The propensity for profanity of certain patients tends to concern family members and nursing staff even though the family might deny that the patient previously used such language publicly.

These disorders result in frustration for the patient because he or she is unable to communicate basic needs adequately to the nursing staff and finds communication attempts difficult even with family members or close friends. Frustration is also evidenced by the listener who wants to aid the patient but does not have the necessary strategies or techniques to ensure successful communication.

Careful sequential assessment of a patient's expressive abilities provides valuable information for treatment guidelines. Although the nurse can perform basic screening functions (Table 15–7), referrals to the speech-language pathologist and other professionals are still necessary. The following assessment considerations are designed to require verbal responses; however, they can be modified to accommodate written and gestural responses as well.

A short oral peripheral examination, evaluating the structure and function of the lips, tongue, cheeks, and palate, is an essential component of assessing expressive capabilities. Particular note is made of any weakness or asymmetry. Dentition, in terms of intact teeth, presence or absence of dentures or partial plates, and alignment, is quickly assessed, and the presence of excessive drooling or insufficient saliva in the oral cavity is documented. Rapid repetition of sound sequences (diadochokinesia) is used to determine the integrity of quick tongue movements in the anterior, middle, and posterior areas of the oral cavity. Clinicians interested in more specific speech mechanism evaluation guidelines should refer to Hodge (1988), who has developed a comprehensive

TABLE 15–6 • COMMON OBSERVATIONS OF PATIENT BEHAVIOR SUGGESTING NEED FOR EXPRESSIVE COMMUNICATION EVALUATION

- Excessive slurring of speech
- Laborious attempts at communicating basic needs
- Significantly reduced speech volume
- Lack of full vocalization during speech attempts
- Facial groping behaviors during communication attempts
- Significant word-finding problems in conversation
- Inability to repeat words of varying lengths
- Inability to speak words when the same words can be effectively sung
- Sound substitutions or distortions
- Tip of the tongue syndrome
- Sudden onset of dysfluent speech
- Perseveration of thoughts or words
- Inability to change topics of discussion without a seemingly mandatory return to previous topic

TABLE 15–7 • EXPRESSIVE SCREENING CATEGORIES

- Oral peripheral screening
  Evaluate structure and function of lips, tongue, cheeks, and palate.
  Evaluate dental status.
- Repetition
  Have patient repeat single sounds, words, and phrases.
- Automatic speech tasks
  Tell the patient, "Count from one to ten."
- Close-ended phrase completion
  Prompt the patient, "The opposite of up is ___________ ." .
- Visual confrontation naming
  Prompt the patient, "Tell me the name of this" (e.g., a telephone).
- Open-ended conversation
  Ask the patient, "Can you tell me why you are in the hospital?"

decision-making process for detailed assessments of the speech mechanism and oral functions.

Once the oral peripheral assessment is completed, the sequence of verbal expression is initiated. Assessment requires the repetition of single sounds, words, and phrases and the production of automatic speech acts (verbal sequences that are overlearned, such as counting from 1 to 10 or naming the days of the week). Close-ended phrases, which include antonyms and synonyms, are generated to assess if the patient can determine closure concepts. Visual confrontation naming tasks are completed, including naming objects, body parts, pictures, and words.

Open-ended conversation is elicited by having the patient describe pictures, tell a story, or explain the sequence of a particular activity of daily living such as brushing teeth. Characteristics of perseveration, echolalia and palilalia, circumlocution, tangentiality, fluency, fluidity of thought, attention, prosody, confabulation, slurring, voice disturbances, and so on are noted in terms of context of occurrence, frequency, and overall effects on functional communication.

A referral to the speech-language pathologist is necessary so that all areas of speech, language, and cognitive performance can be evaluated with appropriate, detailed therapy programs established and implemented. The speech-language pathologist can also recommend various referrals to be completed, depending on the characteristics observed. A referral to an otolaryngologist is made if the patient's voice is hoarse, breathy, excessively soft, or harsh.

A diagnosis of vocal fold pathology can be obtained by the physician and needs to be completed before voice therapy initiation because various ramifications of physiologic and structural components could require modifications of traditional voice therapy procedures (Parks & Shanks, 1983). The otolaryngologist can also examine the hearing mechanism to determine if the patient who speaks softly has a hearing loss that interferes with adequate auditory feedback of verbal messages. The otolaryngologist may then refer the patient to a certified audiologist or hearing aid specialist for evaluation and provision of hearing aids.

A referral is made to the neuropsychologist when the patient's expressive content is disorganized and shows signs of significant confusion. The neuropsychologist will complete tests as described earlier in this chapter. Careful differential diagnosis of language versus cognitive manifestations must be made.

Brookshire (1978) discussed eight principles of therapeutic intervention for patients with acquired neurologic damage affecting speech and language processes (Table 15–8). Although these suggestions are designed with the speech-language pathologist in mind, generalizations for routine nursing intervention can be made.

In collaboration with Brookshire's principles, many other researchers and clinicians point to various modifications and concepts that enhance the patient's ability to communicate basic needs efficiently and effectively. These concepts form the basic touchstones of therapists around the nation.

An example is assigning patients with expressive communication disorders to semiprivate rooms rather than private rooms. Routine nursing procedures can be discussed with the patient, providing numerous opportunities for the patient to attempt communication while participating in his or her own care. Of course, maintenance of proper oral hygiene will extend the potential for the patient to desire to speak.

Whenever possible, speaking behaviors should be modified and directed toward positive speaking situations. Keeping the conversation focused on familiar topics will tend to produce more intact word usage than will conversations about unfamiliar subjects. A patient interested in gardening, for example, will achieve more efficient and effective communication if the discussion includes gardening topics. The nurse should also stress the "can do" approach to rehabilitation by focusing conversations on the speech and language abilities that remain rather than on the patient's deficits. Such focusing will augment the patient's self-esteem and maintain a positive attitude toward communication. As a listener and communication partner, the nurse should try to maintain a positive, accepting attitude toward the patient and praise successful attempts at communication. This is often difficult for nurses and other caregivers to do

TABLE 15–8 • BROOKSHIRE'S EIGHT PRINCIPLES OF INTERVENTION

1. Structure treatment programs so that most of the patient's tasks are at levels of difficulty that cause performance to be slightly deficient but not completely erroneous.
2. Keep stimulus materials used in treatment simple and relevant to the patient's areas of deficit.
3. Elicit large numbers of responses from the patient.
4. Begin each treatment session with familiar tasks in which the patient is generally successful.
5. Introduce new materials and procedures as extensions of familiar materials and procedures.
6. Provide feedback regarding accuracy and appropriateness of the patient's responses when such feedback appears to be beneficial.
7. Show the patient his or her progress.
8. Direct treatment toward general abilities rather than specific responses whenever possible.

From Brookshire, R. (1978). *An introduction to aphasia* (2nd ed.). Minneapolis: BRK Publishers.

because it frequently takes considerably more time to allow the patient to try to communicate on his or her own rather than to anticipate and supply answers. Such patients also tend to exhibit emotional lability, which needs to be accommodated by switching topics of conversation quickly, for if not dealt with quickly and purposefully, emotional lability can be perseverated and thus become more difficult to modify.

The nurse should allow the patient ample time to produce speech. As discussed earlier, human discourse is a cooperative event between two or more people, which involves complex sequencing and patterning of thoughts and words. Many patients can participate effectively if they have enough time to process incoming messages and produce outgoing communication. Encouraging the patient to express his or her thoughts as independently as possible is essential. The nurse speaker must exercise care to support, rather than criticize, the patient's attempts to communicate. This can be done by encouraging the patient to use spontaneous, overlearned speech, such as "Hi," and "I don't know," so that the patient can become part of the communicative and social setting as much as is feasible. Patients can be encouraged to use gestures and printed words or communication charts to augment verbal communicative performance as necessary.

It should be noted, however, that even with significant opportunities presented to the patient to enter into a communicative interchange, successful communication on the part of the patient may not be achieved. A variety of simple procedures may be employed to facilitate patient communication with the nurse or other team members.

Several cuing strategies, including associative, descriptive, phonologic, gestural, and graphic cues, can benefit the patient who demonstrates word-finding difficulties. Associative cues include providing antonyms, synonyms, category members, and overlearned expressions, such as "A cold hand, a warm (heart)." Descriptive cues may focus on physical attributes, such as "It is tall and green and has leaves. It is a (tree)." Functions of objects can be provided to aid in word retrieval, such as "You sleep in a (bed)." Phonologic cues provide the patient with part or all of a word, such as "b" or "bed" given as a cue to the word "bedpan." Pantomiming actions, directions, descriptions, and qualifiers of words or ideas provides gestural cues. The neuroscience nurse may ask the patient to demonstrate the use of an object he or she desires. Cues, such as writing the first letter and leaving spaces for subsequent letters of a word, or writing the entire word, can often elicit the patient's verbal response through the multimodal presentation conceptual framework.

The neuroscience nurse can maximize the patient's expressive capabilities in other ways, including anticipating the patient's needs, expanding the patient's responses, avoiding continual direct confrontation of the patient's speech errors, and determining what is most important for the patient to communicate with expectation and preparation for responses.

The nurse must consider any type of communication as beneficial. Care must be given to verbal, nonverbal, and gestural attempts of the patient. It is important to emphasize and praise any and all attempts, because motivation often waxes and wanes for the patient with communication difficulties. At the same time, the nurse can indicate acceptance and understanding of the patient's communicative difficulties by asking questions that can be answered within the patient's expressive mode and current abilities. For example, if the patient's responses are limited to yes-or-no verbalizations, questions that require exposition, such as "Why don't you feel well?" are inappropriate. Questions such as "Does your head hurt?" and "Do you want a pain pill?" are much better suited to the immediate situation.

Nursing personnel can greatly enhance the patient's ability to generalize communicative success outside the hospital or clinic setting. Superimposed organization with predictable outcomes in the inpatient unit should always be the first step toward generalization. Clearly, as the world does not gravitate toward complete organization and structure, it is important to allow for eventual inclusion of unpredictable scenarios in as many settings as is feasible (Helm-Estabrooks & Albert, 1991). However, patient frustration and tolerance levels must be taken into account throughout this process.

If the patient's expressive difficulties are caused by motor weakness problems, adherence to a few general guidelines can greatly enhance the overall intelligibility of the verbal output. The nurse must remember that transmission of speech involves four distinct but interacting processes: respiration, phonation, articulation, and resonation (Darley, Aronson, & Brown, 1975). Disruption of any of these processes results in reduced intelligibility. Dysarthria and, to a lesser extent, apraxia and dysprosody are primary expressive manifestations of motor speech disorders. These problems can occur singularly but more often compose a group of problems that complicate assessment (Kent & Kent, 1988).

The speech-language pathologist can help by suggesting specific exercises that facilitate stronger and more purposeful interaction of the processes. Generally, the patient with dysarthria should be encouraged to reduce his or her own rate of speech, to attempt to become cognitively attuned to muscle mobility and patterning, and to shorten length of utterance per breath so that speech can be produced clearly with decreased need for repetition. The patient should be taught how significant decreases in overall intelligibility can be minimized by prevention of fatigue.

Realizing that verbal communication involves a complex sequence of linguistic and physical activities alerts the neuroscience nurse to the fact that difficulties in expression can occur and will worsen if not carefully monitored and modified. Frustrations on the part of the patient, family, and medical staff can be effectively reduced if proper evaluation and therapeutic intervention strategies can be implemented in a timely fashion.

AUGMENTATIVE COMMUNICATION SYSTEMS

For purposes of this discussion, *augmentative communication system* refers to any assistive device that enhances functional communication by increasing either comprehension or expression capabilities. The goal of any augmentative communication system is to match the current communicative needs of an individual with the functioning of a specific augmentative device. Current research supports an increase in the public's acceptance of individuals who use augmentative communication systems. This is more evident in young populations (Dale & Gruen, 1992) but is beginning to affect adults and geriatric populations as well since miniaturization and computer interfaces have become more widely used.

A prime focus of augmentative systems is to promote a "conversation" environment between two or more individuals (MacDonald & Gilette, 1989). Intervention must focus on reciprocal communication. The interdisciplinary team, with major input from the patient's nurse to the speech-language pathologist, provides a comprehensive evaluation of a patient's communicative status.

Beukelman and Mirenda (1992) suggested that children with severe congenital or acquired disorders may require specialized systems. For these individuals, intervention must focus on expressing preferences, sensitizing facilitators of communication, responding to spontaneous signals, and teaching routine contexts.

Questions relating to evaluation or potential use of augmentative communicative devices include the following: What is the present communicative need? How long will the patient require the communicative aid? What potential benefits and risks are present with the preferred communicative aid? What is the potential for acceptance of the device as it pertains to the patient, the family, and the neuroscience nurse? Are there sufficient financial resources for obtaining an expensive piece of equipment? Would a handmade, less expensive version be more appropriate? Have the patient's physical and cognitive abilities been evaluated?

Answers to these questions should focus on the patient's motor ability, sensory function, ability to move various body parts, complexity of operation of the device, and overall comprehension abilities (Mast, 1983). Once questions about the patient's abilities and problems are answered, consideration of various types of augmentative communication systems is necessary.

Types of Augmentative Devices

Research and development of augmentative communication systems is a fast-growing, complex specialty. Because most devices are extremely individualized and because a comprehensive list of available devices would rapidly become obsolete, only general information is provided here. Consultation with the speech-language pathologist or rehabilitation engineer is recommended for more patient-specific information.

Generally, augmentative systems can be divided into nonmechanical and mechanical or computerized systems, each of which can provide specific or general help to the patient in his or her endeavor to receive and send messages.

NONMECHANICAL

A communication chart is perhaps the most commonly used nonmechanical communication system in medical settings. Usually a notebook with pictures and words, a lap board with letters or pictures, or a wall hanging may serve as a communication chart. The chart encapsulates specific words or concepts that depict an entire activity that is useful or necessary to the patient. The nurse must ensure that only a limited number of purposeful items are used; cluttered communication charts often result in significant confusion and frustration. The patient usually begins with only a few items, practices using them to communicate basic needs, and gradually adds more items as she or he becomes more adept at using the chart. The simplicity or complexity of the completed communication chart will depend on the motor control, manual dexterity, visual abilities, mode of mobility, method of message indication, type and number of required messages, and amount of time available to make the patient's needs known (Mast, 1983). To keep the communication chart useful for long periods, the nurse may wish to preserve it by covering it with clear plastic or by hanging it on the wall when not in use. Most situations require the chart to encompass orientation information; "yes," "no," and "uncertain" response blocks; and listings of basic needs.

MECHANICAL OR COMPUTERIZED

Mechanical or computerized versions of communication charts are available through most speech suppliers and may be useful for patients who will need to use them for extended periods. These systems usually require preprogramming before patient use. Power sources, including AC line and battery power, generally adapt to available services; batteries must be recharged on a regular basis. Mechanical communication charts are not recommended for patients who will not require them for extended periods because of the cost of purchase, service, and operation.

The letter clock is used infrequently in the modern technological world, but it can be useful for mildly to moderately cognitively impaired children and adolescents. The letter clock has letters of the alphabet located in place of the numbers on a clock face. Using a switch mechanism, the patient rotates a bar similar to an hour hand around the clock face and stops the bar when it reaches the desired letter. Once the letter has been identified, the patient reactivates the system to locate the next letter. Modifications of the letter clock include placing pictures around the face that depict activities of daily living.

Sophisticated computerized augmentative communicative systems are available that can be programmed to produce either visual graphic or auditory messages. The user simply pushes a button or tab to respond to a message. Printers are available for permanent recordings. Miniature typewriterlike devices are used for spelling and printing messages (Fig. 15–1). Adequate fine motor coordination skills are needed for a person to use such systems effectively.

Personal home computers have adaptations for the nonverbal patient's use in communicating. Many large computer companies have special adapters for using computers for communication purposes. Patients with high cervical spinal cord injuries can use a variety of switches, including brow switches, pneumatic devices, and similar methods to control a scanner that produces messages (Fig. 15–2). Many hospital staff members can provide instruction

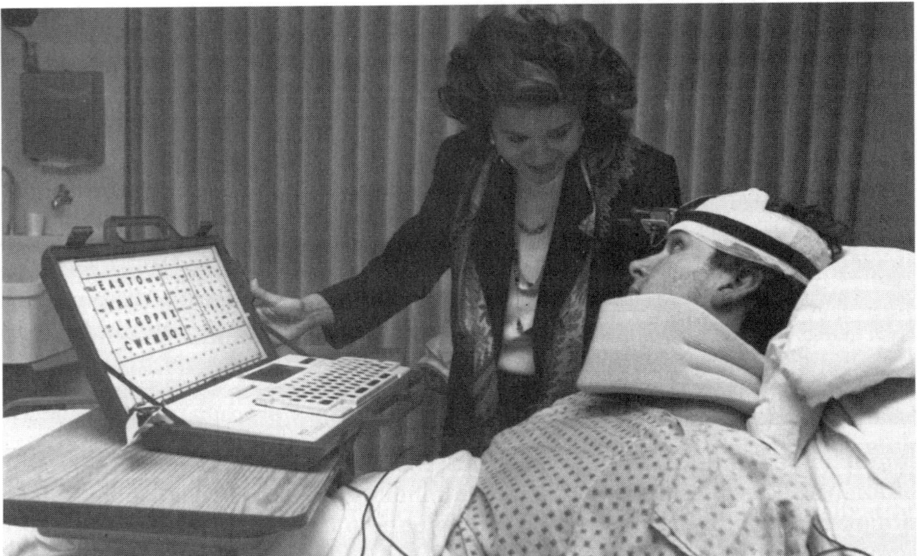

FIGURE 15–1 • A patient regains his ability to communicate by using a small typewriterlike device with a printout record.

and practice, with the result that the patient's behavior will be enhanced by his or her increased ability to indicate basic personal needs. Programs are available that provide activities dealing with memory, abstraction, reasoning, and judgment for the patient who demonstrates cognitive-linguistic deficits.

The artificial larynx is another mechanical device used for nonverbal patients. Although traditionally recommended for use by laryngectomized patients, it has been shown to be effective for patients with endotracheal tubes. The artificial larynx mechanism lends itself to patient maneuverability. A vibratory wave is transmitted through the neck wall into the oral cavity, which simulates laryngeal vibration. When the oral musculature is moved freely and precisely, the artificially produced voice is transformed into purposeful speech. The patient must be able to follow commands consistently, be capable of manipulating articulators with good mobility, and be willing to accept the artificial sound of the voice so produced. Advances in the artificial larynx industry allow for mechanical voices in child, female, and male ranges.

Because many patients in the neurosurgical unit have significant hearing difficulties, a short general discussion of the precautions and problems frequently encountered with hearing aids is appropriate here. More detailed information can be obtained from a certified audiologist. Parks and Shanks (1983) suggested the following precautions:

1. Do not expose the aid to excessive heat.

2. Do not allow the aid to get wet. Patients should remove the aid before showering. If the aid gets wet, take the batteries out immediately. Wipe

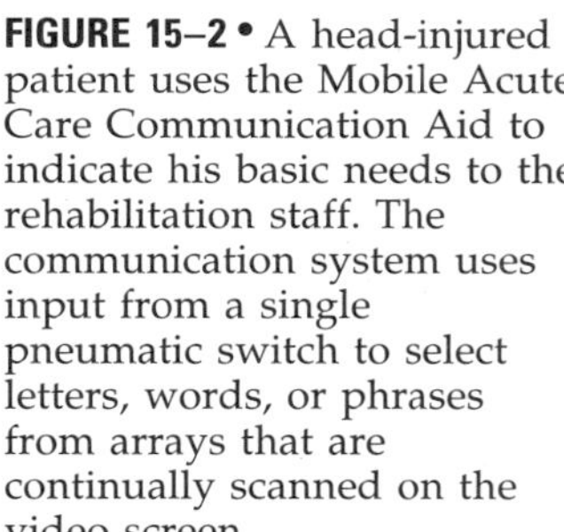

FIGURE 15–2 • A head-injured patient uses the Mobile Acute Care Communication Aid to indicate his basic needs to the rehabilitation staff. The communication system uses input from a single pneumatic switch to select letters, words, or phrases from arrays that are continually scanned on the video screen.

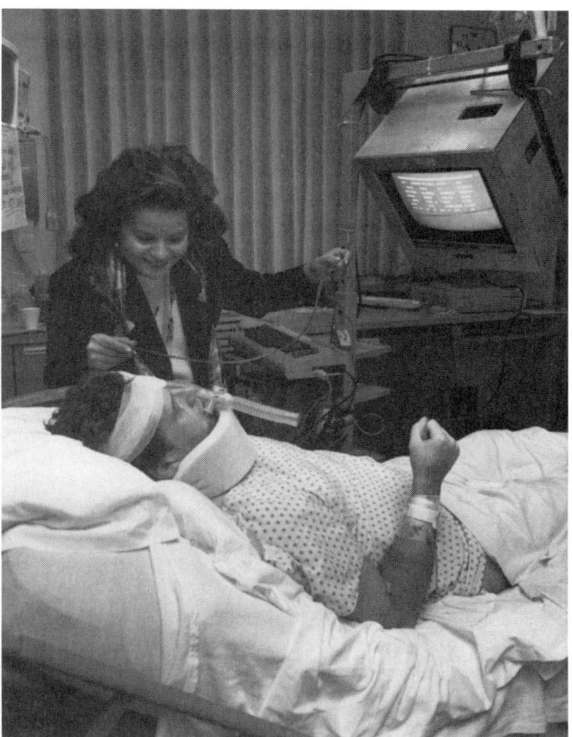

the exterior surface with a dry cloth. Place the aid in a warm (but not hot) place. A hair dryer on a low setting may be used cautiously to dry the aid. Do not place the aid in an oven or microwave oven.

3. Do not use alcohol, acetone, or cleaning fluid on the case.

4. Discard leaking batteries at once.

5. Be sure to remove batteries or open the battery case when the aid is not in use.

Using precautions and good cleaning procedures should extend the functional use of the hearing aid. If, however, the aid does not appear to function properly, the nurse can use the information presented in Table 15–9 from Parks and Shanks (1983) to troubleshoot problems.

Knowing about and using augmentative communication devices can benefit both patient care and service delivery. The nurse should refer patients to a speech-language pathologist whenever functional communication of personal needs is limited because of physical, environmental, or physiologic problems.

TABLE 15–9 • TROUBLESHOOTING HEARING AID PROBLEMS

- If no sound is heard, first check the batteries and be sure to align the positive terminal marking with the appropriate marking on the case. If still no sound is heard, try a new battery.
- If the aid does not appear to be useful to the patient, make sure that the controls are set according to recommendations outlined by the audiologist. Consultation with family members may be required to accomplish this goal. Often the M (microphone) and T (telephone) switches may be set for the wrong listening situation, necessitating adjustment.
- If feedback occurs, the connections of the ear mold and hearing aid should be examined to locate possible cracks or leaks. If any are found, an audiologist or hearing aid specialist should be consulted and a new mold impression taken if indicated. Other sources of feedback problems include dirty or clogged ear molds and internal damage to the receiver. A maintenance check may be required.

From Parker, J., & Shanks, J. (1983). The nurse and voice disorders. In S. Shanks (Ed.), *Nursing and the management of adult communication disorders* (pp. 5–30). San Diego, CA: College Hill Press.

SUMMARY

The nurse is an integral part of the interdisciplinary team. It is not uncommon for the nurse to be confronted with significant needs from patients. The nurse often becomes a spokesperson for the communicatively impaired individual. Knowing, understanding, and implementing the functional framework of detailed behavioral observation, informal assessment, and practical intervention strategies for the patient with communicative or cognitive-linguistic deficits will greatly enhance patient communication, education, and satisfaction.

References

Beukelman, D., & Mirenda, P. (1992). *Augmentative and alternative communication: Management of severe communication disorders in children and adults.* Baltimore, MD: Paul H. Brookes.

Beukelman, D., & Yorkston, K. (1991). *Communication disorders following traumatic brain injury: Management of cognitive, language, and motor impairments.* Austin, TX: Pro-Ed.

Bijur, P. E., Haslum, M., & Golding, J. (1990). Cognitive and behavioral sequelae of mild head injury in children. *Pediatrics, 86*(3), 337–344.

Boss, B. (1984). Dysphasia, dyspraxia, and dysarthria. Distinguishing features, part II. *Journal of Neurosurgical Nursing, 16,* 211.

Brockway, J. (1991). Psychosocial disturbances after head injury. In D. R. Beukelman & K. M. Yorkston (Eds.), *Communication disorders following traumatic brain injury: Management of cognitive, language, and motor impairments* (pp. 111–132). Austin, TX: Pro-Ed.

Brookshire, R. (1978). *An introduction to aphasia* (2nd ed.). Minneapolis: BRK Publishers.

Cummings, J., & Read, S. (1988). Multi-infarct dementia. *Hospital Medicine, 11,* 27–42.

Dale, P., & Gruen, A. (1992). Attitudes toward users of augmentative communication devices. *Voice, 40*(2), 9.

Darley, F., Aronson, A., & Brown, J. (1975). *Motor speech disorders.* Philadelphia: W.B. Saunders.

Gruen, A. (1982). *The effect of presentation rate on the auditory comprehension of adult aphasics.* Unpublished master's thesis, University of Arizona, Tucson.

Gruen, A., & Gruen, L. (1994). *Back into life (book II): The issues of singles.* Eau Claire, WI: Thinking Publications.

Helm-Estabrooks, N., & Albert, M. (1991). *Manual of aphasia therapy.* Austin, TX: Pro-Ed.

Hodge, M. (1988). Speech mechanism: Assessment. In D. Yoder & R. Kent (Eds.), *Decision making in speech-language pathology* (pp. 104–109). Philadelphia: Decker.

Hooper, C., & Dunkle, R. (1984). *The other aphasic person.* Rockville, MD: Aspen.

Kent, R., & Kent, J. (1988). Motor speech disorders. In D. Yoder & R. Kent (Eds.), *Decision making in speech-language pathology* (pp. 154–155). Philadelphia: Decker.

Louis, M., & Poyse, S. (1980). Aphasia and endurance: Considerations in the assessment and care of the stroke patient. *Nursing Clinics of North America, 15,* 265.

Luterman, D. (1991). *Counseling the communicatively disordered and their families.* Austin, TX: Pro-Ed.

MacDonald, J., & Gilette, J. (1989). *ECO: A partnership program.* San Antonio, TX: Special Press.

Mast, D. (1983). Selecting and implementing augmentative communication systems for adults. In S. Shanks (Ed.), *Nursing and the management of adult communication disorders* (pp. 195–224). San Diego, CA: College Hill Press.

Murdoch, B. (1990). *Acquired speech and language disorders: A neuroanatomical and functional approach.* London: Chapman and Hull.

Norman, S., & Baratz, R. (1979). Understanding aphasia. *American Journal of Nursing, 79*(12), 2135–2138.

Ozuna, J. (1984). Alterations in mentation: Nursing assessment and intervention. *Journal of Neurosurgical Nursing, 17,* 66.

Parker, J., & Shanks, J. (1983). The nurse and voice disorders. In S. Shanks (Ed.), *Nursing and the management of adult communication disorders* (pp. 5–30). San Diego, CA: College Hill Press.

Ryan, W. (1982). *The nurse and the communicatively impaired adult.* New York: Springer.

Schwartz-Cowley, R., & Gruen, A. (1986). Rehabilitation assessment of communicative, cognitive-linguistic, and swallowing functions. *Trauma Quarterly, 3*(1), 63–75.

Serbin, S., & Sommers, R. (1984). *Aphasia and associated problems: A family guide.* Kent, OH: Blaca Enterprise.

Weinhouse, S. (1984). Speaking to the needs of your aphasic patient. *Nursing, 11,* 34.

Zasler, N., Kreutzer, J., & Taylor, D. (1991). Coma stimulation and coma recovery: A critical review. *Neurorehabilitation, 1*(4), 33–54.

The authors wish to acknowledge Connie P. Walleck, MS, RN, CNRN, for her contributions concerning nursing diagnoses of cognitive-language disorders in the first edition.

AFFILIATIVE RELATIONSHIPS PHENOMENA

16 | Affiliative Relationships: An Overview

CATHERINE ECOCK CONNELLY • A. SUSAN BIDWELL

Neurologic problems often precipitate major changes in patients' lifestyles and affect ability to function independently. Families, significant others, and close friends struggle with neurologically impaired patients to cope with the illnesses, crises, and grieving processes associated with neurologic disabilities. Empathetic reactions of loved ones usually provide support to patients; at other times, the demands and stress resulting from dealing with and supporting a loved one through an illness can create strain. Families may be so overwhelmed physically, emotionally, or economically that they become less effective in providing social support or may even become barriers to care. Understanding the nature and dynamics of affiliative relationships enables nurses to help families or significant others mobilize their own support systems throughout various crises and stages related to the illness. Such understanding enables neuroscience nurses to perceive patients' responses to illness in the context of their family or affiliative system.

Literature and research in nursing that focus on the impact of family concepts on nursing practice have developed significantly. The American Nurses Association in 1980 and the World Health Organization in 1985 emphasized the importance of family to the health of individuals by identifying the family as the basic unit of care (Duffy, 1988). Whall and Fawcett (1991) acknowledged the growing trend to view the family as the unit of care and proposed modification of nursing's metaparadigm to reflect "nursing's concern with the family as a whole." However, despite the widespread endorsement by nurses of family-oriented approaches to care, Gilliss (1989) noted that there has been little nursing research on nontraditional forms of family.

Social mores and demographic changes have altered the living patterns of Americans, expanding the generally accepted definition of family. This chapter uses the term affiliative relationship and conceptualizes the family from the perspective that the family includes various systems of relationships that, regardless of their biologic or legal basis, exhibit certain characteristics and fulfill deep personal needs flowing from the individual's need for relatedness.

Affiliative relationships are conceptualized as social systems composed of significant, patterned, meaningful relationships characterized by emotional commitment, intimacy, stability, and continuity. This chapter discusses the various forms of affiliative relationships in our society and the ways in which human needs are met through them. A framework for assessment of affiliative relationships is presented.

NATURE OF AFFILIATIVE RELATIONSHIPS

Two basic assumptions underlie the analysis of affiliative relationships. The first assumption is that individuals meet their needs for supportive interpersonal relationships in many forms, not limited to the traditional family structure (Stein, 1977). The significance of these relationships is not necessarily dictated by the biologic or legal status of the relationship, but rather by the importance that the relationship has in the personal lives of the individuals involved.

The second assumption is that the major theoretical frameworks developed to study family relationships are also applicable in assessing other forms of affiliative relationships. This view recognizes that the essence of affiliative relationships lies in the human needs for love, sharing, and communication. Human needs are satisfied by these special relationships in a way that distinguishes affiliative relationships from more casual ones. Realization of these basic needs operates as a dynamic process in family relationships (Spanier, 1981) but is not limited to formalized families. These processes operate in other significant relationships as well (Lindsey, 1981).

Consistent with these two assumptions, Naisbitt (1982) called for a "new definition" of the family. The inclusion of long-standing voluntary relationships in this new definition will lead to "new family models." Trends that characterize the American family are older age of first marriage, delayed parenthood and reduced fertility rates, single households composed of individuals of all ages, dual-career and dual-earner couples, high divorce rates, second marriages, blended families, cohabitation by heterosexual and homosexual couples, single parents, and male homemakers (Staples, 1989).

The demographic shifts in American population, although altering the structure of affiliative relationships, have not decreased the significance of family life in our society. The elderly, particularly those age 85 years and older—the fastest-growing segment of our population—continue to report regular interaction with family and reflect continued reliance on family. Although most older people live independently—only 5% are in institutional settings—the elderly report that they maintain frequent contact with extended family for support (Wilson & Trost, 1978).

Nine of 10 Americans eventually marry, and 80% of divorced people remarry. The increase of 41% in the number of cohabiting couples and the proportion of remarriages and reconstituted families indicates that the search for intimate relationships is a major force in American life (Gilliss, 1989; Spanier, 1981). Skolnik (1991) asserted that the commentary that decries the "decline of the American family" muddles the problem and underestimates the evolution that reflects cultural, psychologic, and economic change. Scanzoni (1983) proposed that a fresh concept of family has the potential for making it a richer institution capable of balancing the interests of society with those of individuals. Orthner (1995) suggested that new forms of family represent new choices and relationships in living arrangements to reflect a transition in family concepts. Howard (1978) concluded that whether the connections are those of choice or chance, the effort people make to create relationships resembling families that provide deep, intimate connections and support is one of the most enduring habits of human beings.

FORMS OF AFFILIATIVE RELATIONSHIPS

Affiliative relationships can be categorized as either legal and biologic or achieved and nonbiologic. An examination of the various forms of affiliative relationships within each category demonstrates the diverse kinds of relationships developed by people to meet their needs for intimacy and relatedness.

Legal and Biologic Families

Legal and biologic families include married couples, nuclear families, extended families, and families of origin. The marriage of a couple without children, whether by choice or not, is the childless dyadic marriage (Friedman, 1998; Kuhn & Janosik, 1980). This may be a temporary stage in the marital relationship for a short or prolonged period or may persist throughout the life of the marriage.

The married childbearing family includes the marital couple and their biologic children, adopted children, or both, even when the children are no longer living in the parental home. This is classified as the family of procreation for the spouses (Heffron & Wolff, 1984). This form, frequently called the traditional or nuclear family, is viewed as having a developmental history based on the age of the oldest child (Duvall & Miller, 1985). The life cycle of the childbearing family is conceptualized in eight stages: (1) the married couple, (2) the childbearing family, (3) the family with preschool-aged children, (4) the family with school-aged children, (5) the family with teenaged children, (6) the family whose children are involved in launching a career, (7) middle-aged parents, and (8) the family whose parents are aged. Duvall and Miller (1985) theorized that each family developmental stage requires the accomplishment of stage-appropriate tasks that characterize the function of the family during that stage.

The single-parent family consists of one parent and his or her biologic children, adopted children, or both (Heffron & Wolff, 1984). Single-parent families are a result of separation, divorce, widowhood, or childbearing or adoption outside marriage. The life-cycle approach proposed by Duvall and Miller (1985) for analyzing the childbearing family is also applicable to understanding single-parent families because of its focus on tasks related to parenting. Despite the arbitrary assignment of family developmental stage to the age of the oldest child, Frude (1991) asserted that describing major family milestones contributes to better understanding of family dynamics.

The extended family includes the nuclear family and other biologically related family members. These may include grandparents, siblings, or other people biologically related to one of the spouses. The extended family sharing the same residence was much more common in the past than it is at present (Heffron & Wolff, 1984). In this age of geographic mobility, extended families tend to be less intensively involved with one another on a regular day-to-day basis. Orthner (1995) concluded that despite separate living arrangements, 50% of Americans with aging parents visit them at least once a month.

The term family of origin refers to the parental family of an individual (Heffron & Wolff, 1984). The maintenance of intense relationships and the role the family of origin plays in the life of an adult vary from individual to individual. For single adults, particularly those who have recently moved away from their nuclear families, the family of origin sometimes remains the primary source of emotional support and relatedness.

Achieved, Nonbiologic Families

Achieved, nonbiologic families are referred to by Lindsey (1981) as chosen families. They exhibit qualities of kinship characterized by love, commitment, and continuity. Chosen or achieved families include those involving cohabitation and those comprising friends as family. The term cohabitation implies a sexual relationship, which can be either heterosexual or homosexual in nature. Common-law marriages can be included in this category.

Lindsey (1981) categorized friends as family as honorary kin, workplace family, and chosen family. Individuals in achieved or chosen families may share the same household, but shared residency is not necessary for achieved or chosen families. Lindsey (1981) described honorary kin as people who, because of their intimacy and emotional ties to the biologic family, become absorbed into and are considered a part of the preexisting family structure. They are frequently chosen by the parents from among their friends and fill roles similar to those of grandparents, aunts, uncles, siblings, or children. Honorary kin are integrated into the family system, and the close relationship continues despite changes and relocation of various family members. They have often played an important role in families in poverty, suggesting that the practical support they provide often precedes and leads to the development of strong emotional ties. Fictive kin, as they are sometimes called, are an integral part of the life of the family and share in major events.

The workplace family develops among people who spend most of their daily time together for extended periods, frequently stretching into years, sharing a common task or goal. Lindsey (1981) observed that the bonds that develop among people who share common commitments and goals in a workplace can often be as intense and enriching as those of the biologic family. Christensen (1992) disagreed, proposing that although work groups seem to fulfill some of the qualities of family, they lack the sense of commitment.

Lindsey (1981) characterized chosen family as relationships that are woven into the fabric of a person's well-being and are deeply emotionally significant despite separations of time and distance. Friends are chosen as family, not always because the biologic family is unavailable or does not satisfy needs for bonding and emotional support, but to expand and extend these meaningful relationships. For many single people, especially those separated by time and distance from their families of origin, chosen families are the source of the deep and enduring emotional support characterized by primary affiliative relationships (Stuart, 1991).

The characteristic of permanence is the essence of affiliative relationships. Such permanence is established through the commitment of members, which is based on strong emotional attachment. Families are said to have a continuity that includes a past, a present, and a future. Kinship involves love, commitment, continuity, and stability amid change, regardless of whether the relationship is based on biologic, legal, achieved, or chosen foundations (Frude, 1991; Lindsey, 1981). We will see, by exploring and analyzing the elements of and the human needs met through affiliative relationships, that these relationships are at the core of the human experience. As such, they set the tone for the life experience of the individual. Any major change in life experience, such as disabling neurologic illness, reverberates throughout the entire affiliative network.

CHARACTERISTICS OF HEALTHY BIOLOGIC OR ACHIEVED FAMILIES

A number of authors have suggested characteristics of heathy families (Frude, 1991; Howard, 1978; Kane, 1988; Pearsall, 1990). First, affiliative or family systems encompass a variety of roles including that of a leader, or prime mover, who is central to the system. Howard (1978) observed that although some families go for generations without a prime mover, clans of all kinds need such a figure. Kane (1988) emphasized the variety and fluidity of relationships in affiliative groups.

Second, affiliative systems include a member who assumes the role of communicator, thus ensuring that other system members are kept informed and up-to-date. Frude (1991) emphasized that openness and clarity of communication are essential ingredients for optimal functioning. The family communicator, according to Howard (1978), is the member who keeps albums and scrapbooks to record the family history.

Third, all members in affiliative systems have extrafamilial concerns and relationships. Their relationships within the system, however, provide essential emotional support and are of greater significance. Pearsall (1990) described the phenomenon of the primacy of the family point of view.

Fourth, members seek close relationships, encourage and support one another, and tend to be hospitable. Good families, suggested Howard (1978), seek to share their relationships and welcome others into their fold. Kane (1988) described the family as available, warm, and sharing, while Pearsall (1990) characterized the family as a ''soul center.''

Fifth, affiliative systems deal with the ''direness'' or the crises of their members. The crises and disasters encountered in life are as much a part of the family's concern as are good fortune and triumphs. They mobilize resources in times of crisis and adversity. Moreover, families demonstrate a tolerance for failure and an ability to forgive (Pearsall, 1990).

Sixth, rituals are an important part of affiliative relationships. Not only do fixed rituals unite a family and deepen the bonds each time they are enacted, but members of families tend to create their own unique rituals to reflect their history and relationships. Kane (1988) describes this phenomenon as a sense of the history marking the developmental epochs in the lives of the members.

Seventh, members in affiliative relationships are affectionate, warm, caring, and responsive toward one another. Families establish their own style of expressing their affection. These expressions range from effusive to restrained; however, the gestures, whatever their form, have a shared meaning for all.

Eighth, affiliative systems share a ''hearth'' or special place for the members. Whether it is the homestead of an extended family or the office of a workplace family, it is a gathering place for the members that is special.

Ninth, members in affiliative relationships develop a sense of posterity and a connection with the past. This is the sense of time and history that expresses cohesive bonds. Pearsall (1990) observed ''family sensation'' demonstrated through a ''family extrasensory perception.''

Tenth, Howard (1978) observed, good biologic or achieved families honor their elders. She noted that there are more grandparents and elderly today as the life span is lengthened and noted the mutual support and special contributions they can make to younger generations.

These characteristics suggest several ways in which nurses can plan to use knowledge of affiliative relationships to enhance care. The communicator and prime mover can be identified and used as primary sources of information and communication. Family rituals can be ascertained and incorporated into care, particularly during lengthy rehabilitation. An institution-based ''hearth'' or gathering place can be provided to help the biologic or chosen family coalesce during crises.

GOALS OF AFFILIATIVE RELATIONSHIPS

Whether they are implicit or explicit, all affiliative relationships have goals. Goals of affiliative or family systems are broadly classified as biologic, psychologic, economic, social, and cultural (Friedman, 1998; Miller, 1980). The broad classification of goals is fundamental to understanding the specific goals established in an affiliative system at any point in time. Goals in affiliative systems are not static, nor are they established in isolation by the members of an affiliative system. The priority given to any of the broad scope of goals and the establishment of specific goals are influenced by a number of factors, including the developmental stage of the family or affiliative system, the environment, the resources available to the members, the societal needs and mores, and the specific circumstances and events in the lives of the members' system (Duvall & Miller, 1985; Friedman, 1998; Miller, 1980).

An example of the relationships among goals in affiliative systems is apparent in the childbearing family. The biologic goals of the family in this stage are focused on ensuring the birth and nurturance of healthy children. The biologic goals of members of affiliative systems in their middle years, however, might be adapting and coping with the physical changes accompanying middle age. Families in poverty need to place a higher priority on economic goals to provide basic necessities. An affluent family easily satisfying biologic goals can focus on psychologic and social goals. In the event of illness in a family member, this family can redirect its focus to biologic goals.

Goals and the priority assigned to them by individual members of an affiliative system are sometimes in conflict, thus causing disruption within the system. This can occur when adopted goals ignore the needs of one or more members. For example, a family of school-aged children continues to prioritize biologic goals at the expense of the social goals that accompany that developmental stage. Goals in affiliative relationships can conflict when individuals set different priorities for the goals. An example is a situation in which one member seeks psychologic and social goals through a lifestyle that diverts monetary resources to the point of interference with the economic goals of other members.

Members of affiliative systems need to take the needs of the individual members as well as those of the system as a whole into consideration when establishing and pursuing goals. Conflict and disruption arise when affiliative systems are unwilling or unable to negotiate and blend individual and system goals. The goals of affiliative systems as they develop and evolve over time, whether conscious or unconscious, serve to support the steady state of the system and set the tone for function and interaction within the system.

Human Needs Met Through Affiliative Relationships

A hierarchy of human needs was proposed by Maslow (1970), including physiologic needs, safety and security needs, love and belonging needs, self-esteem needs, and self-actualization needs. Marston and Chambers (1980), in their proposed eclectic framework for understanding family systems, built on Maslow's hierarchy. Three core human needs were identified in this framework. These core needs are viewed as behavioral motivators and include the concepts of existence, relatedness, and growth (Marston & Chambers, 1980). The Marston and Chambers conceptualization asserts that existence needs encompass material and physiologic needs; safety; security; stability; dependency; protection; freedom from fear, anxiety, and chaos; and a formal structure providing law, order, and limits. Relatedness needs in this framework include emotional gratification, personal happiness, companionship, and support, whereas growth needs include the need for personal growth and self-actualization (Marston & Chambers, 1980). Both the Maslow and the Marston and Chambers models suggest that individuals are free to pursue higher-level needs when more basic ones are satisfied. Marston and Chambers described three resource dimensions that are the domains within which core needs are met in family systems: time, the sequential and developmental dimension of the family life cycle; territory, the bounded and unbounded distance-regulating dimension in which family interaction takes place; and technology, the family's ability to use resources and energy to meet their needs.

Although individuals are enabled and supported in meeting the whole range of human needs in affiliative or family systems, some independent adults appear able to meet their existence and growth needs in relative isolation. We all can think of examples of people who seem to satisfy their needs, who are not living in affiliative relationships. However, shared residence is not necessarily a criterion for these all-important sustaining relationships. Affiliative relationships, whatever their form, seem to facilitate and enhance the satisfaction of basic human needs. The unique dimension that relatedness adds to the quality of human life suggests that, indeed, these aspects are significant motivators in establishing and maintaining affiliative relationships. A summary of the satisfactions and personal fulfillments attributed to family and affiliative relations in the literature underscores the importance ascribed to various relatedness needs by experts in the field. The list includes love and intimacy (Brain, 1976; Dyer, 1979; Friedman, 1998; Frude, 1991); personal happiness (Dyer, 1979; Frude, 1991); emotional gratification and support (Dyer, 1979; Friedman, 1998; Scanzoni, 1983; Spanier, 1981); complementarity and companionship (Dyer, 1979; Stuart, 1991); connectedness, continuity, commitment, and solidarity (Howard, 1978; Lindsey, 1981; Parsons, 1965; Scanzoni, 1983); and psychologic validation of identity (Brain, 1976). The importance of these aspects of affiliative relationships reflects the bonds that cement these relationships, even when more basic needs for existence are threatened. It is the fulfillment and enrichment of relatedness that enable affiliative systems to survive in the face of physical deprivation, illness, or even the death of one of the members.

ISSUES IN ASSESSING AFFILIATIVE SYSTEMS

The multiplicity of factors and variables having an impact on affiliative systems makes assessment of these relationships a complex task. Theoretical frameworks provide an organizing frame of reference that specifies those aspects that are relevant to a particular problem (Fawcett, 1989). The purpose of theoretical frameworks used to study the family is to guide observation and assessment for interpreting and understanding families and other types of affiliative relationships. Frameworks also provide a sound basis for theory development, research, and clinical intervention with families and affiliative systems (Doherty & McCubbin, 1985). Theoretical frameworks to study families are an attempt to produce order from the disorder of family life and to describe the commonalities of all families while recognizing the uniqueness and the individuality of each (Janosik & Green, 1992; Mercer, 1989).

The general systems theory that is used extensively to study the family is effective because it is applicable to individuals, to all forms of affiliative and family relationships, and to society. It views family in context, not separate from its physical, social, economic, geographic, and political environment. Other frameworks, although not as broad in scope because of the detail in which they examine various aspects of family life, also provide useful insight in assessing affiliative relationships. Various family frameworks developed to understand and explain the dynamics of family life differ from one another in the way they define the family and the factors and variables that influence family relationships. Different frameworks suggest different foci for analyzing and assessing the factors and variables operating in family systems. These frameworks are likewise applicable to other forms of affiliative relationships—specifically, chosen or achieved families. Because no single framework explains all the aspects of the dynamics of the family, nurses need to understand the major frameworks and elect aspects from each to guide their assessment of affiliative systems (Friedman, 1998; Frude, 1991; Janosik & Green, 1992; Marston & Chambers, 1980; Mercer, 1989). The following descriptions of the major theoretical approaches to studying the family provide an overview of their focus, assumptions, and implications for assessing affiliative relationships.

MAJOR THEORETICAL FRAMEWORKS

Social Exchange Framework

The social exchange framework is built on the work of Homans (1993). It maintains that interaction between persons is an exchange of material and nonmaterial goods, given and received in transactions that represent rewards and costs to the individuals in the relationship (Mercer, 1989; Nock, 1987). The social exchange framework is based on the following assumptions: (1) human behavior is rational and directed toward maximizing rewards and gains while limiting costs; (2) all behavior, no matter how rewarding, exacts some costs, even if limited only to the time and energy expended in the actual behavior; and (3) past rewards increase the expectation and likelihood of the behavior recurring in the future. Individuals presume reciprocity (i.e., rewards that are extended are expected to be returned in kind); the more of an asset an individual possesses, the less rewarding additional rewards of the same kind are perceived (Nock, 1987; LaRossa & Reitzos, 1993).

Assessment of family dynamics using the social exchange framework emphasizes the give and take operating in any relationship and tends to view family as a series of transactions supported by an atmosphere of quid pro quo.

It seems most appropriate to relationships between and among equals in which terms of the relationship and establishment of priorities incorporate the needs and expectations of the participants. Although this framework captures essential components of mutuality and transactions in relationships, it seems to fail to explain the deferred return, inequalities, and discrepancies in the exchange among intimates and family when there is a disproportionate amount of time, energy, and support given without reciprocation, or the apparent proximate promise of return as demonstrated in relationships with children, the seriously physically or developmentally challenged, and the seriously or terminally ill.

Structural-Functional Framework

The structural-functional approach to family analysis is also primarily a sociologic framework. In this approach, the family is viewed as a social system that functions to meet the basic needs of individuals and society. This framework supplants the institutional approach and examines the structure or makeup of the family at a given point in time (Dyer, 1979; Friedman,1998). It emphasizes the functions or operations needed to meet the individual needs of its members and those of society (Friedman, 1998). The major concepts of the structural-functional approach are based on the following assumptions: (1) certain functional requirements must be met for society to survive, (2) the family is one of the functional subsystems that meets these requirements, (3) the family as a social system has functional requirements that parallel those of society, and (4) the individual family is a small group possessing the basic characteristics of all small groups (Friedman, 1998; McIntyre, 1989).

Assessment in the structural-functional framework examines the various roles that individual family members fulfill. It focuses on the interaction and interdependence of family members seen as necessary for internal family and societal stability (Heffron & Wolff, 1984). The concepts of nuclear and extended family, the instrumental roles (economic and decision making), and the expressive roles (socioemotional function) are factors to be examined in the structural-functional framework (Friedman, 1998; Logan, 1978). The tendency to view adherence to "normal" family structure, function, and roles suggests to some critics that this approach tends to be static (Duffy, 1988; Heffron & Wolff, 1984).

Interactional Framework

The family is viewed in the interactional framework as a social group in which members interact in patterned ways (Dyer, 1979; Mercer, 1989). The interactional framework is a social-psychologic approach often called symbolic interaction (Schvanevelt, 1981). Symbolic interaction refers to socialization processes in which people act in response to individual and environmental events. Specific responses arise from the meaning ascribed to the events and reflect past experiences (Janosik & Green, 1992). The individual is viewed as both actor and observer, with the self-concept developing as a result of consensually validated relationships with significant and generalized others. The self-concept, therefore, enables the individual to choose roles that can be enacted with others, thus learning complementarity of roles. Because of its focus on roles, some writers call this approach role theory (Mercer, 1989; Schvanevelt, 1981). The assumptions on which the interactional framework is based include (1) human life is in a symbolic as well as a physical environment, (2) humans are stimulated by and stimulate others through symbols, (3) humans learn meanings to symbols through interaction with others, and (4) roles are guided and directed by the related meaning of clusters of symbols (Schvanevelt, 1981). Assessment from an interactional perspective focuses on the ways families relate as interacting personalities. Specific aspects included in the assessment are internal dynamics, family roles, status, decision making, communication, and coping patterns (Friedman, 1998). The interactional framework assesses the internal processes in families by observing overt behavior to which symbolic meaning is ascribed as family members enact complementary roles. The interactional approach has been criticized because it fails to take biologic, structural, and environmental factors into account (LaRossa & Reitzos, 1993).

Developmental Framework

The developmental approach to family analysis views the family as a unit of interacting personalities with a life cycle and related developmental tasks that evolve over time (Duvall & Miller, 1985). Duvall and Miller conceptualized an eight-stage life cycle of the family that parallels Erikson's (1963) developmental model. Developmental tasks emerge in each life-cycle stage from physical maturation, cultural pressures and expectations, and individual internal aspirations and values (Duvall & Miller, 1985; Friedman, 1998). The developmental framework is based on the assumption that the family is defined as a nuclear, conjugal unit. Success in accomplishing each developmental task is accompanied by a mastery that facilitates function in successive developmental levels. Tasks are goals, not jobs, and each family member has a unique age-role expectation in reciprocity with those of the other members of the family (Rowe, 1981). Critics have raised issue with the limitations imposed in guiding assessment based on the age of the oldest child because many families do not have offspring and even those who do vary greatly in the timing of the arrival of the firstborn as well as that of later children. Mercer (1989), however, asserts that the developmental approach does provide insight into needs, priorities, and values in families.

Doherty and McCubbin (1985) apply a life-cycle approach to proposing a six-phase "family health and illness" cycle. The family health and illness cycle is not dependent on childbearing or on the age of the individuals or the family. Instead, it follows the group through the sequence encountered in coping with actual or potential interferences with health and illnesses. The six phases include (1) family health promotion and risk reduction, (2) family vulnerability and illness onset, (3) family illness appraisal, (4) family acute response, (5) family's critical decision as to whether or not to enter the health care system and seek care, and (6) family adaptation.

Assessment in the developmental framework looks at the family in a chronologic perspective and examines the extent to which family function, roles, and tasks change over time (Janosik & Green, 1992; Mercer, 1989). It is concerned with the way family function and interaction patterns support the accomplishment of the appropriate life-cycle tasks.

GENERAL SYSTEMS THEORY AND ASSESSING AFFILIATIVE RELATIONSHIPS

Because no single family theoretical framework has been demonstrated to explain and describe all the relevant issues related to affiliative relationships, nurses in their practice tend to incorporate and integrate the different facets from existing conceptualizations in understanding affiliative relationships. The general systems theory provides a broad framework in which to view the open, living affiliative systems and to incorporate the diversity of related phenomena essential to the assessment of affiliative relationships. The general systems theory affords a structure for analyzing elements constituting social systems, including affiliative systems. The general systems theory was developed by Von Bertalanffy (1968) and gained wide acceptance as a framework for organizing and explaining relationships and interactions among elements or parts of a whole. Basic premises underlying the general systems theory include the following: (1) systems are viewed in the context of their environment and as part of a larger system; (2) systems need to be perceived as a whole and are more than and different from the sum of their parts; (3) systems and subsystems can achieve the same goals even when coming from different points and progressing in different ways; (4) anything that affects a part of a system reverberates throughout the system; and (5) causes and effects are interactive and interchangeable, not linear or singular. The general systems theory reflects an innovative way of looking at phenomena, in which attention is focused on multiple variables in dynamic interaction (Friedman, 1998; Frude, 1991; Mercer, 1989). The components of a system that are relevant in assessing affiliative systems include structure, boundaries, function, tension, processes, and equilibrium (Friedman, 1998; Frude, 1991; Heffron, 1984).

The structure of a system refers to the parts that compose the system as a whole and the organization and pattern of the relationship among those parts. Describing the structure of an affiliative system involves identifying the individuals involved and their relationships with each other. The boundary of the system is the perimeter separating it from suprasystems and other systems. The boundaries define who participates in the system. Boundaries may be rigid, with members of the affiliative system relating almost exclusively with each other. Conversely, an affiliative system may have loose boundaries, with relatively few emotional ties between members (Frude, 1991; Miller, 1980).

The function of a system refers to the processes required to achieve its apparent objectives. The function of an affiliative system is influenced by communication patterns, the environment, and available resources (Friedman, 1998; Kuhn & Janosik, 1980). Communication, a key element in the function of a social system, is categorized as affective and instrumental. Affective communication expresses the emotional aspects of relationships within the system, whereas information is exchanged through instrumental communication (Parsons & Bales, 1955). The environment encompasses the physical, social, and emotional conditions in which the system operates. It includes the proximate environment and extends to the social and cultural environment of the suprasystem of which it is a part (Friedman, 1998; Heffron, 1984). The resources available to the affiliative system are part of the environment. These resources are emotional, material, and social, and they influence the extent and ease with which the system achieves its goals.

TABLE 16–1 • FRAMEWORK FOR AFFILIATIVE RELATIONSHIP ASSESSMENT

Structure

Form	What is the form of the affiliative system? Who are the members who compose the system?
Cultural background	What is the cultural orientation of the affiliative system, and how does it relate to the predominant cultural environment of the suprasystem of which it is a part?
Developmental stage	What are the developmental stages of the individual members of the affiliative system, and how do they relate to and shape the developmental stage of the affiliative system?
Educational background	What is the educational background of the members, and how does it influence the affiliative system?

Boundaries

Environmental factors	What are the internal and external environments of the affiliative system, including the physical, social, political, and psychologic factors? To what extent and in what ways do the affiliative system and its members relate to the environment?

Function

Roles	What are the various roles of the members of the affiliative system, and how do these roles fulfill the needs of the individual members and those of the system? How are roles ascribed, achieved, evolved, and changed?
Rules	What are the implicit and explicit rules under which the affiliative system operates? How do they influence system function?

Tension Processes

Input and throughput	What are the communication and output and feedback interaction patterns within the affiliative system and between the system and its members and other systems and suprasystems? How do these patterns influence relationships and functions of the affiliative system?

Equilibrium

Goals	What are the explicit and implicit goals of the affiliative system and those of the individual members? What are the power issues in establishing goals and equilibrium? How do the goals express the values, existence, relatedness, and growth needs of the members?
Coping patterns	What are the coping patterns for dealing with the demands of everyday life as well as the crises that disrupt equilibrium?

Tension refers to the energy in the system that is needed to adjust to the demands of the environment. Input is the process by which energy, matter, and information are introduced into the system from the environment. Throughput is the process by which the energy is transformed and used. Feedback is the process by which the system monitors and regulates its response to internal and external stimuli.

Equilibrium is the dynamic steady state maintained by living systems. Family and affiliative systems maintain a steady state that reflects and supports the needs of the members. Factors and events, internal or external to the system, that threaten to disrupt the steady state are resisted by members of the system.

Assessment of affiliative relationships that uses the general systems theory encompasses evaluation of structure, boundaries, function, tension processes, and equilibrium. Specific factors that might be assessed are shown in Table 16–1.

This overview of the major theoretical frameworks used to study the family highlights the issues and concepts found to influence family relationships. Some of the family frameworks overlap and share concepts and hypotheses, yet each has its own focus and priority for explaining the way various factors influence families and their functions. They provide different dimensions for assessing affiliative relationships. Although some frameworks clearly limit their focus to biologic and legal family relationships, all deal with concepts applicable to all forms of affiliative relationships.

SUMMARY

Individuals meet their need for affiliation and relatedness in a variety of forms of relationships. Recognition of the importance and influence of these relationships in the lives of individuals is essential for assessing the needs of neurologic patients and clients in the context of their affiliative or family systems. A general systems approach provides a framework for assessing relationships and supports the integration of concepts and issues from the major theoretical family frameworks.

References

Brain, R. (1976). *Friends and lovers.* New York: Basic Books.

Christensen, B. J. (1992). The definition of the family should remain limited. In D. L. Bender & B. Leone (Eds.), *Family in America: Opposing viewpoints* (pp. 47–54). San Diego, CA: Greenhaven.

Doherty, W., & McCubbin, H. (1985). Families and healthcare: An emerging area of theory, research and clinical intervention. *Family Relationships, 34*(1), 5–11.

Duffy, M. E. (1988). Health promotion in the family: Current findings and directives for nursing research. *Journal of Advanced Nursing, 13,* 109–117.

Duvall, E. M., & Miller, B. C. (1985). *Marriage and family development* (6th ed.). Philadelphia: Lippincott.

Dyer, E. D. (1979). *The American family: Variety and change.* New York: McGraw-Hill.

Erikson, E. H. (1963). *Childhood and Society* (2nd ed.). NY: WW Norton & Co.

Fawcett, J. (1989). *Analysis and evaluation of conceptual models of nursing* (2nd ed.). Philadelphia: F.A. Davis.

Friedman, M. N. (1998). *Family nursing. Theory and practice* (4th ed.). Stamford, CT: Appleton & Lange.

Frude, N. (1991). *Understanding family problems.* New York: John Wiley & Sons.

Gilliss, C. L. (1989). Family research in nursing. In C. L. Gilliss, B. L. Highly, B. M. Roberts, & I. M. Martinson (Eds.), *Toward a science of family nursing* (pp. 37–63). Reading, MA: Addison-Wesley.

Gilliss, C. L., Highly, B. L., Roberts, B. M., & Martinson, I. M. (1989). What is family nursing? In C. L. Gilliss, B. L. Highly, B. M. Roberts, & I. M. Martinson (Eds.), *Toward a science of family nursing* (pp. 64–73). Reading, MA: Addison-Wesley.

Heffron, P. B. (1984). General systems and adaptation. In J. M. Flynn & P. B. Heffron (Eds.), *Nursing: From concept to practice* (p. 9). Jacksonville, FL: Brady.

Heffron, P. B., & Wolff, E. M. (1984). The family as a system. In J. M. Flynn & P. B. Heffron (Eds.), *Nursing: From concept to practice* (p. 593). Jacksonville, FL: Brady.

Homans, G. C. (1993). *Social behavior as exchange.* Manchester, NH: Irvington Publishers.

Howard, J. (1978). *Families.* New York: Simon & Schuster.

Janosik, E., & Green, E. (1992). *Family life: Process and practice.* Sudbury, MA: Jones & Bartlett.

Kane, C. F. (1988). Family social support: Toward a conceptual model. *Advances in Nursing Science, 10*(2), 18–25.

Kuhn, K., & Janosik, E. H. (1980). Establishment of a family system. In J. R. Miller & E. H. Janosik (Eds.), *Family focused care* (p. 147). New York: McGraw-Hill.

LaRossa, R. & Reitzos, D. C. (1993). Symbolic interaction and family studies. In P. G. Boss, W. J. Doherty, R. LaRossa, R. Schumm, & W. R. Steinmetz (Eds.). *Sourcebook of family theories and methods: A contextual approach.* New York: Plenum.

Lindsey, K. (1981). *Friends as family.* Boston: Beacon Press.

Logan, B. B. (1978). The nurse and the family: Dominant themes and perspectives in the literature. In K. A. Knafl & H. K. Grace (Eds.), *Families across the lifecycle: Studies in nursing* (p. 3). Boston: Little, Brown.

Marston, M. V., & Chambers, B. M. (1980). Development of family conceptual frameworks. In J. R. Miller & E. H. Janosik (Eds.), *Family-focused care* (p. 416). New York: McGraw-Hill.

Maslow, A. (1970). *Motivation and personality.* New York: Harper & Row.

McIntyre, J. (1989). The structural-functional approach to family study. In F. I. Nye & F. M. Bernado (Eds.), *Emerging conceptual frameworks in family analysis* (2nd ed., p. 52). Westport, CT: Praeger.

Mercer, R. T. (1989). Theoretical perspectives on the family. In C. L. Gilliss, B. L. Highly, B. M. Roberts, & I. M. Martinson (Eds.), *Toward a science of family nursing* (pp. 9–36). Reading, MA: Addison-Wesley.

Miller, J. R. (1980). The family as a system. In J. R. Miller & E. H. Janosik (Eds.), *Family-focused care* (p. 3). New York: McGraw-Hill.

Naisbitt, J. (1982). *Megatrends.* New York: Warner Books.

Nock, S. L. (1987). *Sociology and the family.* Paramus, NJ: Prentice-Hall.

Orthner, D. K. (1995). Families in transition: Changing values and norms. In R. D. Day, K. R. Gilbert, K. R. Settles, & W. R. Burr (Eds.). *Research and theory in family science* (pp. 3–19). Pacific Grove, CA: Brooks-Cole.

Parsons, T. (1965). The normal American family. In S. M. Farber, P. Mustacchi, & R. H. L. Wilson (Eds.), *Man and civilization: The family's search for survival* (p. 31). New York: McGraw-Hill.

Parsons, T., & Bales, R. (1955). *Family socialization and interaction.* New York: Free Press.

Pearsall, P. (1990). *Power of the family.* New York: Doubleday.

Rowe, G. P. (1981). The developmental conceptual framework to the study of the family. In F. I. Nye & F. M. Bernado (Eds.), *Emerging conceptual frameworks in family analyses* (2nd ed., p. 198). Westport, CT: Praeger.

Scanzoni, J. (1983). *Shaping tomorrow's family: Theory and policy for the 21st century.* Thousand Oaks, CA: Sage Publications.

Schvanevelt, J. D. (1981). The interactional framework in the study of the family. In F. I. Nye & F. M. Bernado (Eds.), *Emerging conceptual frameworks* (2nd ed., p. 97). Westport, CT: Praeger.

Skolnik, A. (1991). *Embattled paradise. The American family in an age of uncertainty.* New York: Basic Books.

Spanier, G. B. (1981). The changing profile of the American family. *Journal of Family Practice, 13*(1), 61.

Staples, R. (1989). Family life in the 21st century: An analysis of the old forms, current trends and future scenarios. In C. L. Gilliss, B. L. Highly, B. M. Roberts, & I. M. Martinson (Eds.), *Toward a science of family nursing.* Reading, MA: Addison-Wesley.

Stein, P. J. (1977). Singlehood: An alternative to marriage. In P. J. Stein, J. Richman, & N. Hannon (Eds.), *The family: Functions, conflicts and symbols* (pp. 382–395). Reading, MA: Addison-Wesley.

Stuart, M. E. (1991). An analysis of the concept of family. In A. L. Whall & J. Fawcett (Eds.), *Family theory and development in nursing: State of the science and art* (pp. 31–42). Philadelphia: F.A. Davis.

Von Bertalanffy, L. (1968). General systems theory. A critical review. In W. Buckley (Ed.), *Research for the behavioral scientist* (pp. 11–30). Uvalde, TX: Aldine.

Whall, A. L., & Fawcett, J. (1991). The family as a focal phenomena in nursing. In A. L. Whall & J. Faucett (Eds.), *Family theory and development in nursing: State of the science and art* (pp. 7–29). Philadelphia: F.A. Davis.

Wilson, N. R., & Trost, R. (1978). A family perspective on aging and health. *Health Values, 2*(2), 52–57.

Alterations in Affiliative Relationships

CATHERINE ECOCK CONNELLY

ALTERATIONS IN AFFILIATIVE RELATIONSHIPS

Affiliative relationships are conceptualized in this textbook as social systems composed of significant, patterned, meaningful relationships characterized by emotional commitment, intimacy, stability, and continuity. The previous chapter described new forms of affiliative relationships in our society that reflect evolving demographic patterns and changing social mores that lead to new ways for individuals to satisfy their deep human needs for closeness and relatedness. This view contends that the deeply personal aspects and needs satisfied by relationships, not their biologic or legal foundations, are the significant aspects of affiliative relationships. This approach implies an expanded conceptualization of family-centered care that focuses on individuals in the context of their significant personal relationships and recognizes families or affiliative systems based on the meaning of these relationships to the individuals involved. The terms *family* and *affiliative system* are used interchangeably in this chapter to describe these significant relationships.

This expanded conceptualization of family is not without its critics. Serious concerns are raised by individuals and groups about the expanded definition of family, calling for a return to a traditional definition of family (Christensen, 1992). The opponents of eclectic definitions of family assert that expanding the definition of the family devalues the concept of family and weakens or abandons traditional ethical, cultural, social, and political mores. Regardless of the controversy surrounding the acceptability of different lifestyles, neuroscience nurses need to support their patients' choices and facilitate meeting their deeply personal human needs rather than judge the appropriateness or acceptability of clients' and families' relationships. Whatever the nurses' personal values, the importance of significant relationships and their influence on the health and well-being of patients underscores the need for nurses to support patients' and families' choices and lifestyles. Family involvement in planning and implementing care has been demonstrated to enhance both its effectiveness and patient and family satisfaction (Gillis, Roberts, Highly, & Martinson, 1989).

This chapter examines the impact of biologic, technological, social, cultural, economic, and political trends on patients, family systems, and neuroscience nursing and analyzes the psychosocial variables that influence patients' and families' adaptations to alterations resulting from neurologic phenomena. Finally, an exploration of specific examples that illustrate the impact of alterations in affiliative systems on the lives of individuals and their loved ones demonstrates the potential of neuroscience nurses to enhance the quality of life of their patients and their families.

RESHAPING HEALTH CARE

Change in our society is pervasive, or, as Naisbitt and Aburdine (1990) asserted, amount and rate of "change" in our society make it a major variable influencing American life. Not only are individual relationships and affiliative systems in transition, but the entire health care system is undergoing revolutionary transformation, requiring a new organization of nursing practice that has important implications for nursing care for patients and families experiencing neurologic dysfunction. Hickey (1993) described the biomedical and technological, demographic, economic, and social changes that are shaping the current and future health care system in the United States. Great advances in the approaches to and efficacy of new treatments and medications, made possible by an increasingly complex technological system, have improved the practice of neuroscience nursing and medicine dramatically. Patients are not only surviving but are improving and recovering from trauma, illness, and malignancy that would have been hopeless in the past. The technological, biomedical, and pharmacologic armaments available to treat and cope with neurologic dysfunction offer hope and effective therapeutic options to sustain and enhance quality of life for patients and their families. However, these developments are accompanied by escalating costs and bring ethical and legal issues to the fore in health care decisions.

The demographic composition of the population is changing, with increased longevity resulting in a larger percentage of older persons combined with a growing number of individuals and families from other cultures whose languages and customs are diverse. As noted in the previous chapter, patterns of marriage, parenting, and living arrangements are quite varied. The growth in the number and proportion of older Americans is accompanied by a rise in the incidence of certain neurologic problems and diagnoses such as stroke, Alzheimer's disease, and Parkinson's disease.

A combination of sophisticated, technical treatment modalities and growing numbers of Americans experiencing health problems exacerbated or precipitated by age has contributed to skyrocketing health care costs. These factors have augmented sharp increases in health care expenditures and an even sharper rise in the percentage of health care spending in the gross national product. Moreover, a number of unemployed Americans are underinsured or lack access to health care. To avert even greater economic woes, cost containment of health care is essential. Diagnosis-related groups, early discharges, ambulatory treatments and surgery, and home care are strategies that reflect an attempt to reduce health care costs. These and other types of community-based care emphasize the need for neuroscience nursing in an affiliative context.

PARADIGM SHIFT TO CHRONIC CARE

Health care systems are forced, because of biomedical advances and demographic changes, to provide services to an increasing number of chronically ill patients. This increase calls for a paradigm shift in neuroscience nursing, incorporating community, collaborative, and multidisciplinary approaches (Hickey, 1993). Caring for the chronically ill patient requires adaptation to the characteristics of care in chronic illness that changes the emphasis and role of the provider from actually performing interventions to educating, facilitating, and enabling patients and families to be the actual providers of care (Connelly, 1993). Supervision and reinforcement by health care providers and treatment guidelines in chronic illness are often intermittent and sporadic, while the day-to-day support and decision making fall, for the most part, on the patients and their families. Home care punctuated by intervals of treatment in traditional health care settings typifies the evolving model of care in chronic illness (Corbin & Strauss, 1988). Hickey (1993) observed that reliance on significant others for assistance and support by neurologic patients in the community sometimes creates ethical-legal dilemmas when family and affiliative systems are unable or unwilling or become overburdened by demands. Community care definitely underscores the need to be sensitive to and to understand cultural beliefs and systems of patients and families.

HUMAN RESPONSES TO ALTERED AFFILIATIVE RELATIONSHIPS

An accident or a diagnosis of neurologic trauma, illness, or alteration is a major blow to individuals and their families because of its actual or potential interference in their lives. Neurologic alterations are often accompanied by physical and behavioral manifestations and limitations that change the structure and function of the family system. Patients coping with altered ability to fill previous roles may become dependent on significant others for assistance and care, sometimes with even very basic physical needs. Family members who provide support can become exhausted, isolated, weary, and overburdened.

Certain symptoms and sequelae of neurologic alterations can be isolating and embarrassing and can cause stigma for patients and families. Physical, emotional, psychologic, and economic demands drain and divert resources from other family members who may become depleted and overcome. Decisions and choices between and among conflicting needs and requirements of family members are difficult and painful. Sustaining family systems through extended chronic illness and disability drains individuals and the system, sometimes precipitating disruption and disorganization of the family system.

ASSESSMENT OF ALTERATIONS IN AFFILIATIVE SYSTEMS

General Systems Theory

The general systems theory developed by Von Bertalanffy (1968) provides a framework to examine issues and factors that influence and affect family systems' responses to neurologic alterations (presented in Table 16–1 in the previous chapter). Key concepts derived from the general systems theory that are particularly relevant to affiliative systems include open systems (i.e., systems characterized by interaction and interchange with the surrounding environment (Friedman, 1992). Nonsummativity or wholeness implies that a family is different from a collection of individuals and must be considered more than the sum of the parts.

Friedman (1992) used the term *ripple effect* to describe the phenomenon whereby a family system is so intricately connected that an event that affects part of the system reverberates throughout the system. The hierarchy of systems reflects the ranking and relationships among various levels of systems in which the family participates (e.g., neighborhood, community, health care system, educational system). The general systems theory replaces linear causality with the idea that units and variables are interactive, interchangeable, and multivariate (Friedman, 1992). Essentially, a general systems approach to affiliative systems suggests that discrete parts, such as an individual or an event, are viewed in the context of the system, and simple cause-and-effect explanations fail to incorporate the complexity of interactions that influence outcomes.

Family Stress Theory

Hill (1949) developed the ABC model of family stress to describe the factors that influence whether or not a particular event produces a crisis in families. The model is based on the assumption that what may precipitate a crisis for one family does not necessarily precipitate a crisis for another. According to Hill's theory, based on observations of families reunited after World War II, A represents the stressor, B refers to family resources, and C stands for the meaning attributed to the event. Hill's conceptualization differentiated *stressor*, an external event that impinges on the family system, from *stress*, defined as the internal, subjective meaning assigned to the event. Factor X indicated crisis or noncrisis.

McCubbin and Patterson (1982) expanded Hill's early conceptualization of family adaptation to ongoing stress by developing what they called the double ABCX model. The double ABCX model accounts for the multiplicity of interacting situations, events, and stressors, internal as well as external in origin, that continually require adaptation and coping by family members. The double ABCX Model depicted in Figure 17–1 asserts a continuum of outcomes, from "bonadaptation," or healthy response, to maladaptation that results from interacting and balancing capabilities, resources, stressors, and demands over time. Boss (1988) added two concentric circles representing external and internal contexts to the model to reflect the impact of environmental factors. External contextual factors were categorized by Boss (1988) as heredity, developmental factors, economic factors, family history, and culture. Internal variables included structural aspects, psychologic characteristics, and philosophical considerations.

McCubbin and Patterson (1982) described what they termed *pileup,* or the accumulation of a series of situational and developmental demands that deplete family coping resources. According to McCubbin and Patterson, aA represents the accumulation of stressors that affect the family system. These include initial stress and hardships, normative transitions, prior strains, consequences of previous efforts to cope, and ambiguity in intrafamily and society communication. Adaptive resources of individual members as well as shared internal family resources are called bB. This also includes family efforts to activate, employ, and develop new coping mechanisms. Family definitions of events and their meanings are referred to as cC. Factor cC exemplifies the evolution and modification by the family of their perceptions of the total situation and the meaning of stressors. The postcrisis adaptation is denoted xX (McCubbin & Patterson, 1982).

The double ABCX model endorses Lazarus and Folkman's (1984) concept of the importance of cognitive appraisal of events or situations and the extent

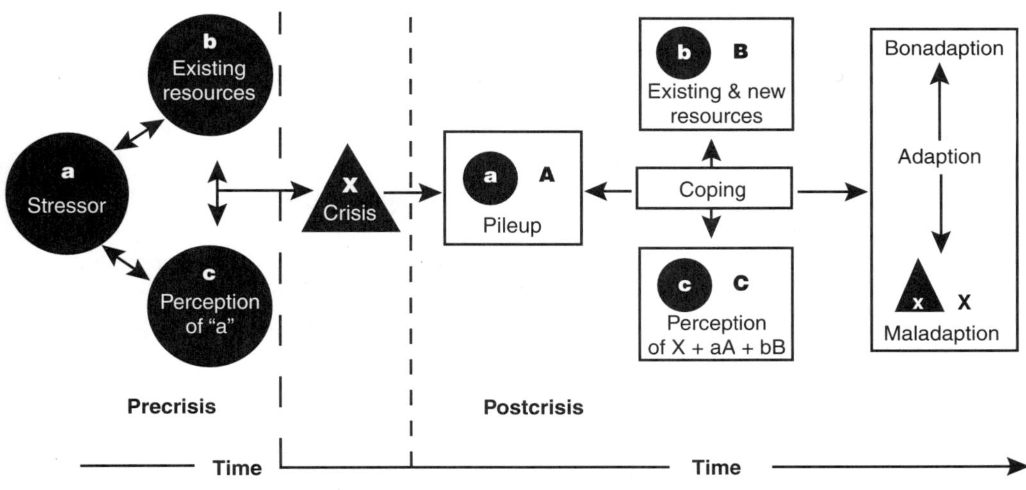

FIGURE 17–1 • Double ABCX model.

to which they are perceived as stressful. The model emphasizes how the idiosyncratic meaning individuals assign to an event determines its impact as a stressor. Boss (1988) described family distortion of events that interfered with perceptual accuracy and adaptation, citing as an example a family that denied alcohol abuse by a member and attributed deviant, aberrant behavior to physical illness.

Family Coping

Family coping includes all the processes and interactions that enable families to fulfill their functions and meet their individual goals (Friedman, 1992). Affiliative systems deal or cope with day-to-day and special events with patterned or habitual responses reflecting their experiences, strengths, and resources. Affiliative systems develop a repertoire of consensually validated and accepted ways of coping that have supported system goals and adaptation in the past.

A major traumatic event or the cumulative effect of stressors on the system may hurl a family system into crisis. Crisis is defined as a situation in which a system's usual ways of coping and adapting become overwhelmed or ineffective in the face of amount or severity of demands on the system. Boss (1988) differentiated family stress from crisis by pointing out that stress is a change in equilibrium and may even be sought, such as a vacation, whereas crisis stems from overwhelming stress in which the family seems immobilized until new coping mechanisms are developed. Crises can stem from developmental or maturational forces such as adolescence or may be precipitated by a specific situation such as an illness or accident. The key issue in the development of crisis is that the system becomes bogged down and unable to adapt.

A single event can be sufficiently traumatic that an affiliative system's coping mechanisms are ineffective. Nurses in the intensive care unit and emergency department all too often see families facing the crisis of death or serious disability of a family member.

Family crises are often precipitated by the interaction of several events that the family may be able to deal with individually but that, when combined, deplete system resources. A common example seen by today's families is coping with and supporting elderly parents or grandparents while simultaneously nurturing a growing, developing family. The "sandwich generation" parents who are expected to provide for the developmental and situational crises of family members across the life cycle reflect affiliative systems actually or potentially in crisis. Nurses working with families in which a member has a chronic neurologic illness often see energy resources and coping ebb and flow as various issues, events, and situations affect family function. Some families appear to move in and out of crises frequently, whereas others are observed to withstand an amazing amount of change and events and continue to cope.

A key issue in the concept of crisis is that usual coping behaviors are not effective and new ways of handling the situation and the accompanying anxiety are attempted. To reduce what often feels like excruciating anxiety, novel approaches are tested. The discomfort and pain that characterize crisis enable individuals and family systems to be open to interventions that offer relief, thus presenting nurses with opportunities to intervene to promote healthy coping strategies. Families that are able to be flexible in roles or to seek external support reflect positive crisis management (Friedemann, 1989).

Conversely, there is an element of risk because some families may embrace maladaptive modes of coping such as blaming or scapegoating. Others become demoralized when their usual coping seems to fail and appears to splinter, and they become unavailable to support an ill or disabled member. Crisis is a critical time when affiliative systems are open to suggestion and intervention to alleviate anxiety and pain. Neuroscience nurses need to be sensitive to the effectiveness of various coping strategies and ready to intervene to promote healthy coping and prevent negative patterns from developing.

FAMILY CARE

Gillis, Roberts, et al. (1989) summarized characteristic features of family care in nursing. First, family care is concerned with the experience of the family over time, it recognizes family history, and it anticipates the family's future. Second, family nursing considers the cultural context and community of the family and seeks to facilitate the interaction between the family and the community, encouraging families to rely on community resources as well as contribute to its community. Third, family care acknowledges the interrelatedness of individuals within the family system and recognizes differences in levels of wellness and adaptation of various members over time. Fourth, family care deals with family systems in illness and health and assumes that the degree of illness or health of individual family members is not a measure of overall family health.

Fifth, although family nursing care is often provided in settings where the focus is on physical and psychologic health problems, nurses offer family care in the context of the interaction of health problems of all members of the family group. Sixth, family nursing recognizes that change in the health status of any member reverberates throughout the family system, influencing each of the members. Seventh, family nursing suggests enabling and facilitating interaction among family members. Eighth, family care recognizes that the individual who seems to need the most attention changes over time as family health and illness responses vary in the course of care. Ninth, family nursing builds on the assets and strengths of the individual members and promotes the mutual solidarity and strength of the family unit.

Locus of Care

Patients experiencing neurologic alterations receive care in acute care hospital settings, in rehabilitation and long-term care settings, and in their communities and homes. The variations for providing care to patients coping with neurologic alterations reflect advances in science and technology that enable effective interventions in hospital or community settings or a combination of both. Leavitt (1989) described a trend in which patients with chronic illness are hospitalized episodically, often when family resources for care become depleted.

Interventions with Affiliative Systems in Acute Care Settings

The multiple needs and stressors of individuals and families whose significant others are critically ill has demonstrated the complexity and diversity of responses. Lynn-McHale and Smith (1991) conducted a comprehensive assessment of families of the critically ill. Citing the stress precipitated by uncertainty about their loved one's condition and prognosis, Lynn-McHale and Smith found that families were distressed about a wide range of anxieties and uncertainties. Families' concerns included potential role changes, isolation and loneliness, loss of the family member, failure to meet their own basic physical needs, financial worry, and transportation difficulties. Families can potentially contribute valuable support in care of the critically ill, yet Lynn-McHale and Smith (1991) acknowledged the risk of families' becoming overpowered and developing dysfunctional coping strategies in the face of critical of life-threatening illness of one of their members.

Lynn-McHale and Smith (1991) categorized areas for assessing families' needs when a loved one is critically ill. First is the need for accurate, timely information about the patient's condition and what is currently happening as well as what is anticipated or planned. Second, significant others need to have the opportunity to visit their critically ill loved one and be supported during visits. Knowing what to expect and when they can see a loved one is crucial to families and facilitates their support for the patient. An important consideration in acknowledging the importance of different forms of relationships to people is that rules limiting visits to biologically or legally defined categories may in fact deny a patient access to the individuals who are most meaningful to his or her psychologic well-being.

Another area to which nurses need to be sensitive is the psychologic impact of the situation, events, and circumstances surrounding the crisis and the patient's condition. Families often need areas for privacy for communication, expression of feelings, and reflection. Families, according to Lynn-McHale and Smith (1991) need to be informed and supported in ways that enable them to keep their hope alive.

Moreover, families need to be informed about and have access to institutional support services, such as social services, chaplains, and financial consultation, that are available. The basic physical needs of significant others when maintaining a vigil for a critically ill family member include places to obtain food, restrooms, and lounges. Attention to environmental factors, especially providing comfortable chairs that offer rest to anxious family members during long, painful vigils, is important.

Interventions with Affiliative Systems in the Home

Home care for patients experiencing neurologic alterations continues to reflect social, cultural, policy, and economic trends. Reliance on technologies such as ventilators and intravenous medications is no longer seen as an adequate reason for hospitalization. Provision of acute and chronic care in the home requires additional support for family members who are called on to actually implement and monitor highly sophisticated interventions. The need for effective patient and family education and mastery of technical aspects of care is essential. Supporting and facilitating patients and families to render and sustain the level of care required by complex regimens are increasing responsibilities for neuroscience nurses. Problems of noncompliance, resulting from overburdened and exhausted family resources, interfere with a family's ability to persevere with costly, time-consuming treatments in the home and are major concerns for families and health care providers.

The difficulties encountered by family caretakers of patients with Alzheimer's disease exemplify some of the challenges faced by families and the nurses who provide support for them. Wilson (1989) used a grounded theory methodology to explore and describe the experiences of caretakers of patients with Alzheimer's disease. Family care providers, often elderly spouses, described three stages of "surviving the brink." Initially, families portrayed a self-dialogue accompanied by attempts to seek support and unburden in what Wilson termed "taking it on." Next, caregivers recounted "going through it"; in the face of the increasing demands and the loved one's deterioration from the illness, they tried to attend to the family member's needs and allocate, protect, and stretch resources. Finally, caregivers described "turning it over," when they realized they could no longer continue to keep their loved one at home. One respondent's comment, "Instead of asking about the patient, nurses and physicians should ask how the caregiver is doing," poignantly captures the depth of distress experienced by families coping with chronic neurologic alteration at home (Wilson, 1989).

Long-Term Care Settings

Patients with neurologic alterations often receive extended treatment, rehabilitation, or prolonged care in long-term care facilities. These settings, while offering the specialized services needed for various types of interventions, often create barriers and restrictions for relationships, intimacy, and communication among members in affiliative systems. Long-term care settings are often a distance from the community in which the patients and family reside, thus accentuating all the problems experienced by families supporting a loved one in an acute care setting, but doing so over a protracted period of time. Issues related to separation, need to maintain normal family processes, and demands while attempting to extend support to the patient sometimes burden families to the point of disruption or abandonment of the patient. Sustaining a loved one through a long and trying rehabilitation can severely strain or devastate a family system's coping.

Buckwalter, Cusack, Kruckeberg, and Shoemaker (1991) tested a collaborative speech–nursing family intervention among communication-impaired residents in a long-term care facility. The authors described neglect of the creative potential for family contribution to adaptation. Deterioration of family and staff relationships results when families are perceived as interfering and respond by relinquishing care to staff. The study compared outcomes of an intervention aimed at replacing competition with collaboration with outcomes of the usual staff-oriented communication training program. Although the results did not support the efficacy of the collaborative program for improving progress related to speech, participating family members expressed significantly increased satisfaction with the care their loved ones received, thought they would be more willing to have the patient return home, and expressed positive perceptions of staff concerns for the patients (Buckwalter et al., 1991).

• C A S E   S T U D Y   1

Mrs. P is a 49-year-old woman admitted through the emergency department, suffering a stroke. She awakened during the night and experienced seizures, confusion, right-sided weakness, and impaired verbal communication. Magnetic resonance angiography indicated an obstruction of the left common carotid artery.

Mrs. P experienced severe headaches during the week immediately before the stroke but attributed the headaches to tension and stress and did not seek medical attention. Mrs. P, who had been in apparent good health before this episode, is perimenopausal, has no history of hypertension, does not smoke, and rarely uses alcohol. Mrs. P, who is employed full-time as an elementary school teacher, is accompanied by her husband, also 49 years old, who is a police officer in the mid-sized city where they live and work. Also in the home are the couple's two children, a daughter, 14 years, and son, 12 years. Mrs. P's 19-year-old son by a previous marriage lives in the dormitory of the state college 100 miles from the home. Mrs. P's 73-year-old widowed mother, who has chronic obstructive pulmonary disorder, and depends on the family for assistance with activities of daily living and financial support, also lives with the family.

There are seven nursing diagnoses that describe the alterations in the affiliative relationships and the related human responses Mrs. P and her family experienced as a result of the diagnosis of stroke and subsequent treatment and rehabilitation.

Nursing Diagnoses for the Patient

ANXIETY RELATED TO UNCERTAIN PROGNOSIS, ALTERED ROLE PERFORMANCE, IMPAIRED PHYSICAL MOBILITY, AND IMPAIRED VERBAL COMMUNICATION

Mrs. P's nursing diagnoses reflected the uncertainty that the stroke created for her current responsibilities and lifestyle as well as for her future and her family's future. *Anxiety* is a state of mental discomfort or uneasiness related to threat (Murray, Pinnell, Leonard, & Zentner, 1985). Before dealing with the other nursing diagnoses, it was essential to enable Mrs. P to cope with the anxiety and uncertainty of her prognosis. Outcomes for Mrs. P include minimizing restlessness, apprehension, feelings of tension, and uneasiness and increasing her ability to focus and communicate with members of her family and the health care team.

Defining characteristics of the anxiety include uneasiness, vague fears, and feelings of impending doom that appear to be a direct response to the physiologic and personal crisis precipitated by the stroke. Table 17–1 lists the activities included in the nursing intervention for anxiety reduction (McCloskey & Bulechek, 1992). Outcomes of anxiety reduction intervention for Mrs. P include ability to accurately understand and verbalize her health status, evaluate her treatment options, and describe her feelings and concerns for herself and her family. Also, the abilities to relax, rest, and concentrate are important outcomes from anxiety reduction interventions.

Defining characteristics of the nursing diagnoses related to Altered Role Performance, Impaired Physical Mobility, and Impaired Verbal Communication include expressions of anxiety, tension, apathy, depression, or withdrawal. Mrs. P's attempts at verbal expression and use of her weak right arm and leg trigger reactions of frustration when these efforts are difficult and ineffective. The effect appears to intensify her fears about her future ability to resume her family, social, and occupational roles. Mrs. P's perseverance in her attempts to communicate verbally and ambulate with assistance further define and influence these nursing diagnoses and selection of interventions.

Communication Enhancement and Counseling are two nursing interventions that will enable Mrs. P to cope with anxiety, continuing uncertainty, and tension during her rehabilitation (McCloskey & Bulechek, 1992). Communication Enhancement facilitates interaction with a patient who has difficulty delivering and receiving communication. Counseling is defined as an interactive helping process focused on the patient's needs and concerns to facilitate coping, problem solving, and interpersonal relationships (McCloskey & Bulechek, 1992). Tables 17–2 and 17–3 detail nursing activities for executing the nursing interventions Communication Enhancement and Counseling.

Outcomes of Communication Enhancement include the ability to express needs, feelings, and thoughts and to participate in interaction with others. Anxiety reduction, reinforcement of speech therapy, and encouragement to the

TABLE 17–1 • DEFINING ACTIVITIES FOR NURSING INTERVENTION: ANXIETY REDUCTION

Use a calm, reassuring approach.
Explain all procedures in advance.
Reduce extraneous environmental stimuli.
Seek patient's perceptions of situation.
Provide factual information re: diagnosis, treatment, prognosis.
Encourage verbalization of fears, concerns, and feelings.
Encourage family visits.
Express empathy and concern for patient.
Provide back rub.

From McCloskey, J.C., & Bulechek, G.M. (1992). *Nursing interventions classification (NIC)*. St. Louis: Mosby–Year Book.

TABLE 17–2 • DEFINING ACTIVITIES FOR NURSING INTERVENTION: COUNSELING

Establish therapeutic relationship.
Demonstrate empathy, concern, and care.
Establish goals and time limits.
Use technique of reflection and clarification to facilitate expression of feelings.
Provide privacy, and ensure confidentiality.
Assist patient to define problems and related factors.
Assist patient to prioritize options and alternatives.
Assist patient to identify strengths, and reinforce these.
Determine how family behaviors influence patient.

From McCloskey, J.C., & Bulechek, G.M. (1992). *Nursing interventions classification (NIC).* St. Louis: Mosby–Year Book.

patient and the family in combination with appropriate medical therapy interact to enable improvement in Mrs. P's ability to send and understand verbal communication. Outcomes of the counseling include Mrs. P's ability to develop an accurate appraisal of her health status, collaborate with members of the health team in establishing goals, and participate in planning for and compliance with rehabilitation including physical, occupational, and speech therapy. Additional and no less important outcomes include Mrs. P's ability to cope and deal with her own and her family's emotional responses to her illness and its sequelae and implications to all of them.

Nursing Diagnoses for the Family

INEFFECTIVE FAMILY COPING, ALTERED FAMILY PROCESSES, AND ALTERED PARENTING

Defining characteristics of Ineffective Family Coping include expressions of anxiety, fear, and confusion and expressions of conflict among Mrs. P's three

TABLE 17–3 • DEFINING ACTIVITIES FOR NURSING INTERVENTION: CRISIS INTERVENTION

Provide supportive atmosphere.
Encourage nonthreatening expression of feelings.
Assist in defining the parameters of the family crisis.
Support discussion of family dynamics and coping patterns.
Facilitate identification of strengths and resources.
Facilitate information gathering and problem solving.
Provide opportunities for expressing and coping with feelings.
Encourage development of goals, plans, and course of action.
Provide information on resources and support services.
Reinforce positive coping mechanism.

From McCloskey, J.C., & Bulechek, G.M. (1992). *Nursing interventions classification (NIC).* St. Louis: Mosby–Year Book.

children. Additional components include the problem of who will provide care and support to Mrs. P's dependent, elderly mother. Mr. P expressed concerns about the financial impact of Mrs. P's potential income loss on her health care costs and the ongoing financial needs of the entire family.

Crisis intervention is the appropriate immediate nursing intervention (Bulechek & McCloskey, 1992). Crisis intervention is the systematic application of problem-solving strategies to resolve the immediate psychologic turmoil and return the family to at least the precrisis level of functioning. Timely support for the individuals experiencing the emotional trauma is essential to enabling the outcomes of active adaptation and coping (Kus, 1992; Murray, Luetje, & Zentner, 1985). Outcomes of effective family crisis intervention include development of novel, effective coping strategies and return to the precrisis level of functioning. Additional behavioral indicators of effective intervention include clear, open communication among family members, respect for expression of feelings and concerns of each member, reduction in interpersonal tension, and expression of solidarity and mutual support.

Defining characteristics of Altered Family Processes and Altered Parenting include confusion among family members about who will assume the multifaceted roles Mrs. P performed in the family, including care for her dependent mother; supervision of the adolescent children while Mr. P works weekend, evening, and night shifts; and organization and implementation of general housekeeping including shopping, food preparation, cleaning, and doing laundry. The interpersonal conflict among the children and the confusion among the children, grandmother, and father emphasized the loss of Mrs. P's role in running the household and facilitating effective communication among family members.

Self-help and peer support groups are demonstrated to be effective vehicles to enable individuals and families to cope and develop strategies to manage problems and ongoing concerns resulting from developmental or situational crises or health or other problems (Table 17–4). Support groups reinforce feel-

---

TABLE 17–4 • DEFINING ACTIVITIES FOR NURSING INTERVENTION: FAMILY SUPPORT GROUP

Assess family's perceptions of and reactions to the situation.
Foster realistic hope.
Encourage expression of feelings, concerns, and questions.
Promote respect and trust among members.
Identify other sources of family support.
Orient family members to health care system and settings.
Provide information on patient's situation and options.
Promote family communication and decision making.
Foster family assertiveness.
Provide accurate feedback on family coping activities.
Promote sharing of experiences and successes.
Promote group cohesiveness.

From McCloskey, J.C., & Bulechek, G.M. (1992). *Nursing interventions classification (NIC)*. St. Louis: Mosby–Year Book.

ings of self-worth, provide emotional support and opportunities for expression of feelings and concerns, reduce isolation and feelings of loneliness in facing problems and challenges, and enable sharing of information and experiences among people with the same challenge or problem. Underlying the supportive dynamics are reinforcement of self-esteem and self-determination when patients and families acknowledge that they are coping as well as they can and are not alone in experiencing anxieties, fears, and even negative feelings. Key elements in the effectiveness of support groups are emotional support, group solidarity, and exchange of practical solutions to day-to-day problems encountered in coping with short-and long-term rehabilitation while maintaining and sustaining family cohesiveness and solidarity.

Outcomes of the ongoing family support group include adaptation and flexibility in negotiating effective family, social, and professional and occupational relationships; group problem solving; and the ability of the family to accept differences between and among members.

SUMMARY

Alterations in affiliative relationships resulting from or accompanying neurologic dysfunctions or disorders require nurses to incorporate and assimilate factors and variables related to the affiliative system and its members, the community of which it is a part, and the health care system. A general systems approach moves beyond simple linear causality, recognizes the interaction and interdependency of the hierarchy and of the systems of which it is a part, and guides assessment and interventions to promote the health and optimal function of the affiliative systems. Individuals grow and flourish in the context of the deeply personal affiliative systems of which they are a part that enable them to meet their needs for security, connectedness, and belonging. Nurses, recognizing the importance of these relationships in the lives of their patients and their families, provide care in the context of the family system.

References

Boss, P. (1988). *Family stress management*. Thousand Oaks, CA: Sage.

Buckwalter, K.C., Cusack, D. Kruckeberg, T., & Shoemaker, A. (1991). Family involvement with communication impaired residents in longterm care settings. *Applied Nursing Research, 14(2),* 77–84.

Bulechek, G.M., & McCloskey, J.C. (1992). Future directions. In G.M. Bulechek & J.C. McCloskey (Eds.), *Nursing interventions; Essential nursing treatments* (2nd ed., pp. 602–609). Philadelphia: W.B. Saunders.

Burr, W. (1973). *Theory construction and the sociology of the family*. New York: John Wiley & Sons.

Caplan, G. (1964). *Principles of preventative psychiatry*. New York: Basic Books.

Christensen, B.J. (1992). The definition of the family should remain limited. In D.L. Bender & B. Leone (Eds.), *Family in America: Opposing viewpoints* (pp. 47–54). San Diego, CA: Greenhaven Press.

Connelly, C.E. (1993). An empirical study of a model of self-care in chronic illness. *Clinical Nurse Specialist, 7(5),* 247–253.

Corbin, J.M., & Strauss, A. (1988). *Unending work and care: Managing chronic illness at home.* San Francisco, CA: Jossey-Brown.

Friedemann, M.L. (1989). Closing the gap between grand theory and mental health practice with families. Part 1: The framework of systemic organization for nursing of families and family members. *Archives of Psychiatric Nursing 3*(1), 10–19.

Friedman, M.M. (1992). *Family nursing: Theory and practice* (3rd ed.). New York: Appleton-Lange.

Gillis, C.L., Roberts, B.M., Highly, B.L., & Martinson, I.M. (1989). What is family nursing? In *Toward a science of family nursing* (pp. 64–73). Reading, MA: Addison-Wesley.

Gillis, C.L., Rose, D.B., Hallburg, J.C., & Martinson, I.M. (1989). The family and chronic illness. In C.L. Gillis, B.M. Roberts, B.L. Highly, & I.M. Martinson (Eds.), *Toward a science of family nursing* (pp. 287–299). Reading, MA: Addison-Wesley.

Hickey, J.V. (1993). The changing health care system: Neuroscience nursing practice in the 1990's. *Journal of Neuroscience Nursing, 25*(2), 73–77.

Hill, R. (1949). *Families under stress.* New York: Harper & Row.

Kus, R.J. (1992). Crisis intervention. In G.M. Bulechek & J.C. McCloskey (Eds.), *Nursing interventions: Essential nursing treatments* (2nd ed., pp. 179–190). Philadelphia: W. B. Saunders. 1992.

Lazarus, R.S., & Folkman, S. (1984). *Stress, appraisal and coping.* New York: Springer.

Leavitt, M.B. (1989). Transition to illness. The family in the hospital. In C.L. Gillis, B.M. Roberts, B.L. Highly, & B.L. Martinson (Eds.), *Toward a science of family nursing* (pp. 262–283). Reading, MA: Addison-Wesley.

Lynn-McHale, W., & Smith, A. (1991). Comprehensive assessment of families of the critically ill. *Critical Care Nursing 2*(2), 195–209.

McCloskey, G.M., & Bulechek, G.M. (1992). *Nursing interventions classification (NIC).* St. Louis: Mosby–Year Book.

McCubbin, H., & Patterson, J. (1982). The family stress process: The double ABCX model of adjustment and adaptation. In H. I. McCubbin, M. Sussman, & J. Patterson (Eds.), *Social stress and the family* (pp. 26–47). Wheeling, IL: Hawthorne.

Murray, R.B., Luetje, V., & Zentner, J.P. (1985). Crisis intervention: A therapy technique. In R.B. Murray & J.P. Zentner (Eds.), *Nursing concepts for health promotion* (3rd ed., pp. 307–368). Paramus, NJ: Prentice Hall.

Murray, R.B., Pinnell, N.N., Leonard, B., & Zentner, J. (1985). Basic considerations in health and illness. In R.B. Murray & J. Zentner (Eds.), *Nursing concepts for health promotion* (3rd ed., pp. 1–35). Paramus, NJ: Prentice Hall.

Naisbitt, J., & Aburdine, P. (1990). *Megatrends 2000: Ten new directions for the 1990's.* New York: William Morrow & Co.

Von Bertalanffy, L. (1968). General systems theory. A critical review. In W. Buckley (Ed.), *Research for the behavioral scientist.* Glenside, PA: Aldine.

Wilson, H.S. (1989). Family caregiving for a relative with Alzheimer's dementia: Coping with negative choices. *Nursing Research, 38*(2), 94–98.

MOBILITY PHENOMENA

18 | Human Mobility: An Overview

KATHRYN S. BRONSTEIN

The ability to move freely is basic to the essence of humanity. Through movement, we express feelings and emotions, carry out work activities basic to life support, and reflect our ability to think as we act on decisions made. Not all mobility is voluntary; for example, vital life processes associated with movement are regulated through the autonomic nervous system as we take in food, eliminate waste, and engage in sexual acts. To be human, to be alive, implies constant movement both within the internal environment of the self and in the external environment surrounding us.

The inability to move has a great impact on the concept of self; for example, 50 patients with chronic spinal pain that resulted in limited mobility had scores below normal on the Tennessee Self-Concept Scale, a physical self subscale, at initial testing before a chronic pain program. After a treatment program that included increasing mobility, self-concept scores at discharge and follow-up were not significantly different from those of the normative population (Bechnan, Axtell, Noland, & West, 1985).

Altered body image as related to the sexual self can be a major problem when immobility is present. Because movement is an integral part of sexual expression in all human beings, those with restricted movement or hypermobility must be assessed to determine the effect that altered mobility has on current and previous styles of physical participation during sex. The nurse must be able to counsel the client in alternative techniques and use of supportive devices to enhance sexuality (Hodges, 1977, 1978; Weinberg, 1982).

The relationship between movement and ability to conduct activities inherent to a chosen occupation is well exemplified in all disorders leading to immobility. The inability to pursue an occupation for which one is trained can greatly reduce a person's standard of living and force retraining in a less desirable and less economically rewarding career.

The ability to put thought into action is associated with mobility. Indeed, educational theorists have defined learning as a change in behavior (Tyler,

1949). Because behavior occurs through movement, a smile, a frown, or a movement toward or away from an object or a person gives the observer information about the individual's cognitive processes, values, and emotions. In conditions that retard or inhibit normal movement, such as those producing bradykinesia or dyskinesia, the patient's intellectual ability may be judged by observers as less than adequate. People in the individual's environment may respond inappropriately to the less mobile person and thus compound the associated problems of poor self-concept and low self-esteem.

Movement is the means by which we humans interact with our environment. For people to be mobile, three essential elements must be present: (1) the ability to move (an intact neuromuscular system or compensated movement), (2) the motivation to move, and (3) a free, nonrestrictive environment in which to move.

The inability to move a major portion of the body or even one arm or leg impairs one's overall interaction with the environment. Unfortunately, when dealing with neurologic injury and disease, alteration in physical mobility is common. In fact, it is ranked as the most frequently used diagnosis in rehabilitation settings. Additionally, neuromuscular impairment also leads to diagnoses related to self-care deficit, decreased activity tolerance, impaired skin integrity, social isolation, and health management deficit (Swain & Heard, 1992).

ABILITY TO MOVE

If normal movement is to occur, the person must have intact voluntary and autonomic neuromuscular systems. In the absence of these, voluntary movements can occur through assistive devices, such as wheelchairs, canes, and walkers, and involuntary movements, such as breathing, can be aided by machines such as the respirator.

Neuroanatomy and Neurophysiology of Movement

The anatomic elements necessary for the generation of normal movement include the muscles themselves, their afferent and efferent innervations, and the segmental spinal cord connections made by these peripheral nerve fibers. Within the spinal cord, descending motor tracts carry information from higher components of the motor system to influence activity at the spinal segmental level. The higher central nervous system elements in the motor system include the cerebral cortex, certain brain stem nuclei, the basal ganglia, and the cerebellum (Atwood & Mackay, 1989; Barr & Kieran, 1983; Hickey, 1992). Dysfunction in any one of these elements can produce alterations in movement or mobility.

The organization of the neuronal elements involved in human mobility gives rise to the terms *suprasegmental* and *segmental motor neurons*, also referred to as upper and lower motor neurons, respectively. The motor neurons of the brain stem cranial nerves and of the ventral horns of the spinal cord are referred to as segmental motor neurons. These neurons directly innervate skeletal muscles and are essential for muscle contraction. The segmental motor neurons receive and integrate activity impinging on them from sensory fibers, local interneurons, and descending and ascending spinal cord tracts. For this reason, the segmental motor neuron is also called the *final common pathway.*

The segmental motor neuron is essential for any muscle movement, and the suprasegmental motor neuron is essential for voluntary movement. Suprasegmental motor neurons give rise to the descending pathways that influence the segmental motor neurons. Many of the suprasegmental motor neurons originate in the primary motor cortex of the cerebrum, whereas others originate within the brain stem. The activity within these suprasegmental motor neurons is influenced and modified by the basal ganglia and the cerebellum (Landau & O'Leary, 1983).

SKELETAL MUSCLE

The basic element in human mobility is muscle contraction. Skeletal muscle is composed of individual muscle fibers or cells. A muscle fiber is largely made up of myofibrils that contain the filamentous contractile proteins actin and myosin, as well as the regulatory proteins troponin and tropomyosin. In striated muscle, actin and myosin are highly organized into sarcomeres, the functional units of contraction (Nagy & Samaha, 1984). When stimulated to contract, the actin filaments slide past the myosin filaments and thus cause shortening of the sarcomere and muscle contraction (Fig. 18–1).

The interaction between actin and myosin filaments is accomplished by formation of crossbridges between the two types of proteins. Structurally, these

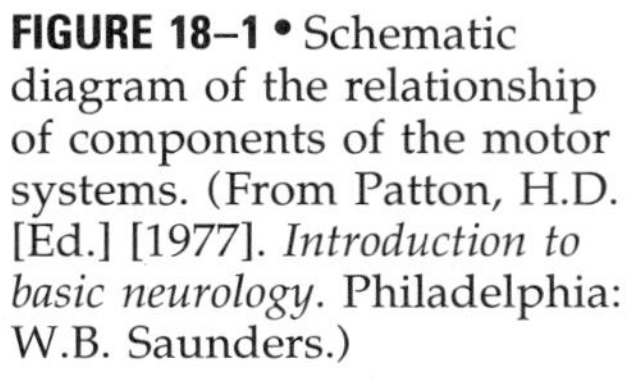

FIGURE 18–1 • Schematic diagram of the relationship of components of the motor systems. (From Patton, H.D. [Ed.] [1977]. *Introduction to basic neurology.* Philadelphia: W.B. Saunders.)

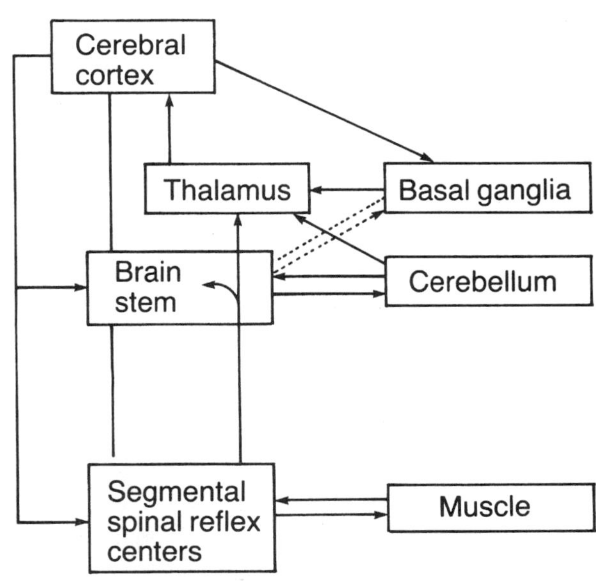

crossbridges are part of the myosin filaments and will interact spontaneously with binding sites on the actin molecules if allowed to do so. This interaction, combined with splitting of adenosine triphosphate (ATP), results in either the movement of actin past myosin and muscle shortening or the crossbridge formation with generation of muscle tension rather than shortening. The presence of the regulatory proteins troponin and tropomyosin normally prevents crossbridge formation and muscle contraction. The inhibitory effects of the regulatory proteins are removed, however, when the concentration of free calcium around the sarcomeres increases. Conversely, a decrease in the calcium concentration around the sarcomeres causes muscle relaxation (Bullock, Boyle, Wang, & Ajello, 1984).

The key to muscle contraction, therefore, is an increase in free intracellular calcium. In skeletal muscle fibers, free calcium concentration in the cytoplasm is normally very low, but the calcium concentration increases dramatically and becomes sufficient to allow contraction in response to motor neuron excitation of the muscle fiber's membrane. In resting muscle, most of the calcium is stored in a specialized form of smooth endoplasmic reticulum, the sarcoplasmic reticulum. When an electrical impulse is generated on the surface of the muscle fiber's membrane, the wave of excitation spreads across the surface of the fiber and penetrates into the interior of the cell via a system of transverse tubules, or T-tubules. The T-tubules bring the wave of excitation near to the sarcoplasmic reticulum, which then triggers the release of stored calcium into the cytoplasm, causing contraction (see Fig. 18–1). This entire process is called excitation-contraction coupling. Active transport systems pump the calcium out of the cytoplasm back into the sarcoplasmic reticulum, and contraction ceases (Nagy & Samaha, 1984).

Diseases that affect the structural and functional integrity of muscle fibers, such as the muscular dystrophies, congenital myopathies, and inflammatory muscle diseases, can interfere with these muscle mechanisms and produce abnormalities in mobility (Guyton, 1987; LiVolsi, Merino, Neumann, & Duray, 1984; Robbins, Cotran, & Kumar, 1984).

NEUROMUSCULAR JUNCTION

The action potential on the muscle membrane triggers muscle fiber contraction and occurs in response to an action potential on the motor neuron that innervates the muscle fiber. The bridging step between these two distinct electrical impulses involves the release of a transmitter at the neuromuscular junction, a process referred to as neuromuscular transmission.

The transmitter at the neuromuscular junction is acetylcholine. Acetylcholine is stored in membrane-bound synaptic vesicles in the axon terminals of the motor neuron. When an action potential invades the nerve terminal, acetylcholine is released by a calcium-mediated exocytotic process. Acetylcholine diffuses across the synaptic cleft, the space between the axon terminal and the muscle membrane, and binds to specific receptors on the muscle membrane

(Fig. 18–2). The interaction of acetylcholine with its receptor changes the membrane's permeability to ions. The resulting fluxes of potassium and sodium produce a local depolarization, the endplate potential. This potential brings the muscle fiber to threshold and initiates a muscle action potential that subsequently causes muscle contraction (Penn, 1984).

The effect of acetylcholine at the neuromuscular junction is short-lived. Some of the released transmitter randomly diffuses away from the synaptic cleft, although most of the transmitter is rendered inactive through the action of an enzyme, acetylcholinesterase, which is also found in the synaptic cleft. Rapid inactivation of acetylcholine is necessary to have precise neural control of muscle contraction. If acetylcholine remains in the synaptic cleft, it can repeatedly stimulate the muscle. Such repeated stimulation initially causes hyperexcitability but ultimately causes muscle paralysis.

The neuromuscular junction is a site for the alteration of muscle activity by pharmacologic manipulations, toxins, and disease processes. For example, botulinum toxin causes a decreased fusion of synaptic vesicles with the presyn-

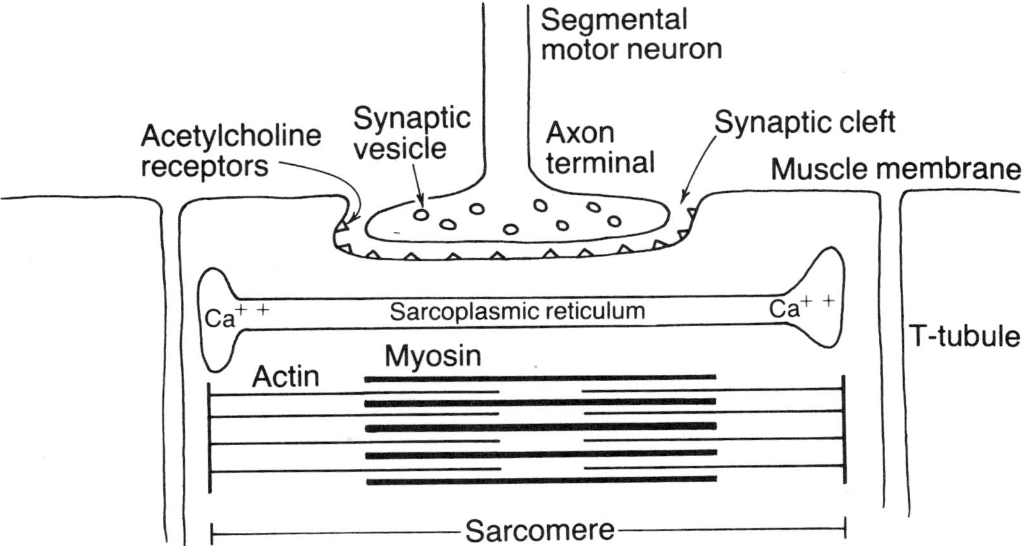

FIGURE 18–2 • Elements involved in neuromuscular transmission. An action potential on the segmental motor neuron causes release of acetylcholine from synaptic vesicles in the axon terminal. The acetylcholine diffuses across the synaptic cleft and binds to specific receptors on the muscle membrane. The interaction of acetylcholine with its receptors alters muscle membrane ion permeability and ultimately results in an action potential, which invades the muscle fiber via the T-tubule system. Calcium is released from the sarcoplasmic reticulum and binds to receptors on regulatory proteins associated with actin. Contractile proteins actin and myosin respond to the change in calcium and interact to produce muscle contraction. T-tubule, transverse tubule.

aptic membrane. Thus, the amount of transmitter released is diminished, creating muscle weakness and paralysis (Walton, 1981). In myasthenia gravis, there is a deficiency of acetylcholine receptors on the postsynaptic membrane. This deficit is believed to be due to an autoimmune condition that results in antibody-mediated destruction of the receptors. The deficiency of receptors decreases the ability of acetylcholine to depolarize the muscle endplate sufficiently to generate an action potential on the muscle membrane. Consequently, the major clinical feature of myasthenia gravis is muscle weakness. Some organophosphate compounds that are used as insecticides can inhibit acetylcholinesterase irreversibly. The resulting prolonged action of acetylcholine at the endplate membrane produces a depolarizing blockade that also effectively inhibits neuromuscular transmission (Penn, 1984).

MOTOR NEURONS

Each muscle fiber has one neuromuscular junction, usually located near the center of the fiber. An individual motor neuron, however, branches out near its distal end, with each branch forming a neuromuscular junction with a single muscle fiber. When an individual motor neuron is excited, the impulse spreads into the axon terminals, causing all the muscle fibers innervated by that axon to contract. A single motor neuron and all the muscle fibers it innervates is called a *motor unit.*

Skeletal muscles are innervated by alpha motor neurons, which have their cell bodies in the ventral horn of the spinal cord. Such neurons are not spontaneously active but must be brought to threshold by the summation of synaptic inputs converging onto them. These motor neurons receive their input from local sensory fibers, local interneurons, and descending and ascending fibers in the spinal cord. Basically, the alpha, or segmental, motor neurons can be excited either by input originating locally and involving activity within the immediate spinal cord segments or by descending input originating in the brain stem and cortex (Bullock et al., 1984).

MUSCLE SPINDLES AND TENDON RECEPTORS

Both proprioceptive and exteroceptive sensory fibers that enter the spinal cord can influence motor neuron activity. Most of the proprioceptive fibers carry information that originates in sensory organs located within the muscle itself. These muscle sensory organs are the muscle spindle fibers and Golgi's tendon organs, and they are found in all voluntary muscles. The muscle spindle fibers, or intrafusal fibers, lie parallel with the main muscle mass, or extrafusal fibers. The sensory fibers arising from the spindle organs are called intrafusal a (Ia) afferent fibers, and they are stimulated by stretch. On entering the spinal cord, the afferent fibers make direct connections with the alpha motor neurons supplying the same muscle (Fig. 18–3). This spinal cord connection constitutes the monosynaptic stretch reflex. Stretch of the muscle will stimulate the sensory ending on the muscle spindle and will initiate impulses on the Ia fibers. These afferent impulses directly excite the alpha motor neurons that innervate the muscle fibers. The ultimate consequence of stretch of the muscle, therefore, is reflex contraction of the same muscle. The deep-tendon reflexes elicited during a neurologic examination indicate the intactness of these reflex pathways (Bates, 1987).

The Ia afferent fibers branch on entering the spinal cord. In addition to making direct synaptic connections with the alpha motor neurons, collaterals from the Ia fibers synapse onto interneurons that are inhibitory to muscles that oppose the contraction. This process is reciprocal inhibition. The Ia collateral fibers also synapse onto interneurons that are excitatory to muscle contraction. Information from Ia afferents is transmitted along ascending pathways to inform higher centers—the brain stem, the cerebellum, and the cerebral cortex—of the length, or contractile state, of the muscles.

Because of the parallel relationship between the extrafusal and intrafusal fibers, it might seem that during muscle contraction the spindle fibers would slacken and be unable to generate important sensory information for movement control. This is not the case, however, because the muscle spindle fibers themselves receive innervation from gamma motor neurons. Motor innervation of

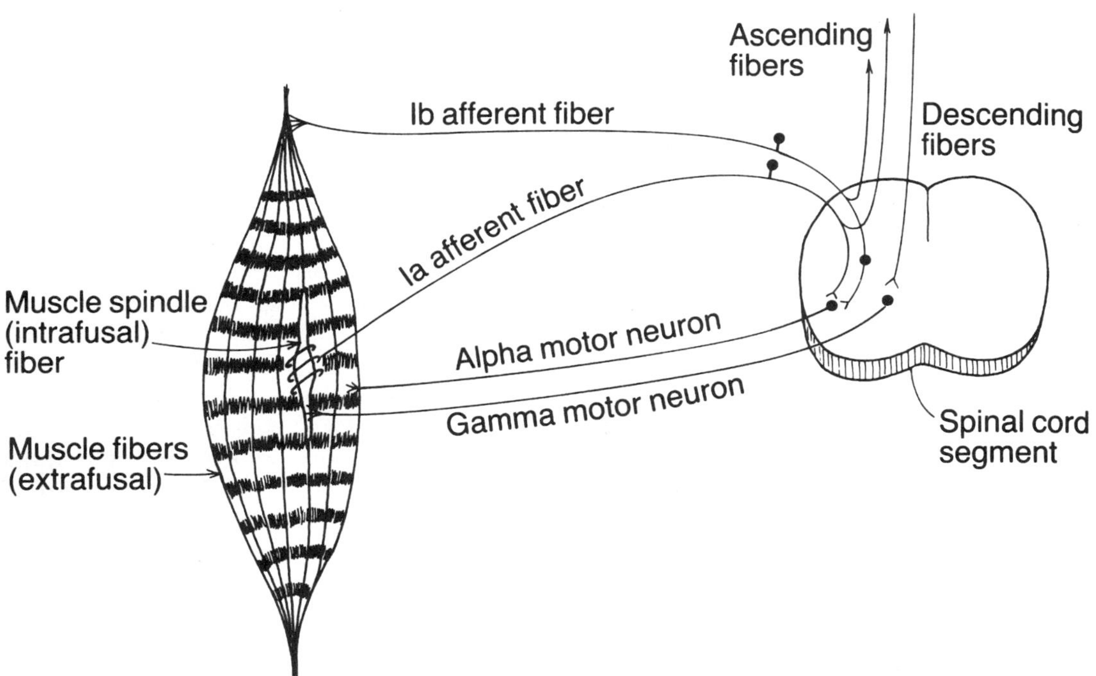

FIGURE 18–3 • Relationship among muscle, its receptors, and the spinal cord segment.

the spindle fibers causes them to contract during extrafusal muscle contraction and thereby permit the sensory organs to remain responsive even as the muscle shortens. During the usual course of voluntary contraction, descending commands excite both the alpha and the gamma motor neurons to a muscle, causing contraction of both the extrafusal and the intrafusal fibers to the muscle. This coactivation of the motor neurons allows sensory input from the muscle during the act of contraction.

Golgi's tendon organs are sensory structures located at the tendon endings of the muscle. The receptors for the afferent fibers originating from Golgi's tendon organs, the intrafusal b (Ib) afferent fibers, are also stimulated by stretch, but because of their location, muscle contraction increases activity on these sensory structures (see Fig. 18–3). These receptors, therefore, respond to the force generated by the muscle as it contracts. The information from the Ib fibers affects neurons locally within the spinal cord and is transmitted along ascending pathways to provide higher centers with important information about the contractile status of the muscles. The information from the Ia and Ib fibers is important to the central nervous system in determining if motor commands were carried out appropriately. If the actual signal generated from the muscles does not match the intended motor movement, a correcting signal can be sent out. Thus, a feedback mechanism for the appropriateness of muscle movements exists using these sensory organs in the muscle.

SEGMENTAL SPINAL CORD ORGANIZATION

Analysis of the synaptic connections made by muscle afferents onto muscle efferents, either direct or indirect, makes it easy to appreciate how excitation of one pathway can result in the production of a stereotyped movement—that is, a reflex. Other spinal cord reflexes can be initiated by activity generated onto exteroceptive fibers. These latter reflex pathways can be stimulated by pain but also by other sensory stimuli, such as touch and pressure. The principal reflex involving these afferent inputs is the flexor withdrawal reflex. The spinal cord connections in this reflex are far more intricate, involving not only the flexor muscles of the affected limb but also the extensor muscles in the contralateral limb. Noxious stimuli will cause the affected limb to withdraw but the opposite limb to extend. Because this reflex can be initiated by stimuli other than noxious stimuli, it is likely that it may normally be elicited during such activities as walking and running, as well as in withdrawal from painful stimuli.

Although local reflex control of spinal motor neurons exists in humans, the nervous system has evolved to the point where the descending pathways dominate the expression of these reflexes and, consequently, motor activity. This is demonstrated by the observation that immediately after transection of the cervical spinal cord, all reflex activity within the cord is suppressed, and the patient suffers spinal shock. Presumably, descending excitatory input to the spinal cord interneurons is necessary for sufficient stimulation of the alpha motor neurons. In time, however, the cord reflexes reappear and may even be expressed in a hyperactive form.

SPINAL CORD TRACTS

In addition to the reflex neuronal connections within the spinal cord, the cord provides a vehicle by which information from higher neuronal centers is conveyed to the spinal motor neurons. These descending pathways affect muscle movement either directly by synapsing onto alpha motor neurons or indirectly by synapsing onto interneurons or gamma motor neurons. The descending pathways can be grouped into two categories, the lateral and the medial systems.

Descending in the lateral system are the corticospinal and rubrospinal tracts. Some of the fibers in the corticospinal tract make direct synaptic connection with alpha motor neurons that control the distal musculature. This tract, therefore, is largely concerned with fine independent movements, especially of the fingers and thumbs. The rubrospinal tract is largely concerned with control of the distal musculature. The medial system contains fibers that originate in the vestibular nuclei, the reticular formation, and the tectum. These descending pathways are primarily concerned with controlling the neck and trunk muscles and the more proximal muscles of the limbs (Netter, 1983).

MOTOR CORTEX

The corticospinal fibers arise in part from the primary motor cortex, which is located in the frontal lobe anterior to the central sulcus. Direct electrical stimulation of the motor cortex causes discrete muscle movements on the contralateral side of the body. Mapping of the motor cortex in this manner demonstrates the motor homunculus, an image of the body projected on the cortex. The area of the motor cortex devoted to any individual body part is proportional to the degree of cortical influence over that structure rather than to the size of the part. Consequently, the hand has a disproportionately large cortical representation. The leg is represented on the medial surface of the motor cortex, followed by the trunk, arm, and hand. The cortical area controlling the face is located laterally (Fig. 18–4). As mentioned, the cerebral cortex, via its projections in the corticospinal tract, is involved in the control of the distal musculature and is, therefore, involved with those movements that are least automated. It mediates fine hand movements.

The effect of lesions in the primary motor cortex depends specifically on the location and extent of the damage. Primary motor cortex lesions or damage isolated to the corticospinal or pyramidal tract, however, gives rise to signs typically associated with suprasegmental (upper motor neuron) lesions. In general, there is weakness of the involved muscles, loss of skilled movements, and unwillingness to use the affected limb. The involved muscles may initially demonstrate decreased tone but will eventually become spastic. This hyperexcitability is presumably due to loss of inhibitory inputs that normally originate in the suprasegmental motor neurons to influence the alpha motor neurons. With cortical lesions, there is the appearance of pathologic reflexes, such as Babinski's reflex, that are caused by the increased excitability of the alpha motor neurons.

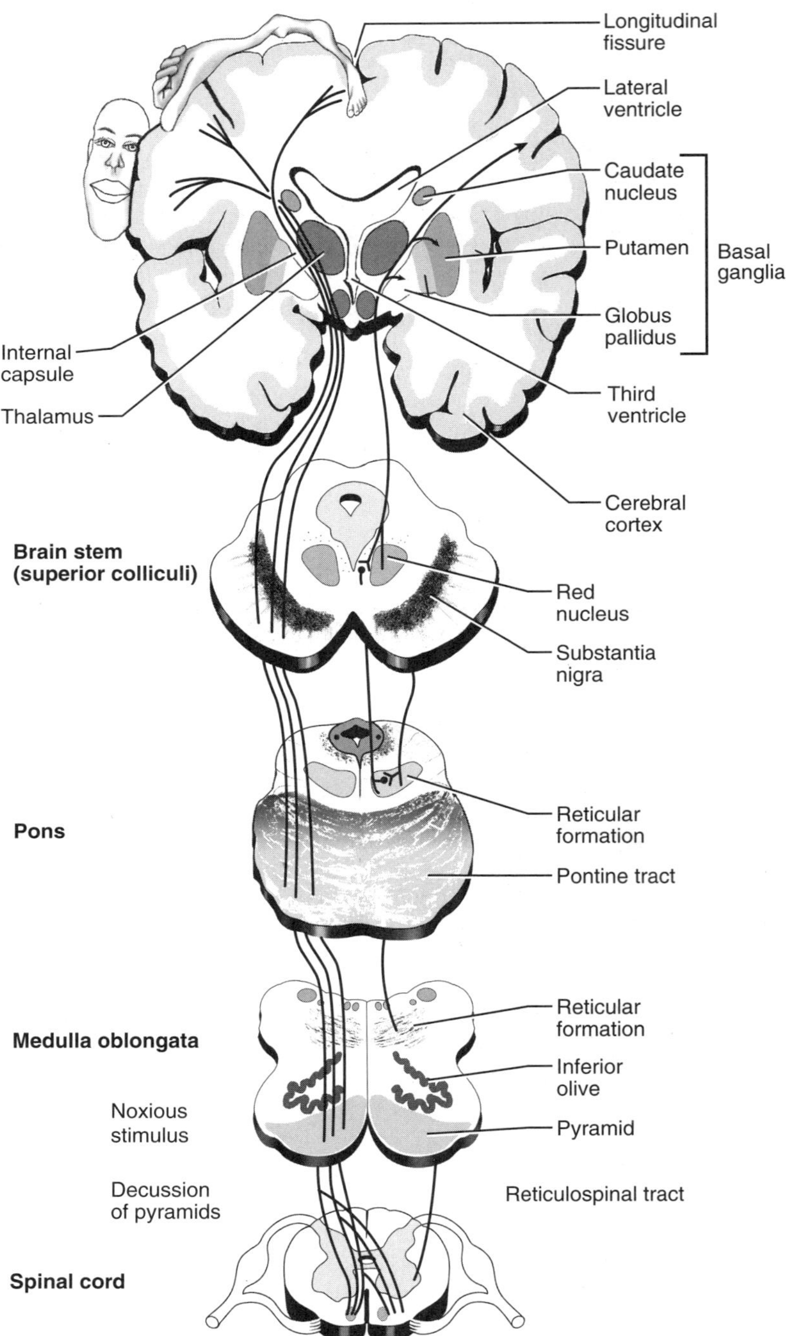

FIGURE 18–4 • *See legend on opposite page*

BRAIN STEM NUCLEI

The rubrospinal tract originates mainly from the red nucleus in the midbrain. The axons from this nucleus cross the midline immediately, then descend the spinal cord in the posterolateral funiculus just anterior to the lateral corticospinal tract. These axons predominantly influence the motor neurons supplying the distal musculature and synapse on interneurons that facilitate both gamma and alpha motor neurons. The red nucleus itself receives the majority of its input from the cerebral cortex and the cerebellum.

Neurons in the brain stem that project to the spinal cord via reticulospinal tracts originate in the pontine and medullary reticular formation. The pontine neurons project via the medial reticulospinal tract and are predominantly facilitatory to flexor motor neurons and those neurons innervating proximal and axial muscles. In the medullary reticulospinal system, most of the fibers terminate on interneurons. The exact function of these neurons is not known, but in general they are not concerned with fine, skilled, voluntary movements but rather with instinctual reactions and postural adjustments.

BASAL GANGLIA

The basal ganglia are groups of neurons located at the base of the cerebrum that are organized into pairs of nuclei, the caudate nucleus, the putamen, and the globus pallidus and that functionally include the subthalamic nuclei and the substantia nigra. These structures, along with the cerebellum and their various connecting pathways, are generally referred to as the extrapyramidal motor system. The basal ganglia receive their afferent input from the cerebral cortex, the thalamus, and the substantia nigra. The major output from the basal ganglia is to the substantia nigra and to the thalamus and from there to the cerebral cortex and to reticular formation in the brain stem.

The connections of the basal ganglia are complex. They do not project directly to the spinal cord; therefore, their influence on motor activity is indirect and the exact function of the basal ganglia is not clearly worked out. Lesions in the basal ganglia give rise to movement disorders—either too much or too little movement—and to disturbances in muscle tone. An excess of movement can be called hyperkinesia or dyskinesia. Deficiency of movement can be called bradykinesia, akinesia, or hypokinesia and is generally present in parkinsonism.

Output from the basal ganglia plays an important role in the initiation of movement. The basal ganglia are also important in determining the balance of alpha and gamma motor neuron activity. Consequently, disorders of the basal

---

FIGURE 18–4 • Pyramidal and extrapyramidal tracts. (From American Association of Neuroscience Nurses [1996]. *Core curriculum for neuroscience nursing* [p. 1637]. Chicago: Author.)

ganglia may be manifested as inability to initiate movements, as excessively slow movements, as abnormalities of muscle tone, or as tremor. The basal ganglia are necessary for the smooth coordination of voluntary movements, the maintenance of posture and muscle tone, the regulation of postural reflexes, and the conduction of automatic movements.

Parkinson's disease provides a good and clinically important example of basal ganglia dysfunction. Parkinson's disease is associated with the degeneration of neurons in the substantia nigra. The substantia nigra is the source of neurons that synthesize the transmitter dopamine. Dopaminergic fibers project to the caudate nucleus and putamen and appear to exert a modulator effect on the level of excitability there. One of the consequences of dopamine depletion in the striatum is that the output from neurons in the globus pallidus occurs chonically rather than physically with movement. This enhanced discharge from the globus pallidus is presumably responsible for symptoms seen in Parkinson's disease, which include rigidity, hypokinesia, and tremor at rest (Fahn, 1984).

CEREBELLUM

The cerebellum is necessary neither for sensory perception nor for the initiation of movement, but it plays an integral role in motor control. The cerebellum is involved in timing, duration, and strength of movements and is essential for fine coordination of movements and ability to judge distances.

The cerebellum receives afferent information from the vestibular system, from proprioceptors and exteroceptors in the limbs, from the brain stem, and indirectly from the cerebral cortex via relays in the pons. The efferent pathways from the cerebellum project to the brain stem and thalamus and via these areas influence activity in the cerebral cortex and spinal cord. Basically, the cerebellum monitors both ongoing afferent information and ongoing information within the motor system. The cerebellum compares the intended signal with what is actually happening. If the two sets of information do not match, the cerebellum sends a signal to correct the ongoing motor activity and makes it appropriate. Lesions in the cerebellum, therefore, produce abnormalities in movement that may be related to interference with vestibular function and cause difficulties with equilibrium and gait, or ataxia. Cerebellar dysfunction may also impair the ability to produce smooth, coordinated movements. With cerebellar damage, there may be decomposition of movement such that muscles act in an isolated rather than a coordinated manner, producing clumsiness in motion. The ability to stop movements accurately at the appropriate time can be affected, causing dysmetria. Difficulties with timing and sequencing of movements in cerebellar damage may produce an intention tremor. Also affected by cerebellar damage is the ability to produce rapidly alternating movements, or adiadochokinesia (Lothmann & Montgomery, 1984).

AGING AND MOTOR FUNCTION

During the aging process, many characteristic changes take place in the motor system. Elderly persons often assume a flexed posture and display muscle rigidity, tremor, and slowness in movements. Disease processes often compound the normal processes of aging, making it difficult to delineate normal changes from abnormal changes while adding to the functional motor deficits.

Among the known structural alterations that occur with increasing age are a decrease in brain weight and a decrease in the number of synapses. The neuronal loss is not uniform throughout the central nervous system, and certain areas of the nervous system are involved more frequently in the degenerative changes than are other areas. The affected areas commonly include the caudate nucleus, the putamen, the substantia nigra, and the dentate nucleus of the cerebellum (Teravinen & Calne, 1983). The neuronal degeneration in these motor centers presumably contributes to the decline in the motor performance seen in the aged. Among the motor areas affected by aging are those areas also affected in Parkinson's disease. Consequently, some of the motor deficits commonly seen in aging are personified in parkinsonism. The decline in the number of synapses, along with a decrease in the maximum conduction velocity of peripheral nerves, may contribute to the prolonged reaction time and movement time also characteristic of the elderly. Once again, however, it is difficult to separate the effects of the normal aging process from the effects of physical inactivity.

As more research is carried out on healthy, elderly individuals, the effects of normal aging on motor function will be distinguished from the effects of physical inactivity. Identification of the normal process may then open avenues for research into the prevention of degenerative nervous system changes that impair motor functions in the elderly.

Compensated Movement

When an individual has a disruption of the neuromuscular system that results in loss of movement, compensated movement can occur through assistive devices or assistance by others in the environment. According to data from the National Health Survey, 6.5 million people require 8 million assistive devices to increase mobility (National Health Interview Statistics, 1980). The determinants for using these devices should include a comprehensive assessment of the combined neurologic, orthopedic, and functional aspects affecting the body during ambulation. Assistive devices can help improve ambulation by the use of a better gait pattern and stance phase of gait (Rinehart, 1983).

More than 645,000 people in our society rely on wheelchairs to increase their mobility and functioning. An investment of more than $500 million in wheelchairs was reported in 1983, with the average cost of each chair estimated at approximately $800 (Kohn, Enders, Preston, & Matlock, 1983). Such costs require that equipment be adapted as precisely as possible to the person and to the environment so that maximum benefit can be realized.

Major considerations in the purchase of assistive devices are the degree of limited movement for which the device will be used, the size and style of the assistive device, and the environment in which the device must be maneuvered. Additional considerations include further growth of the individual, course of the disease, accessibility to repair shops, proximity to rehabilitation or medical facilities, and changes in housing and caretaker arrangements (Kohn et al., 1983).

When the individual is unable to move himself or herself, the nurse or family member may compensate for the lack of movement through a number of activities. To prevent and treat disuse phenomena associated with immobility, people in the disabled individual's environment can participate in (1) body positioning, (2) joint-mobility exercises, (3) muscle-conditioning exercises, and (4) environmental structuring (Mitchell & Loustau, 1981). The degree and use of specific measures by people in the environment are directly related to the patient's ability and the nature of the immobility phenomenon. These measures are discussed in more detail in Chapters 20 and 21.

ROLE OF MOTIVATION IN MOBILITY

In many cases, the inability of a person to move in a normal fashion can be related to a lack of motivation. The lack of motivation may result from a temporary change in equilibrium, from an adaptive response to demands operating in the environment, or from the presence of emotional-motivational blocks.

A lack of motivation to move is often associated with psychologic disequilibrium. A common symptom of depression is limited movement, termed *psychomotor retardation.* Severely depressed people often take to their beds and must be forced to participate in physical activity. Perhaps the classic example of immobility associated with mental disequilibrium is found in people in a catatonic state (Stuart & Sudeen, 1983).

Normal patterns of increased and decreased activity are associated with temporary changes in equilibrium. During periods of minor illness, a decrease in activity is a natural response as the body tries to conserve energy needed for healing. After intense emotional, social, or physical activity, fatigue–our body's signal to rest—decreases our motivation for activity. Activities that conserve energy help restore our physical bodies and emotional and psychologic reserves. A reduction in movement can bring back a sense of equilibrium with the environment.

Often, movement declines as a mechanism of adaptation to environmental changes. When there is a discrepancy in the amount of energy a person has and the demand an environment requires for interaction, the person with limited energy must decrease movement in order to cope. For example, a stroke victim with a weak left side who lives on the second floor may decrease movement in the environment because it is no longer possible to maneuver the stairs without severe fatigue. When an environment is characterized by overwhelming psychologic or social demands, the person usually withdraws. By decreasing physical movement and interaction with others, stress is reduced and energy is restored.

Emotional-motivational blocks in children have been cited as a major cause of poor motor functioning (Stott & Moyes, 1985). In these children, a physical handicap may be the primary reason for poor motor performance. A fear of failure, however, magnifies the effects of the physical handicap. The vicious cycle that follows takes on different forms in accordance with the child's personality. The child who lacks confidence may exhibit a frozen inhibition; the child who is easily distracted has difficulty following instructions and thinking ahead about the steps in a task. The end result in both types of children is a defeatist attitude: "I can't do it." Strategies to help overcome these emotional-motivational blocks are necessary to encourage maximum mobility in a child with a physical handicap.

ENVIRONMENT AND MOBILITY

In some instances, restricted movement can be related to barriers in the environment. A person may have an intact neuromuscular system and the motivation to move about but be faced with an environmental restraint to movement. Examples include the patient in traction, the person with a cast, and those confined to bedrest.

Barriers to movement commonly exist as a component of buildings and structures. However, many of these barriers have come down because of the passage of a series of federal laws aimed at enhancing the quality of life for disabled Americans (DeJong & Lifchez, 1983). A major piece of legislation, the Architectural Barrier Bill, was signed into law by President Johnson on August 12, 1968. This law provides full access to any facility wholly or partly financed by federal funds and intended for public use. The law also includes buildings to be used for employment or as residences of disabled persons. In 1973, the Rehabilitation Act was passed. This law extends to America's disabled citizens all programs, services, and benefits that are federally funded. Access to education and job-teaching programs were written into the regulations.

The Americans with Disabilities Act (ADA) was signed into law (Channing, 1992). This act is intended to prohibit discrimination against disabled individuals by guaranteeing equal opportunities in such areas as employment, access to public buildings, public transportation, availability of telecommunication devices, and services and programs provided by the government. The law is meant to apply to individuals with either physical or mental disability.

For those persons with limited mobility, this law guarantees that employers must modify the work environment to accommodate such things as wheelchairs and walkers so that individuals will be able to do their jobs. In addition, the law states that businesses that provide services or entertainment, such as restaurants, hotels, movie theatres, and banks, must be accessible to people in wheelchairs and if structures can't be modified, then the businesses need to provide their services in another manner. Perhaps the most beneficial aspect of the bill is the section that mandates that railways and buses provide access for the disabled or that an alternative system of transportation be available, such as door-to-door service. An additional aspect of the law is the provision that programs supported by state and local funds cannot exclude individuals with disabilities. Individuals who require these special services or accommodations cannot be charged an additional fee or be charged a higher rate than nondisabled individuals.

A barrier-free environment includes the concept of freedom from physical barriers and psychologic barriers. Perhaps one of the greatest barriers to movement is the attitude of others in a person's space. According to Lombana (1980), negative attitudes toward people with disabilities are common throughout all areas of our society. Elliott and Byrd (1982) cited television as one media source that reinforces negative attitudes through misinformation about disabilities and dramatization of negative disability stereotypes.

Livneh (1982) developed a classification system according to the sources of negative attitudes toward the disabled. He concluded that because of the complexity of factors interacting in the creation of negative attitudes, short-duration interventions aimed at attitude change were futile.

In our efforts to intervene in the environment to create freedom for mobility, political strategies and public education are needed. The attitude of the family, the neighbors, and those in the community must be positive if disabled people with limited mobility are to overcome isolation and find freedom of movement within others' space. Efforts to influence policy at the local, state, and federal levels should be viewed as part of nursing intervention in the community if immobilized people are to live in a barrier-free world.

SUMMARY

The ability to move with purpose and freedom within the environment is dependent on an intact neuromuscular system, the presence of assistive aids and people to help when physical limitations are present, a desire to move, and a free, nonrestrictive environment. Absence of any of these components can result in disuse syndrome and the resulting consequences of immobility. Because nursing encompasses Florence Nightingale's philosophy of nursing the patient as well as the environment, a comprehensive assessment of each of these components inherent in the concept of mobility is needed if appropriate nursing interventions are to be instituted. Chapter 19 provides a general framework for assessing mobility, Chapter 20 delineates appropriate nursing interventions in the care of people responding to conditions causing acute immobility, and Chapter 21 discusses those who live with chronic immobility as a part of their daily lives.

References

Atwood, H.L., & Mackay, W.E. (1989). *Essentials of neurophysiology.* Hamilton, ON: B.C. Decker.
Barr, M., & Kieran, J. (1983). *The human nervous system: An anatomical viewpoint* (4th ed.). Philadelphia: Lippincott-Raven.

Bates, B. (1987). *A guide to physical assessment* (4th ed). Philadelphia: J.B. Lippincott.

Bechnan, C., Axtell, L., Noland, K., & West, J. (1985). Self-concept: An outcome of a program for spinal pain. *Pain, 22,* 59.

Bullock, J., Boyle, J., Wang, W., & Ajello, R. (1984). *Physiology.* New York: John Wiley & Sons.

Channing, L. (1992). *About the Americans with Disabilities Act.* New York: Bete Co.

DeJong, G., Lifchez, R. (1983). Physical disability and public policy. *Scientific American, 248,* 6.

Elliott, T.R., & Byrd, E.K. (1982). Media and disability. *Rehabilitation Literature, 43,* 348.

Fahn, S. (1984). Extrapyramidal system. In E.D. Frohlich (Ed.), *Pathophysiology: Altered regulatory mechanisms in disease* (p. 771). Philadelphia: J.B. Lippincott.

Guyton, A.C. (1987). *Basic neuroscience: Anatomy and physiology.* Philadelphia: W.B. Saunders.

Hickey, J. (1992). *The clinical practice of neurological and neurosurgical nursing.* Philadelphia: J.B. Lippincott.

Hodges, L. (1977). *Body image and bladder care in cord injured.* Unpublished master's thesis. Emory University, Atlanta, GA.

Hodges, L. (1978). Human sexuality and the spinal cord injured: Role of the clinical nurse specialist. *Journal of Neurosurgical Nursing, 10*(3), 125.

Kohn, J., Enders, S., Preston, J., & Matlock, M. (1983). Provision of assistive equipment for handicapped persons. *Archives of Physical Medicine and Rehabilitation, 64,* 378.

Landau, W.M., & O'Leary, J.L. (1983). Disturbances of movement. In R.S. Backlow (Ed.), *MacBryde's signs and symptoms: Applied pathologic physiology and clinical interpretation* (6th ed., p. 669). Philadelphia: J.B. Lippincott.

Livneh, H. (1982). On the origins of negative attitudes toward people with disabilities. *Rehabilitation Literature, 43*(11–12), 338.

LiVolsi, V.A., Merino, M.I., Neumann, R.G., & Duray, P.H. (1984). *Pathology.* New York: John Wiley & Sons.

Lombana, J. (1980). Fostering positive attitudes toward handicapped students: A guidance challenge. *School Counseler, 27*(3), 176.

Lothmann, E.W., & Montgomery, E.B. (1984). Control of motor activity in the cerebrum and cerebellum. In E.D. Frohlich (Ed.), *Pathophysiology: Altered regulatory mechanisms in disease.* (3rd ed, p. 741). Philadelphia: J.B. Lippincott.

Mitchell, P., & Loustau, A. (1981). *Concepts basic to nursing.* New York: McGraw-Hill.

Nagy, B., & Samaha, F.J. (1984). Physiology of normal and diseased muscle. In E.D. Frohlich (Ed.), *Pathophysiology: Altered regulatory mechanisms in disease* (p. 805). Philadelphia: J.B. Lippincott.

National health interview statistics: Use of special aids. 1977 Vital and health statistics, Series 10, Number 135 (October, 1980) (DHHS Publication No. [FHS] 81–1563). Rockville, MD: U.S. Department of Health and Human Services.

Netter, F.H. (1983). Functional neuroanatomy. In E.D. Grohlich (Ed.), *Nervous system. Part I. Anatomy and physiology* (pp. 68–71). CIBA.

Penn, A.S. (1984). Neuromuscular junction. In E.D. Frohlich (Ed.), *Pathophysiology: Altered regulatory mechanisms in disease* (p. 789). Philadelphia: J.B. Lippincott.

Rinehart, M.A. (1983). Consideration for functional training in adults after head injury. *Physical Therapy, 63*(12), 1975.

Robbins, S.L., Cotran, R.S., & Kumar, V. (1984). *Pathologic basis of disease* (3rd ed). Philadelphia: W.B. Saunders.

Stott, D.H., & Moyes, F.A. (1985). Treatment strategies for emotional-motivational blocks to motor functioning in childhood. *Physical Therapy, 65*(6), 915.

Stuart, B., & Sudeen, S. (1983). *Principles and practice of psychiatric nursing.* St. Louis: Mosby–Year Book.

Swain, D., & Heard, L. (1992). Nursing diagnoses used most frequently in rehabilitation nursing practice. *Rehabilitation Nursing, 17*(5), 256.

Teravinen, H., & Calne, D.B. (1983). Motor system in normal aging and Parkinson's disease. In R. Katzman & R. Terry (Eds.), *The neurology of aging* (p. 85). Philadelphia: F.A. Davis.

Tyler, R. (1949). *Basic principles of curriculum and instruction.* Chicago: University of Chicago Press.

Walton, J.N. (1981). Neurology. In L.H. Smith & S.O. Thieu (Eds.), *Pathophysiology: The biological principles of disease.* Philadelphia: W.B. Saunders.

Weinberg, J. (1982). Human sexuality and spinal cord injury. *Nursing Clinics of North America, 17*(3), 407.

Assessment of Human Mobility

ANN D. HOLLERBACH

Movement may be defined as a form of voluntary and automatic coordinated skeletal muscle activity that is essential for carrying out the tasks of daily living. It is a highly complex process involving the interaction of a human being with the environment. The musculoskeletal system provides structure, support, stability, and protection for movement, and the central nervous system provides the necessary neural innervation. The capability for movement is facilitated by the individual's internal motivation and a free, nonrestrictive environment.

Therefore, physiologic, psychosocial, and environmental components must be considered when assessing mobility (Fig. 19–1). A holistic approach to assessment should be used, including a thorough nursing history, a neuromuscular examination related to functional status of mobility, and an assessment of the individual's role-related activities.

FUNCTIONAL ASSESSMENT

Lawton (1971) defined functional assessment as "any systematic attempt to measure objectively the level at which a person is functioning in any of a variety of areas such as physical health, quality of self maintenance, quality of role activity, intellectual status, social activity, attitude toward the world and toward self, and emotional status" (p. 466). Sarno, Sarno, and Lurta (1973) emphasized that the level of the individual's physical function is not a true indicator of the individual's ability to function in life.

Although many instruments have been developed to assess specific mobility functions, a systematic approach to functional assessment of mobility is lacking in the literature. Specific instruments developed for functional assessment in conjunction with the physical examination can be grouped into three categories: (1) global instruments, which focus on a comprehensive assessment of an individual's functional status, such as PULSES and the Functional Life Scale (FLS); (2) the activities of daily living (ADL) scales, such as the Katz

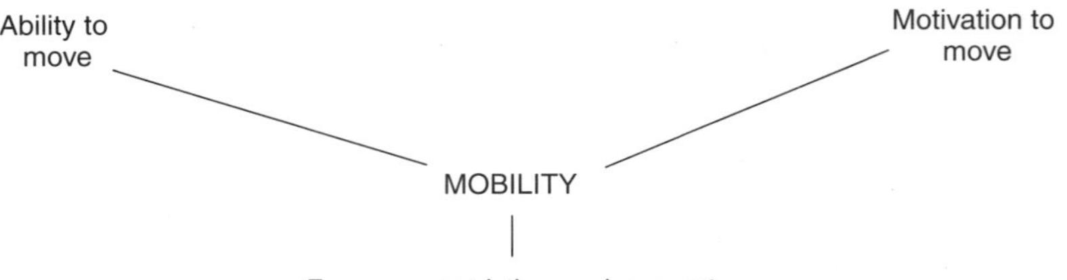

FIGURE 19–1 • Three elements essential to mobility.

Index of ADL and the Barthel Index; and (3) functional profiles, which enable one to assess a particular disease or condition or to evaluate a single functional parameter, such as the Jebsen Test for Hand Function (Granger & Gresham, 1984; Jebsen, Taylor, & Trieschmann, 1969; Katz, Ford, & Moskowitz, 1963; Mahoney & Barthel, 1965; Sarno et al., 1973). The ADL scales are used most frequently to assess mobility functions.

Recently, health care team members have recognized that one problem with developing a comprehensive tool has been a lack of standard terminology and classification for the term *disability*. Granger and Gresham (1984) expanded on Townsend's presentation of five distinct meanings for disability.

1. Anatomic, physiologic, or psychologic abnormality
2. Chronic clinical condition altering or interrupting normal physiologic or psychologic processes
3. Functional limitation of ordinary activity
4. Pattern of behavior of a socially deviant kind
5. Socially defined position or status, usually of inferiority (p. 7)

Nagi (1965) concluded that the pattern of disabling behavior is influenced in three ways:

1. The effect of the pathologic condition
2. The individual's perception of the situation
3. The perception of the situation by the family, significant others, and health care professionals

Granger (Granger, Demis, Peters, Sherwood, & Barrett, 1979; Granger & Gresham, 1984) developed a conceptual model (Fig. 19–2) for functional assessment based on the Nagi (1965) and Wood and Badley (1978) disability models. This model is helpful in synthesizing a framework for assessing the functional status of mobility.

Granger's (Granger & Gresham, 1984) model focuses on collecting data to gain a profile of the whole person, including medical status, status in performance of tasks, and fulfillment of social roles, together with knowledge of the

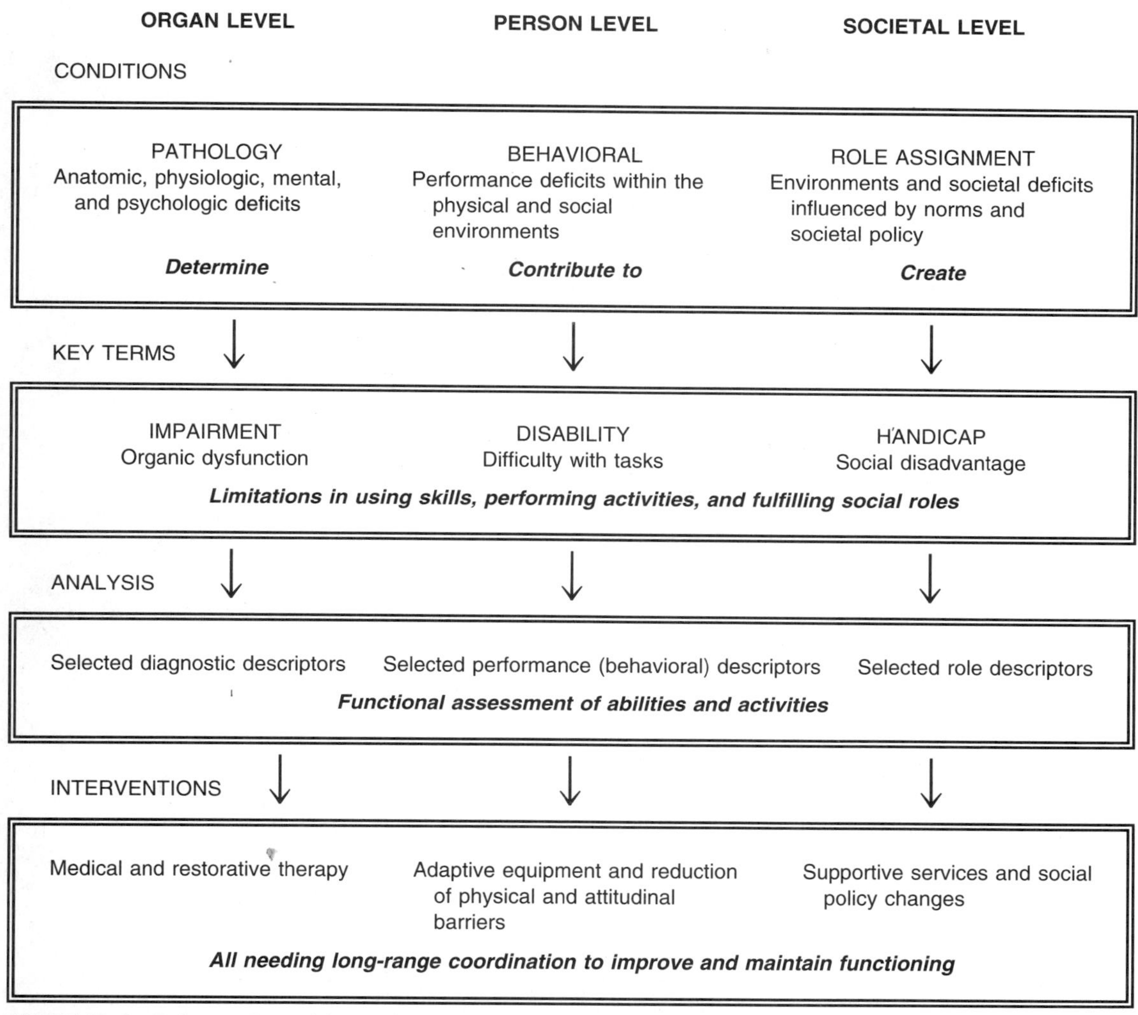

FIGURE 19–2 • Relationship of functional assessment to the impairment, disability, and handicap model. In the upper half of the diagram, concepts are related horizontally across the three levels of concern: the organ, person, and societal levels. Pathology, manifested as various forms of deficits, determines IMPAIRMENT, DISABILITY is the central person concept, and HANDICAP is the social disadvantage consequent to impairment and disability. The lower half of the figure illustrates functional assessment related to this modified version of Nagi's (1965) and Wood and Badley's (1978) disability models. The most important measure is that of performance related to impairment, disability, and handicap. (From Granger, C.V. [1984]. A conceptual model for functional assessment. In C.V. Granger & G.E. Gresham [Eds.], *Functional assessment in rehabilitation medicine* [p. 14]. Baltimore: Williams & Wilkins.)

TABLE 19–1 • ACTIVITIES OF DAILY LIVING ASSESSMENT FOR GERIATRIC CLIENTS

A. Self-care
   1. Dressing, undressing, maintaining clothing
      a. Keeping clothes in good repair (mending)
      b. Having access to clothes
      c. Getting into and out of underwear (bra, girdle, underpants, pantyhose, stockings, garter belt)
      d. Putting on and removing pants
      e. Getting arms in sleeves
      f. Managing zippers, buttons, snaps (especially in back), ties
      g. Putting on socks and shoes, tying laces
      h. Applying prostheses (e.g., glasses, hearing aids)
   2. Grooming and hygiene
      a. Washing, drying, and brushing hair
      b. Brushing teeth
      c. Cleaning and putting in dentures
      d. Shaving
      e. Nail care (feet and hands)
      f. Applying makeup
      g. Preparing bath water and testing temperature
      h. Getting into and out of tub or shower
      i. Reaching and cleaning all body parts
   3. Elimination
      a. Altering position for urination or sitting on toilet
      b. Ability to wipe self
B. Mobility
   1. Difficulty climbing or descending stairs (Is bedroom or bathroom on upper level? How many stairs or flights to apartment or house?)
   2. Sitting up, rising from bed
   3. Lowering to or rising from chair
   4. Walking (short and long distances; describe necessity for walking)
   5. Opening doors
   6. Reaching items in cupboards
   7. Necessity for lifting (and any difficulty)
C. Communication
   1. Dialing telephone
   2. Reading numbers
   3. Hearing over telephone
   4. Answering door
   5. Immediate access to neighbors, help
D. Eating (see nutritional section for details about appetite, weight, food consumption)
   1. Access to market
   2. Preparing food (opening cans and packages; using stove; reaching dishes, pots, utensils)
   3. Handling knife, fork, spoon (e.g., cutting meat)
   4. Getting food to mouth
   5. Chewing, swallowing
E. Housekeeping, doing laundry, house upkeep
   1. Making bed
   2. Sweeping, mopping floors
   3. Dusting
   4. Cleaning dishes
   5. Cleaning tub, bathroom
   6. Picking up clutter (to client's satisfaction)
   7. Taking out trash, garbage
   8. Use of basement (stairs, cleaning)

TABLE 19–1 • ACTIVITIES OF DAILY LIVING ASSESSMENT FOR GERIATRIC CLIENTS
Continued

   9. Laundry facilities (in home or near residence, washtub, clothesline)
  10. Yard care—garden, bushes, grass
  11. Other home maintenance concerns (e.g., access to fuse box, storm windows, furnace filters, painting)
F. Medications
   1. Large number of prescriptions
   2. Difficulty remembering
   3. Ability to see labels and directions
   4. Medications kept in one area
G. Access to community
   1. Busline
   2. Walking
   3. Driving (by self or by service from others)
   4. Church, dry cleaning agency, drugstore, bank, health care facility, dentist, other community agencies
H. Other
   1. Caring for spouse/relative/companion
   2. Financial management (able to write checks, make payments, cash checks)
   3. Care of pets

From Thompson, J.M., & Bowers, A.C. (1984). *Clinical manual of health assessment* (2nd ed.). St. Louis: C. V. Mosby.

individual's level of social supports. This database provides a framework for an orderly review of the needs at organ, person, and societal levels. These needs are important to the use of skills, the accomplishment of tasks, the fulfillment of social roles, and a satisfactory quality of life.

Functional assessment of the aged patient is a particular concern for nurses, and Granger's model is applicable for evaluating ADL if it is expanded to include instrumental activities, such as housekeeping, taking of medications, arranging of transportation, financial management, and care of pets. Thompson and Bowers (1984) have presented an ADL assessment for geriatric clients that is inclusive of many of the instrumental activities. It is a helpful adjunct for identifying needs of the aged patient (Table 19–1).

The examiner must assess not only the individual's reaction to the impairment or disability but also the effect it has on the individual's performance. Essential components of a functional assessment tool for mobility include (1) determination of any neuromuscular disabilities; (2) evaluation of independence in self-care and mobility; (3) evaluation of social support, including environmental factors (housing, architectural barriers, transportation) and financial resources; (4) evaluation of social interactions and performance of social roles or obligations, psychologic outlook and coping techniques, and support of family or significant others; and (5) evaluation of work or educational training.

Mitchell and Irvin (1977) proposed a model for the neurologic assessment that goes beyond the medical model used to identify and diagnose neurologic dysfunction. The instrument is used to assess the functional abilities of the patient in relation to neurologic status. The instrument is directed specifically at the nurse's primary purpose, which is to determine (1) the presence of neurologic dysfunction and (2) the effect that the dysfunction has on the individual's ability to perform self-care as well as the effect on self-image and safety. The model consists of six functional categories: (1) consciousness, (2) mentation, (3) movement, (4) sensation, (5) regulation, and (6) coping with disability (Mitchell, Ozuna, Cammermeyer, & Woods, 1984). This model is used to focus on the basic assessment of movement of the stable, conscious patient. The integrated functions of seeing, speaking, moving, and walking are fully evaluated (Table 19–2). Because the focus of this examination is primarily on the individual's function in relation to self-care, the cranial nerves (CNs) and motor reflexes are integrated into the functions they serve.

This model does not specifically assess skills and activities, so the Barthel Index, which is a simple index of independence in self-care and mobility, is integrated into the assessment (Mahoney & Barthel, 1965; Mitchell et al., 1984). The Barthel Index (Table 19–3) is a reliable and valid clinical tool for establishing a functional baseline for the patient, monitoring improvement throughout rehabilitation, and identifying the point of maximum benefit therapy. The Barthel Index consists of 10 weighted ADL variables and has a maximum score of 100 for functional competence. The value assigned to each item is determined by

TABLE 19–2 • ASSESSMENT OF MOVEMENT

Functional Category	Anatomic Correlates	Tests
Head		
Seeing (motor aspects)	Oculomotor (III), trochlear (V), and abducens (VI) nerves and brain stem pathways, cerebellum	Extraocular movements
Eating Chewing	Trigeminal (V) and hypoglossal (XII) nerves	Chewing, jaw opening, moving tongue
Swallowing	Glossopharyngeal (IX) and vagal (X) nerves	Swallowing
Expressing	Facial (VII) nerve	Facial movements (eye closing, smile, frown)
Speaking Articulating	Facial (VII), glossopharyngeal (IX), vagal (X), and hypoglossal (XII) nerves and the cerebellum	"Ma," "La," "Ca"
Phonating*	Vagal (X) nerve	Vocal sounds, "Ah," soft palate elevation
Body		
Walking	Cortex, basal ganglia, pyramidal and extrapyramidal systems, cerebellum	Observation of gait—arm swing, rhythm, symmetry, coordination
Activities of daily living	As above	Muscle strength testing, assessment of bulk and tone, observation of movement excesses or deficits (involuntary movements, bradykinesia)
Coordination	Cerebellum	Finger-nose, heel-shin, rapid alternating movements, tandem walking, Romberg's test.

*The above functions involve 8 of the 12 cranial nerves.
From Mitchell, P.H., Ozuna, J. Cammermeyer, M. & Woods, N.F. (Eds.) (1984). *Neurological assessment for nursing practice.* Paramus, NJ: Reston.

TABLE 19–3 • ADAPTATION OF CRITERIA FOR BARTHEL INDEX AS MODIFIED BY THE NEW ENGLAND REHABILITATION HOSPITAL, OCTOBER 1973

Index Item	Description of Functional Ability	Score Weight
Feeding	Independent. Able to apply any necessary device. Feeds in reasonable time.	10
	Needs help (e.g., for cutting).	5
Bathing	Performs without assistance.	5
Personal toilet (grooming)	Washes face, combs hair, brushes teeth, shaves (manages plug if electric razor).	5
Dressing	Independent, ties shoes, fastens fasteners, applies braces.	10
	Needs help but does at least half of task within reasonable time.	5
Bowel control	No accidents. Able to use enema or suppository if needed.	10
	Occasional accidents or needs help with enema or suppository.	5
Bladder control	No accidents. Able to care for collecting device if used.	10
	Occasional accidents or needs help with device.	5
Toilet transfers	Independent with toilet or bedpan. Handles clothes, wipes, flushes or cleans pan.	10
	Needs help for balance, handling clothes or toilet paper.	5
Chair-bed transfers	Independent, including locks of wheelchair and lifting footrests.	15
	Minimum assistance or supervision.	10
	Able to sit but needs maximum assistance to transfer.	5
Ambulation	Independent for 50 yards. May use assistive devices, except for rolling walker.	15
	With help for 50 yards.	10
	Independent with wheelchair for 50 yards, only if unable to walk.	5
Stair climbing	Independent. May use assistive devices.	10
	Needs help or supervision.	5
Total score		

From Granger, C.V., Demis, L.S., Peters, N.C., Sherwood, C.C., & Barrett, I.E. (1979). Stroke rehabilitation: Analysis of repeated Barthel index measures. *Archives of Physical Medicine and Rehabilitation, 60*, 14.

the amount of help given in self-care activities and mobility if the person is unable to perform the activity unassisted. The patient's ability to perform each activity is scored, and the 10 items are tallied. The index is a beneficial adjunct for periodic assessment of self-care activities, such as feeding, bathing, personal toilet, bowel and bladder control, and mobility, such as transfers, ambulation, and stair climbing. A major disadvantage to those with a holistic approach to nursing is that the Barthel Index does not include psychosocial or environmental factors. It has, however, been stressed that the evaluator should recognize that these factors can have an effect on the client's score. Any psychosocial or special requirements should be documented, because they can cause a lower score—for example, if the bathroom door is not wide enough for easy access by wheelchair.

For purposes of this discussion, three essential elements for mobility are required: (1) the ability to move (an intact neuromuscular system or compensated movement), (2) the motivation to move, and (3) a free, nonrestrictive environment in which to move. A workable framework for assessing mobility would include (1) the physical dimensions of mobility (voluntary, involuntary, and compensated) related to functional ability, (2) the psychosocial dimension (motivational aspects), and (3) the environmental dimension (assessment of the environment for barriers, assistive devices, and ease of passive movement).

PHYSICAL DIMENSION OF MOBILITY

The assessment should begin with gathering of pertinent health history data. Biographic data, such as age, are important parameters, because some neurologic disorders occur most commonly within certain age groups. For example, Parkinson's disease occurs most commonly in people older than 40 years. Family history is important, because some neurologic disorders may be inherited, and a genogram may be helpful to fully visualize the family history. Other helpful history data regarding musculoskeletal and neurologic function, nutritional status, and cardiopulmonary status should be assessed (Table 19–4). The variations in the neuromuscular assessment for children from birth to 6 years will be discussed at the completion of the discussion of the physical dimension.

Equipment needed for the examination includes (1) tape measure, (2) goniometer (optional), (3) percussion hammer, (4) Snellen's chart or reading material, (5) penlight, (6) cotton swab, and (7) tongue depressor. An overall screening examination of neurologic function can be conducted in approximately 5 minutes if no abnormalities are identified (Table 19–5). This is invaluable in assessing functional abilities as well as dysfunction and its location.

If abnormalities in movement are identified, a thorough mobility assessment is needed. The examination proceeds in a systematic head-to-toe fashion, focusing on the integrated functions of seeing, eating and speaking, and moving and walking (see Table 19–2).

Seeing

The sensory components of seeing (pupillary response, visual acuity, and visual fields) are described in Chapter 23. For practical reasons, they are examined at the same time as are the motor components.

Extraocular muscle function is tested by examination of corneal light reflex, cover-uncover test, and assessment of six cardinal fields of gaze. To test the client's corneal light reflex, the examiner stands in front of the client and shines a penlight, held 12 to 15 in away, between the eyes. The bright dot reflected on the cornea should be located in the same spot on each eye, indicating a symmetrical reflex. If there is an asymmetrical reflex, a muscular imbalance could be causing the deviating eye.

TABLE 19–4 • HISTORY DATA

Parameter	Data
Musculoskeletal function	Past or present problems with muscle strength, tone, reflexes, range of motion, motility, muscle control, or physical endurance.
	Perceptual-motor problems: soft signs, such as clumsiness, impaired fine motor coordination, increased or decreased general activity or level of minimal brain dysfunction, hyperkinesis, learning disability.
	Activity level.
	Aids.
	Safety factors related to age or impaired mobility. Assistance required in activities of daily living.
	Description of current muscular impairment or limitation in range of motion.
	Current medications that interfere with or enhance muscular functions.
	Special needs related to age or impaired functions.
Nervous system	Past or current problems with intellectual functions, sensation, movement, or pain.
	Past or present problem that was inherited or in other family members.
	Communication and speech patterns.
	Special needs related to age or disease process.
Cardiovascular functions	Activity endurance or fatigability.
	Medications used that enhance or inhibit cardiovascular functions.
Respiratory functions	Past or present respiratory problems.
	Shortness of breath (precipitating factors, frequency, measures that relieve symptoms, and effect on activities of daily living).
	Medications used that enhance or inhibit respiratory function.
Nutritional patterns	Evaluate adequacy and intake of basic four food groups and liquids.
	Special needs related to disease or age.

From Conway-Rutkowski, B.L. (1982). *Carini & Owen's neurological and neurosurgical nursing* (8th ed.), St. Louis: C.V. Mosby.

TABLE 19–5 • SCREENING EXAMINATION OF NEUROLOGIC FUNCTION*

Examination Stimulus	Function or System Tested
Observe gait, symmetry	Motor, cerebellar, position sense
Ask: Why are you here? Has your ability to take care of yourself changed?	Perception, expectations, orientation, self-care to change, coping
Read headline, tell meaning, recall later	Seeing, recall, language
Take glass of water, swallow, hand back to examiner (or any act across midline, with three components)	Swallow, right-left orientation, concentration, sensory, coordination
Dress or undress	Motor, sensory, cerebellar
Simultaneously observe language, eye movement	Language, seeing

*If no abnormality is present, this entire examination can be performed in 5 minutes.

From Mitchell, P.H., Ozuna, J., Cammermeyer, M., & Woods, N.F. (Eds.). (1984). *Neurological assessment for nursing practice*. Paramus, NJ: Reston.

The cover-uncover test is used to evaluate the client's ability to maintain parallel gaze, which is essential for binocular vision. The examiner asks the client to gaze at a specific point. The left eye is covered with an opaque card, and the examiner observes the right eye to see if it moves to fixate on the object. If it does move, it was not in straight alignment. The left eye is then uncovered, and if it jerks into position to again rest on the object, the eye has drifted while resting. This is usually indicative of a muscular imbalance.

The movement of the eyes through the six cardinal fields of gaze is assessed with the examiner being certain to direct the eyes to the extremes of each field. The examiner asks the client to follow with the eyes the tip of a pen or a penlight. Nystagmus or abnormal eye movement should be noted.

Eating and Speaking

These integrated functions require the same intact structure of the peripheral nervous system for normal functioning. For articulation, the facial (seventh), glossopharyngeal (ninth), vagal (10th), and hypoglossal (12th) CNs and the cerebellum must be intact. For chewing and swallowing, these nerves and the trigeminal (fifth) nerve must be intact. If a client articulates, chews, and swallows without difficulty, it can be assumed that these nerves are intact. If any difficulties are noted, the various parameters of speech and ingestion must be evaluated to determine the CN precipitating the dysfunction. Each CN can be individually assessed by evaluating the results of various tests.

FIFTH CRANIAL NERVE

The motor component of the fifth CN (trigeminal) serves the muscles of mastication. To test this nerve, the examiner asks the client to clench all teeth and then palpates the masseter and temporal muscles bilaterally, noting symmetry and strength. Absent or weak contractions of the masseter and temporal muscles may indicate a lesion of the fifth CN. Bilateral weakness may result from upper and lower motor neuron involvement. (The absence of teeth obviously complicates interpretation of this test.) To observe symmetry and strength of the pterygoid muscles, the examiner asks the client to open the mouth slightly and press the jaw laterally against the examiner's hand. Any atrophy or deviation of the jaw to one side is rated, and deviation indicates that the muscles of the jaw on the side to which it deviates are stronger than those on the opposite side. Movement will be noted to the opposite side of the paralysis or weakness, not to the paralyzed side.

SEVENTH CRANIAL NERVE

The seventh CN (facial) is the motor component that innervates the facial muscles bilaterally. A sensory component to the taste perception of the anterior two thirds of the tongue is also part of the facial nerve.

To assess the function of the seventh CN, the examiner should inspect the face for symmetry at rest and during conversation. The client is asked to raise the eyebrows, frown, and then close both eyes tightly while the examiner tries to open them. The client is then instructed to show teeth, smile, and puff out the cheeks to assess facial muscle strength, symmetry, or abnormal movements. Muscle weakness may be indicated by drooping of one side of the mouth, flattening of the nasolabial folds, or laxity of the lower eyelid.

NINTH AND TENTH CRANIAL NERVES

The ninth (glossopharyngeal) and 10th (vagus) CNs are clinically tested as a unit, because they are closely related both anatomically and physiologically and are similar in function. The motor component of the ninth CN innervates the stylopharyngeus muscle used in swallowing; and the sensory fibers innervate the mucous membranes of the pharynx, posterior one third of the tongue, middle ear, and eustachian tube. The motor fibers of the 10th CN innervate the pharynx, larynx, palate, and thoracic and abdominal visceral organs. The sensory fibers of the vagus innervate the heart, lungs, and aortic bodies.

The client is assessed for any hoarseness or nasal speech. The soft palate is inspected for symmetry or any deviation. The client is asked to say "Ah," with the examiner noting if the palate rises symmetrically. Unilateral weakness is indicated by drooping of the palate on the affected side. The palate fails to rise at all if a bilateral lesion of the 10th CN is present. To assess the palatal reflex, the mucous membrane of the soft palate is stroked with a cotton swab, and the stroked side should rise promptly. When the posterior pharyngeal wall is touched with a tongue depressor or cotton swab to elicit the gag reflex, the palate should elevate and the pharyngeal muscles should contract. This reflex may be diminished or absent in some normal people.

Swallowing is assessed by giving the client a glass of water and requesting that the client take a few sips. The examiner observes the swallowing, noting any abnormalities. Ice chips can be used if there is any concern that swallowing may be impaired.

TWELFTH CRANIAL NERVE

The 12th CN (hypoglossal) is responsible for normal tongue movements involved in speech and swallowing. The examiner inspects the tongue for size, symmetry, and fasciculations in its resting state. Then the client is asked to stick out the tongue; it should be midline without deviating to one side and should be devoid of fasciculations. A tongue blade is pressed against one side of the tongue to assess muscle strength; then the other side is assessed. Rapid alternating movements, such as moving the tongue rapidly in and out and from side to side, are assessed for symmetry. Diminished or slowed alternating movements may be caused by upper motor neuron disease.

The seventh, ninth, 10th, and 12th CNs must be intact for speaking. If the individual articulates clearly and without difficulty, the CNs are intact. If an abnormality is noted, a more detailed examination must be performed to determine which sounds are abnormal. If a deficit is noted in any of these sounds, the related CN should be evaluated (Mitchell et al., 1984, p. 45).

Abnormality	Cranial Nerve
Disrupted labial sounds ("mee, bee")	Seven
Disrupted lingual sounds ("la")	Twelve
Disrupted guttural sounds ("ka, ga")	Nine and Ten
Hoarseness	Ten
Nasal speech	Ten

Moving and Walking

Six areas to observe closely when assessing motor function, excluding the face, are (1) posture, (2) muscle coordination, (3) muscle mass and tone, (4) muscle strength, (5) reflexes, and (6) abnormal movements.

The presence or absence of movement, as well as the quality of movement, is always assessed, and motor responses in symmetrical body parts are compared. When interpreting findings, the examiner must consider alterations as a result of age or unrelated disease or injury.

POSTURE AND MUSCLE COORDINATION

In assessing gait and posture, movement of body parts, symmetry of gait, stance, cadence, steadiness of movement, coordination, and type of steps taken if gait is abnormal must all be noted. If possible, the client should be observed walking, sitting in a chair, or performing ADL without the client's being aware of the observation. The need for assistive devices should be determined. The client is asked to walk heel to toe in a straight line and to walk on the toes and then on the heels. The ability to do this is impaired in cerebellar disease.

Coordination is further assessed in the lower extremities by (1) rapid rhythmic alternating movements, such as tapping the examiner's hand with the ball of the foot alternately, and (2) point-to-point testing, in which the client places the foot on the opposite knee and slides it down that shin to the great toe. Note any slowness, hesitation, or awkwardness with both maneuvers.

MUSCLE MASS, TONE, AND STRENGTH

The examiner first inspects muscle mass, comparing symmetrical body parts, and then flexes and extends upper and lower extremities bilaterally to assess tone and resistance to movement. Muscle rigidity or spasticity is noted as increased muscle tone or increased resistance. Decreased resistance denotes decreased muscle tone or flaccidity.

To assess muscle strength of the major muscle groups, the examiner puts them through the normal range of motion, initially against gravity and then against active resistance. The strength of muscles is graded 5 to 0 based on the following standard scale:

Grade	Strength
5	Full range of motion against normal resistance and gravity
4	Full range of motion against moderate resistance and gravity
3	Full range of motion against gravity only
2	Full range of motion with gravity eliminated
1	Slight muscle contraction palpable, but no movement noted
0	No visible or palpable contraction; paralysis of limb

Generally, the person is considered to have a disability if muscle strength is rated below grade 3.

REFLEXES AND ABNORMAL MOVEMENTS

Assessment of reflexes includes both superficial reflexes, graded 0 to 1+ (absent or present), and deep tendon reflexes, graded 0 to 3+.

Superficial Reflex Grades

0	Absent
±	Barely present
1+	Normally active

Deep Tendon Reflex Grades

0	Absent
1+	Present but diminished
2+	Normal; increased but not necessarily pathologic
3+	Hyperactive with or without clonus present

Superficial and deep tendon reflexes give the examiner information about upper motor neuron function and lower motor neuron function, respectively. The muscle groups that innervate specific reflexes are shown in Tables 19–6 and 19–7.

Superficial reflexes are elicited by stroking the superficial skin surface with a dull object—for example, a tongue depressor. Deep tendon reflexes are elicited by applying a brisk stimulus with the reflex hammer to a partially stretched tendon, bone, or joint. Reflexes should be symmetrical.

After the physical examination, the client's overall motor function should be described quantitatively. The focus is then directed to how the client's impairments are reflected in ADL.

The nurse must be cognizant of the nursing framework for neuromuscular examination focusing on movement. With this combined framework, the nurse is able to determine nervous system dysfunction, alterations in ADL, safety, self-concept, and coping behaviors. Based on the initial history and the physical examination, specific nursing diagnoses should be stated. Examples of alterations in movement based on the Mitchell et al. (1984) model include the following:

1. Impaired verbal communication related to impaired articulation

2. Impaired swallowing related to alteration in gag and swallowing reflex

TABLE 19–6 • SUPERFICIAL REFLEXES

Reflex	CNS Level	Test and Response
Upper abdominal	Thoracic 7, 8, 9	Test: The client lies supine. With the handle of the reflex hammer, the examiner strokes the skin from the upper abdominal quadrants toward the umbilicus, observing the movement of the umbilicus. Normal response: Umbilicus moves up and toward area being stroked. Slight abdominal muscle contraction observable.
Lower abdominal	Thoracic 11, 12	Test: The client lies supine. With the handle end of the reflex hammer, the examiner strokes the skin from the lower abdominal quadrants toward the umbilicus, observing the movement of the umbilicus. Normal response: Umbilicus moves down and toward area being stroked. Slight abdominal muscle contraction observable.
Cremasteric (males)	Thoracic 12 Lumbar 1, 2	Test: With the client supine, the examiner strokes the medial side of the upper thigh, using the handle end of the reflex hammer. Normal response: Contraction of the cremaster muscle, which pulls the scrotal sac upward on the side stroked.
Gluteal	Sacral 3, 4, 5	Test: With the client lying prone, the examiner separates the buttocks and strokes the perianal skin with the handle end of the reflex hammer. Normal response: Contraction of the external and anal sphincter muscles.
Plantar	Sacral 1, 2	Test: The examiner runs the handle end of the reflex hammer from the heel of the foot up the lateral border of the sole, turning medially and going across the ball of the foot underneath the great toe. Normal response: Flexion of the toes. Before the age when a child walks, the normal response is extension and fanning of the toes.

CNS, central nervous system.

From Fields, W.L., & McGinn-Campbell, K.M. (1983). *Introduction to health assessment* (p. 176). Paramus, NJ: Reston.

TABLE 19–7 • DEEP TENDON REFLEXES

Reflex	CNS Level	Test and Response
Biceps	Cervical 5, 6 (primarily C5)	Test: The examiner places the client's arm over the opposite forearm and holds client's elbow. The client is instructed to relax the arm completely. The examiner places the thumb at the insertion of the biceps tendon superior to the antecubital fossa and taps the thumbnail with the narrow rubber end of the reflex hammer. Normal response: Contraction of the biceps muscle, resulting in slight flexion of the forearm at the elbow joint. Normally, the examiner sees or feels a slight jerk of the biceps muscle.
Triceps	Cervical 6, 7, 8 (primarily C7)	Test: The examiner supports the client's arm in the same manner used to test the biceps reflex. The examiner taps at the insertion of the triceps tendon superior to the olecranon with the narrow rubber end of the reflex hammer. Normal response: Contraction of the triceps muscle, resulting in extension of the arm at the elbow joint.
Patellar	Lumbar 2, 3, 4 (primarily L4)	Test: The examiner instructs the client to sit on the edge of the examining table with the legs dangling free, palpates the soft tissue depression on both sides of the patellar tendon, and taps the tendon with the flat rubber end of the reflex hammer. Normal response: Contraction of the quadriceps muscle, resulting in extension of the leg at the knee joint.
Achilles	Sacral 1, 2 (primarily S1)	Test: With the client sitting on the edge of the table with the legs dangling, the examiner dorsiflexes the foot slightly. The insertion of the Achilles tendon is located by palpating the soft-tissue depressions on both sides of it. The tendon is then tapped with the flat rubber end of the reflex hammer. Normal response: Contraction of the triceps surae muscle, resulting in planter flexion of the foot.

CNS, central nervous system.

From Fields, W.L., & McGinn-Campbell, K.M. (1983). *Introduction to health assessment* (p. 174). Paramus, NJ: Reston.

3. Impaired physical mobility related to neuromuscular impairment, intolerance to activity, perceptual or cognitive impairment, or pain and discomfort

4. Dressing or grooming self-care deficit related to neuromuscular and musculoskeletal disorder

5. Self-evaluation of self-concept, body image, self-esteem, role performance, and personal identity

6. Ineffective individual coping related to situational crises, inadequate support systems, and verbalization of inability to cope (North American Nursing Diagnosis Association, 1999).

Special Considerations for Infants and Children

The neuromuscular assessment of children from birth to 6 years necessitates a careful and accurate evaluation of neuromuscular status and neuromuscular progress and skills. A critical component of newborn assessment focuses on evaluation of the infant for actual or potential impairments of physical mobility.

The assessment of the physical dimension of the client and the family is essentially the same with the following modifications and additions, as well as with modifications for the child's level of understanding.

The newborn is carefully inspected, and gestational age is established (Bellack, 1992). The Dubowitz Clinical Assessment is a standardized scale useful in evaluating the neonate's gestational age within 48 hours of birth, based on 11 physical characteristics and 10 neuromuscular signs (Table 19–8) (Dubowitz, Dubowitz, & Goldberg, 1970).

The infant's fetal growth pattern and size for gestational age are then determined using standard intrauterine growth curves. The infant is then classified as small, appropriate, or large for gestational age by percentile curve placement for weeks of gestation (Seidel, Ball, Dains, & Benedict, 1992, p. 67). Infants are classified as follows:

Classification	Weight Percentiles
Appropriate for gestational age	10th to 90th
Small for gestational age	<10th
Large for gestational age	>90th

An increased incidence of morbidity and mortality is associated with infants who are large or small for gestational age. Being either preterm or postterm further increases the infant's risks (Seidel et al., 1992).

The infant is further assessed for the musculoskeletal abnormalities of congenital clubfoot and congenital hip dysplasia and for evidence of injury to the musculoskeletal system during birth, such as fracture of the clavicle.

An evaluation of the newborn's reflexes (Table 19–9) and the infant's response to painful stimuli is for assessment of neurologic functioning. Absence of a reflex may be due to abnormality of the central or peripheral motor functions, whereas persistence of a reflex may be due to a lesion of the central nervous system or a developmental delay (Behrman, Kliegman, Nelson, & Vaughn, 1991). The method for neonatal reflex testing is described in Table 19–9, as are the normal and abnormal responses.

A withdrawal of all limbs from painful stimuli, such as a light pinprick to hands and feet, provides a measure of sensory integrity. This tests the intactness of peripheral pain fibers and pathways to the thalamus (Behrman et al., 1991; Seidel et al., 1992). Other aspects of sensory function are not routinely tested.

There may also be some unexpected findings in the school-age child that would be normal in the younger child. These neurologic soft signs are nonfocal, functional neurologic findings that often provide subtle clues to an underlying central nervous system deficit or a neurologic maturation delay. Soft signs can be found

TABLE 19–8A • SCORING SYSTEM OF PHYSICAL AND NEUROLOGIC SIGNS FOR ASSESSMENT OF GESTATIONAL AGE*

External Sign	0	1	2	3	4
Edema	Obvious edema of hands and feet, pitting over tibia	No obvious edema of hands and feet, pitting over tibia	No edema		
Skin texture	Very thin, gelatinous	Thin and smooth	Smooth, medium thickness. Rash or superficial peeling	Slight thickening, superficial cracking and peeling, especially of hands and feet	Thick and parchmentlike, superficial or deep cracking
Skin color	Dark red	Uniformly pink	Pale pink, variable over body	Pale pink only over ears, lips, palms, or soles	
Skin opacity (trunk)	Numerous veins and venules clearly seen, especially over abdomen	Veins and tributaries seen	A few large vessels seen clearly over abdomen	A few large vessels seen indistinctly over abdomen	No blood vessels seen
Lanugo (over back)	No lanugo	Abundant, long and thick over whole back	Hair thinning especially over lower back	Small amount lanugo and bald areas	At least half of back devoid of lanugo
Plantar creases	No skin creases	Faint red marks over anterior half of sole	Definite red marks over >anterior half, indentations over <anterior third	Indentations over >anterior third	Definite deep indentations over >anterior third
Nipple formation	Nipple barely visible, no areola	Nipple well defined, areola smooth and flat, diameter <0.75 cm	Areola stippled, edge not raised, diameter <0.75 cm	Areola stippled, edge raised, diameter >0.75 cm	
Breast size	No breast tissue palpable	Breast tissue on one or both sides, <0.5 cm diameter	Breast tissue both sides, one or both 0.5–1 cm	Breast tissue both sides; one or both >1 cm	
Ear form	Pinna flat and shapeless, little or no incurving of edge	Incurving of part of edge of pinna	Partial incurving whole of upper pinna	Well-defined incurving whole of upper pinna	
Ear firmness	Pinna soft, easily folded, no recoil	Pinna soft, easily folded, slow recoil	Cartilage to edge of pinna, but soft in places, ready recoil	Pinna firm, cartilage to edge, instant	
Male genitals	Neither testis in scrotum	At least one testis high in scrotum	At least one testis		
Female genitals (with hips half abducted)	Labia majora widely separated, labia minora protruding	Labia majora almost cover labia minora	Labia majora completely cover labia minora		

*Follow directions for assessment of each of the 11 external signs and assign a score.

TABLE 19–8B • GESTATIONAL AGE IN WEEKS FOR SUM OF SCORES*

Total Score	Weeks of Gestation	Total Score	Weeks of Gestation
0–9	26	40–43	35
10–12	27	44–46	36
13–16	28	47–50	37
17–20	29	51–54	38
21–24	30	55–58	39
25–27	31	59–62	40
28–31	32	63–65	41
32–35	33	66–69	42
36–39	34		

*Add the scores from the signs and compare the total with this table to determine the neonate's gestational age in weeks. Note the age of the neonate at the time of assessment.
From Seidel, H., Ball, J., Dains, J., & Benedict, G. (1992). *Mosby's guide to physical examination* (2nd ed., pp. 66–67). St. Louis: Mosby–Year Book.

in gross motor, fine motor, sensory, and reflex functional areas. Table 19–10 describes neurologic soft sign findings and the age at which you should become concerned if still present. Children with multiple soft signs are often found to have learning problems (Seidel et al., 1992, p. 670).

A comprehensive plan of care for the infant or child and the family necessitates a full assessment of the child and the family members to determine what concerns they have about the child's neuromuscular and developmental status. They should also be asked to fully describe their concerns, what problems they anticipate, and the factors that make the problem better or worse. The assessment should accomplish the following:

1. Validate that the child is developing normally or detect problems early
2. Provide an opportunity to plan appropriate anticipatory guidance and counseling for the child and the parents
3. Help the parents understand the child's behavior
4. Identify the child's fears and concerns
5. Foster optimal development (Sperhac, 1990, p. 432)

A practical plan for screening infants, toddlers, and preschoolers is recommended for early identification of children with developmental delays (Fig. 19–3). Procedures recommended are based on age, risk, and previous developmental screening.

The Prescreening Developmental Questionnaire (PDQII) is a 105-item questionnaire that is written at the sixth-grade reading level. The tool is administered at home or in the waiting room by the parents. Research has shown that parents with a high school education accurately report the child's developmental status with this tool (Frankenburg, 1992).

If one delay is identified, a rescreening with the PDQII is recommended 1 month later with age-appropriate activities recommended. If one or more

TABLE 19–9 • NEONATAL REFLEXES*

Reflex	Method of Eliciting Reflex from Infant	Normal Response	Abnormal Response
Rooting	Stroke cheek near corner of mouth.	Head turns toward side being stroked, and sucking movements appear.	Persistence beyond 12 months.
Sucking	Place examiner's finger or nipple in infant's mouth.	Rhythmic sucking movements; usually disappears 3–4 months; best noted in a hungry infant.	Persistence as a reflex beyond 12 months.
Extrusion	Touch tip of tongue.	Tongue pushes out of mouth.	Persistence beyond 4 months.
Grasp palmar	Place examiner's finger in palm of infant's hand.	Fingers flex around examiner's hand; becomes voluntary about 6 months.	Persistence beyond 6 months as an involuntary response.
Grasp plantar	Place examiner's finger on sole of infant's foot at base of toes.	Toes flex toward examiner's finger.	Absent in defects of lower spine (meningomyelocele); persistence beyond 8–12 months.
Stepping (dancing)	Hold infant in vertical position with soles of feet lightly touching firm surface.	Flexion and extension of alternate legs as though to simulate walking movements.	Persistence beyond 6 weeks.
Babinski's reflex	With fingertip, stroke lateral aspect of sole of foot from midpoint at heel, forward and across the ball of the foot to the great toe.	Great toe flexes dorsally while remaining toes fan outward.	Persistence beyond 12–18 months.
Tonic neck	Quickly turn head to left or right.	Extension of arm and leg on side to which face is turned. Opposite arm and leg flex.	Continuous posturing; persistence beyond 46 months.
Moro	Hold in supine position. Permit head to fall back about 3 in, taking care not to cause too great an extension.	Extension and abduction of arms. Extension and fanning of fingers, except thumb and forefinger, which form a ''C'' shape. Legs flex and adduct.	Persistence beyond 4 months.
Startle	Clap hands loudly.	Arms abduct and flex at elbows; hands are clenched.	Persistence beyond 4 months.
Landau	Suspend in horizontal prone position with head raised actively or passively.	Appears about 4–6 months; lifts head, extends legs and spine.	Absence may signify cerebral palsy; exaggerated in hypertonic infants; persistence beyond 12–24 months.
Parachute	Hold under armpits in vertical position. Move body downward at head-first angle.	Appears about 7–9 months; arms extend in a protective motion.	Absence may signify cerebral palsy.

*One unsuccessful attempt at eliciting the reflex does not mean the reflex is not present. Absence, depression, or asymmetry of response may signal neurological deficit.

From Bellack, J., & Edlund, B. (Eds.) (1992). *Nursing assessment and diagnosis* (2nd ed., p. 421). Sudbury, MA: Jones & Bartlett.

TABLE 19–10 • ACTIVITIES FOR EVALUATING NEUROLOGIC SOFT SIGNS IN CHILDREN, THE ASSOCIATED SOFT SIGN, AND THE AGE AT WHICH THE FINDING SHOULD NO LONGER BE OBSERVED

Activity	Soft Sign Findings	Latest Expected Age of Disappearance (yr)
Walking, running gait	Stiff-legged with a foot-slapping quality, unusual posturing of the arms	3
Heel walking	Difficulty remaining on heels for distance of 10 ft	7
Tiptoe walking	Difficulty remaining on toes for a distance of 10 ft	7
Tandem gait	Difficulty walking heel to toe, unusual posturing of arms	7
One-foot standing	Unable to remain standing on one foot longer than 5–10 sec	5
Stopping in place	Unable to rhythmically hop on each foot	6
Motor stance	Difficulty maintaining stance (arms extended in front, feet together, and eyes closed), drifting of arms, mild writhing movements of hands or fingers	3
Visual tracking	Difficulty following object with eyes when keeping the head still, nystagmus	5
Rapid thumb-to-finger test	Rapid touching of thumb to fingers in sequence is uncoordinated, unable to suppress mirror movements in contralateral hand	8
Rapid alternating movements of hands	Irregular speed and rhythm with pronation and supination of hands patting the knees	10
Finger-nose test	Unable to alternately touch examiner's finger and own nose consecutively	7
Right-left discrimination	Unable to identify right and left sides of own body	5
Two-point discrimination	Difficulty localizing and discriminating when touched in one or two places	6
Graphesthesia	Unable to identify geometric shapes drawn in child's open hand	8
Stereognosis	Unable to identify common objects in own hand	5

delays are noted on rescreening, the client is referred for screening with the Denver II test. If two delays are noted, the client is referred for the Denver II with age-appropriate activities suggested.

The Denver II test is a standardized tool that screens for developmental problems in children from birth to 6 years (Frankenburg et al., 1992a, 1992b). The four areas tested are as follows:

1. Personal-social: Getting along with people and caring for personal needs

2. Fine motor-adaptive: Eye-hand coordination, manipulation of small objects, and problem solving

3. Language: Hearing, understanding, and using language

4. Gross motor: Sitting, walking, jumping, and overall large muscle movement (Frankenburg et al., 1992a, 1992b)

Complete instructions for administering and scoring the Denver II test are available in the *Denver II Screening Manual* (Frankenburg et al., 1992a, 1992b). The test results are interpreted as noted in Figure 19–4.

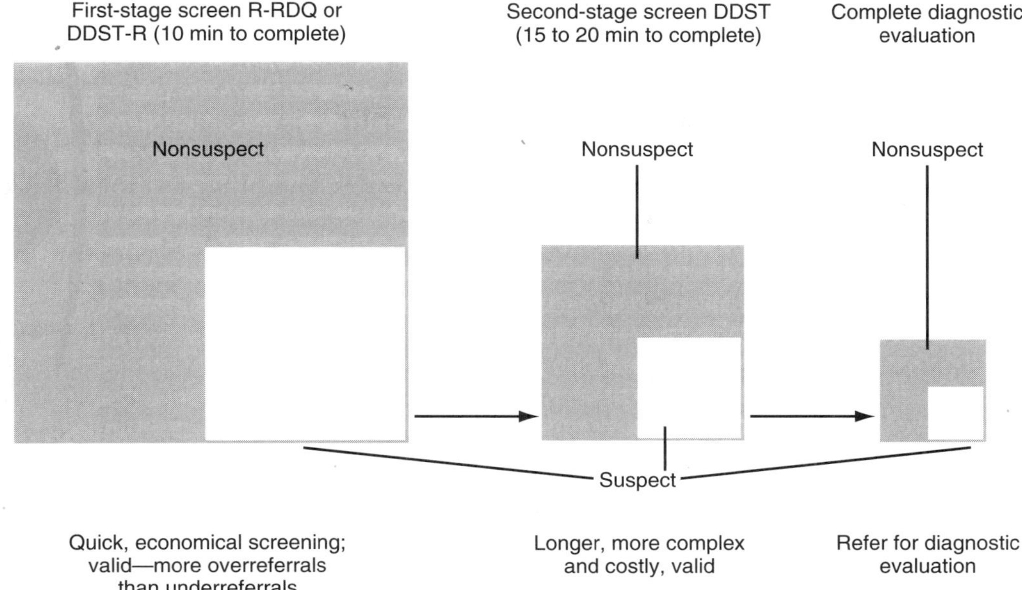

FIGURE 19–3 • Two-stage screening process. (Adapted from Blackman, J.A. [1992]. Developmental assessment: Infant and preschool developmental screening. In M.D. Levine, W.B. Carey, & A.C. Crocker [Eds.], *Developmental behavioral pediatrics* [p. 31]. Philadelphia: W.B. Saunders.)

NORMAL
  No delays and a maximum of one caution.
  Conduct routine rescreening at next well-child visit.

ABNORMAL
  Two or more delays.
  Refer for diagnostic evaluation.

QUESTIONABLE
  One delay or two or more cautions, or both.
  Offer the parent suggestions on improving the child's knowledge or skills in delay or caution areas, and rescreen in 3
    months or at the next well-child visit, whichever comes first. If, on rescreen, the child's score is again questionable
    or has become abnormal, refer for diagnostic evaluation.

UNTESTABLE
  Interpret depending on the number of refusals that would be delays or cautions if scored failures.
  If the test would be abnormal, rescreen in 2 to 3 weeks. If the rescreen is also untestable abnormal, refer for diagnostic
    evaluation. If return for rescreen is unlikely, refer directly to diagnostic evaluation.
  If the test would be questionable, follow-up is the same as for questionable, above.

REFERRAL CRITERIA
  Although initial referral criteria might be those listed above, the final criteria for referral must be determined locally on
    the basis of everything one knows about the child and local eligibility for various types of services.

FIGURE 19–4 • Denver II test interpretation.

Assessment data obtained regarding neuromuscular status, developmental progress, and skills are analyzed, and nursing diagnoses are identified. Some possible diagnoses are as follows:

1. Altered growth and development related to effects of disability

2. Impaired physical mobility related to decreased muscle strength or limited range of motion

PSYCHOSOCIAL DIMENSION OF MOBILITY

Humans are unique, biopsychosocial beings in constant interaction with the changing environment. To cope with the environment, humans use various mechanisms to maintain homeostasis. The ease of adaptation or ability to cope depends on one's individual characteristics, the influence of others in the environment, and other available resources, such as support systems, finances, and so on.

Because the ability to move about in the environment is so intricately related to all our activities and to perception of self, a functional assessment of mobility would be incomplete without a full understanding of the psychosocial dimension of the individual. Movement not only provides a way for us to express ourselves but also facilitates the attainment of our goals and life pursuits.

Psychosocial aspects, focusing on the motivation to move, are integrated into the overall assessment as follows: (1) self-perception and self-concept patterns; (2) individual strengths and weaknesses; (3) coping patterns, including independency and dependency needs; (4) available support systems; and (5) emotional and social adjustment.

Self-Concept and Self-Perception

Smitherman (1981) stated that self-concept is never static: "Throughout life it is continually changing, being altered and expanded to adapt to changes of the self and changes in the environment" (p. 338). She suggested that self-concept consists of three components: (1) the existential self, (2) the physical self, and (3) the psychologic self. The existential is the most basic of the three components and can be stated as "I exist," or "I am." The physical self correlates with body image and focuses on the "individual's conscious and unconscious beliefs and thoughts about his [or her] body—external and internal" (Smitherman, 1981, p. 337). This might be stated by the individual as "I am short," or "I am male." The third component, the psychologic self, focuses on attitudes the individual holds pertaining to self, such as "I am intelligent," or "I am organized."

People with an alteration in mobility are often confronted with an alteration in self-concept. "The [client's] psychological self may be threatened ('Can I master this?'), his [or her] physical self ('Is my body intact?'), or his [or her] very existence ('Will I survive?')'' (Smitherman, 1981, p. 337). This offers a unique challenge to the nurse to recognize threats to the self-concept and assist the individual to adapt to changes.

Smitherman (1981) also categorized into three areas various events that have the potential for altering one's self-concept. She stated that changes can occur because of altered appearance, functioning, or control. Because each individual attaches special significance to the physical appearance of the self, it is difficult to predict how an individual will respond to a change in body image. Changes can be sudden or chronic, temporary or permanent, visible to others or easily camouflaged. The individual's response to this threat will depend on individual strengths and weaknesses, the meaning attached to appearance, and others' reactions to altered appearance. The face, especially the eyes, is usually identified as the most significant aspect of self in relation to physical appearance (Smitherman, 1981).

In addition to altered appearance, events can lead to altered function, which can have an effect on an individual's self-concept. This altered function may be an actual event, or it could be a perceived change. Either way, it will threaten the individual's self-concept and can lead to anxiety, frustration, and decreased self-esteem. The client with Parkinson's disease has an altered appearance—for example, masklike facial expression, akinesia, and loss of posture control. The perception of self, as well as the perception the person believes others hold, can have a profound effect on the self-concept. The person with Parkinson's disease experiences altered function because of difficulty ambulating, change in gait, and tremors. This alteration in mobility may affect the individual's self-concept, leading to a change in the psychologic self.

Information about the client with an alteration in function should include (1) the typical daily schedule with the usual health status and with the current problem, (2) assistance required in ADL, and (3) the effect that illness as a problem has on pursuit of life goals, ADL, and ability to support oneself.

Some events may cause the individual to experience altered control of the body, thus creating a threat to the self-concept. In our normal daily routine, we perform many activities without consciously thinking about them. With an illness or mobility problem, the individual focuses energy on the problem and its effect on ADL. This often causes the individual to focus on body changes that can be threatening to the self-concept. Information related to altered control includes (1) ideal versus real roles, (2) usual methods for coping with stress, (3) effectiveness of coping technique, (4) level of independence in ADL, and (5) priority setting and goals. Alterations in appearance, function, and control can thus occur singly or in any combination. When two alterations occur, it is more problematic for the client. The nurse must be aware of this and assist the client in coping with the changes.

Individual Strengths and Weaknesses

People are motivated by specific goals to meet basic needs and to develop to the fullest potential. An understanding of the relationship between basic needs and motivation theory, along with their impact on ADL, is essential to understanding the psychosocial dimension.

Maslow's (1970) hierarchy of basic human needs assists the nurse in identification of the psychologic parameters affecting mobility. This list of basic needs includes physiologic, safety, love, esteem, and self-actualization needs. They usually emerge in that order when lower-level needs have been gratified. Gratification of needs has an important role in motivation of the individual.

In limited or absent mobility, the individual is placed in a dependent and somewhat vulnerable position because of reliance on another for such basic physiologic needs as food and water, elimination, activity, and exercise. Mobility can also have an effect on safety and security needs. The person may feel vulnerable and insecure if unable to protect himself or herself from threatening physical and psychologic situations in the environment. Changes in roles and expectations can occur as a result of impaired mobility, leading to an alteration in established patterns of social interaction with family and friends. The role changes often lead to insecurity because the stability of past patterns has been altered. A regression to an infantile state, accompanied by ego regression, may be noted.

Alterations in physical abilities and appearance may lead to fear of rejection by significant others and may hinder fulfillment of love and belonging needs. According to Maslow (1970), we all have a need or tendency to flock together or belong to a group. Lack of fulfillment of this need can have a profound effect on self-worth as a self-perception, including self-concept and body image. The individual's sense of value and usefulness may be diminished.

Self-actualization needs are dependent on meeting all lower-level needs successfully. Because impairment in mobility can hamper achievement of lower-level needs, self-actualization may not be achieved. The nurse's goal is to help the individual develop to her or his full potential by assisting in the fulfillment of needs.

Coping Patterns

The concept of human uniqueness is paramount in understanding the impact of neurologic disability or impairment on ADL. Because each person is unique, the psychosocial significance of a mobility problem depends on the characteristics of the individual, the influence of the environment, and the availability of resources (Carlson, 1980).

According to Carlson (1980), to understand the psychosocial significance of a neurologic disorder, the nurse must have knowledge of the neurologic condition and the physical effects resulting from that condition. The nurse must assess the impact of the neurologic condition on the psychologic self— body image, self-esteem, coping—taking into account the individual's social network or environment in relation to the situation.

Some common psychosocial consequences of neurologic conditions that should be considered when dealing with a client with altered mobility include (1) alteration of life patterns, (2) changes in self-perception, (3) visibility of the

TABLE 19–11 • BASIC EXAMINATION: COPING WITH DISABILITY

Self-care competence	Observation: Adaptive aids, deficits
Role competence	History: Effect of disorder
Coping	Observation: Congruence of verbalizations, body language, body posture, expression, adaptive aids
	Interview: Coping style

From Mitchell, P.H., Ozuna, J., Cammermeyer, M., & Woods, N.F. (Eds.). (1984). *Neurological assessment for nursing practice* (p. 112). Paramus, NJ: Reston.

physical condition, (4) disruption in the method of coping, and (5) impact on significant others (Carlson, 1980, p. 312).

Specific data collection of methods of coping with a disability or an alteration in mobility assists in identifying patterns of coping with stressful situations. Mitchell et al. (1984) presented a basic examination for assessing coping behaviors (Table 19–11) that can be completed in an interview or by a paper-and-pencil questionnaire. Some helpful parameters to assess coping style that are built into Mitchell et al.'s model include assessment of problems created by the illness or disability, methods for handling the problem, and support from significant others.

ENVIRONMENTAL DIMENSION OF MOBILITY

The environment has an impact on the individual's mobility status at various points on the health-illness continuum throughout the life cycle. Stairs may be a problem, for example, for a person with a full-leg cast. Having to maneuver between two levels of a home to carry out ADL will be extremely difficult, as well as exhausting. Even placement of furniture and decorative items, such as throw rugs, can be a safety or environmental hazard for the person trying to maneuver on crutches or with an unsteady gait.

The nurse's responsibility to each client varies greatly depending on the setting of the client and his or her physical and mental capabilities (Mitchell & Loustau, 1981). The client with a recent stroke, for example, will need more assistance to maintain safety than will another person who has adapted to the changes created by a disability. Whether the individual is in the hospital or at home will greatly influence the impact the nurse can have. Changes are often easier to initiate in the hospital than in the home, because the nurse is the primary caretaker in the hospital. The nurse must work with the support system in all phases of care and adapt the plan accordingly.

Environmental areas (Table 19–12) that must be included in the overall assessment include the following:

1. Physical barriers or obstacles to mobility (work, living environment including neighborhoods, access to transportation)

TABLE 19–12 • ENVIRONMENTAL DIMENSIONS

Physical barriers or obstacles
   Description of home (stairs, layout, conveniences)
   Description of work setting
   Description of neighborhood (proximity, relationships with neighbors, environmental)
   Alterations to improve client health care
Assistive devices
   Rails, ramps, widened doors
   Crutches, prostheses
Safety factors
   Developmental level
   State of mobility
   Potential hazards
   Sensory deficits
   Use of prosthetic and other supportive devices
Available support systems
   Family and significant others

2. Assistive devices in the environment (e.g., rails, ramps, widened doorways)

3. Safety factors

4. Available support systems from family units or significant others

5. Adequate environmental stimulation

6. Financial resources

7. Community resources

When assessing the external environment for physical barriers or obstacles, the examiner fully assesses the home and work environments to determine if the client has freedom of movement within those settings. Both areas must be described fully regarding layouts, number of floors, stairs if they are a problem, and so on. The examiner should assess the client's neighborhood, focusing on location, whether it is urban or suburban, relationship with neighbors, and influence from industrial sites.

An assistive device is often the only aid the person requires to make him or her independent and not in need of assistance in ADL. All devices need to be selected for proper fit for the individual and existing environment. Clients should be instructed in proper travel with a wheelchair and in how to use crutches and a prosthesis correctly.

Throughout the life span, safety is a concern. Each developmental level must be considered in terms of expected patterns and variations. As mobility increases with growth and development, the individual is confronted with a variety of hazardous situations. Consider the toddler who has increased opportunities to explore through mobility. Electrical outlets may be a safety problem because they are now accessible.

Sensory deficits caused by either disease or physiologic changes associated with aging—for example, decreased vision and a less sensitive balance center—have a profound effect on the mobility plan. Sensory stimulation may be inadequate because of primary sensory changes or because mobility is too limited for the disabled individual to join in activities. Such a person is in a socially restricted environment as a result of physical disabilities and living conditions. Aged people are the primary group who experience a restricted environment because of their physical or emotional inability to move. People who are in situations with monotonous environments devoid of sensory stimuli suffer from social limitations. People who are depressed and who choose not to associate with others and people with chronic debilitating conditions are included in this category (Mitchell & Loustau, 1981).

Therapeutically, restricted environments are also a concern. A patient on a Strykerframe, in Buck's traction, or on bedrest is in an environment that is restricted because of immobility, and sensory stimulation can be greatly decreased. In contrast, in the intensive care unit, an overload of sensory stimuli that are meaningless to the individual may occur and affect psychologic homeostasis (Mitchell & Loustau, 1981).

Other areas to assess include financial resources. Does the client have health insurance or funds adequate to maintain health? Does the recently diagnosed paraplegic or his or her family have insurance or funds necessary for hospitalization and rehabilitation? Will they be able to sustain its effect without severely damaging the family unit? Even brief illnesses can have a great impact on an individual and family who have a limited income. Insurance may pay the major cost of hospitalization, but the loss of income and child care costs while significant others attend to the client are an added burden and create potential problems.

Knowledge of services available for assistance is important for assessing community resources. If the individual lacks knowledge of services, the nurse should guide the individual and the family.

One final area to assess is transportation. Can the individual travel by community bus, car, walking, or service of others? This issue can greatly restrict a person who would otherwise be mobile.

SUMMARY

The ability to move about in the environment is intricately related to one's ability to move, the motivation to move, and a free, nonrestrictive environment. An alteration in movement or mobility will occur if there is a dysfunction in any of these three essential elements. Therefore, assessing the concept of mobility from physiologic, psychosocial, and environmental perspectives offers the nurse a more comprehensive framework for making accurate nursing diagnoses and developing appropriate nursing strategies.

References

Bickley, L.S. (1999). *Bate's guide to physical examination* (7th ed.). Philadelphia: J.B. Lippincott.
Behrman, R., Kliegman, R., Nelson, W., & Vaughn, V. (1991). *Nelson's textbook of pediatrics* (14th ed.). Philadelphia: W.B. Saunders.

Bellack, J. (1992). Assessment of the neonate. In J. Bellack & B. Edlund (Eds.), *Assessment and diagnosis* (2nd ed.). Sudbury, MA: Jones & Bartlett.

Blackman, J.A. (1992). Infant and preschool developmental screening. In M.D. Levine, W.B. Carey, & A.C. Crocker (Eds.), *Developmental behavioral pediatrics* (2nd ed.). Philadelphia: W.B. Saunders.

Carlson, C.E. (1980). Psychosocial aspects of neurologic disability. *Nursing Clinics of North America, 6,* 309.

Conway-Rutkowski, B.L. (1982). *Carini & Owens' neurological and neurosurgical nursing.* St. Louis: C.V. Mosby.

Dubowitz, L., Dubowitz, V., & Goldberg, C. (1970). Clinical assessment of gestational age in the newborn infant. *Journal of Pediatrics, 77,* 1.

Edlund, B. (1992). Activity-sleep assessment. In J. Bellack & B. Edlund (Eds.), *Nursing assessment and diagnosis* (2nd ed., pp. 482–512). Sudbury, MA: Jones & Bartlett.

Fields, W.L., & McGinn-Campbell, K.M. (1983). *Introduction to health assessment.* Paramus, NJ: Reston.

Frankenburg, W.K., Dodds, J., Archer, P., Bresnick, B., Mascha, P., Edelman, N., & Shapiro, H. (1992a). *Denver II screening manual.* Denver, CO: Denver Developmental Materials.

Frankenburg, W.K., Dodds, J., Archer, P., Bresnick, B., Mascha, P., & Edelman, N.H. (1992b). *Denver II technical manual.* Denver, CO: Denver Developmental Materials.

Granger, C.V., Demis, L.S., Peters, N.C., Sherwood, C.C., & Barrett, J.E. (1979). Stroke rehabilitation: Analysis of repeated Barthel index measures. *Archives of Physical Medicine and Rehabilitation, 60,* 14.

Granger, C.V., & Gresham, G.E. (Eds.) (1984). *A conceptual model for functional assessment in rehabilitation medicine.* Baltimore: Williams & Wilkins.

Jebsen, R.H., Taylor, N., & Trieschmann, R.B. (1969). An objective and standardized test of hand function. *Archives of Physical Medicine and Rehabilitation, 51,* 311.

Katz, S., Ford, A., & Moskowitz, R. (1963). Studies of illness in the aged. The index of ADL. *JAMA, 185,* 914.

Konikow, N. (1985). Alterations in movement: Nursing assessment and implications. *Journal of Neurosurgical Nursing, 17,* 61.

Lawton, M.P. (1971). The functional assessment of elderly people. *Journal of the American Geriatrics Society, 19,* 465.

Mahoney, F., & Barthel, D. (1965). Functional evaluation: The Barthel index. *Maryland State Medical Journal, 14,* 61.

Malasanos, L., Barkauakas, V., Moss, M., Stoltenberg-Allen, K. (1986). *Health assessment* (3rd ed.). St. Louis: Mosby–Year Book.

Maslow, A. (1970). *Motivation and personality* (2nd ed.). New York: Harper & Row.

Mitchell, P.H., & Irvin, N.J. (1977). Neurological exam: Assessment for nursing purposes. *Journal of Neurosurgical Nursing, 9*(1), 23.

Mitchell, P.H., & Loustau, A. (1981). *Concepts basic to nursing* (3rd ed.). New York: McGraw-Hill.

Mitchell, P.H., Ozuna, J., Cammermeyer, M., & Woods, N.F. (Eds.) (1984). *Neurological assessment for nursing practice.* Paramus, NJ: Reston.

Nagi, S.Z. (1965). Some conceptual issues in disability and rehabilitation. In M.B. Sussman (Ed.), *Sociology and rehabilitation.* Columbus, OH: Ohio State University Press.

North American Nursing Diagnosis Association. (1999). *NANDA nursing diagnoses: Definitions and classification 1999–2000.* Philadelphia: Author.

Sarno, J.E., Sarno, M.T., & Lurta, E.L. (1973). The functional life scale. *Archives of Physical Medicine and Rehabilitation, 54,* 214.

Seidel, H., Ball, J., Dains, J., & Benedict, G. (1992). *Mosby's guide to physical examination* (2nd ed.). St. Louis: Mosby–Year Book.

Smitherman, C. (1981). *Nursing actions for health promotion.* Philadelphia: F.A. Davis.

Sperhac, A.M. (1990). Developmental assessment. In S. Mott, S.R. James, & A.M. Sperhac (Eds.), *Nursing care of children and families* (2nd ed., pp. 432–435). Reading, MA: Addison-Wesley.

Thompson, J.M., & Bowers, A.C. (1984). *Clinical manual of health assessment* (2nd ed.). St. Louis: Mosby–Year Book.

Wood, P.H., & Badley, E.M. (1978). Setting disablement in perspective. *International Rehabilitative Medicine, 1,* 32.

Abrupt Alterations in Mobility

JEANETTE C. HARTSHORN

Abrupt changes in mobility can result from a variety of disturbances in the neurologic structures and functions of the systems responsible for normal movement. Diseases and disorders that create these abrupt changes in mobility occur in the brain or spinal cord or in the fiber tracts that connect the higher structures with the segments of the spinal cord that ultimately send messages to move to the muscles. Responses to abrupt losses of movement range from hemiplegia to quadriplegia. Although the pathologies that precipitate abrupt loss of movement differ, the disuse syndrome is common to all. In this chapter, acute injuries (spinal cord injury and stroke) and their impact on mobility are discussed.

NEUROANATOMIC CORRELATES OF ABRUPT LOSS OF MOBILITY

Impairments in mobility occur as a result of suprasegmental (upper motor neuron) or segmental (lower motor neuron) lesions. A suprasegmental lesion can occur at any level within the brain or spinal cord; cerebral lesions can be cortical, subcortical, in the internal capsule, or in the brain stem. Spinal cord lesions occur at any segmental level.

Suprasegmental Disruption

Cortical lesions usually involve fewer upper motor neurons because of the wide surface distribution of the fibers. A cortical lesion will, therefore, usually cause a monoplegia or paralysis of the face, with little or no disruption of the adjacent cortex (Bannister, 1992).

Subcortical lesions that occur in the corona radiata involve more fibers because they are closer together than in the cortex. A subcortical lesion causes a greater degree of impairment, usually contralateral hemiplegia or hemiparesis. One limb may be affected more seriously than the others. A lesion of the internal capsule is even more devastating because of the denser distribution of the upper motor neurons. Damage to the internal capsule causes hemiplegia.

Brain stem lesions can cause either hemiplegia or quadriplegia, because the corticospinal tracts lie so close together. Hemiplegia from a brain stem lesion can be differentiated from capsular hemiplegia by associated signs of nearby structures. For example, hemiplegia with involvement of the cranial nerve nuclei would indicate brain stem damage, because the cranial nerves are in close anatomic proximity to the corticospinal tracts. Suprasegmental (upper motor neuron) lesions have certain common characteristics. A group of muscles, rather than an individual muscle, is affected. If any movement is possible, the appropriate functional relationship of the muscle groups, whether agonist, antagonist, synergist, or fixator, remains intact. Paralysis never includes all the muscles on one side of the body, no matter how severe the hemiplegia may be. Bilateral movements, such as of the eyes, jaw, pharynx, larynx, neck, thorax, and abdomen, are scarcely affected, if at all, because of bilateral cortical innervation of these structures (Adams & Victor, 1993).

Suprasegmental lesions above the pons usually produce deficits that are greater in the arm and hand than in the leg, and the muscles of the tongue and lower face are severely affected. Flexor muscles of the arm and extensor muscles of the leg are usually the most severely involved. The muscles exhibit an increased reactivity to a stretch stimulus (Adams & Victor, 1993). The clasp knife phenomenon can be elicited by quick stretching of the muscle of the affected extremity. Continuous passive extension of the spastic arm can follow a distance, stopping abruptly and then continuing its motion of extension. Slow extension of the same arm causes little or no change in muscle tone. Muscle wasting is minimal, compared with that of a lower motor neuron lesion. A slight reduction of muscle mass is due to muscle disuse over time.

Segmental Disruption

Disorders that may cause abrupt loss of segmental function include poliomyelitis and spinal cord injury. A segment can be defined as a portion of the brain stem or spinal cord that includes activity from the reflex arc to the individual muscle innervated. When an injury involves a segment, therefore, functions affected include reflex aspects of movement, cranial nerve and muscle stretch reflexes, integration of autonomic nervous system functions, pure motor or sensory functions with respect to the muscle group innervated, and trophic input to the muscles.

When a direct injury to the spinal cord occurs, the functional loss experienced depends on the degree of spinal cord damage. Upper and lower extremities are impaired with a lesion above the cervical enlargement. Lower extremities are affected if the lesion is below the cervical enlargement. Because of the varying degrees of spinal shock, however, loss may not correspond directly to the vertebral level, particularly in the thoracolumbar and sacral levels.

There are eight cervical spinal cord segments, which are named for their corresponding vertebrae. When damage occurs to the first two cervical segments, the individual will suffer total quadriplegia and respiratory paralysis. The third, fourth, and fifth cervical segments innervate the diaphragm via the peripheral phrenic nerve. Therefore, segments C3–C5 offer functional control over diaphragmatic excursion. Damage to C3–C4 causes total quadriplegia, a weak diaphragm, and absent intercostal movement. In addition to the diaphragm, C5 also innervates the trapezius muscle along with the spinal accessory nerve (the 11th cranial nerve) and regulates the individual's ability to shrug a shoulder.

The fifth and sixth cervical segments innervate the deltoid, biceps, brachioradialis, and triceps muscles. The innervation includes the axillary, musculocutaneous, and radial nerves, which allow arm elevation, forearm supination, and neutral forearm flexion. Segmental damage to C5 and C6 causes quadriplegia with retention of gross arm movements. The diaphragm may be impaired initially, but function may return with time. The sixth cervical segment, in conjunction with the seventh and eighth, controls forearm and wrist extension. Specifically, the extensions of carpi radialis and ulnaris muscles are innervated. The seventh and eighth cervical segments also control wrist flexion. Damage to C6–C7 causes quadriplegia, with biceps and deltoid function but no triceps function. Damage to C7–C8 causes quadriplegia, with triceps function but no intrinsic hand function.

Grip and finger spreading are controlled by the C8 and T1 segments. The adductor pollicis and dorsal interossei muscles are innervated through these segments, as are the peripheral median and ulnar nerves. The first through the 12th thoracic segments innervate the intercostal, rectus abdominus, and oblique muscles. These segments involve thoracic and lumbocervical peripheral branches and influence respiration through intercostal muscles. In addition, the segments influence the muscles of the trunk.

Damage to T1–T5 produces paraplegia with diaphragmatic breathing and loss of leg, bladder, and bowel function. Arm function is intact, and sensation is present to the nipple line. When there is damage to T6–T12, the individual is paraplegic, with no abdominal reflexes at T6 and all abdominal reflexes at T12. Generally, with this level of injury, there is spastic paralysis of the lower limbs. Damage to T12 is usually accompanied by sensation present to the groin area.

The first three lumbar segments control hip flexion through innervation of the iliopsoas muscle and the peripheral femoral nerve. Knee extension is controlled through L2–L4. These segments innervate the quadriceps femoris muscle involving the peripheral femoral nerve. The fourth lumbar through the second sacral segment control foot dorsiflexion and knee flexion. This control originates through innervation of the extensor hallucis, digitorium, biceps femoris, and hamstring muscles, including the peripheral deep peroneal and sciatic nerves. Hip flexion through the gluteus maximus muscle and plantar flexion through the gastrocnemius muscle are controlled through L5–S2.

When damage occurs to a segment below the level of L2, the individual may present with mixed sensorimotor loss and bladder, bowel, and sexual loss depending on the nerve roots damaged. Should the conus medullaris be damaged, there is bowel and bladder sphincter dysfunction, lower leg weakness, hypoesthesia of the sacral dermatome or anesthesia, and back pain. If the cauda equina is involved, there is asymmetric, atrophic, and areflexic paralysis, indicating involvement of the lower motor neurons. Sensory root loss causing decreased sensation in the outer aspect of the legs, ankles, posterior lower limbs, and saddle area will occur. Damage to the cauda equina also causes sphincter dysfunction.

Sacral segments innervate the sphincter muscles through the pudendal peripheral nerves. Damage to sacral segments 1–5 causes loss of bladder, bowel, and sexual function, and some foot displacement may be present. Loss of sensation caused by this type of injury involves the saddle area, the scrotum, the perineum, the penis, the anal area, and the upper third of the posterior aspect of the thigh.

If the segment is not damaged but cannot receive input from the suprasegmental tracts, such symptoms as spasticity may be seen. Spinal shock is an example of how this type of disruption may occur. Spinal shock occurs as early as 30 to 60 minutes after cord injury and involves the complete or nearly complete suppression of all reflex activity below the level of the injury. Tendon reflexes diminish or disappear, and temperature control and vasomotor tone are lost. Bladder and bowel paralysis resulting in urinary retention, ileus, and fecal retention may also occur. Spinal shock occurs because of the sudden loss of impulses from the descending pathways, which normally maintain the cord neurons in a ready state of excitability. With loss of the constant flow of impulses, the resting excitability of the cord is reduced greatly. Occasionally, in a patient with complete cord transection, sacral reflexes may be present immediately after transection. These reflexes show a diminished response, and commonly reflex activity returns after recovery from spinal shock. Without the modulating influence of the central cortex, reflexes are hyperactive. There is a wide variation in the duration of spinal shock, with some cases resolving in several days and others requiring several months for resolution. No specific medical treatment has been identified for spinal shock (Hickey, 1992).

PATHOPHYSIOLOGY OF COMMON CONDITIONS PRODUCING ABRUPT IMMOBILITY

Spinal cord injury and stroke are two examples of acute disorders that can damage suprasegmental and segmental structures abruptly. These disorders cause disruption of the structures previously discussed and result in partial or complete loss of voluntary movement, involuntary movement, balance, coordination, and postural reflexes.

Pathophysiology of Stroke

Stroke occurs when acute neuronal and vascular changes in the brain result in ischemia or infarction. Stroke can be classified into two major categories: occlusive and hemorrhagic.

Occlusive disease is caused by an obstruction of the lumen of a vessel, resulting in an infarction of the brain tissue. Occlusion may be caused by abnormalities in the vessel wall, such as arteriosclerosis or inflammation. It can also result from red blood cell deformities, platelet aggregation, increased blood viscosity, dehydration, fever, and hemodynamic changes, which cause thrombosis or embolism. Arteriosclerosis is the most common source of thrombosis. Emboli frequently result from cardiac sources, such as valvular lesions, cardiac arrhythmias, and prosthetic valves. They also may originate in extracranial vessels from atherosclerotic plaque. Infarction by embolus frequently progresses to a hemorrhagic stroke. Regional phenomena that occur during infarction include cytotoxic and vasogenic edema and vasomotor paralysis.

Intracranial hemorrhage may occur into the brain substance itself, the subarachnoid space, and the potential spaces below and above the dura. The cause of hemorrhage can be hypertension, ruptured aneurysm, arteriovenous malformation, trauma, blood dyscrasia, or brain tumor; the hemorrhage can also be of unknown origin.

After occlusion of a cerebral vessel, damage to autoregulation occurs. Zones of hypoperfusion or hyperperfusion are a result of the degree of autoregulatory damage to the adjacent areas. Hemorrhages appear in the cortex, and ischemic necrosis occurs in the underlying white matter. There is widespread destruction of nerve cells, nerve fibers, and glial tissue (except microglia). Infarction can cause so much swelling that signs of increased intracranial pressure occur. An embolus usually causes vasospasm or cerebral abscess and may be followed by mycotic aneurysm formation.

Intracerebral hemorrhage acts as a space-occupying lesion, which compresses surrounding tissue and becomes edematous.

Pathophysiology of Spinal Cord Injury

Acute lesions of the spinal cord affect both the corticospinal tracts (upper motor neuron) and the segmental reflex. Such lesions cause not only a paralysis of voluntary movement, but also a temporary loss of reflexes below the level of the lesion because of spinal shock. After a time, this flaccid paralysis gives way to spasticity, with a hyperactivity of tendon reflexes and Babinski's reflex. Spasticity is the result of loss of descending inhibitory input and maintained activity of facilitatory influences (Adams & Victor, 1993).

Several events occur during a spinal cord injury that interfere with voluntary movement. Vascular damage has been identified as a component of spinal cord injury. After injury, a hemorrhagic lesion forms, involving primarily the central gray matter. Chromatolysis, vacuolation, and alterations in cytoplasmic density and stainability are observed. Minimal edematous changes in white matter, more marked in internal than in external layers, have been identified. The mechanical distortion of spinal cord tissue after compression trauma promotes not only intrinsic biochemical changes within the injured cells but also related changes involving extraneural tissues, particularly the blood vessels supplying the cord tissue. Thus, the infiltration by platelets and red blood cells into the perivascular spaces serves to worsen the intraneural damage normally accompanying the tissue distortion.

After extravasation of the blood elements, polymorphonuclear leukocytes leak into the cord tissue, heralding various degrees of cellular necrosis. Moderately severe impact lesions of this type involve infractions of the myelin sheath, leading to neuronal degeneration in the central gray matter. Within 24 to 48 hours after this type of injury, fibrocytes increase substantially. Moderate to severe cavitation of the central gray matter occurs after stabilization of the injury. Distal to the site of trauma, wallerian degeneration with demyelination of the axon sheath occurs. This change is characterized by swelling of the myelinated axon, which then breaks into fragments and finally disappears from the tissue. When the axon regrows in limited circumstances, the glial processes retract, and if synaptic contact is restored between cells, sensorimotor function may return completely or to a degree. The way in which the healing of the injury proceeds is directly influenced by the severity and the site of the injury, by the time elapsed since trauma, and by the observed physiopathologic changes.

HUMAN RESPONSES TO ACUTE IMMOBILITY

Acute Disuse Phenomena

Acute disuse phenomena occur when mobility is affected by the abrupt loss of functional neurons as a result of a suprasegmental or segmental lesion. Acute disuse phenomena have an impact on all body systems, contributing to multisystem complications.

Responses of the cardiovascular, pulmonary, gastrointestinal, and integumentary systems to nervous system injury only serve to compound the deleterious effects of the insult suffered by the patient.

CARDIOVASCULAR EFFECTS

As a result of acute immobility, there is an increased workload on the heart. Cardiac output and stroke volume are increased because of the loss of gravity's effect on blood return to the heart. Heart rate increases as a result of cardiac muscle fatigue. Immobility of the lower extremities causes sluggish venous blood return to the heart. This pooling of blood combined with hypercoagulability of the blood increases the risk of deep venous thrombosis and pulmonary embolism. In stroke, the risk of deep venous thrombosis in the paralyzed leg is as high as 75%, whereas in the nonparalyzed leg it is approximately 7% (National Institutes of Health, 1986).

RESPIRATORY EFFECTS

With immobility from any cause, there is an increase in the work of breathing, an increase in intraesophageal pressure, and a slight increase in tidal volume.

The end result is that more effort is required to expand the lungs and exchange gas. Immobility can be complicated by decreased strength of the muscles of respiration, which leads to decreased chest expansion. The pressure of the bed against the chest decreases expansion, predisposing the person to shallow breathing. Lack of activity decreases the normal stimulus to deep breathing. All these factors lead to stasis of the normal secretions of the lung, creating a medium for bacterial growth. When a person is supine, the effects of gravity tend to draw the mucus present in a bronchiole toward the bottom, leaving a dry upper epithelium, which is more vulnerable to bacterial invasion. This can lead to pneumonia. Atelectasis may occur if static secretions become thick and block a bronchiole. If a person is unable to cough, being too weak, unconscious, or in pain, pneumonia is possible.

Patients with high-level cervical cord injury have reduced lung volume and capacity, poor oxygen exchange, and carbon dioxide retention. Each patient demonstrates a variable cough, a progressive decrease in thoracic compliance, and an elastic recoil of the lungs because of decreased volume. The cough reflex is impaired significantly by paralysis of the intercostal and abdominal muscles. These people require total respiratory support, at least for a prescribed period.

METABOLIC EFFECTS

Immobility leads to a multitude of metabolic and digestive changes, including a decrease in basal metabolic rate and oxygen consumption. These decreases reflect a lower energy requirement of the body.

Negative nitrogen balance may occur with immobility. Normally, anabolism (protein synthesis) is in balance with catabolism (protein breakdown). During immobilization, catabolism increases, as reflected in a marked increase in excretion of urinary nitrogen (urinary nitrogen is a byproduct of protein metabolism). The marked urinary excretion of nitrogen results in a negative nitrogen balance, indicating a depletion of stores for protein synthesis, which is necessary in tissue healing after trauma or surgery. Maximal loss occurs from the fourth to eighth day after injury (Halm, 1990).

Immobility may affect the calcium balance adversely. Normally, calcium is released in the process of bone resorption, and the body uses what it needs and excretes the excess. During immobilization, however, calcium is retained in the urine, and because the volume of urine rises only slightly, the calcium concentration is increased. Because the citric acid concentration in the urine does not change, the calcium–citric acid ratio is altered, and the pH of the urine rises, indicating reduced acidity. This combination of factors creates the possibility of calcium precipitation and stone formation (Mitchell & Loustau, 1981).

ELIMINATION EFFECTS

Paralytic ileus may occur with immobility. During the acute stage after spinal cord injury, many patients experience loss of bowel sounds and abdominal distention from the loss of peristaltic movements in the intestines. Peristaltic activities are mediated by the parasympathetic nervous system, and the exact cause of paralytic ileus in these patients is generally the sudden paralysis and interruption of impulse pathways. Severe gastric dilation from a paralytic ileus can interfere with diaphragmatic functioning. Vomiting can occur, putting the patient at risk for aspiration.

Immobile clients can suffer from alteration in elimination for a number of reasons. One of the most common forms of this alteration is constipation, and several anatomic and physiologic principles explain this. The large bowel musculature has its own neural center within the intestinal wall that responds to distention caused by the fecal contents. Although this type of innervation is usually not greatly affected in stroke or spinal-cord–injured patients, the client may suffer from loss of the sensation of fullness in the lower bowel, loss of awareness of bowel evacuation, loss of ability to control the rectal sphincter, and loss of ability to contract the abdominal muscles and to expel the stool (Halm, 1990).

Other causes of constipation in the immobile patient include restricted diets with inadequate amounts of roughage and fluids, insufficient muscle strength to pass stool, and weakened perineal and abdominal muscles as a result of bedrest.

MUSCULOSKELETAL EFFECTS

Acute immobility leads to a rapid loss of both muscle strength and muscle mass. As a result of the decrease in muscle strength, the patient experiences a decrease in tolerance for exercise and adapts to the situation by cutting back on activity, which further decreases muscle strength, and the cycle continues.

When muscles and joints are not used to their full capacities, there is a change in metabolic activity that leads to further loss of mobility. Normal mobility depends on the free movement of the joints and muscles and the ability of the loose network of connective (collagen) fibers to stretch to accommodate the full range of motion. When motion is limited, the collagen network becomes dense and rigid, resulting in fibrosis. Muscles become progressively shorter and pull the joints, creating contractures, which can be permanent. Although permanent contractures occur more frequently with paralysis, deformed posture may result from poor positioning during prolonged bedrest.

During immobilization, the bones are not performing their specific functions of weight bearing and motion. This disturbs the balance between bone formation (osteoblastic activity) and bone resorption (osteoclastic activity). Osteoclastic activity increases, and the bone matrix becomes thin and porous, resulting in osteoporosis. Increased osteoclastic activity also degrades collagen fibrils and causes minerals, particularly calcium and phosphorus, to be released and excreted. The osteoporosis of immobilization is usually reversible when the period of immobilization is over, although it can become pathologic with excessive bone and mineral loss.

If a bone that has become porous because of immobility is subjected to weight bearing, pathologic fracture may result (Mitchell & Loustau, 1981).

INTEGUMENTARY EFFECTS

A major problem for the immobilized patient is the need to maintain the integrity of the skin. Pressure sores or decubitus ulcers are commonly seen in immobilized people. The lack of muscle tone, voluntary movement, and perception of pain are factors in the development of pressure sores. The most important factor, however, is the lowered tissue resistance to pressure caused by interruption of the vasomotor pathways. Decubitus ulcers involve cutaneous and subcutaneous tissue and occur in areas of the body subjected to unrelieved pressure, such as the back of the head, the sacrum, the heels of the feet, and the trochanters. Skin and subcutaneous tissue die, slough away, and leave areas of ulceration. Cells in these tissues die because sufficient nutrients cannot diffuse from the capillaries to them, and their waste products cannot be carried away. Pressure on the tissues is greater than the hydrostatic pressure in the capillaries, and this pressure difference effectively opposes diffusion from the capillaries, leading to tissue ischemia. Prolonged tissue ischemia leads to the production of pressure sores. These sores develop much more rapidly in denervated or paralyzed tissues because of the decrease in trophic factors.

CASE STUDIES

Acute immobility-related nursing diagnoses are examined here through an evaluation of three case studies. These case studies include one patient with a cervical spinal cord injury, one patient with a stroke, and one patient with peripheral nerve injury.

• C A S E S T U D Y 1

Cervical Spinal Cord Injury

Mr. J, a 21-year-old active-duty serviceman, was drinking heavily at a party. He left the party, driving his motorcycle. Shortly after leaving, he remembered that he had forgotten his helmet, but because he was tired, he decided to continue rather than return for the helmet. While traveling on a darkened road, he hit an oncoming vehicle head on and was thrown onto the pavement. He landed squarely on top of his head and immediately lost consciousness. Within 10 minutes, the emergency medical services team arrived and transported him to the local trauma center.

On admission, his words were garbled, but he was able to respond to some commands. He had lost sensation from the nipple line down and was experiencing respiratory difficulty. An x-ray examination confirmed the diagnosis of a C4 fracture. After stabilization of the fracture in the trauma center, Mr. J was transferred to the neurologic intensive care unit.

On admission to the unit, Mr. J was found to be unable to move any extremities and unable to breathe. He was placed on a volume ventilator shortly after admission. Mr. J's intercostal muscles were paralyzed, although some diaphragmatic function remained intact. Once his respiratory status was stabilized, it was necessary to begin interventions to stabilize the cervical injury. Cervical tongs were inserted while he was under local anesthesia. Seven pounds of traction were added to stabilize the fracture.

Twelve hours after admission to the neurologic intensive care unit, Mr. J was awake but very frightened. He demonstrated signs of acute anxiety and was unable to recall the events of the accident that caused his injury. Throughout his stay in the neurologic intensive care unit, Mr. J's cardiovascular activity was monitored.

• C A S E   S T U D Y   2

Stroke

Mr. F, a 52-year-old father of three children, was admitted to the neurosurgical intermediate intensive care unit, with an admitting diagnosis of a left stroke. He was accompanied by his wife, from whom a history of the present illness and a past medical history were obtained.

Mrs. F stated that her husband had a 20-year history of high blood pressure and blamed this on his job. He was a successful attorney and averaged 10 to 12 hours of work per day (including most Saturdays and Sundays) at the office. He had been involved in an $18 million lawsuit for the past year, so "he felt especially pressured." He was 35 lb overweight and smoked a pack of cigarettes a day. Mr. F had been followed by an internist for his medical care plan. He had taken various medications for his hypertension, with limited success, primarily because "he wouldn't bother to take them as the doctor prescribed." Mr. F had not been able to stop smoking or lose weight. Mrs. F was distraught, saying, "I'm at my wits' end. I've seen this coming for years."

Mr. F had no history of cardiac disease, neurologic disease, diabetes mellitus, or other major medical problems. He had had the usual childhood diseases without complications and had not undergone any surgical procedures. There was a family history of vascular disease. His mother had died of a stroke at the age of 76 years, and his brother had survived a myocardial infarction 6 years earlier.

Mr. F had suffered his first transient ischemic attack (TIA) about 4 months before the hospital admission. He had come home late from the office. While he was sitting and reading the paper, he suddenly experienced right-arm weakness and heaviness and felt as if a "curtain covered his left eye." This lasted approximately 1 minute and resolved spontaneously. He did not mention this incident to his wife until he experienced the same symptoms twice in one day 2 months later. Mrs. F convinced Mr. F to see his internist the following morning.

Mr. F's evaluation at the internist's office for his TIAs revealed a carotid bruit and decreased carotid pulse on the left side. Periorbital directional Doppler studies suggested compromise of circulation on the left internal carotid artery. No neurologic deficits were noted, and no evidence of cardiovascular involvement was found. The laboratory results showed his usual hypercholesterolemia. In view of the two recent attacks and the risk factors predisposing him to cerebrovascular disease, it was recommended that Mr. F be hospitalized to undergo further evaluation for possible carotid endarterectomy. Mr. F was scheduled for admission to the hospital in 2 weeks and was started on a regimen of aspirin and dipyridamole (Persantine) in conjunction with chlorthalidone (Hygroton) and furosemide (Lasix) for hypertension. Mr. F was unexpectedly detained out of town during the time he was to be hospitalized. "I begged him to reschedule his tests, but he always said he was too busy. Then he woke up this morning with his right side paralyzed and couldn't speak," said Mrs. F.

The medical evaluation at the time of this admission to the emergency department included a physical examination, 12-lead electrocardiogram (ECG), chest x-ray, blood test (including complete blood count, clotting profiles, electrolytes, triglycerides, cholesterol, blood urea nitrogen, creatinine, glucose, and uric acid), routine urinalysis, and computed tomographic (CT) scan. The medical diagnosis of left stroke of probable thrombotic origin of the left internal carotid, with emboli to the left middle cerebral artery, was suggested. Mr. F was transferred to the neurosurgical intermediate intensive care unit with an intravenous catheter, 40% misted oxygen via face tent, and a Foley catheter in place.

On admission to the unit, the nursing assessment showed that Mr. F had clear but shallow respirations at 24 breaths per minute. His blood pressure was 170/110, and the apical heart rate was 110. His peripheral pulses were thready and equal. Capillary refill was less than 1 second, and no jugular venous distention or peripheral edema was noted. His skin was slightly diaphoretic and pale but warm to touch. His Foley catheter was draining an adequate amount of clear yellow urine. A thorough neurologic assessment was done. Mr. F was lethargic; he opened his eyes to the examiner's voice but was unable to respond appropriately to orientation questions. He was able to verbalize "yes" and "no" with difficulty; otherwise, his words were unintelligible. Sensory evaluation was deferred because of his aphasia. The motor examination showed marked hemiparesis on the right side. The right upper extremity was assessed to be 1/5, and the right lower extremity was 2/5 on the universal scale. The left side was 5/5 for both upper and lower extremities, and coordination was intact. Asymmetry was noted in Mr. F's face, and, on closer examination, weakness was found on the right side when he was asked to puff out his cheeks and to smile. When assessing speech, the nurse found consistent articulation errors. Difficulty with lingual and labial sounds was evident. Deviation of the tongue to the right side (the weaker side) was present. Mr. F was uncooperative when he was asked to open his mouth to assess motor function of the 9th and 10th cranial nerves. Gag reflex testing was deferred. The patient was unable to swallow his own saliva. He was also noted to have a conjugate gaze preference to the left.

• C A S E   S T U D Y   3

Peripheral Nerve Injury

Mrs. C was a 50-year-old woman who was admitted to the neurology nursing unit with a chief complaint of tingling in her hands and feet and progressive weakness in both legs and arms for the past 2 weeks. She had fallen the day before her admission, which prompted her to consult her family physician. She had suffered an intestinal flu approximately 2 weeks before the onset of these symptoms.

Mrs. C's admission assessment showed a well-developed, well-nourished woman in no apparent distress. She was alert, oriented, pleasant, and relaxed during the interview. Her blood pressure was 110/68, her pulse 76, her respirations 16 and regular, and her temperature 37°C. Her breath sounds were clear, and chest excursion was normal. She denied feeling short of breath. There was no evidence of cardiac abnormalities, and peripheral pulses were equal and strong. Mrs. C denied problems with diet or elimination.

Neurologically, Mrs. C's mental status examination was within normal limits. The first through 12th cranial nerves were intact. Motor strength was diminished to 4/5 bilaterally in the legs and 5/5 in the arms. Mrs. C complained of some tenderness in her muscles to deep palpation. Proprioception was intact, and vibration was slightly impaired. Heel to shin showed a mild ataxia. Finger-to-nose and rapid alternating hand movements were performed without deficit. Mrs. C was unable to stand from a sitting position without assistance. She exhibited a widebase stance and gait. Sensation was grossly intact. Deep tendon reflexes were diminished bilaterally. Babinski's reflex was absent. Mrs. C's blood work, ECG, and chest x-ray were within normal limits. Lumbar puncture showed a mild elevation in proteins.

Two days after admission, Mrs. C developed respiratory difficulty and, by that evening, had flaccid paralysis of her legs and increased weakness of her arms. Sensation remained intact. A lumbar puncture was again performed, which showed a rise in cerebrospinal fluid proteins to 160 mg per 100 mL and 10 lymphocytes. Nerve conduction velocity studies showed a significant slowing. The medical diagnosis of Guillain-Barré syndrome was made on the basis of these findings. Mrs. C was transferred to the intermediate neurologic intensive care unit for observation.

The following day, Mrs. C become more dyspneic. Her arterial blood gases showed hypoxemia, a moderate respiratory alkalosis, and a decreased oxygen saturation, and her vital capacity was decreased to 800 mL. She was intubated, and ventilatory support was instituted.

Mrs. C progressed to complete quadriplegia and areflexia by her fifth hospital day. A facial diplegia was present, showing involvement of the seventh cranial nerve. Autonomic function was impaired by evidence of urinary incontinence, lability in blood pressure, sinus bradycardia, and profuse diaphoresis.

Nursing Diagnoses Related to the Individual

Patients with acute disruptions in mobility have common nursing diagnoses regardless of the specific cause of the disruption. In this chapter, diagnoses appropriate for the acute phase are discussed. Each of the conditions discussed in this chapter has both acute and chronic components, and, in Chapter 21, nursing care for the chronic aspects is discussed.

INEFFECTIVE BREATHING PATTERNS

Changes in innervation to the muscles of breathing, resulting from the injury and from the problems specifically caused by immobility, make the patient a likely candidate for ineffective breathing patterns, defined as rate, rhythm, or depth of breathing insufficient to support adequate oxygen–carbon dioxide exchange. Whether or not a patient with a spinal cord injury develops respiratory complications is dependent also on the level of injury.

Initial assessment of the respiratory function of the immobile patient should include assessment of respiratory rate and respiratory excursion. Lung sounds are assessed for the degree of movement of air and the presence of adventitious sounds. Specific respiratory parameters, such as tidal volume and vital capacity, are measured. Arterial blood gases are assessed for levels of oxygen, carbon dioxide, and pH in the blood.

One of the major goals in caring for the immobile client with ineffective breathing patterns is to support ventilation. In addition to the assessment parameters already described, it may be necessary to implement such procedures as suctioning, caring for an artificial airway, and ventilator therapy. A second goal is to prevent respiratory infection or atelectasis. Interventions that help in this area include frequent turning, coughing and deep breathing, increasing fluids, and suctioning as necessary. The patient must be monitored for elevations in temperature.

Two types of special beds have been developed to assist in the respiratory care of the immobile patient. The rocking bed is a regular hospital bed attached to a framework with a motor that allows the ends of the bed to move alternately up and down. The rocking action takes advantage of gravity; as the head lowers, the abdominal viscera fall lower in the abdominal cavity, allowing the diaphragm to flatten and increasing the thoracic space and volume of air inhaled. The patient is taught to inhale as the head rises and to exhale as the head lowers. Both the speed and the degree of tilt of the bed can be adjusted. The speed is set to correspond to the rate of desired respirations; the tilt is adjusted to get the desired tidal air volume. The total rocking arc of most beds is between 40 and 44 degrees.

Another bed with similar characteristics is the kinetic bed. This type of bed provides automated position movement over a 124-degree range. Because of continuous postural changes, lung secretions are mobilized, allowing for easier expulsion of secretions and better respiratory exchange. In addition to assisting with respiratory care, these beds are useful in preventing other consequences of immobility, such as skin breakdown.

IMPAIRED PHYSICAL MOBILITY

Physical mobility is impaired for a number of reasons in the spinal-cord–injured patient. Loss of voluntary movement and involuntary movement and the presence of environmental barriers have been discussed. The major characteristic of the immobile person is an inability to move purposefully within the physical environment, including mobility, transfer, ambulation, and locomotion. The degree of impairment of physical mobility is related to the level of injury.

In assessment of the immobile client, it is necessary to check frequently the range of motion of all extremities. Muscle strength and tone can be similarly checked on a routine basis. To test muscle tone, the nurse notes whether rigidity (increased resistance throughout range of motion of the joint), spasticity (increased muscular resistance to brisk movement of the joint), and clonus (oscillation between flexion and extension of the foot when back pressure is applied to the sole) are elicited by passive motion. Muscles are palpated for tenderness or spasm.

Muscle strength is tested in several ways. To test the shoulder girdle, the examiner presses on the patient's arms after he or she abducts them to shoulder height. Upper extremities are tested by evaluating biceps, triceps, wrist dorsi-flexion, hand grasps, and strength of finger abduction and extension. Lower extremities are tested through hip flexors, abductors and adductors, knee flexors and extensors, foot dorsiflexion, invertors, and evertors. Muscle strength is graded as normal, minimal, or moderate strength; severe weakness; or paralysis.

A major goal in caring for the immobile patient is to prevent complications, such as contractures, through nursing interventions. Both active and passive range-of-motion exercises are needed on a frequent basis. Because the patient is maintained on bedrest, proper positioning is essential. Extremities should be supported at all times. Frequent turning and repositioning of the patient help in maintaining proper alignment. When voluntary muscle contraction is possible, the nurse may assist the patient in performing muscle-conditioning exercises. Setting exercises in which the muscle is contracted as hard as possible for 10 seconds and then released are a type of isometric exercise that may be helpful. Resistive exercises, in which the muscle contracts in pushing or pulling against a stationary object, can be used to help maintain strength.

Associated Diagnoses

A variety of nursing diagnoses occur secondary to the impaired mobility of individuals who have suffered such traumas as stroke, spinal cord injury, and peripheral nerve injury. Although these phenomena are discussed in detail in their corresponding chapters, they are summarized here to emphasize the primary role that mobility plays in all aspects of human response to illness.

SELF-CARE DEFICIT

Self-care tasks are performed daily to meet bodily needs and to participate in society. Dependence in this area can impede one's participation in society. Most self-care activities require a significant amount of upper-extremity func-tion, which poses obvious problems for patients with cervical cord injury.

The immobile patient with a spinal cord injury can suffer from varying levels of self-care deficit. During assessment, inability to move in bed and to transfer from bed to chair, difficulty in grasp and grip, and difficulties using tools and utensils indicate the presence of self-care deficits. Nursing interven-tions are planned to minimize the deficit to the greatest extent possible. The goal of nursing care with this diagnosis is to ensure that feeding, bathing, dressing, and toileting occur with as much assistance as possible from the patient. It is critical that the patient be involved in his or her own care, maintain-ing independence for as long as possible.

As the patient nears discharge from the acute care unit, several options for assistance are available. In particular, the occupational therapist can be consulted for assistance in developing new types of utensils that can be used by a patient with a weakened grasp. Occupational therapists can teach the patient ways of dressing despite the restrictions imposed by the injury. This phenomenon is discussed in detail in Chapters 32 and 33.

ALTERATION IN ELIMINATION

Any immobile patient may suffer from problems with urinary elimination. Those with spinal cord injury may suffer additional problems as a result of the flaccidity of the bladder that occurs during spinal shock. Depending on the level of injury, control over bladder function may return. Specifically, in upper motor neuron lesions, reflex activity below the cord lesion returns. Chapters 27 and 28 discuss the diagnosis of alteration in urinary elimination. Bowel elimination is also impaired with acute spinal cord injury, during the stages of spinal shock as well as chronically. Constipation may occur as a result of decreased activity. Chapters 27 and 29 discuss bowel elimination problems.

POTENTIAL IMPAIRMENT OF SKIN INTEGRITY

Prevention of pressure sores is a top priority in caring for an immobile client. Skin assessment is made at least every 8 hours. Generally, one the first signs of skin breakdown is the presence of reddened areas. Once noted, these areas should be protected immediately. Assessment of the skin should include all areas of the body, with particular attention to the elbows, earlobes, sacrum, and heels of the feet.

Other parameters to assess include the nutritional status of the patient and other medical problems present at the same time. Wound healing is slowed in those suffering from poor nutritional status. These individuals, therefore, are more likely to suffer from pressure sores. Medical problems, such as diabetes mellitus, may also lead to skin breakdown. While assessing these parameters, the nurse can build a picture of the risk an individual patient may run for development of pressure sores. Other factors that contribute to the development of ulcers include debilitated conditions, edema, anemia, and trophic skin changes. A study suggests that initial treatment of acute spinal cord injures should include the use of pressure-relieving maneuvers or devices as soon as possible, particularly in patients with anticipated extensive immobilization (Cury & Casady, 1992).

Several interventions are helpful in both the prevention and the treatment of pressure sores. The patient should be repositioned to relieve pressure on body parts at least every 2 hours. The skin should be kept clean and dry, particularly in areas prone to the development of pressure sores. Reddened areas are massaged with lotion, and linen should be kept clean, dry, and wrinkle free.

Specific treatment of pressure sores varies from institution to institution. Specialized beds may be of assistance in keeping the patient off the pressure areas. Other preventive measures, such as sheepskin, air mattresses, egg-crate mattresses, and heel and elbow pads, are useful. The use of an occlusive plastic film has gained some popularity. This film covers the area, keeps bacteria out, and allows granulation tissue to develop. A number of antibacterial creams have been recommended for different types of pressure sores, and periodic application of heat may be useful in treatment of existing areas of skin breakdown. More severe pressure sores may require surgical débridement and plastic surgery. Research continues in this area, and the nurse should consult the current literature for the latest information on the problem of pressure sores.

SEXUAL DYSFUNCTION

Immobile clients may suffer from sexual dysfunction. Those with spinal cord injury will probably have some change in sexual activity related to the level of cord injury. Chapters 30 and 31 discuss sexual dysfunction.

POTENTIAL FOR INEFFECTIVE COPING

Immobility from any cause leads to multiple problems for an individual. Immobility resulting from spinal cord injury may cause the patient to confront several additional problems. Reactions that can be expected include denial, anger, and depression. Each nurse works with the patient to help in developing methods for dealing with all the feelings relating to the injury. Studies of the individual's reaction to immobility are based on two major concepts: grief and crisis theory.

Psychologic support of the patient should begin at the time of the injury. As the patient moves through different physical stages, the emotional reactions can vary considerably. For example, in the acute stage of the injury, the patient may be so concerned with holding onto life that there is no opportunity to think about the future in any detail. As he or she becomes more physically stable, the patient may experience some denial of the extent of the injury and eventually some depression. As an understanding develops about the extent of injury and what that means in terms of overall functioning, anger may result. Feelings of inferiority, inadequacy, powerlessness, lack of self-worth, and despair may also occur.

As the patient goes through each of these stages, nursing interventions include encouraging expression of feelings. The nurse can learn about the patient's perception of his or her condition and his or her expectations. Education at this point will help the patient maintain a realistic view of the future. Goals can be set mutually by the nurse and the patient so that the patient can achieve and experience the satisfaction that comes with goal attainment. Nurses can do much by repeatedly expressing confidence in the patient's ability to perform successfully, always emphasizing the positive. Working toward maintaining open and honest communication and being sensitive to the patient's need for acceptance are interventions that are frequently successful in working with these patients.

There are times, however, when the nurse is not the best person to help the patient work through these problems. In this situation, the nurse should consider asking for consultation with a clinical nurse specialist in psychiatric nursing or some other health care provider who can establish a relationship with the patient and offer the needed support.

POTENTIAL FOR INJURY

With limited mobility because of hemiplegia or hemiparesis, being cared for in unfamiliar surroundings, and visual defects, the patient with an acute disruption in mobility is at risk for injury. Careful assessment of visual acuity and visual fields is critical. Issues of room safety, such as placement of the bedside table and accessibility of the call bell or urinal, should be assessed, keeping visual and mobility deficits in mind. Objects should be placed within the visual field. Patients can be taught methods to compensate for visual field cuts. Keeping the bed in the lowest position and keeping the patient oriented to the environment will help protect the patient from injury.

ALTERATION IN NUTRITION

The caloric needs of the immobile client are increased. Several factors related to immobility, such as stress, preexisting nutritional problems, and associated multisystem problems, influence the extent of nutritional needs in the individual (Blissitt, 1990).

An overall nutritional assessment, including history, physical examination, and biochemical data, should be completed and used as a basis for development of the nutritional plan.

Nursing Diagnoses Related to the Family and Significant Others

POTENTIAL FOR FAMILY CRISIS

As the patient works through various stages of anger, depression, and denial, so does the family. A multitude of factors combine to help form the attitudes of the family toward the situation. For example, the family may suffer from guilt, thinking that they may have been able to do something to prevent the injury. The length of time required for hospitalization of the patient may produce an additional strain on the family. Members may disagree about the best decisions to be made on behalf of their family member. For example, once discharge is planned, some would prefer that the patient return to the home setting, whereas others within the same family may ask that the patient be taken to an extended care facility for further rehabilitation.

One of the major goals in dealing with families at this time is to maintain satisfactory family relationships. In assessing the family relationship, it is important to accept the family as they are. The approach to the family should be one of determining how they are coping, not trying to impose any personal beliefs. The nurse must assess the family dynamics, coping strategies, knowledge of disease process, and attitudes.

Interventions for the family parallel those for the individual. Initially, it is important to give the family the opportunity to express their feelings. During the early days after the injury, the family may require constant reassurance and explanations. As time progresses, they may feel more trust for the staff and require fewer explanations. They will continue to require a way to express their feelings, however. Support groups for families may assist in this process. Family assessment and interventions are discussed in detail in Chapter 17.

Nursing Diagnoses for the Community

POTENTIAL FOR INADEQUATE COMMUNITY RESOURCES

Many changes in community resources for the disabled have taken place. Buildings, services, and activities that were off-limits some years ago are more accessible to the disabled. Yet, more changes are required and should be considered before the patient's discharge. Although the traditional picture of an individual with a spinal cord injury is that of a young person, with improving technology we are seeing more and more older people surviving significant injuries. These individuals present needs that are very different from those of younger individuals (Roth, Lovell, Heinemann, Lee, & Yarkony, 1992; Weingarden & Graham, 1992).

Perhaps one of the most fundamental issues when the spinal-cord–injured person is returned to the community is that of role change. Only some spinal-cord–injured clients will return to their original jobs after the injury. Vocational rehabilitation programs will help some people return to the community. Generally, vocational rehabilitation programs are funded with federal money and, as such, are always subject to potential decreased funds. Nurses can help in this area by impressing on their legislators the importance of vocational rehabilitation programs.

Communities may not have the employment opportunities available to help the individual move back into society. Disabled people must have a realistic impression of the types of positions they can fill within the community, and employers must be helped to see the types of jobs within their businesses that can be filled by disabled people. If a patient is discharged from the health care institution without any thought being given to potential employment opportunities, it is likely that the individual's adjustment to being home will be unsuccessful.

Access throughout the community remains a problem. Although more buildings have been made accessible to those with altered mobility, many buildings continue to be inaccessible. Again, legislative efforts are most likely

TABLE 20–1 • FREQUENT WARNING SIGNS FOR STROKE (BRAIN ATTACK)
• Sudden numbness or weakness of face, arm, or leg, especially on one side of the body
• Sudden confusion, trouble speaking or understanding
• Sudden trouble seeing in one or both eyes
• Sudden trouble walking, dizziness, loss of balance or coordination
• Sudden severe headache with no known cause

Source: *National Stroke Association* (1999). http://www.stroke.org

to influence this situation. A change in the attitude of society with respect to the worth of disabled people will help in this type of legislative effort.

Implications for the community with respect to the patient who has had a stroke are similar. Stroke ranks third as a cause of death in the United States and is one of the leading causes of disability. Approximately 1.5 million strokes are diagnosed in a year, and at any one time 2.5 million people have suffered strokes in varying degrees. Both U.S. and international data indicate that roughly 70% of stroke victims will survive the first 30 days. Ten percent of those who survive the first month will recover without discernible neurologic deficits. Forty percent have mild residual deficits, another 40% have severe deficits requiring special care, and the remaining 10% require institutional care (Aho et al., 1980; Posner, Gorman, & Woldow, 1984). It is clear that stroke is one of society's leading health problems.

Education of the public is paramount in the prevention of stroke. Information about risk factors, the nature of the disease, prevention, and general care of the stroke patient should be disseminated on an ongoing basis. Education should be available to all age groups, high-risk groups, and the disadvantaged. The general population may be reached through printed material distributed at schools, doctors' waiting rooms, grocery stores, and places of employment. Television, radio, and newspapers are also effective means of disseminating information.

Prevention of stroke requires the awareness of health care personnel. Screening programs can identify people at risk for stroke and refer them to specialists for diagnosis and treatment. Screening programs can also identify people who have warning signs of impending stroke, such as TIAs (Table 20–1). Community resources should be identified and used by patients who have survived the acute stage of stroke. If the patient is at home, resources—such as a visiting nurse, a visiting physician for emergency and follow-up care, a physical therapist, special assistive devices, homemaker or household assistance, and financial assistance—should be available. Public transportation suitable for the handicapped should be easily accessible. Architectural barriers at home and in the community should be eliminated. Whether long-term care is given in the hospital, in ambulatory settings, at home, or in other institutions, emphasis must be placed on rehabilitation and prevention of recurring stroke, which poses an added financial burden on the patient and society.

References

Adams, R. B., & Victor, M. (1993). *Principles of neurology* (5th ed.). New York: McGraw-Hill.

Aho, K., Harmson, P., Hatano, S., Marquardson, J., Smirnov, V. E., & Strasser, T. (1980). Cerebrovascular disease in the community: Results of a WHO collaborative study. *Bulletin of the World Health Organization, 58*(1), 113–130.

Bannister, R. (1992). *Brain's clinical neurology* (7th ed.). New York: Oxford University Press.

Blissitt, P. A. (1990). Nutrition in acute spinal cord injury. *Critical Care Nursing Clinics of North America, 2*(3), 375–384.

Brott, T., & Reed, R. L. (1989). Intensive care for acute stroke in the community hospital setting: The first 24 hours. *Stroke, 20,* 694.

Cury, K., & Casady, L. (1992). The relationship between extended periods of immobility and decubitus ulcer formation in the acutely spinal cord–injured individual. *Journal of Neuroscience Nursing, 24*(4), 185–189.

Halm, M. A. (1990). Elimination concerns with acute spinal cord trauma: Assessment and nursing interventions. *Critical Care Nursing Clinics of North America, 2*(3), 385–398.

Hickey, J. V. (1992). *The clinical practice of neurological and neurosurgical nursing.* Philadelphia: J.B. Lippincott.

Mitchell, P. H., & Loustau, A. (1981). *Concepts basic to nursing* (3rd ed.). New York: McGraw-Hill.

National Institutes of Health (NIH) (1986). Prevention of venous thrombosis and pulmonary embolism. NIH Consensus Conference. *JAMA, 256,* 744.

Posner, J. D., Gorman, K. M., & Woldow, A. (1984). Stroke in the elderly: I. Epidemiology. *Journal of the American Geriatrics Society, 32*(2), 95.

Roth, E. J., Lovell, L., Heinemann, A. W., Lee, M. Y., & Yarkony, G. M. (1992). The older adult with a spinal cord injury. *Paraplegia, 30,* 520–526.

Weingarden, S. I., & Graham, P. (1992). Young spinal cord injured patients in nursing homes: Rehospitalization issues and outcomes. *Paraplegia, 30,* 828–833.

Chronic Alterations in Mobility

CHERYL S. DEELEY • CATHERINE A. KERNICH

Altered mobility is a common problem for patients with a number of neurologic disorders. The specific pathophysiology may arise from (1) lack of neurotransmitter substances in brain structures (as in Parkinson's disease), (2) altered transmission of electrical signals along motor fibers (as in multiple sclerosis), (3) deficient neurotransmission at the neuromuscular junction (as in myasthenia gravis), (4) destruction of the motor neuron (as in amyotrophic lateral sclerosis) and other portions of the central nervous system (as in stroke or spinal cord injury), or (5) disorders of the muscles themselves (as in muscular dystrophy). Although the pathophysiology determines the pattern of altered mobility, there are a number of responses to altered mobility that people with chronic changes have in common, including decreased endurance for activities of daily living (ADLs), potential needs for adaptive mobility aids, potential for social isolation and altered coping ability, and potential for respiratory and nutritional disorders. People with chronic disorders that affect mobility make up a large segment of patients requiring prolonged care. Many of these disorders are progressive. Nurses can encounter patients with chronic illness and associated mobility difficulties in numerous settings including community health practices, outpatient clinics, inpatient units, long-term care facilities, and rehabilitative settings. Nurses may encounter patients of all ages, and each patient will have his or her own unique developmental issues that require consideration. The evolving role of nurses, particularly in light of widespread health care changes, affects their ability to meet care needs of patients with chronic disorders.

CHRONIC ILLNESS AND MOBILITY

Chronic illness can be defined as a condition that interferes with daily functioning for longer than 3 months in 1 year, causes hospitalization for longer than

1 month in a year, or at the time of diagnosis is likely to do either (Hobbs, Perrin, Ireys, Moynihan, & Shayne, 1984). Severity of illness is much more difficult to measure. Several disease-specific assessment tools are available to help rate the severity and impact of illness. The Unified Parkinson's Disease Rating Scale incorporates psychologic features, a functional activities scale, an examination of parkinsonian signs, an assessment of complications, a slightly modified Hoehn-Yahr Scale (assesses disease severity and distribution), and the Schwab and England Activities of Daily Living Scale (Lang & Fahn, 1989). The Tufts Quantitative Neuromuscular Examination (TQNE) is designed to quantify neuromuscular deficit and rate of disease progression in amyotrophic lateral sclerosis (Andres, Skerry, & Munsat, 1989). Functional level for Huntington's disease is evaluated using the Huntington's Disease Functional Capacity Scale (HDFC). The HDFC incorporates the categories of occupational function, financial function, domestic function, self-care, and level of care (Shoulson et al., 1989). The Kurtzke Expanded Disability Status Scale is used for multiple sclerosis; it assesses functional systems individually and then assigns a disability score (Poser, 1989). The Fahn-Marsden Scale is a quantitative assessment for torsion dystonia that incorporates a movement scale and a disability scale that is based on the patient's subjective impairment in ADLs (Fahn, 1989). The Sickness Impact Profile is designed to assess the functional status of patients with chronic disease and assesses both physical and psychosocial dimensions. Although it is not disease specific, its utility has been demonstrated specifically with Parkinson's disease (Longstreth, Nelson, Linde, & Munoz, 1992). Several more general rating scales are also available to evaluate neurologic impairment as well as disability. The five components suggested to measure the impact of chronic illness in childhood might also be applied to the concerns of adults. These concerns are (1) financial burden (out-of-pocket expenses greater than 10% of family income); (2) restriction of physical development; (3) impaired ability to engage in accustomed and expected activities; (4) significant emotional problems expressed as maladaptive coping strategies; and (5) disruption of family life, as evidenced by increased marital friction and sibling behavior disturbances (Hobbs et al., 1984).

There have been several attempts to describe theories of chronicity and the adjustment process patients and families go through as they cope with chronic illness. Kodadek (1985) summarized an application of crisis theory to chronic illness, including three stages of adaptation and resulting tasks that must be addressed. The first phase is the diagnostic or initial stage, in which there is a period of disorganization and disequilibrium. The second, or chronic stage, is that of reorganization; it can be crucial, because this stage is when patients and families learn to manage their chronic illness. The adaptive tasks seen during this second phase include the need to learn to (1) function normally, (2) adapt to ongoing change, (3) interact productively with various health care providers and the health care system in general, (4) manage role shifts, and (5) develop communication channels to prevent isolation. The third stage, that of resolution, involves accepting the chronicity associated with the illness or its terminal nature. The stages described can overlap and change as the nature of the illness changes (Kodadek, 1985). The length of time required to move through these stages can also vary considerably.

Neurologic nurses caring for patients with chronic neurologic problems that impair mobility need a broad understanding of the nursing care measures that these disorders have in common. The importance of early diagnosis and intervention; the rehabilitative focus on abilities; and assisting the patient with problem solving, adjusting to chronicity, and learning to control his or her own life are common themes. A clear understanding of the natural history of these chronic disorders assists the nurse in setting appropriate goals with the patient and the family. Patients with chronic neurologic disorders, such as multiple sclerosis, muscular dystrophy, Parkinson's disease, and amyotrophic lateral sclerosis, can have widely different abilities that cannot be predicted from an incomplete or biased knowledge of prognosis. For example, optimal function for one patient may be to learn to accept a wheelchair for mobility; for another, it may be to avoid dependence on it.

Common Movement Problems in Chronic Neurologic Conditions. Weakness is a common finding in chronic disorders and is one of the most common complaints in outpatient practice. Weakness is characterized by the inability of the muscle to exert its normal force and can arise from dysfunction of any component of the motor system that is involved with voluntary muscle movement. Weakness may be objective, subjective, local, generalized, acute, or chronic. True muscle weakness is secondary to lesions in the upper motor neuron or lower motor neuron pathway and can be present in a wide variety of neurologic diseases.

Subjective complaints of weakness may actually represent a different sort of problem. Patients often use the term weakness to refer to fatigue or lassitude. Complaints of weakness may represent extrapyramidal dysfunction characterized by rigidity and postural instability (Bernat & Vincent, 1987). Local weakness can be seen with spinal cord nerve root impingement; generalized weakness is apparent with myasthenia gravis. Disorders such as multiple sclerosis and myasthenia gravis are often associated with an abrupt onset of weakness followed by some improvement. Disorders such as strokes and spinal cord injuries usually have an abrupt presentation followed by some marginal improvement and achievement of a static state of deficit. Chronic disorders, such as Parkinson's disease, amyotrophic lateral sclerosis, and the muscular dystrophies, have a more insidious course that can span years. Fatigue is commonly seen in muscle weakness or is caused by overwork of limited available musculature. Fatigue can immobilize a person of normal strength and cardiovascular conditioning. For a patient with chronic immobility, minimal activity can often be a stress that produces muscle weakness and profound fatigue. For patients with myasthenia gravis, Parkinson's disease, and multiple sclerosis, this weakness can be accentuated by nerve or neurotransmitter fatigue. In muscular dystrophy or amyotrophic lateral sclerosis, this condition can be a result of specific muscle weakness or imbalance. Changes in muscle tone, associated movements, gait, and tremor can alter mobility in patients with Parkinson's disease or Huntington's disease. Spasticity is characterized by increased muscle tone resulting from an upper motor neuron lesion and can be both immobilizing and painful. For the infant or child with spasticity associated with cerebral palsy, contractures may develop and further interfere with developmental milestones. Spasticity can also be problematic for patients with strokes, amyotrophic lateral sclerosis, and multiple sclerosis by interfering with movement and transfers and by creating pain. Immobility resulting from severe muscle weakness and change in muscle tone can result in contractures and atrophy of the affected muscle group. The effects of deconditioning associated with a lack of physical activity may be apparent in a matter of days; the normal individual on bedrest loses strength from baseline levels at a rate of 3% a day. Patients with nerve or muscle pathology are subject to the effects of disuse as well as the intrinsic effects of their disease. The immobilized patient can have weakness of respiratory muscles and muscles of speech and swallowing as well as altered visual perception. Disorders such as spinal cord injury and multiple sclerosis can be associated with sensory abnormalities that can interfere with perception and comfort. The neurologic disorders associated with chronic immobility may be viewed as affecting the upper and lower motor neurons.

Neurologic disorders affecting mobility are caused by lesions in upper or lower motor neuron pathways. The lower motor neuron carries impulses from the cell body in certain cranial nerves and the anterior horn cells of the spinal cord to the muscle. The lower motor neuron is referred to as the final common pathway or the final linkage between the central nervous system and the peripheral nervous system. Signs and symptoms of lower motor neuron diseases include flaccid paralysis, muscle atrophy, and loss of muscle tone and reflexes.

The upper motor neuron originates in higher brain centers and influences the activity of the lower motor neuron via central nervous system pathways. The role of the upper motor neuron is to facilitate and inhibit muscle contraction. Loss of this inhibition by diseases of the upper motor neuron leads to spasticity, increased muscle tone, and hyperreflexia. Examples of lower motor neuron diseases include spinal cord injury and polio. Examples of upper motor neuron diseases include Parkinson's disease and Huntington's disease. Amyotrophic lateral sclerosis affects both upper and lower motor neurons.

HUMAN RESPONSES TO CHRONIC ALTERATIONS IN MOBILITY

The patient with chronic alterations in mobility because of muscle weakness or fluctuations in strength will face many changes, gradual and abrupt, throughout life. Coping with limitations in daily activities can be the most significant problem facing patients with chronic neurologic disorders. Additionally, patients can be acutely immobilized during three situations: (1) in the initial diagnostic period; (2) when a treatment is initiated (such as corticosteroids, immunosuppressants, or temporary drug abstinence); and (3) when a crisis occurs (e.g., respiratory infection, surgery, ventilatory failure). For many patients, these three situations may require hospitalization to resolve. To assess the patient's degree of immobility, the nurse will need to make frequent checks of reliable indicators.

The patient may be immobilized both physically and emotionally during crises but function at a near-normal level days later. Monitoring vital signs or the patient's subjective perceptions may be of assistance, although in some cases these measures will not allow the nurse (or the newly diagnosed patient) to make reliable judgments about the patient's true functional ability. An experienced patient may be able to describe the symptoms vividly but rarely with the sophistication of quantitative objective measures. Quantitative measures a nurse can employ to assess the patient's status are discussed as they relate to specific nursing diagnoses. A flow sheet (Fig. 21–1) to simplify recording data obtained from patient assessment is very helpful to monitor long-term changes or to signal abrupt deterioration in many chronic neurologic disorders.

Patients should be familiar with the assessment methods used in the hospital, long-term care facility, or outpatient setting and be encouraged to monitor themselves by keeping a symptom diary that can be useful during telephone calls and outpatient visits.

Date: Time	FVC	Count/1 Breath	SW	DBL vision	Arm hang	Med
4:00 PM	2.00 L	20/1 breath	3/5	R lat gaze	30 sec R	Mestinon 60
8:00 PM	1.00 L	9/1 breath	1/5	R lat gaze ptosis bilat	10 sec R	Could not swallow med

A

Date: Time		Worse	Parkinson	Best	Dyskinesias	Worse	Med/dose
	Scale:	0%	−50%	100%	+50%	0	
5:00 PM			−70				Sinemet 20/200
7:30 PM					+15 (Freezing noted)		Sinemet 10/100
10:00 PM			−95		(Mild)		Sinemet 20/200

B

FIGURE 21–1 • Bedside flow sheet for monitoring (A) status of patients with myasthenia gravis and (B) mobility in patients with Parkinson's disease.

Nursing Diagnoses Related to Individuals

The following diagnostic categories frequently have chronic altered physical mobility as the main etiology: potential for injury, activity intolerance, self-care deficit, ineffective breathing patterns, inadequate nutrition, constipation, altered communication, altered vision, sexual dysfunction, discomfort, ineffective coping, social isolation, knowledge deficit, impaired home maintenance management, and alterations in health maintenance.

Case studies are used to illustrate several of these diagnoses.

• C A S E   S T U D Y   1

Chronic Immobility Associated with Parkinson's Disease

Mr. Earl is a 76-year-old man who has had symptoms of parkinsonism for at least 25 years. He was forced into early retirement at age 52 years because his parkinsonism interfered with his ability to perform his job as the proprietor of a newsstand. Treatment with levodopa almost completely restored his mobility, although the positive effects were marred by nausea and brief periods of tremor and weakness. Occasionally, he would awaken at night choking on his saliva. These episodes were accompanied by stertorous respirations (labored breathing) that were relieved by walking. In 1974, he switched to Sinemet; this formulation of levodopa eliminated his nausea. With Sinemet, he began to notice slight dyskinesias—periods of (chorealike) extra movements characterized by grimacing, swaying on standing, or, when sitting, a kicking, restless-leg movement. These movements were not bothersome, and Mr. Earl usually did not notice them unless a family member drew his attention to them. They often accompanied times when he felt the most mobile, relaxed, and energetic. After 5 years of treatment with Sinemet, Mr. Earl's dyskinesias began to occur unpredictably throughout the day rather than only after each dose of Sinemet. In addition, attempts to improve mobility by altering the dosing schedule and increasing the amount of Sinemet did not improve mobility and resulted in increased dyskinesias. The dyskinesias on a higher dose were so pronounced that they caused profuse sweating and dehydration. On one occasion, Mr. Earl developed fever and constipation, which prompted hospitalization. On a lower daily dose of Sinemet, he noticed less relief of symptoms of immobility and continued to have unpredictable periods of improved movement. Swallowing occurred only with effort, even during relatively mobile times. Mr. Earl lost 10 lb, to weigh 105 lb.

Constipation was treated with laxatives, stool softener, suppositories, and enemas. Burning sensations affecting his forearms and the soles of his feet interfered with his ability to be comfortable at night and obtain needed rest. Aching pain in his shoulders and arms was relieved with frequent range-of-motion exercises during the day and the night. Mrs. Earl was becoming frustrated and overwhelmed with her husband's needs for assistance with all activities; her sciatica was recurring and interfering with her ability to obtain a full night's rest. Mr. and Mrs. Earl could not afford to hire help, and they could not receive reimbursement for Mr. Earl's health care expenses. After several failed attempts to involve him in day activities for the elderly, several falls, increasing weight loss, and recurring constipation, Mr. Earl was admitted to the hospital for medication adjustment and evaluation and treatment of a chronically distended abdomen. Although Mr. Earl has many diagnoses, his case is used to discuss the diagnosis of potential for injury, including potential for falls and potential for skin breakdown.

POTENTIAL FOR INJURY

Physical safety is the most basic of human needs. The potential for injury is defined as a state in which the individual is at risk for or has experienced damage to body tissues because of perceptual or physiologic deficit, lack of awareness, or maturational age (Carpenito, 1993). Amyotrophic lateral sclerosis, stroke, muscular dystrophy, multiple sclerosis, and many of the chronic motor disorders can cause one's ability to move to be so disturbed that potential injury is a severe threat. Patients with Parkinson's disease, in particular, have difficulty because of the unpredictability of the degree and the timing of response to the levodopa therapy that reduces bradykinesia and rigidity. This occurs in patients who have had parkinsonism for several years and have been receiving levodopa therapy usually for longer than 5 years (Lusis, 1997; Riley & Lange, 2000). These responses to levodopa may be characterized by involuntary movements (dyskinesias) or by lack of movement (akinesia or bradykinesia). Dyskinesias place the individual at risk for being thrown off balance or out of chairs. Off periods are times without satisfactory mobility and may occur gradually or suddenly.

Additional problems include reduced position sense and slowing of one's ability to correct a loss of balance through movement. This can lead to injury or falls. Reduced sensitivity of the autonomic system can be accentuated by some of the medications used to treat Parkinson's disease, as well as being an independent symptom. Orthostatic hypotension can contribute to loss of balance. Shuffling or short steps of low amplitude associated with parkinsonism is caused by bradykinesia and rigidity and can lead to tripping and falls. The patient with footdrop resulting from muscular dystrophy or multiple sclerosis is also in danger of falling without proper intervention. The fatigued or weakened individual, such as the person who suffers from a chronic neurologic disorder, is at risk for injury, because he or she experiences reduced strength and mobility related to prolonged inactivity.

Defining characteristics of the diagnosis of potential for injury include evidence of environmental hazards or lack of knowledge about environmental hazards, history of accidents, and lack of knowledge about safety precautions. Impaired mobility and sensory deficits contribute to the diagnosis of potential for injury. The activity level may be consciously or unconsciously altered in an effort to compensate for slight but definite changes in mobility and strength affecting safety as well as self-care capabilities.

Assessment for potential for injury should include (1) Romberg's sign, (2) gait, (3) orthostatic blood pressure, (4) posture, (5) muscle strength, (6) coordination, (7) uncontrolled involuntary movements, (8) ability to recover position when forcibly displaced (retropulsion test), (9) body position sense, and (10) sensation. Information obtained from the client should include the number, the precipitating factors, and the frequency and type of any injuries or falls. It is important to know if mobility aids are being used properly and successfully. The expected outcome for this diagnosis is that the patient be able to maintain maximal independent mobility without physical injury.

Nursing interventions for the person with impaired mobility focus on teaching that person to associate particular symptoms with a potentially injurious situation. Examples of these situations and the precautions that can be taken follow.

POTENTIAL FOR FALLS

For lightheadedness or orthostasis, the person should change position slowly; moving from a supine position to sitting or standing may need to be done over 5 minutes or more. Blocks under the bed's headframe may reduce orthostasis by placing the person in the reverse Trendelenburg position to minimize the difference between the lying and upright positions. Waist- or thigh-high elastic support hose may also help minimize severe orthostasis. Persons should avoid standing for prolonged periods in one position. Additionally, the patient should take great care to maintain sufficient fluid intake and avoid dehydration and intake of heavy meal portions. Marked dyskinesias in persons with Parkinson's disease or choreoathetosis in persons with Huntington's disease, may necessitate temporary retirement to a chair or bed to prevent loss of balance or injury to the legs or arms from flailing movements. Shuffling steps reduce the size and thus the stability of one's base for standing and can lead to tripping. Leather-soled, well-supported shoes with low heels are recommended for carpeted areas. Sandals, slippers, or slip-on shoes should be avoided. Women, particularly, need to avoid high heels as these further add to poor posture and center of gravity displacement. Parallel strips of tape about 1 ft apart on the floor provide visual input that paradoxically reduces freezing for the person with parkinsonism.

Mr. Earl required assistance for balance in ambulation most of the time; this was accomplished by having someone walk backward holding onto both of his hands and facing him. He was unable to use a walker because of a tendency to fall backward (retropulsion). For others, using a wheeled walker with brakes or walking behind and pushing a wheelchair can be helpful in providing support and stability. When Mr. Earl returned home, a public health nurse reviewed the home situation for anticipation of potential hazards, such as proper rug placement, presence of grab bars in the bath, family plans to cope with falls, and use of appropriate transfer techniques. The nurse noticed that Mr. and Mrs. Earl's furniture was comfortable and did not create barriers, that they did not have a gas stove, and that their equipment was in good repair. The nurse discussed the correct method of using the wheelchair and of going up and down ramps safely and reinforced the importance of using a seatbelt in the car.

Some homes may require modification, particularly those with bathrooms only on the second floor or steep stairwells that the mobility-impaired patient finds difficult or impossible to climb. The mobility-impaired patient who gets up frequently at night to use the bathroom will need to have this problem addressed to prevent falls. A bedside commode or urinal may reduce the need for nighttime trips to the bathroom. Ramps, mechanical lifting devices, and other home modifications can prevent accidents and injuries to the patient or to the family member who lifts or transfers the patient. This family member should be included in care planning.

The dangers in stair use for the person with reduced mobility are the potential for loss of balance backward or forward or the inability to complete stair climbing because of weakness. The tendency to fall backward can be caused by other situations that challenge position sense, such as reaching or gazing upward, stepping backward when opening a door, moving suddenly to avoid injury, or performing more than one activity simultaneously. Patients should be cautioned to use additional reference points in space to increase their awareness of position. Examples of common methods of support are touching furniture or walls when walking, having the back against a wall, or leaning into a sink even slightly when standing for long periods. Those individuals with right-sided strokes need to learn to rethink automatic activities, such as getting out of bed, to include their compromised left side. After they learn which situations can precipitate injury, patients may be more willing to try independent activities with more self-confidence and should continually increase and challenge these skills.

POTENTIAL FOR SKIN BREAKDOWN

The patient with spinal cord injury or multiple sclerosis may have reduced sensory awareness below the level of the lesions that interferes with awareness of ischemic pressure areas. This person must be checked and must learn to check herself or himself periodically, every 2 to 3 hours, for areas of skin blanching, redness, or breakdown. The person with a hemispheric stroke needs to also be conscientious in monitoring for skin breakdown of the affected side. For others with intact sensation, such as patients with Parkinson's disease, amyotrophic lateral sclerosis, or myasthenia gravis, periods of immobility or weakness may hamper their ability to shift position and thus predispose them to skin breakdown. Equipment such as an overhead bed trapeze or an automatic recliner with a lift seat may allow increased independence and the ability to shift position to relieve pressure. Excessive involuntary movements of dyskinesia or chorea can contribute to bruises and abrasions of the extremities. Equipment or furniture may need to be padded with sheepskin, foam, or linen to prevent injury. Frequent repetitive movement can quickly cause a pressure sore where none existed previously, especially at the sacrum, heels, elbows, or ankles. Lastly, profuse diaphoresis is a common complaint for people with Parkinson's disease and for those with autonomic dysfunction. This can also be a predisposing factor for skin breakdown. Lightweight, breathable clothing and frequent changes to dry clothing as well as meticulous hygiene can help minimize this risk.

• C A S E   S T U D Y   2

Immobility Associated with Myasthenia Gravis

Mrs. X was on her way to class; in 2 weeks she would graduate from community college with an associate's degree in nursing with an A average. It did not seem like it had been just 9 years since the birth of her seventh child. She had been only 33 years old and had felt very frightened. Immediately after the uncomplicated birth, the intense fatigue, hoarse voice, and catch in her throat she had experienced over the preceding 3 months worsened. She was unable to swallow saliva, her eyelids drooped, she saw two of everything, and, worst of all, she could not catch her breath.

The next 3 days were a blur of intravenous tubes, infusions, medications, and being on and off the ventilator. Pneumonia complicated her hospitalization. Finally, edrophonium chloride was used to diagnose a disease Mrs. X had never heard of, myasthenia gravis. During the years that followed, she had to modify her activities considerably. Mrs. X was not able to climb the two flights of stairs in her home more than once a day and could hold the baby only while sitting down. She was able to rely on her older children to run many errands in the house, such as going up and down the stairs and doing the laundry. Managing a home with seven children did not afford her much rest, however, and she frequently had to call on friends and relatives for assistance. Her husband could not cope with the limitations imposed on him by the disease and ultimately abandoned the family. After several years of treatment, which included thymectomy and alternate-day corticosteroids, she was slowly able to resume her usual busy schedule. When her vision and strength stabilized, she resumed driving again. This enabled her to have a great deal more independence. She became involved with the local volunteer ambulance squad and enrolled in nursing school. After 10 years of treatment, she commented, ''I know a lot more about nursing now and hope that I can help patients as much as I was helped through those awful years.'' The diagnosis illustrated by her case is activity intolerance.

ACTIVITY INTOLERANCE

Activity intolerance can be related to fluctuations in neurotransmitters, failure of neuromuscular transmission, muscle weakness or atrophy resulting from loss of nerve or muscle fibers, prolonged inactivity, depression, and fear. For patients with myasthenia gravis and multiple sclerosis, heat, particularly hot baths, can increase weakness. Physical exercise, stress, and infection can also exacerbate symptoms. The central feature of this diagnosis is that the patient is unable to tolerate an increase in activity.

Defining characteristics include shortness of breath and fatigue after activity, specific patterns of muscle weakness in tested muscle groups, and reports of self-care deficits that may vary throughout the day. Being unable to climb stairs or ambulate for long distances, as well as avoiding usual activity patterns or exercise, is common.

Assessment should include identification of subjective and objective measures of activity tolerance. The patient may describe an inability to initiate or complete ADLs or to ambulate independently. The patient should be asked to review daily and weekly activity patterns, including activity related to occupation, leisure, rest, and exercise. Knowledge of other environmental factors, such as changes in the weather, the number of stairs in the home, and the distance traveled walking from work to home or to the car, may assist in understanding the baseline activity tolerance. The nurse should record subjective complaints of shortness of breath and results of objective tests of strength. Strength and functional ability can vary from hour to hour or consist of a more subtle change in activity pattern in a previously active patient. The activity pattern seen before the onset of illness will influence the patient's expectations. A young adult who ran or jogged several miles a day will experience different expectations and ability to adapt to changes in activity tolerance than will a less active or aged client. The expected outcome of this diagnosis is that the patient will adapt to varying levels of strength to pursue a full range of satisfying activities.

Nursing interventions for patients having severely reduced activity tolerance include scheduling activities during periods of maximal strength. This can occur at peak doses of medications, such as levodopa or anticholinesterases, or, for some patients, in the morning hours when they are fully rested. This may mean a change in the patient's previous activity patterns. Working with the patient to develop a plan for each day can be of assistance. Encouraging the patient to pretend to be an executive with a predetermined daily schedule that incorporates periods of rest has been suggested (Myasthenia Gravis Foundation, 1979). This was important to Mrs. X, because she was able to enlist her older children to help supervise the younger children during naps and to do the laundry. In many cases, the patient should double the amount of time he or she would normally expect to prepare for an activity, both to provide a rest period and to allow for unanticipated problems. Asking the patient to rehearse the day also assists in setting realistic goals. A cane or walker provides support; walkers with front-leg wheels provide support without necessitating picking up the walker and reduce energy requirements for weakened or fatigued persons.

Patients with severe proximal weakness and resultant difficulty in stair climbing will need to consider alternative methods of climbing stairs. These considerations need careful advance planning in patients with progressive disorders who have homes that may become inaccessible as time goes on. Home adaptations need to be considered with this in mind. Stair rails on both walls and wall grips or handles at landings can be helpful. Rails in the shower and bath, as well as bath benches and handheld shower hoses, must be considered. The patient with footdrop that interferes with mobility should be fitted with lightweight plastic short leg braces, also called ankle-foot orthoses.

When the patient is completely immobilized, which can occur in muscular dystrophy, amyotrophic lateral sclerosis, and spinal cord injury, range-of-motion exercises are necessary to maintain joint mobility. Some patients with neuromuscular disease will eventually require a wheelchair to maintain normal activities. Many chairs have features attractive to the patient with a chronic mobility disorder. Some chairs are lightweight and have the added feature of being able to have a motor attached (Fig. 21–2). Consideration should also be given to a wheelchair that has removable armrests and footrests to facilitate transfers.

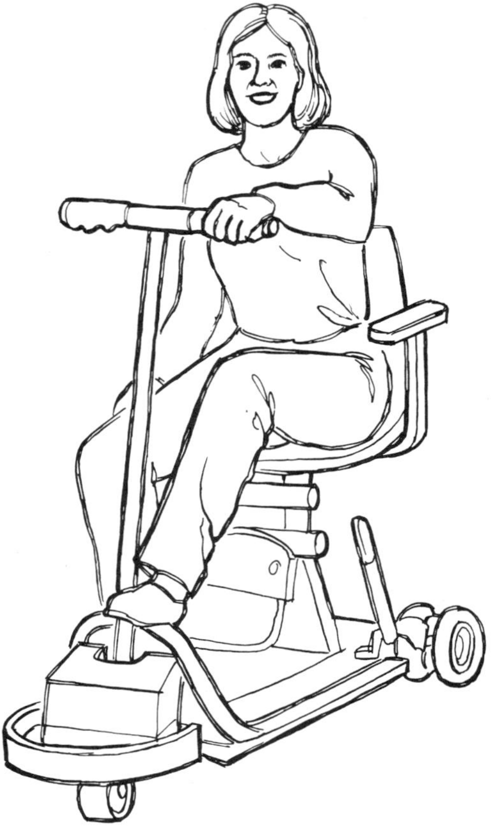

FIGURE 21–2 • Motorized scooter. (From Maloney, F. P., Burks, J. S., & Ringel, S. [1985]. *Interdisciplinary rehabilitation of multiple sclerosis and neuromuscular disorders.* Philadelphia: J.B. Lippincott.)

For the patient with less variability in symptoms and potential for improving strength, consideration should be given to designing an exercise program. Specific exercise programs that improve flexibility and endurance as well as increase strength have many benefits (Cobble & Maloney, 1985). Most patients avoid exercise because it is perceived as a significant stressor. Indeed, many aerobic programs are inappropriate for patients with severe muscle weakness and fatigue. There has been renewed interest in designing individual exercise programs for patients with chronic mobility disorders. A successful study of patients with multiple sclerosis demonstrated positive effects on strength, endurance, work, and muscle power by using an aquatic fitness program (Gehlsen, Grigsby, & Winant, 1984). Another study examining the benefits of a home exercise program for patients with Parkinson's disease suggested exercise as a factor in promoting self-care in ADLs (Hurwitz, 1989). Before beginning any exercise program, patients should request the assistance of their health care providers to monitor its effects on their strength and functional ability. Individual exercise prescriptions that address the patient's age, strength, interests, and functional ability can do much to improve the patient's well-being as well as motor strength, flexibility, and endurance.

Lack of transportation and accessibility have been deterrents for wheelchair-bound patients. Several ambulatory patients have reported that participation in a graduated exercise program is possible. In fact, several symptomatic patients with myasthenia gravis and multiple sclerosis have continued exercise programs that include weightlifting, swimming, stationary rowing, and jogging. One patient with myasthenia gravis reported completing a marathon. Many handicapped patients benefit from participation in handicapped sports, such as wheelchair basketball, baseball, bowling, and field hockey. Empirical studies of the benefits of exercise in the patient with chronic mobility problems are urgently needed. Until they are completed, each patient needs to be individually considered and carefully monitored. For the extremely weak patient, performing ADLs will provide all the exercise they need to maintain strength, and energy should be conserved for these activities.

• C A S E   S T U D Y   3

Chronic Immobility Associated with Muscular Dystrophy

Mike was 5 years old when his parents realized that he was not keeping up with his peers. Subsequently, they have always felt the worst period in their lives was the time when they were told that he had muscular dystrophy. He has been cared for in a comprehensive multidisciplinary clinic practice since the diagnosis was made at age 6 years. By age 10 years, Mike's balance was so precarious that he began to fall frequently. The wheelchair that his parents formerly dreaded came as a relief. He continued to be able to stand for several hours a day with the assistance of long leg braces and a standing table. His parents wanted him to be treated like any other child, and he enjoyed attending a mainstream school with his older sister. At first, he found it difficult to ask his friends to assist him, especially with toileting. To assist him with this and other problems, a plan was developed each year with the assistance of the clinic staff and school nurse to coordinate transportation between classes, appropriate physical education activities, note taking, and social activities. Mike graduated from college with an associate's degree in computer science. A work-study program gave him experience as a computer programmer; however, he was not able to find a job when the family moved.

Although always described as quiet, Mike had many friends. His family was active with the local chapter of the Muscular Dystrophy Association. His mother attended a mothers' group that served to share problems and concerns. They offered such practical advice as how to use assistive devices, mechanical lifting devices, commodes, and wheelchairs. Health care providers from the clinic were often invited guests.

Mike always had trouble getting over upper respiratory infections. At age 19 years, he had his first severe pneumonia that required hospitalization. He was treated with postural drainage and cupping, using intermittent positive-pressure breathing with a bronchodilator before and after the treatment. Broad-spectrum antibiotics and hydration were continued during his 14-day hospital stay. This was a stressful time for Mike. He was secure in his usual home routine and was fearful that the nurses would not understand his needs. Because of his severe contractures, it would often take extended periods to position him correctly. Some nurses were patient; others could not understand why he continuously asked for repositioning. He was fearful that he would drop his call bell or that someone would not hear him if he called. He had great difficulty feeding himself while he was in the hospital. The hospital overbed tables were awkward, and unless he was positioned just right he could not feed himself. His forced vital capacity (FVC) was 700 mL during the acute episode and increased to 1 L several months later. After this episode, Mike began asking questions about his breathing, and options for future ventilatory support were discussed. Self-care deficit and impaired respiratory function are the diagnoses discussed in relation to Mike's case.

SELF-CARE DEFICIT

Self-care deficit can be related to the severity of muscle weakness and its resultant immobility. This may occur as a static or fluctuating problem in patients with many of the chronic mobility disorders, depending on the extent of involvement.

Defining characteristics of self-care deficit include inability to feed or bathe oneself independently and to complete other aspects of hygienic care (care of hair, nails, teeth, and skin; makeup application). The patient may manifest difficulty getting on and off the toilet as a result of proximal muscle weakness. Many patients with severe muscle weakness as seen in muscular dystrophy, spinal cord injury, and amyotrophic lateral sclerosis develop contractures in a specific pattern associated with weakness of specific muscle groups. For patients with multiple sclerosis, stroke, and spinal cord injury, contractures are usually due to severe spasticity and become a significant problem in patient self-care management.

Assessment includes physical assessment of the patient's strength and functional ability as well as assessment of daily self-care routines. The goal for this diagnosis is to develop an individualized plan of care that is flexible enough to respond to changes in the patient's abilities and yet promotes maximum independence and positive coping.

Nursing interventions may include providing assistance in ADLs as the patient directs. The hospital care plan should reflect the patient's home routines as closely as possible to allow the nurse to assess the patient's safety during transfers and the degree of symptom control and to allow the patient to feel "in charge." For patients with disorders in which fatigue is a factor, such as myasthenia gravis and multiple sclerosis, specific considerations must be made. Hospital routines rarely reflect the effort that home activities require. The patient who is not taxed in the hospital or does not participate in care that reflects home requirements may have further difficulties on discharge. While assisting patients in self-care activities or developing a care plan, the nurse should encourage the fatigued patient not to overextend himself or herself and to plan rest periods throughout the day. Discussing how the patient will manage the same activities at home can be accomplished at this time. A community health nurse can continue with assessment and interventions in the home.

For patients with Parkinson's disease, myasthenia gravis, or multiple sclerosis, meals and activities should always be scheduled at periods of peak strength or flexibility. This typically occurs at peak dose time of medications. The nurse could use these times of hospitalization or rehabilitation to teach the patient to use energy-saving routines, such as dressing and combing the hair while lying down. In addition, for patients with static or more slowly progressing disorders, energy-saving devices, such as a bath bench, handheld shower hose, and easy-grip eating utensils, can be suggested for use at home. Special utensils or equipment to maximize use of motor capabilities will save energy, facilitate communication, and allow independence. For patients with severe weakness, positioning may be a key factor in allowing self-feeding. A ball-bearing orthosis attached to the wheelchair will allow patients with severe shoulder weakness yet sufficient biceps strength to feed themselves (Fig. 21–3). Other devices, such as wrist splints and built-up utensils, enable the patient with a weakened grip to manage meals independently. An occupational therapist should be consulted to evaluate the patient for these devices. Only in unusual circumstances should the nurse feed the patient with chronic immobility. Feeding oneself may be the only measure of independence such people have, as in Mike's case. For many patients with chronic immobility, bathroom modifications may be necessary. Use of a mechanical lifting device, a raised toilet seat, and a wheelchair-accessible shower should be considered. Velcro closures can allow some patients ease in dressing, although they may need the assistance of another if they are pressed for time by school or employment in the morning. Many retail stores carry lines of adaptive clothing for those with mobility disorders. These can also be readily ordered through catalogues. Additional devices or techniques can be obtained from other patients and from literature provided by support groups such as the Myasthenia Gravis Foundation, the Amyotrophic Lateral Sclerosis Society, the Multiple Sclerosis Society, and the several Parkinson's disease organizations.

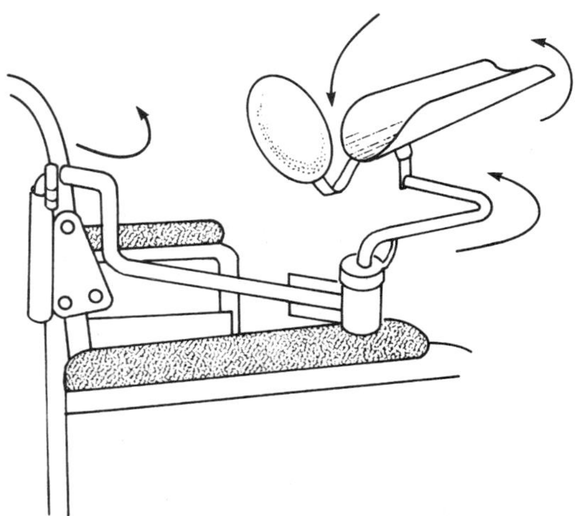

FIGURE 21–3 • Assistive devices: Ball-bearing feeder. (From Maloney, F. P., Burks, J. S., & Ringel, S. [1985]. *Interdisciplinary rehabilitation of multiple sclerosis and neuromuscular disorders.* Philadelphia: J.B. Lippincott.)

IMPAIRED RESPIRATORY FUNCTION

The patient with impaired respiratory function has reduced airway clearance or ineffective breathing patterns. These are present in the acutely ill patient with myasthenia gravis but are most frequently seen during the late stages of muscular dystrophy, amyotrophic lateral sclerosis, and Huntington's disease and are often precipitated by respiratory infection. Patients with high cervical (above C3) lesions also contend with ventilatory failure.

Patients with chronic mobility disorders rarely have significant blood gas abnormalities on a chronic basis as a defining characteristic unless obstructive disease is present. Blood gas abnormalities consistent with alveolar hypoventilation usually follow significant changes in pulmonary function tests or occur only in the presence of respiratory infections. Before the 1960s, many patients with respiratory dysfunction as a result of neurologic disease died secondary to pulmonary compromise. Patients with myasthenia gravis often experience respiratory crisis precipitated by upper respiratory infections, surgery, significant dysarthria and dysphagia, and aspiration (Donohoe, 1994; Sanders & Howard, 2000). Patients with neuromuscular diseases, such as muscular dystrophy, amyotrophic lateral sclerosis, and late stages of multiple sclerosis, have severely reduced objective pulmonary function indicators. Respiratory insufficiency as a result of a decline in pulmonary function is a common cause of death in muscular dystrophy and amyotrophic lateral sclerosis (Brooke, 2000; Mitsumoto, 2000). Atelectasis and aspiration pneumonia are frequent causes of hospitalization in advanced multiple sclerosis and are often terminal events. For those multiple sclerosis patients who have large lesions on the medulla or spinal cord, acute loss of voluntary respiration may occur, with apnea and acute respiratory failure. In these situations, ventilatory support may be necessary (Smeltzer, Utell, Rudick, & Herdon, 1988). Respiratory compromise is the most frequent cause of death in Huntington's disease patients and is thought to be related to dysphagia and aspiration secondary to the involuntary movements affecting swallowing (Riley & Lange, 2000). Studies in patients with parkinsonism have revealed both restrictive and obstructive components to their pulmonary function. Reduced vital capacity and more consistently reduced maximal flow rates were closely correlated with the degree of tremor and rigidity in these patients. The flow rates were postulated to be reduced in relation to the parasympathetic overactivity (Neu, Connolly, Schwestley, Lodwig, & Brody, 1967).

Assessment of patients with potential for impaired respiratory function should include (1) tests of pulmonary function, particularly FVC, maximum static pressures, maximum expiratory pressure (MEP), and maximum inspiratory pressure (MIP); (2) estimate of counting in one breath; (3) evaluation of ability to cough and swallow; (4) assessment of presence of pharyngeal secretions; (5) patient description of subjective sensations of shortness of breath or choking; (6) observation of chest expansion; and (7) assessment of breath sounds. The goal for the patient with impaired respiratory function is maintenance of the air passage through the respiratory tract and exchange of gases between the lungs and the vascular system. Another goal is prevention of aspiration.

Specific interventions include monitoring of pulmonary function at frequent intervals. If possible, the nurse should calculate percent predicted FVC, minimum ventilatory volume, MEP, and MIP for height and age to determine the extent of abnormality. The patient should be monitored while asymptomatic to establish a baseline. With myasthenia gravis, pulmonary function tests and other assessments should be made at intervals to correspond with the anticholinesterase dosage to observe the effects of the medication and to determine the lower limit of the patient's strength.

Patients with chronic immobility should be monitored closely because of their potential to change unpredictably and briskly. Patients with muscle weakness rarely show retraction or tachypnea; as their fatigue increases, their muscles become increasingly weak. This may prevent them from asking for assistance or from exhibiting the usual signs of pulmonary compromise, such as restlessness and tachypnea.

Nursing intervention also includes patient teaching. The patient should receive instructions on deep breathing, preventing infection, treating infection early, and monitoring for signs of respiratory fatigue. The patient should know how to take his or her temperature and to notify the physician at the first sign of respiratory infection. Many medications and antibiotics affect the neuromuscular junction and should be avoided in patients with myasthenia gravis. These patients should take medications, including over-the-counter medications, only on the advice of their neurologist. The patient should be aware of the need to increase fluid consumption to at least 2 L or more per day during an upper respiratory infection. Patients with chronic mobility disorders should receive the pneumonia vaccine (Pneumovax) and a yearly flu shot to prevent pneumonia and influenza.

The patient with poor pulmonary function, that is, anyone with FVC less than 1 L or less than 10 to 15 mL/kg body weight, may need tracheotomy and ventilatory support after severe respiratory infections or surgery because of anticipated disease worsening such as occurs in myasthenia gravis. Appropriate explanations of procedures and sensations to be experienced should be discussed. Many patients recover from these crises to resume their previous activity level; others may not be able to be weaned from ventilatory support. This should be anticipated and discussed well before the acute episode in chronic progressive disorders. For those patients who have difficulty handling secretions, suction equipment is required. The patient may be able to learn how to clear oral secretions; however, it is also important that the family learns this as well, particularly if a tracheostomy is in place.

Ventilatory support for patients with chronic mobility disorders is not a new phenomenon, yet technology has changed the options for these patients. The poliomyelitis experience of the 1940s and 1950s demonstrated the utility of providing ventilatory support in the hope that the patient would stabilize and improve. The intensive care unit, first described in the literature in 1955, originated from the concept of clustering patients in polio wards to consolidate those who required highly skilled nursing care (Cadmus, 1980). Today, providing extraordinary means of support has been simplified by the availability of compact portable systems for positive pressure. A newer technology of pressure-support ventilation may also delay the need for tracheostomy and continual respiratory support (Difilippo & Jenkins, 1988). Although the negative-pressure devices used in the poliomyelitis era have been used in the home with success, their availability is declining, and portable positive-pressure systems are becoming an attractive option (Griggs & Donohoe, 1985; Splaingard, Frates, Jefferson, Rosen, & Hardson, 1985).

Negative-pressure ventilators in use include the cuirass, the wrap or raincoat ventilator, and the iron lung. The cuirass is a plastic shell that fits over the anterior chest wall and can be molded to conform to a scoliotic curvature. The wrap ventilator, also called the raincoat, has a metal cage that spans the chest and supports a heavy plastic raincoatlike material away from the body. The tank or iron lung ventilator can be used to simulate inspiration and promote air exchange. It is very heavy, may require home modifications, and is reported to be in short supply (Curran, 1981). The pneumobelt is another noninvasive device. It has a plastic inflatable bladder attached to a corset that fits around the abdomen. It serves as an expiratory assist; with inflation, the abdomen is compressed and the diaphragm is pushed upward. The patient must be sitting to use it comfortably.

Positive-pressure devices are the next most frequently used ventilatory support systems. They can be used intermittently, such as for intermittent positive pressure breathing (IPPB) treatments, or continuously, with mouthpiece or tracheotomy. Some patients can use mouth positive pressure comfortably. Most patients with severe respiratory weakness require tracheotomy. The compact portable systems (such as the LP10 by the Aegitron Corporation, the PPV by Life Care, the Puritan Bennett Companion, and the Bear system) have also been used successfully for home care. When these systems are used, the use of patient glossopharyngeal breathing to augment vital capacity has been suggested. This procedure requires that the patient take a series of deep breaths without exhaling and has been used by poliomyelitis and spinal-cord–injured patients successfully to give the patient time off the ventilator (Alexander, Johnson, Petty, & Stauch, 1979). The BiPAP S/T Ventilatory Support System uses pressure support for delivery of intermittent positive-pressure ventilation. It is a small, lightweight, pressure-support ventilator used for those persons able to breathe spontaneously and for those who require ventilatory assistance rather than continual ventilatory support. Positive pressure is provided in response to a spontaneous breach. Positive-pressure support allows continual use of the respiratory muscle and thus helps prevent the atrophy of disuse.

Intermittent positive-pressure ventilation has been demonstrated to be an effective form of management for individuals with respiratory muscle weakness, particularly for nighttime ventilation. This system can be used with tracheostomy, face or nasal mask, or mouthpiece (Difilippo & Jenkins, 1988). The need for tracheostomy may be deferred under these circumstances, particularly as nighttime use of system and mouthpiece or mask does not significantly interfere with eating, drinking, and talking. Multiple manufacturers have products available for ventilatory support.

Patients with neuromuscular disease often have pneumonias and retained secretions. Postural drainage and cupping have always been used in conjunction with appropriate antibiotics, hydration, and, if necessary, supplemental oxygen and intermittent positive-pressure breathing for treatment of this problem. Intermittent positive-pressure breathing or other methods provide sighs and hyperexpansion in the patient with hypoventilation as a result of muscle weakness. The method of postural drainage described in most texts is laborious and time-consuming. Few studies have documented its worth on empirical grounds, although it makes sense on practical grounds for patients who cannot produce a sufficient cough, cannot bring up retained secretions, or fatigue rapidly in an effort to do so. Some practitioners and the authors have found that a simpler method is effective and is tolerated better by patients (Callahan, 1985; Lavigne, 1979). This method consists of draining the lungs in two positions, with patients lying on their right side and then their left side with the hips elevated above the head in the Trendelenburg position (Fig. 21–4). The position is maintained on each side for a minimum of 30 to 45 minutes. The patient should be comfortably positioned to tolerate this time. Patients with diaphragmatic weakness or severe respiratory insufficiency will need to be on the ventilator during postural drainage and cupping. Other patients will need sighs or intermittent positive-pressure breathing before and after the procedure. Although it takes an hour, the thoroughness of this procedure reduces the necessity of its performance more often than every 4 hours, and it is well tolerated by patients at home (Callahan, 1985).

Mike and his family successfully learned the postural drainage and cupping procedure during his first hospitalization for pneumonia and subsequently used it once a day with intermittent positive-pressure breathing to prevent

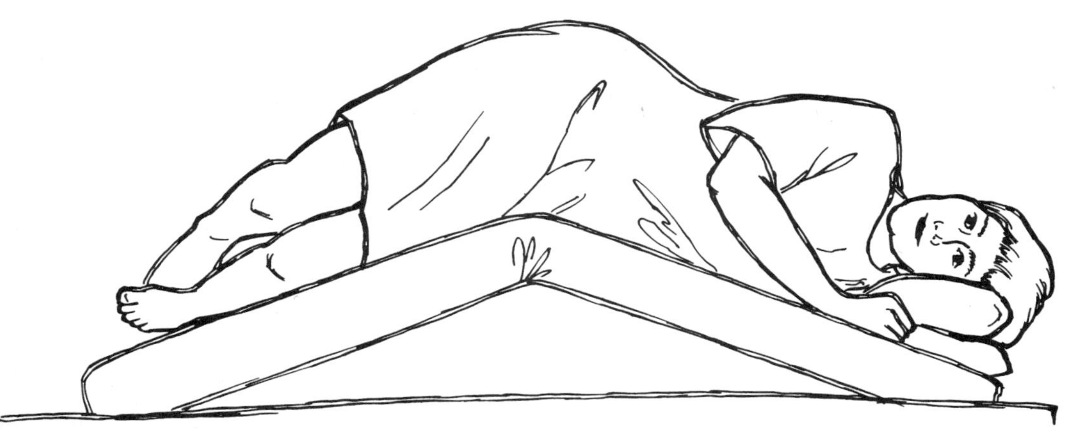

FIGURE 21–4 • Patient in the correct position for postural drainage.

atelectasis and to facilitate secretion removal. Community health nurses can expect an increase in the number of persons requiring extensive pulmonary toilet and home ventilatory support as services expand to accommodate extensive home care needs and hospitals look for alternatives to expensive long-term maintenance.

Associated Nursing Diagnoses

Chronically altered mobility serves as an etiology for a number of other nursing diagnoses. The relationship of these diagnoses to chronically altered mobility is discussed briefly here.

INADEQUATE NUTRITION RELATED TO DYSPHAGIA

Inadequate nutrition can be related to reduced swallowing and chewing ability, as in the case study of Mr. Earl, as well as to other chronic mobility disorders. In fact, any one or all of the five phases of ingestion may be affected. An inability to prepare food can affect the person with weakness or fatigue. The inability to chew and to swallow food is a severely distressing state. Fear of choking or fear of making a mess prevents attempts to eat. Family members or significant others are hesitant to assist the patient because they are afraid of being unable to manage choking episodes effectively. Mealtimes may take an inordinate amount of time and valuable energy. Additionally, increased caloric consumption is often necessary as a result of the increased physical demands required to move or as a result of involuntary movements such as dyskinesia in Parkinson's disease or chorea in Huntington's disease. Persons with Huntington's disease, for example, may require 4000 to 6000 calories a day to maintain their weight (Hunt & Walker, 1989). This increased caloric need coupled with dysphagia may jeopardize the patient's nutritional state. Small bites of soft or pureed foods that are high in calories and nutritional value can help ensure sufficient intake. Nutritional supplements may also be indicated.

Placement of a feeding tube helps ensure sufficient nutritional intake and hydration as well as minimizes the risk of choking, or aspiration. Additionally, for those with limited energy resources, valuable time that would be used in feeding oneself can be available for other types of activities. Percutaneous endoscopic gastrostomy feeding tubes are typically placed when the patient is under local anesthesia and have a shortened recovery time as compared with the traditional gastrostomy tubes placed surgically and with the patient under general anesthesia. For those patients with severe gastroesophageal reflux and high risk for aspiration, a jejunostomy feeding tube may be preferable (Guenter, 1989).

Generally, balanced diets incorporating the four food groups are recommended for those with chronic mobility disorders. Some illnesses have specific dietary recommendations. People with advanced Parkinson's disease and its associated motor fluctuations benefit from a protein-redistribution diet or a diet that keeps a five-to-one ratio of carbohydrates to protein (Berry, Growden, Wurtman, Caballero, & Wurtman, 1991; Karstaedt & Pincus, 1992). People with multiple sclerosis should incorporate increased amounts of vitamin C in their diets to acidify the urine and reduce the likelihood of urinary tract infections. Diet claims of illness cure need to be carefully examined and shared with a health care provider who can help validate or disclaim accordingly. Defining characteristics, assessment, and interventions for this diagnosis are found in Chapter 22.

CONSTIPATION RELATED TO DECREASED ACTIVITY

Constipation is defined as the state in which the individual experiences or is at high risk of experiencing stasis in the large intestine, resulting in hard, dry feces and infrequent elimination. All neurologic disorders resulting in chronic immobility place the individual at risk for this problem.

As the body's activity level slows, the movement of material through the gastrointestinal track also becomes slower. With slowing, more fluid is extracted from the feces, and it becomes more compact. This process makes elimination even more difficult for the weakened patient. Medications can contribute to the presence of constipation by slowing bowel function further—for example, the anticholinergics used in the treatment of movement disorders such as Parkinson's disease. Difficulty in chewing and swallowing can lead to inadequate fluid intake, and reliance on fast, prepared, or pureed foods that have little fiber can lead to constipation. Obesity, which can develop easily in the immobile patient, can hinder bowel and abdominal muscle function. Hospitalization or the need for assistance with elimination removes privacy. Irregular patterns may develop because of these factors. In an effort to treat irregularity, laxatives and enemas may be employed; chronically, these make the bowel musculature lazy and further contribute to constipation. The older person experiences reduced motility of the gastrointestinal tract related to normal aging. Defining characteristics, assessment, and intervention for this diagnosis are found in Chapter 29.

ALTERED COMMUNICATION RELATED TO DYSARTHRIA AND DYSPHONIA

The patient with chronic immobility resulting from many mobility disorders may have poor communication because of dysarthria, dysphonia, and limb and hand muscle weakness. Communication is also impaired when a tracheostomy is in place. The patient who is quadriplegic secondary to spinal cord injury, multiple sclerosis, muscular dystrophy, or amyotrophic lateral sclerosis, for example, is limited in the ability to communicate verbally or with the extremities. For someone with amyotrophic lateral sclerosis, the eye muscles may be the only muscles preserved, and thus eye movements serve as a means of communicating. Advances in computer technology have increased the number and type of alternative communication devices available. For the hospitalized patient, a pressure-sensitive call bell under the head may help relieve anxiety and ensure that help can be summoned.

Most patients with chronic neurologic disorders with fatigable weakness, such as myasthenia gravis, Parkinson's disease, or multiple sclerosis, have no difficulty with comprehension. For these patients, dysarthria and dysphonia are evident in prolonged conversation. A patient can be tested for fatigue by being asked to read aloud. Shortness of breath or ineffective breathing patterns will also interfere with verbal communication. Assessment and interventions for this diagnosis are found in Chapters 14 and 15.

ALTERED VISION RELATED TO OCULAR MUSCLE WEAKNESS

Altered vision can be associated with a chronic immobilizing disorder and can contribute to immobility. Contributing factors include pathophysiologic, situational, and maturational changes. In myasthenia gravis, altered vision can be related to fatigue of ocular muscles at the neuromuscular junction or structural ophthalmologic dysfunction. Ptosis, a drooping of the eyelids, also interferes with vision. In Parkinson's disease, reduced ocular accommodation can contribute to blurred vision, and fatigue of the muscles involved in eye movements can interfere with reading or other close work. Slowed eye movements in Huntington's disease can slow receipt of information and increase the effort involved in daily activities, such as driving, reading, and housekeeping. Multiple sclerosis can cause diplopia, scotomas, blurred vision, and nystagmus. Optic neuritis is often the presenting symptom of multiple sclerosis.

Defining characteristics of altered vision include difficulty reading; accomplishing ADLs; driving; doing fine work with the hands; and watching television, movies, or plays. Severe difficulty with spatial orientation secondary to diplopia, ptosis, or other oculomotor dysfunctions is another characteristic.

Assessment includes evaluation of the patient for signs of ptosis and diplopia and performance of tests of visual acuity. The presence of cataracts should be considered when assessing blurred vision. The goal is to maximize the patient's visual abilities with supportive devices or to supplement sensory perceptions by using other senses. These methods, it is to be hoped, will reduce the potential for reduced mobility resulting from fear and instability.

Interventions include using eyelid tape or crutches that support the drooping eyelid or wearing sunglasses to protect the eyes from the sun's glare (particularly if the patient is bothered by heat). Diplopia can be relieved by patching one eye. If one eye is covered with a patch, the patient will notice a decrease in depth perception and should be warned that this may impair driving ability. The patient should alternate patches frequently to prevent disuse in the patched eye. The acutely ill patient may benefit from having someone read newspapers and letters aloud. Large-print books, talking books, and tape-recorded letters from friends and family can add to the patient's enjoyment. Treatment of cataracts is of great help to patients with diminished activity and is usually recommended when the cataracts interfere with functional abilities (e.g., driving, reading).

SEXUAL DYSFUNCTION

Sexual dysfunction can be a result of physiologic changes associated with illness or the related problems of immobility; fatigue; decreased endurance; cognitive, sensory, and communication deficits; depression; and concerns about self-image. Medications may also contribute to sexual dysfunction. There is no reported physiologic disturbance to impair enjoyment of sexual response in patients with muscular dystrophy or myasthenia gravis. A physiologic disturbance that impairs the sexual response is seen with spinal cord injury. The level and completeness of the lesion determines erectile function and ejaculatory ability after spinal cord injury. Sexual dysfunction in multiple sclerosis occurs frequently. Seventy-five percent of men with multiple sclerosis have sexual problems, and two-thirds complain specifically of erectile dysfunction (Stenager, Stenager, & Jensen, 1992). Other sexual problems reported include impotence, decreased sensation, fatigue, decreased libido, difficulty with arousal, and impaired fertility (Dewis & Thornton, 1989; Hanak, 1992; Weiss, 1992). Fifty percent of women complain of sexual dysfunction, noting, in particular, change in sensation in the thighs and the genital area (Stenager et al., 1992). Women also report fatigue, decreased libido, problems with orgasm, difficulty with arousal, and reduced vaginal lubrication (Hanak, 1992; Weiss, 1992). Symptoms may occur early in the disease process and may increase as the disease severity worsens. Subsequent studies have supported a high frequency of sexual dysfunction in both sexes and at all stages of the disease (Dewis & Thornton, 1989; Hanak, 1992; Weiss, 1992). Persons with multiple sclerosis also need to contend with bladder dysfunction, which may esthetically interfere with sexual functioning.

Males with amyotrophic lateral sclerosis may have erection and ejaculation dysfunction as well as impaired fertility and libido in the later stages of illness (Hanak, 1992). Sexual dysfunction in Parkinson's disease has been documented; however, knowledge in this area continues to be limited. Lipe, Longstreth, Bird, and Lind (1990) studied married men with Parkinson's disease and found that sexual dysfunction in elderly patients is related to age and to illness-related disability. Koller et al. (1990) studied sexual dysfunction in men and women with Parkinson's disease. They also assessed for the presence of depression, medication use, and autonomic dysfunction. Nearly half the men noted decreased interest in sex, reduced drive, and inability to achieve erection. Sixty percent did not have nocturnal erections, and 67% did not have morning erections. Seventy-one percent of the women had reduced sexual interest, and 62% had reduced drive. Nearly 40% were unable to achieve orgasm, and an equal percentage complained of vaginal dryness during intercourse. These results, when compared with historical references, indicate a higher incidence of sexual dysfunction compared with the general population. This could not be clearly attributed to depression or to medication use; however, autonomic dysfunction was common (69%) in this patient population and may well have been a significant factor (Koller et al., 1990). The change in sexual behavior characterized by increased libido and greater coital frequency seen during levodopa therapy is usually thought to be the result of improved motor activity and affect (Bowers & VanMoert, 1972). Inappropriate sexual expression, including hypersexuality, has been documented in Parkinson's disease, Huntington's disease, and multiple sclerosis, but it is infrequent (France, 1993; Stenager et al., 1992; Wermuth & Stenager, 1992). The prevalence and etiology of the dysfunctions are not well understood in Huntington's disease. Defining characteristics, assessment, and interventions are found in Chapters 30 and 31.

DISCOMFORT

The state in which a patient feels an uncomfortable sensation in response to a noxious stimulus is discomfort. Reduced ability to shift positions, exercise, or even participate in ADLs leads to pressure area formation, increased muscle stiffness, reduced joint mobility, and contractures. Additional features such as dystonia, rigidity, spasticity, and sensory dysesthesia add to feelings of discomfort. Involuntary movements can lead to repeated trauma to body parts and to discomfort. Dysesthesias in Parkinson's disease, spinal cord injury, and multiple sclerosis can become disabling. These may include burning or tingling sensations. Warm or cool temperature intolerances may also be present. Postural changes that accompany Parkinson's disease and muscular dystrophy can create strain and back discomfort, particularly in the lumbar region. Reduced muscle tone also interferes with proper support, while sitting contributes to feelings of discomfort. Often, people with mobility problems request frequent and sometimes prolonged repositioning to relieve discomfort.

The defining characteristic is the patient's report of pain or discomfort. For the person with multiple sclerosis or spinal cord injury, the pain may be localized to a referred place. Pain with multiple sclerosis is reported by as many as 70% of patients. This pain is often chronic in nature (Clark, 1991). A guarded position, facial expression of pain, or crying and moaning suggest the presence of some discomfort even though the client may not be able to express this problem verbally. Additionally, there may be evidence of autonomic responses to acute pain, such as increased blood pressure, pulse, and respirations; diaphoresis; and dilated pupils.

The assessment of discomfort is accomplished by determining pattern, location, onset, duration, aggravating factors, characteristics, relieving maneuvers, and treatments. The goal in any problem characterized by discomfort is to maximize comfort. The nurse does this by correctly determining the cause of the discomfort whenever possible.

Discomfort related to immobility is relieved by the nursing interventions of repositioning of the limbs or the body, passive range-of-motion exercises, or such active exercises as walking, swimming, or active range-of-motion exercises. Movement relieves pressure at bony prominences and restores circulation. Water pillows, Gelfoam mattresses, foam-rubber pads, or cushions reduce pressure over prominences and relieve discomfort. Spasticity can be a tremendous source of discomfort for several conditions including multiple sclerosis, cerebral palsy, amyotrophic lateral sclerosis, spinal cord injury, and stroke. Passive and independent stretching exercises can relieve spasticity as well as cramping and feelings of stiffness. These exercises can be particularly helpful before bedtime to promote comfort and sleep. Massage and relaxation may also be beneficial. Applications of heat, cold, or both applied in an alternating fashion can be helpful for relief of pain associated with dystonia, or cramping. Back braces or supports may help truncal stability, particularly while the patient is sitting, and improve comfort level. Dysesthesias in Parkinson's disease are thought to be especially bothersome in the more immobile patient. If activity can be increased, there may be at least partial relief of this problem.

Pharmacologic agents can play a significant role in the relief of general discomfort and spasticity. Analgesics are helpful for relief of general muscle or joint discomfort. The pain of general or focal dystonia can be relieved with tricyclics or anticholinergics. Botulinum toxin injections into the overactive muscles can be more effective than oral medications in relieving pain associated with focal dystonia. Botulinum toxin causes a temporary chemical denervation by disrupting the function of the neuromuscular junction, resulting in muscle weakness. Frequently, these injections are used to treat cervical dystonia; however, the effect is temporary, and reinjection is required about every 3 months (Jankovic & Schwartz, 1990). Surgical intervention, such as selective peripheral denervation, is also an option; however, these procedures are irreversible, the results variable, and relapse possible (Jankovic & Brin, 1991). The dystonia associated with Parkinson's disease can be treated with antiparkinsonian medications or, if related to medication side effects, a lowering of the medication dosage. Spasticity can be treated with medications such as oral dantrolene, tizanidine, and baclofen. Baclofen is considered to be the most effective medication for relieving spasticity (Gianino, 1993). Intrathecal baclofen may be an option for those patients with severe spasticity that does not respond to more conservative measures including oral administration. Intrathecal baclofen administration is used for treatment of spasticity that is of spinal origin such as in spinal cord injury and multiple sclerosis. Intrathecal baclofen administration results in improved function, characterized by improved independence with ADLs, and ability to transfer resulting from the relief of hyperactive flexion reflexes that interfere with smooth, voluntary movement. Spinal stimulation, chemical neurolysis, and ablative surgical measures such as open neurectomies, muscle and tendon lengthening, and release of fixed contractures may also be used when more conservative measures fail (Gianino, 1993). The use of botulinum toxin injections for the treatment of spasticity in multiple sclerosis and hemiplegic stroke has also been documented. The adductor muscles in patients with multiple sclerosis and the biceps and forearm flexor muscles in patients with stroke were successfully injected, with relief of spasticity and some functional improvement documented. These were short-term studies, and further investigation is required (Tim & Massey, 1992).

POTENTIAL FOR INEFFECTIVE COPING

Selye (1976) described coping as the process by which adaptation occurs. Skills developed during the early stages of illness assist the patient in coping with subsequent stages of illness (Moos & Schaefer, 1984). Unfortunately for many patients with chronic disorders and for their families, early diagnosis is the exception and not the rule. This is the overwhelmingly stressful period of many patients' experience (Latham, Bresnan, & Sollee, 1983). The diagnosis of a chronic, often progressive illness can be devastating and can create feelings of uncertainty about the future. The associated stressors can be tremendous. Beulow (1991) reported a positive correlation between uncertainty about the future and fatalistic coping style in a correlation study of 20 adults with multiple sclerosis who were hospitalized. For some disorders, such as muscular dystrophy, amyotrophic sclerosis, and Huntington's disease, a shortened life expectancy is the rule. Changes in body image and self-concept and fluctuations in strength and functional ability make coping a difficult task. The nurse should be aware of factors that influence coping ability, such as age, sex, temperament, intelligence, presence of chronic adversity, and proximity of social relationships and support. Rapidity of change is another important factor in the patient's ability to cope. Timing in the life cycle can be a significant variable for the different concerns at each stage. Patients who develop a chronic disease in childhood or adolescence have different developmental needs and require different coping strategies than do those who are affected by illnesses with onset in middle age. Younger patients can be more severely affected (Singer, 1974). Witte (1987) indicated that parents of adolescents with muscular dystrophy are often not aware of the child's emotional and personal needs because of their own levels of anxiety concerning the illness. Often, as a result, parents become overprotective and form a closed family system, perhaps in an effort to protect themselves and the child from the disease. Coping with a disease that is progressive and chronic, lasting many years, is different from coping with an illness in which the deficit is static. Depression related to feelings of being overpowered by physical limitations may arise (Lambert & Lambert, 1987). The degree of disability a person experiences may be determined by the effectiveness of his or her coping methods. Poor coping strategies limit an individual's ability to reach an optimal level of functioning (Buelow, 1991). It is important to keep in mind that, although many of these chronic motor disorders are incurable, they are not untreatable. Factual, honest information about the disorder, its course, and its treatment can help the patient and family cope by reducing fear and uncertainty of the unknown.

Defining characteristics include reduced or increased verbalization and inability to make decisions. The presence of confused roles, inability to relinquish control, or inability to meet basic needs can be a clue to inadequate coping.

Assessment should include the patient's previous experiences with illness, particularly how he or she made decisions and coped with adversity in the past. This could also include changes in lifestyle or problems unrelated to health. Present and anticipated stressors as well as specific coping methods employed by the patient should be identified and an assessment made of their impact and effectiveness. The goal is to promote coping skills that improve the patient's ability to function.

Interventions include supplying accurate information in a way that clarifies the patient's understanding of his or her illness. During the initial diagnostic phase, education should be designed so that it is not an overwhelming process. The nurse should draw on the patient's past experience and coping ability to provide complete information in small, easily digestible segments. Adequate time should be allowed for patient discussion and clarification. Asking the patient to discuss previous accomplishments and future plans will assist the nurse in fostering the patient's coping abilities. The use of positive coping strategies should be reinforced, or assistance should be provided for the development of new coping strategies. Helping the patient cope with chronic illness is not something that can be done in one appointment or during an initial hospitalization. The outpatient or community health nurse can assess patient response over time. The patient should feel that she or he has easy access to her or his health care provider through frequent appointments or telephone conversations to clarify questions. Praise regarding positive problem-solving ability and achieving of realistic goals should be liberally distributed. Rehearsals of how the patient will deal with crises or changes in performance often help the patient structure his or her responses in an appropriate way. All life-cycle concerns should be addressed at some point, including information about childbearing, marriage, occupational choice, and leisure activities. The patient should know how these concerns will interact in the face of fatigue and changes in strength and mobility.

The patient should be encouraged to participate actively in his or her care to have more control over the illness, particularly while hospitalized. Attempts to give power or control over the immediate environment may also be helpful. Persons who rely on large amounts of daily medication to have movement, as with Parkinson's disease or myasthenia gravis, may feel their bodies are being particularly assaulted. In addition to friends and family, another source of support is a peer group. Discussing how one feels with others who have been through similar situations is perceived as very useful. There are support groups under the auspices of the Multiple Sclerosis Society, various Parkinson's disease associations, the Myasthenia Gravis Foundation, and independent living centers in many areas. Many patients and families learn that their responses to crises are not always unique and are comforted to know that others live through this period in their lives and progress to achieve their goals (Latham et al., 1983). Further research is necessary to clarify the most efficient and effective ways of counseling patients with chronic disorders.

SOCIAL ISOLATION

Social isolation is a state in which the patient has a need or desire for contact with others but is unable to make that contact. The loss of function of one or more extremities, of verbal skills, or of sensory stimulation can contribute to social isolation and contribute to further immobility. For others, news of a diagnosis deemed to be devastating leads to isolation and a reluctance to inform friends, employers, and family members. In a study of 169 people with Parkinson's disease, Singer (1974) noted "premature social aging" characterized by isolation from interpersonal contacts when those people were compared with age-matched healthy controls. People with Parkinson's disease were less likely to work, to participate in household management, or to enjoy a circle of close friends (Singer, 1974). Loss of bladder control associated with multiple sclerosis has also been shown to result in altered self-image and social isolation (Ahearn & Schwetz, 1985). With illness and disability come loss of income, job, and previous lifestyle. For children, adolescents, and young adults, schooling can be disrupted. One's occupation, whether as student or employee, is an important source of socialization as well as recognition. Inability to maintain contact with others can lead to depression and reduced motivation to improve one's situation in other ways (Hyman, 1972). The patient usually becomes dependent on others for some part of socialization. Dependence on a wheelchair or the embarrassment resulting from outward appearance of involuntary movements or unusual gait are other examples of barriers to socialization and features that can contribute to social isolation (Lambert & Lambert, 1987).

The defining characteristics of this state include expressed feelings of abandonment, underactivity, or uselessness. Inability to make decisions, irritability, anxiety, failure to interact with others nearby, change in eating or sleeping habits, and change from a previous state of good health can signal depression as a consequence of social isolation. In time, anxiety about going out socially when the opportunity is available may interfere with efforts to treat this problem.

Assessment should include a determination of the frequency and level of social interaction that the patient experienced before the illness or its worsening. When this information is compared with the patient's current social activities, the nurse is alerted to the person at risk for problems and learns those activities the patient may return to most easily. It is important to know if the patient perceives himself or herself as needing more socialization. The goal for this diagnosis is the maintenance of sufficient contact with others despite immobility.

Nursing interventions should include supporting the patient in maintaining the premorbid lifestyle, if possible, including occupation, hobbies, and other forms of social interaction. Those persons who adjust to the physical and emotional demands of their illness are more likely to maintain a higher level of employment than are those who are unable to adjust in a satisfactory manner. Changes in the type or responsibilities of occupation may be required, and occupational retraining may or may not be feasible (Lambert & Lambert, 1987). If the patient cannot continue in his or her occupation, it is important to do some anticipatory planning about activities that may occupy time productively during a period of disability. Workshops, day care centers, day programs, exercise programs, and volunteer work are some of the options available to the disabled and help to reduce social isolation.

The opportunities available can often be increased immensely with the addition of transportation; mobility-impaired people may be taught to drive or to use special equipment. In one city, volunteers have been organized to visit people in the community weekly who are socially isolated (Compeer; Rochester, NY). When anxiety secondary to depression or fear of becoming isolated occurs, the patient needs a supportive individual to help him or her initiate social activities. At these times, the professional may have more influence than a close family member.

KNOWLEDGE DEFICIT

Knowledge deficit can be seen during any stage of the disease process, particularly following diagnosis. The patient will need to learn about her or his illness and perhaps learn new psychomotor skills. Defining characteristics of this diagnosis include the patient's verbal report of difficulty understanding or the patient's communication of inaccurate information. Lack of compliance with desired or prescribed treatments and the presence of anxiety are important factors to assess.

Initially, the nurse should assess the patient's knowledge of his or her illness. This includes any previous knowledge of the disorder as well as problems encountered during experiences with the health care system in the past. It is important to ascertain whether the patient knows anyone else with the illness. The goal is to provide the patient with complete information to allow him or her to independently manage the problems of immobility resulting from illness.

The patient should be encouraged to learn at his or her own pace. The nurse should take into account situational and developmental needs as well as anxiety levels. Interventions should include a complete discussion of pathophysiology and etiology of the current understanding of the disorder and its effect on functional ability. The patient should know measures that improve and limit strength; for example, the patient with myasthenia gravis should know that rest and timing of anticholinesterases will improve strength and that some medications, such as aminoglycosides, beta blockers, and others, will increase weakness. The patient should be encouraged to consult with his or her specialist before initiation of any new medication. The patient should wear a Medic Alert tag for identification, particularly if unable to communicate. Patients should receive thorough instructions about their medications and how these influence their symptoms. Patients receiving corticosteroids or immunosuppressives should understand how these influence pathophysiology and the side effects associated with their use.

Patients may feel overwhelmed by the amount of information they need to learn. Having contact with other patients or participating in a support group can be a great benefit to a patient. During these initial stages of therapy, the nurse should test the patient's knowledge and not rely solely on head shakes as a measure of understanding. Many patients with chronic disorders are motivated learners and often scour the literature and the Internet in an attempt to master their illness. Literature, newsletters, and Web sites from national or local disorder-related organizations are typically written for the layperson and also enable one to keep abreast of new information and helpful hints for living. In addition, publication of new and ongoing research findings in the field can provide a sense of optimism for the future. For those who ask few questions and appear to deny their illness, the nurse must judge if this is a typical response pattern for that patient or if this coping mechanism is getting in the way of care. For some patients, denial is a comfortable mechanism, particularly when the illness is threatening and the consequences are overwhelming.

HOME MAINTENANCE MANAGEMENT DEFICIT

Home maintenance management can be a potential problem in a patient with chronic immobility and can require that a patient radically change previous living patterns. During a crisis, many families alter their responsibilities, but when the crisis is over, patients may be burdened with responsibilities they are no longer able to handle.

Defining characteristics include the expression of difficulty by individual family members in accomplishing all activities related to home maintenance. The expectations can be altered significantly by the developmental stage of the family. The spouse or parent will display evidence of anxiety or lack of understanding about the patient's illness or will avoid contact with the care providers. They may show signs of overtaxing the patient with trivial concerns.

The nurse should assess the patient's ability to manage self-care activities, occupational concerns, exercise, financial management, home repairs, meal preparation, and leisure activities. The nurse should determine who usually performs these activities and who the patient expects to perform them if he or she needs help. Family meetings for discharge planning should begin shortly after hospital admission and should include all members of the multidisciplinary team. The goal is to maintain family functioning during changes and fluctuations in the patient's abilities.

Interventions are dependent on the individual's physical and emotional developmental stage and the family constellation and their status. The nurse should discuss how the patient might organize the day and accomplish daily needs. The patient should be encouraged to organize himself or herself and the surroundings to prevent wasting energy, such as going up and down stairs. Simple tips, such as sitting on a high stool instead of standing while working in the kitchen and using a portable shopping cart to carry heavy items in the store and to and from the house, can save energy expenditure. A motorized three-wheeled scooter can serve the patient with limited strength on long shopping trips (see Fig. 21–2). Encouraging the patient to use telephone, mail-order, and Internet shopping and grocery-delivery services can be important.

For the patient with severe impairment in mobility, supports such as Meals on Wheels, public health nurses, home health aides, or even private housekeepers can be employed as short-term solutions.

Patients with long-term chronic disorders require extensive home care planning. Financial counseling should be provided, particularly regarding occupational choice, disability concerns, tax planning, and health insurance. Seeking support from family members is necessary. The nurse can assist the patient in learning negotiation strategies to accomplish tasks and to distribute tasks according to the family members' interests and desires. The patient and family should renegotiate responsibilities at frequent intervals to account for changes in the patient's abilities. Patients have considerable difficulty allowing others to complete tasks that they know they could do better than their helpers. The nurse should allow patients to express these feelings and let them know that this is a normal reaction. In some cases, consideration as to the feasibility of keeping the patient at home needs to be addressed.

Independent living centers teach handicapped patients to live on their own or to find housing that offers the degree of support necessary so that they may live alone. Such housing can vary; among the options are living in an apartment with an emergency call system, living as a boarder with a supportive family, or living in a group home. If the patient requires assistance and further education to maintain mobility and overcome environmental barriers, admission to a rehabilitation facility can prove beneficial. Osberg, Corcoran, Dejong, and Ostruff (1983) stated, "Our disabled patients are handicapped only to the extent that we are unable to provide them with enhanced personal abilities, diminished environmental demands, and suitable interface devices to operate or manipulate their environment." The rehabilitation milieu is often an excellent experience for patients who view their illness in terms of deficits; it gives them a chance to concentrate on their strengths. Many rehabilitation facilities offer weekend and evening outings that serve to maintain the patient's links to the real world and keep the treatment program oriented to reality (Osberg et al., 1983). For some, nursing home placement may be an option and should be planned for before the time of crisis. The need for placement may simply reflect the unavailability of resources and is dependent on both the individual family unit and the geographic area. Some localities are moving toward the formation of programs designed specifically for keeping people at home with services as opposed to placing them in long-term care facilities. However, even this is often limited if a reliable backup—family member or friend—is not available for the home.

HEALTH MAINTENANCE

Problems with health maintenance can be seen in the patient with problems of immobility resulting from acute or chronic illnesses when the patient considers his or her disabilities to be overwhelming. The perception that the primary illness is the only impediment to happiness fosters delay of return to previous health practices and reflects a lack of acceptance of the problem. The patient may express inadequate knowledge of preventive health behaviors.

Defining characteristics include noticeably poor oral and body hygiene, obesity, sleep disturbances, poor exercise habits, and visual and hearing problems. Patients who are frequent users of the emergency department or those who lack a consistent source of health care are also at risk for this problem. Those who have frequent minor illnesses related to their immobility that evolve into illnesses requiring hospitalization, such as a cold leading to pneumonia or an injury leading to infection, are experiencing difficulty with health maintenance. Patients with chronic motor disorders can also be at risk for cancer and other chronic diseases because of such risk factors as family history, smoking, poor diet, and, for patients with myasthenia gravis or multiple sclerosis, immunosuppressive therapy. Contributing factors include knowledge deficit about health care practices, previous negative experiences with health care providers, and lack of financial means or transportation to continue to use one's chosen health care source. Patients with multiple health care providers may be confused about who should provide their care. Some patients have differing beliefs and cultural systems that cause them to reject accepted health care practices.

Assessment measures include recording whom the patient identifies as the usual source of health care and how frequently he or she uses that source. The patient should be asked about his or her knowledge of health and health care practices, particularly those health problems consistent with age and developmental level. The goal is to prevent further health care problems and to assist the patient in optimizing health.

Interventions include clarifying the roles of the patient's primary and specialty providers, including the nurse's role, and the services unique to each. The nurse should praise the patient for attempting to improve his or her health through diet and exercise plans, dental visits, and ophthalmologic examinations. All women should know preventive health care practices, such as breast examination and the importance of Papanicolaou smears. Men should be taught the technique of testicular examination. Detailed health maintenance plans are outlined in many sources (Breslow & Somers, 1977; Frame & Carlson, 1975). The nurse should consult these sources to develop an appropriate plan of care related to developmental level and age.

Nursing Diagnoses for the Family and Significant Others

ALTERATION IN FAMILY PROCESSES AND POTENTIAL FOR INEFFECTIVE COPING

Ineffective family coping can occur during the initial diagnostic period or at any time during the patient's course of illness. These problems can be related directly or indirectly to the patient's immobility. There are many reactions to the diagnosis of a chronic disorder. Families have been known to react initially to the diagnosis of myasthenia gravis with relief, taking comfort that there is a specific cause and that medicine will control the problem (Sampson & Cosley,

1983). Other families have more difficulty adjusting and are unprepared to cope with the unknown future. Problems may arise when the family or significant others deny the reality of the disease. If the prognosis is poor, it can be extremely difficult to learn how to encourage a family member to live when he or she is dying. Initially, family members may be angry because the patient has few noticeable signs of weakness or because the illness carries with it the likelihood of other family members being similarly affected, as in Huntington's disease and some of the muscular dystrophies. Mothers who are presumed carriers of Duchenne's disease can suffer from guilt and severe stress from within and outside the family. If the patient is unable to communicate adequately with family members, both the patient and the family can become frustrated and perhaps resentful. Individual family member's needs and abilities need to be assessed. Not all family members can be or want to be caregivers. Middle-aged individuals and spouses may be particularly affected by the impact of chronic illness because this is typically a time when increased responsibilities of social, economic, and career parameters are expected. Caregiving spouses feel overwhelmed with new roles and responsibilities. Role conflict and overload are contributing factors to caregiver burden. Accordingly, the health of the caregiver may be affected. O'Brien (1993) studied health-promoting behaviors of spousal caregivers of people with multiple sclerosis. The health-promoting behaviors of the caregiver decreased as the dependency needs of the spouse with multiple sclerosis increased. This was particularly true for male caregivers as the dependency needs of the female were found to be greater. This potentially limits the caregiver's ability to continue in the role of caregiver. Nurses may need to assist the caregivers with the development of interventions to ease their caregiving load and maintain their own health (O'Brien, 1993). Alternatives for providing the care that the patient requires may need to be examined so as to help the family remain as functional as possible. Defining characteristics, family assessment, and interventions are discussed in Chapter 17.

KNOWLEDGE DEFICIT

Although many families report that they have heard of chronic disorders such as multiple sclerosis, muscular dystrophy, amyotrophic lateral sclerosis, and Parkinson's disease before their family member was diagnosed, few know the ramifications of the disorders. It is particularly vital that the family become well informed if the afflicted family member is a dependent or if cognitive difficulties or dementia accompany the illness, as in Huntington's disease or, potentially, Parkinson's disease and multiple sclerosis. Defining characteristics of this diagnosis include the family's expressed lack of knowledge, their misconceptions, or their lack of support.

The nurse will need to assess the family's level of understanding as well as their knowledge of the therapeutic regimen and the potential genetic implications for such disorders as muscular dystrophy and Huntington's disease. The family may have misconceptions about the limitations imposed by the disease and its treatment. Contributing factors are language and cultural differences and interpersonal problems, such as anxiety, depression, denial, and lack of motivation. The goal for this diagnosis is to provide the family with sufficient information to allow them to support the patient throughout her or his illness.

Interventions can include developing an educational plan for the family that parallels that of the patient. The patient's feelings should be consulted, and, if possible, the patient should be present during all educational family meetings. Many patients like to assist the nurse when educational plans are discussed. This can be a good time to verify the patient's knowledge base. Various organizations have patient and family pamphlets to reinforce teaching plans about medications, symptom control, disease process, and management. Families should have a clear idea of how to handle problems, particularly emergencies. Many would benefit from instructions about cardiopulmonary resuscitation and the Heimlich maneuver and should know emergency phone numbers. The educational process should not be confined to the initial hospital admission and needs to continue on an ongoing basis. The family should be encouraged to voice their questions and should have a clear idea of when to ask for assistance. This is particularly important for patients with neurodegenerative illnesses because symptoms and care needs vary but typically progress with time.

Nondirective genetic counseling should initially be scheduled as part of the educational program for those families affected by diseases with an inheritable pattern, such as the muscular dystrophies, Huntington's disease, spinal muscular atrophies, Wilson's disease, the dystonias, and Tourette's syndrome. For some families, tests to determine if a person carries the gene for an illness—for example, Huntington's disease, Wilson's disease, and some forms of muscular dystrophy—are available with varying degrees of certainty. This topic is usually a complex one to discuss with those who are uninformed and requires repetition over several sessions and written materials for reference and review at home.

Nursing Diagnoses for the Community

KNOWLEDGE DEFICIT

Our society values independence, strength, and athletic and competitive ability, all of which are affected in chronic motor disorders. Immobility is seen as a threat to independence. Because many patients state that their most stressful period is during the initial diagnostic process, improving public recognition of these diseases may facilitate early diagnosis. Reducing the obscurity of the disease may decrease the fear and anxiety that a chronic neurologic diagnosis carries. Although it is the purpose of nonprofit organizations, such as the Huntington's Disease Society of America, the Myasthenia Gravis Foundation, the Muscular Dystrophy Association, and the various Parkinson's disease associations, to increase public and professional awareness of the diseases, they cannot do this alone. As nurses, we must continue to educate all health care providers, as well as patients and families. Nurses should encourage positive public attitudes toward the handicapped person by looking beyond the wheelchair and focusing on the patient's strengths, not her or his handicaps. Nurses should become more active in lay organizations that advocate for handicapped people.

The Myasthenia Gravis Foundation has formed a national nursing advisory board to coordinate educational efforts for patients and professionals. A scholarship program has been planned to further nursing research on the care of the patient with myasthenia gravis, and educational programs and pamphlets have been developed. In other organizations, such as the Multiple Sclerosis Society and several of the Parkinson's disease organizations, nurses are involved actively in patient programs and educational activities.

BARRIERS TO MOBILITY

There are innumerable physical and social barriers to mobility for patients with chronic immobilizing disorders. These barriers are most easily appreciated for the wheelchair-bound person. The efforts of groups of disabled patients and their advocates have led to legislation or contingencies linking accessibility to facilities with continued funding. Ramps, wide doorways, and low curbs have been added to building codes. Much more needs to be done, but the process of change is slow.

Barriers to mobility are associated with society's lack of appreciation of the person behind the disability and with society's history of isolating those who are different from the accepted norm. The effects of social isolation limit the potential of the handicapped individual. For the vast majority of people, disability means minimal income. Expenses related to medications, special equipment, nursing assistance for daily care needs, and transportation, including specially equipped vans and ramps, often are not covered by insurance. Therefore, financial barriers are another source of limitations to reaching individual potential. The state offices of vocational rehabilitation offer skills evaluation and training or schooling scholarships and generally facilitate the reentrance of disabled people into the job market. Increased visibility of disabled individuals can help expedite change and relieve barriers.

INSUFFICIENT COMMUNITY RESOURCES

The community must address many needs in the case of patients with chronic mobility disorders and immobility. One of the most important questions is, who will pay for the chronic care necessary to maintain the quality of life of these patients? The problems of the expense of transportation and personal attendants must be overcome to allow these patients to become useful and productive members of the community. In many cases, rehabilitation can make these patients independent, at least for a time. These services must be accessible and supported by the community at large. Many families need respite care to allow them to continue to support their affected family member. The U.S. Government

Accounting Office reports that 20% to 40% of patients in nursing homes could be cared for at home if sufficient resources were available (Allen, 1993). This not only is cost-effective but also allows individuals to carry out their lives in their own environments.

The development of exercise programs would allow patients to participate in activities outside their homes, to make gradual improvements in strength, and to reduce disuse atrophy. Patients with muscle weakness and fatigue have been excluded from many exercise programs because of their disability or lack of access to many facilities. The success of cardiac rehabilitation and exercise programs for cerebral palsy, Parkinson's disease, and multiple sclerosis patients lends support to the notion that the chronically ill population should not be overlooked for rehabilitation.

Society must change its values to include the needs of those who are less independent. A renewing of the focus of one's life activities to include community support projects does not apply just to nurses. In the years to come, attention to community needs should become an expectation and not an exception for all citizens. The work of established health organizations and coalitions of these groups is necessary to lobby for the rights of the disabled if a change in the government support of the needs of the chronically ill is to be effected. This type of work requires energy above and beyond that necessary just to meet the daily needs of the patient. Many patients and families may not have this energy and expertise and will need to elicit the support of friends, health care providers, and elected officials. Community and home-based care, as opposed to institutional care, should be the priority.

FUTURE OF HEALTH CARE

Widespread change in our health care delivery system is anticipated. The goal is to provide universal health care to all Americans. The role of the nurse will likely change to incorporate the newly identified needs of the country. The focus of care is shifting back toward primary care with more emphasis on health and preventive maintenance. Treatment locales are also shifting away from acute care settings and back to the community and home. Accordingly, resources will have to change to meet this shift. The community and the home have been longstanding sites for nursing care delivery. Therefore, nurses may well find themselves in positions of leadership in a new health care delivery system and in expanded roles for delivery of patient care.

SUMMARY

The problems of people with chronically impaired mobility can affect every area of their functioning. Limitations imposed by their physical disabilities can be significant and may be accompanied by or result in psychosocial limitations in functioning. As a society, it is our responsibility to minimize any limitations within our jurisdiction as expeditiously as possible and in the most cost-effective manner. Change in society's values may be apparent only in generations to come. It will be facilitated only by the rapid manner in which knowledge of current events can be shared around the world.

References

Ahearn, J., & Schwetz, K. (1985). Comprehensive supportive therapy in multiple sclerosis. *Seminars in Neurology, 5*(2), 146.

Alexander, M. A., Johnson, E. W., Petty, J., & Stauch, D. (1979). Mechanical ventilation of patients with late stage Duchenne muscular dystrophy: Management at home. *Archives of Physical and Medical Rehabilitation, 60,* 289.

Allen, S. (1993, March). Time to fight for a single payer system. *American Nurse, 4,* 6.

Andres, P. L., Skerry, L. M., & Munsat, L. (1989). Measurement of strength in neuromuscular diseases. In L. Munsat (Ed.), *Quantification of neurologic deficit* (pp. 87–100). Woburn, MA: Butterworth-Heinemann.

Bernat, J. L., & Vincent, F. M. (1987). *Neurology: Problems in primary care.* Montvale, NJ: Medical Economics Company.

Berry, E. M., Growden, J. H., Wurtman, J. J., Caballero, B., & Wurtman, R. J. (1991). A balanced carbohydrate:protein diet in the management of Parkinson's disease. *Neurology, 41,* 1295–1297.

Boller, F., & Frank, E. F. (1982). *Sexual dysfunction in neurologic disorders.* Lancaster, CA: Raven Press.

Bowers, M. B., & VanMoert, M. H. (1972). Sexual behavior during L-dopa treatment of Parkinson's disease. *Medical Aspects of Human Sexuality, 1,* 88.

Breslow, L., & Somers, A. R. (1977). The lifetime health-monitoring program. *New England Journal of Medicine, 296*(11), 601.

Brooke, M. H. (2000). Disorders of skeletal muscle. In W. G. Bradley, R. B. Daroff, G. M. Fenichel, & C. D. Marsden (Eds.), *Neurology in clinical practice* (3rd ed., pp. 2167–2185). Boston: Butterworth-Heinemann.

Buelow, J. M. (1991). A correlational study of disabilities, stressors and coping methods in victims of multiple sclerosis. *Journal of Neuroscience Nursing, 23*(4), 247–252.

Cadmus, R. (1980). Intensive care reaches silver anniversary. *Hospitals, 54,* 98.

Callahan, M. (1985). A prudent pulmonary rehabilitation program. *American Journal of Nursing, 85*(12), 1368.

Carpenito, L. J. (1993). *Nursing diagnosis: Application to clinical practice.* Philadelphia: J.B. Lippincott.

Clark, C. (1991). Nursing care for multiple sclerosis. *Orthopaedic Nursing, 10*(1), 21–32.

Cobble, N. D., & Maloney, F. P. (1985). Effects of exercise in neuromuscular disease. In F. P. Maloney, J. Burkes, & S. Ringel (Eds.), *Interdisciplinary management of multiple sclerosis and neuromuscular disease* (p. 228). Philadelphia: J.B. Lippincott.

Curran, F. J. (1981). Night ventilation by body respirator for patients in chronic respiratory failure due to late stage Duchenne muscular dystrophy. *Archives of Physical and Medical Rehabilitation, 62,* 270.

Dewis, M. E., & Thornton, N. G. (1989). Sexual dysfunction in multiple sclerosis. *Journal of Neuroscience Nursing, 21*(3), 175–179.

Difilippo, N. M., & Jenkins, A. J. (1988). Pressure support ventilation. *American Family Physician, 38*(2), 147–150.

Donohoe, K. M. (1994). Autoimmune disorders. In E. Barker (Ed.), *Neuroscience nursing* (pp. 559–590). St. Louis: Mosby–Year Book.

Edmonds, C. E. (1966). Huntington's chorea, dysphagia and death. *Medical Journal of Australia, 2,* 273.

Fahn, S. (1989). Assessment of the primary dystonias. In T. L. Munsat (Ed.), *Quantification of neurologic deficit* (pp. 241–270). Woburn, MA: Butterworth-Heinemann.

Frame, P. S., & Carlson, S. J. (1975). A critical review of periodic health screening using specific screening criteria. *Journal of Family Practice, 2,* 29, 123, 189, 283.

France, J. K. (1993, August). Huntington's disease: Helping the patient retain function. *American Journal of Nursing, 93,* 62–64.

Gehlsen, G. M., Grigsby, S. A., & Winant, D. M. (1984). Effects of aquatic fitness program on muscular strength and endurance in patients with multiple sclerosis. *Physical Therapy, 64*(5), 653.

Gianino, J. (1993). Intrathecal baclofen for spinal spasticity: Implications for nursing practice. *Journal of Neuroscience Nursing, 25*(4), 254–264.

Griggs, R. C., & Donohoe, K. M. (1985). Emergency management of neuromuscular disease. In R. J. Henning & D. Jackson (Eds.), *Handbook of critical care neurology and neurosurgery* (p. 251). Westport, CT: Praeger.

Griggs, R. C., Donohoe, K. M., Utell, M. J., Goldblatt, D., & Moxley, R. T. (1981). Evaluation of pulmonary function in neuromuscular disease. *Archives of Neurology, 38,* 9.

Grob, D., Brunner, N. C., & Namba, T. (1981). The natural course of myasthenia gravis and effect of therapeutic measures. *Annals of the New York Academy of Science, 377,* 652.

Guenter, P. (1989). Percutaneous endoscopic gastrostomy feeding tube in neuroscience patients. *Journal of Neuroscience Nursing, 21*(2), 122–124.

Hanak, M. (1992). *Rehabilitation nursing for the neurological patient.* New York: Springer Publishing.

Hobbs, N., Perrin, J. M., Ireys, H. T., Moynihan, L. C., & Shayne, M. W. (1984). Chronically ill children in America. *Rehabilitation Literature, 45*(7–8), 206.

Hunt, V. P., & Walker, F. O. (1989). Dysphagia in Huntington's disease. *Journal of Neuroscience Nursing, 21*(2), 92–95.

Hurwitz, A. (1989). The benefit of a home exercise regimen for ambulatory Parkinson's disease patients. *Journal of Neuroscience Nursing, 21*(3), 180–184.

Hyman, M. (1972). Sociopsychological obstacles to L-dopa therapy that may limit effectiveness in parkinsonism. *Journal of the American Geriatrics Society, 20,* 200.

Jankovic, J., & Brin, M. F. (1991). Therapeutic uses of botulinum toxin. *New England Journal of Medicine, 324*(17), 1186–1194.

Jankovic, J., & Schwartz, K. (1990). Botulinum toxin injections for cervical dystonia. *Neurology, 40,* 277–280.

Karstaedt, P. J., & Pincus, J. H. (1992). Protein redistribution diet remains effective in patients with fluctuating parkinsonism. *Archives of Neurology, 49*(2), 149–151.

Kodadek, S. M. (1985). Working with the chronically ill. *Nurse Practitioner, 10*(3), 45.

Koller, W. C., Vetere-Overfield, B., Williamson, A., Busenbark, K., Nash, J., Pardsh, D. (1990). Sexual dysfunction in Parkinson's disease. *Clinical Neuropharmacology, 13*(5), 461–463.

Lambert, V. A., & Lambert, C. E. (1987). Adaptation to chronic illness. *Nursing Clinics of North America, 22*(3), 327–533.

Lang, A. T., & Fahn, S. (1989). Assessment of Parkinson's disease. In T. L. Munsat (Ed.), *Quantification of neurologic deficit* (pp. 285–309). Woburn, MA: Butterworth-Heinemann.

Latham, E. E., Bresnan, M. J., & Sollee, N. L. (1983). Psychosocial issues in raising a child with Duchenne muscular dystrophy: A parent group ethnography. In L. Charash, S. G. Wolfe, A. H. Kutscher, R. E. Lovelace, & M. S. Hale (Eds.), *Psychosocial issues of muscular dystrophy and allied diseases* (p. 221). Springfield, IL: Charles C Thomas.

Lavigne, J. (1979). Respiratory care in neuromuscular disease. *Nursing Clinics of North America, 14,* 110.

Levine, J. S. (1985). Bowel dysfunction in multiple sclerosis. In F. P. Maloney, J. S. Burks, & S. Ringel (Eds.), *Interdisciplinary rehabilitation of multiple sclerosis and neuromuscular disorders* (p. 62). Philadelphia: J.B. Lippincott.

Lipe, H., Longstreth, W. T., Jr., Bird, T. D., & Lind, M. (1990). Sexual function in married men with Parkinson's disease compared to married men with arthritis. *Neurology, 40,* 1347–1349.

Longstreth, W. T., Jr., Nelson, L., Linde, M., & Munoz, D. (1992). Utility of the sickness impact profile in Parkinson's disease. *Journal of Geriatric Psychiatry and Neurology, 5*(3), 142–148.

Lusis, S. A. (1997). Pathophysiology and management of idiopathic Parkinson's disease. *Journal of Neuroscience Nursing, 29*(1), 24–31.

Maloney, F. P., Burks, J. S., & Ringel, S. (Eds.) (1985). *Interdisciplinary rehabilitation of multiple sclerosis and neuromuscular disorders.* Philadelphia: J.B. Lippincott.

Marsden, C. D., Parkes, J. D., & Quinn, N. (1982). Fluctuations of disability in Parkinson disease— Clinical aspects. In C. D. Marsden & S. Fahn (Eds.), *Movement disorders* (p. 96). Woburn, MA: Butterworth-Heinemann.

Mitsumoto, H. (2000). Disorders of upper and lower motor neurons. In W. G. Bradley, R. B. Daroff, G. M. Fenichel, & C. D. Marsden (Eds.), *Neurology in clinical practice* (3rd ed., pp. 1985–2018). Boston: Butterworth-Heinemann.

Moos, R., & Schaefer, J. (1984). The crisis of physical illness: An overview and conceptual approach. In R. Moos (Ed.), *Coping with physical illness: New perspectives* (p. 3). Reading, MA: Plenum.

Myasthenia Gravis Foundation (1979). *Patient to patient memo.* New York: Author.

Neu, H. C., Connolly, J. P., Schwestley, F. W., Lodwig, H. A., & Brody, A. W. (1967). Obstructive respiratory dysfunction in parkinsonian patients. *American Review of Respiratory Diseases, 95,* 33.

O'Brien, M. T. (1993). Multiple sclerosis: Health-promoting behaviors of spousal caregivers. *Journal of Neuroscience Nursing, 25*(2), 105–112.

Osberg, S., Corcoran, P. J., Dejong, G., & Ostruff, E. (1983). Environmental barriers and the neurologically impaired patient. *Seminars in Neurology, 3*(4), 180.

Poser, S. (1989). Disability rating scales for the assessment of multiple sclerosis. In T. L. Munsat (Ed.), *Quantification of neurologic deficits* (pp. 163–169). Woburn, MA: Butterworth-Heinemann.

Riley, D. E., & Lange, A. E. (2000). Movement disorders. In W. G. Bradley, R. B. Daroff, G. M. Fenichel, & C. D. Marsden (Eds.): *Neurology in clinical practice* (3rd ed., pp. 1889–1930). Boston: Butterworth-Heinemann.

Sampson, R., & Cosley, S. (1983). Physical, emotional, social, and family interactions in childhood myasthenia gravis. In L. I. Charash, S. G. Wolfe, A. H. Kutscher, R. E. Lovelace, & M. S. Hale (Eds.), *Psychosocial aspects of muscular dystrophy and allied diseases* (p. 183). Springfield, IL: Charles C Thomas.

Sanders, D. B., & Howard, J. F. (2000) Disorders of neuromuscular transmission. In W. G. Bradley, R. B. Daroff, G. M., Fenichel, C. D. Marsden (Eds.), *Neurology in clinical practice* (3rd ed., pp. 2167–2185). Boston: Butterworth-Heinemann.

Selye, H. (1976). *The stress of life.* New York: McGraw-Hill.

Shoulson, I., Kurlan, R., Rubin, A. J., Goldblatt, D., Behr, J., Miller, C., Kennedy, J., Bamford, K. A., Caine, E. D., Kido, D. K., Plumb, S., & Odoroff, C. (1989). Assessment of functional capacity in neurodegenerative movement disorders: Huntington's disease as a prototype. In T. L. Munsat (Ed.), *Quantification of neurologic deficit* (pp. 271–283). Woburn, MA: Butterworth-Heinemann.

Singer, E. (1974). Premature social aging: The social-psychological consequences of a chronic illness. *Social Science Medicine, 8,* 143.

Smeltzer, S. C., Utell, M. J., Rudick, R. A., & Herdon, R. M. (1988). Pulmonary function and dysfunction in multiple sclerosis. *Archives of Neurology, 45*(11), 1245–1249.

Splaingard, M. L., Frates, R. C., Jefferson, L. S., Rosen, C. L., & Hardson, G. (1985). Home negative pressure ventilation: Report of 20 years of experience in patients with neuromuscular disease. *Archives of Physical and Medical Rehabilitation, 66,* 239.

Stenager, E., Stenager, E. N., & Jensen, K. (1992). Sexual aspects of multiple sclerosis. *Seminars in Neurology, 12*(2), 120–124.

Tim, R., & Massey, J. M. (1992). Botulinum toxin therapy for neurologic disorders. *Botulinum Toxin Therapy, 91*(6), 327–334.

Weiss, J. (1992). Multiple sclerosis: Will it come between us? Sexual concerns of clients and their partners. *Journal of Neuroscience Nursing, 24*(4), 90–193.

Wermuth, L., & Stenager, E. (1992). Sexual aspects of Parkinson's disease. *Seminars in Neurology, 12*(2), 125–127.

Witte, R. (1987). Private worlds of Duchenne muscular dystrophy adolescents. In L. L. Charash, R. E. Lovelace, S. G. Wolf, A. H. Kutscher, D. P. Roye, & C. F. Leach (Eds.), *Realities in coping with progressive neuromuscular diseases* (pp. 133–145). Philadelphia: Charles Press.

Alterations and Management of Neurologic Swallowing Disorders

ROBERTA SCHWARTZ-COWLEY
• ANDREW K. GRUEN

Varying degrees of swallowing dysfunction (dysphagia) are found in patients who demonstrate acquired neurologic deficits. It is widely accepted that swallowing problems can be associated with many disease processes such as stroke, Parkinson's disease, Huntington's disease, amyotrophic lateral sclerosis, encephalitis, meningitis, anoxia, demyelinating disease, traumatic brain injury, brain stem tumor or trauma, metabolic myopathy, carcinoma, and hypopharyngeal and esophageal webs. Swallowing difficulties can result from certain complications following implants or surgical interventions in the oropharyngeal and esophageal areas.

With an increasing emphasis placed on facilitation of functional improvement and desired outcomes in patients, swallowing assessments and treatment programs are available in most progressive medical environments. Still, clinicians suggested that many exceptions could be found, especially in settings designed for acutely ill patients. Zimmerman and Oder (1981) suggested that some patients were left undiagnosed and untreated because of a general lack of understanding of dysphagia and its effects on normal feeding and nutritional support of patients.

Patients at risk for nutritional deficits can often display a number of behaviors that are indications for positive action on the part of the neuroscience nurse and other involved caregivers. An early assessment from the registered dietician is often helpful to provide a baseline of nutritional status and support as needed during the course of recovery from many conditions. Table 22–1 outlines common observations that could be considered at-risk behaviors for nutritional concerns.

The careful evaluation and treatment of neurologically based swallowing disorders requires a consistent interdisciplinary team approach. The American Speech-Language-Hearing Association (1992, pp. 73–74, 85–86) has furnished preferred practice patterns for the interdisciplinary assessment and treatment of swallowing dysfunctions. In many facilities, a dysphagia or swallowing team

513

TABLE 22–1 • COMMON NUTRITIONAL AT-RISK BEHAVIORS AND OBSERVATIONS

- Presence of nasal, oral, or gastric feeding tubes
- Observed choking during swallowing
- Chewing problems
- Decreased level of consciousness
- Regular complaints of hunger
- Dental problems
- Substantial weight loss
- Inadequate intake
- Recurrence of vomiting or regurgitation
- Residual food particles in oral cavity

---

is led by a swallowing therapist (often a speech-language pathologist or an occupational therapist) with input from the patient's physician, nurse, dietician, and radiologist.

NORMAL SWALLOWING

Before effective evaluation and therapy procedures can be applied to the patient with a swallowing disorder, the neuroscience nurse should review the normal process of swallowing. It is essential to understand the role cranial nerves play in the entire swallowing process. Table 22–2 outlines cranial nerve involvement for eating and swallowing.

An excellent review of anatomy and physiology of the pharynx, an essential component of the swallowing process, can be found in the work of Donner, Bosma, and Robertson (1985). A brief physiologic review of swallowing follows.

TABLE 22–2 • CRANIAL NERVE INVOLVEMENT IN THE EATING AND SWALLOWING PROCESSES

Olfactory (first cranial nerve): Detects and transmits olfactory information (smells) to the brain; an important component in the identification of and the personal satisfaction achieved from foods

Trigeminal (fifth cranial nerve): Sensory input from the mouth and nose, including pain, touch, and temperature; motor innervation of muscles of mastication (chewing)

Facial (seventh cranial nerve): Sensory input from taste from anterior two thirds of the tongue and soft palate; visceral sensation; motor innervation of facial muscles and salivation

Glossopharyngeal (ninth cranial nerve): Sensory input from taste, membranes of the tonsils and pharynx, and posterior one third of the tongue; visceral sensation; motor innervation for swallowing movements (stylopharyngeus muscle) and salivation

Vagus (10th cranial nerve): Sensory input from pharynx, larynx, and epiglottis; visceral sensation (gastrointestinal tract); motor innervation for swallowing movements, including those of the pharynx and larynx

Hypoglossal (12th cranial nerve): Motor innervation of tongue muscles

---

Leopold and Kagel (1983) suggested an anticipatory phase to the swallowing process. This phase includes the decisions made by an individual before eating. Considerations include amount, type, form, and rate of feeding and swallowing. More traditional viewpoints of the feeding process begin at the oral preparatory phase, the point at which a piece of food is bitten or chewed using the teeth, tongue, cheeks, and lips. The bolus is formed by mixing the food particles with saliva. The lips close to form a seal that prevents the bolus from escaping. When chewing is completed, the tip of the tongue rises to the hard palate, and the bolus is thrust to the posterior portion of the pharynx by action of the cheeks and tongue. The tongue acts as a barrier to prevent the bolus from returning to the anterior oral cavity.

Blonsky, Logemann, Bosches, and Fisher (1975) reported transit time from the oral stage to the pharyngeal stage of swallowing to be approximately 1 second. Reflexive action takes over as the bolus enters the pharyngeal stage. Respiration temporarily stops, and the larynx receives protection by the upward and forward movement caused by muscle contraction and covering by the epiglottis, which folds down over the laryngeal area. The hyoid bone displaces upward and posteriorly. The bolus, which has been displaced to the posterior pharyngeal area, stimulates pharyngeal sphincter peristalsis. Sequential contractions and relaxations of the sphincter muscles propel the bolus down the pharynx, around the epiglottis, which is folded over the laryngeal area, and down to the cricopharyngeal segment. Transit time from the pharyngeal to the esophageal phase is approximately 1 second (Blonsky et al., 1975).

In most individuals, the swallowing reflex is a critical component of the pharyngeal phase of swallowing. The reflex is triggered at the anterior faucial area. However, in some patients, the bolus must contact the aryepiglottic folds or enter the pyriform sinuses to trigger the reflex (Logemann, 1983). Thermal stimulation procedures, strongly advocated by clinicians such as Logemann, focus on cold stimulation of the lower faucial arches in the anticipation that such stimulation will elicit or facilitate the swallowing reflex. Table 22–3 lists at least eight physiologic activities that occur as the result of a triggered swallowing reflex. The swallowing reflex not only is essential for movement of the

TABLE 22–3 • EIGHT PHYSIOLOGIC ACTIVITIES CAUSED BY TRIGGERED SWALLOWING REFLEX

1. Upward and backward movement of the velum
2. Closure of the velopharyngeal port
3. Rhythmic propulsion of the bolus down the pharynx to the cricopharyngeal sphincter
4. Upward movement of the larynx
5. Closure of the epiglottis and aryepiglottic folds
6. Closure of the false vocal folds
7. Closure of the true vocal folds
8. Relaxation of the cricopharyngeal sphincter for passage of the bolus to the esophagus

Data from Logemann, J. (1983). *Evaluation and treatment of swallowing disorders.* San Diego, CA: College Hill Press.

bolus from the oral cavity to the esophagus, but also allows for initiation of several components of airway protection during eating and swallowing.

The esophageal phase begins when the cricopharyngeal segment relaxes and the bolus move into the esophagus. Through the process of peristalsis (and, to a lesser extent, gravity), the bolus is transferred through the esophagus and through the gastroesophageal sphincter into the stomach. Mandelstam and Leiber (1970) suggested a transit time of 8 to 20 seconds for this process to be completed. The interested reader should review the works of Logemann (1983), Donner et al. (1985), Miller (1986), and Lazarus (1991) for more comprehensive information about neural and physiologic aspects of normal swallowing.

The successful swallowing process depends on a rapid sequence of finely tuned muscle movements in voluntary and reflexive control mechanisms. Logemann (1983) suggested that the relationship and codependency between the voluntary initiation of swallowing and the swallowing reflex are not completely understood. Roueche (1980) stated that "both voluntary and reflex components are involved in the normal swallow. Neither mechanism alone is capable of producing swallowing with the regularity and immediacy which is necessary during the normal process or oral feeding."

Disorders or disruptions can be found in any phase of swallowing and can significantly affect the patient's ability to take food orally and to maintain adequate nutrition. It is essential that the neuroscience nurse carefully monitor the patient's ability to feed and swallow. Clear documentation of behaviors observed, referral for a complete bedside or radiographic evaluation, and implementation of a reasonable, effective management program are necessary to ensure a successful and functional feeding program for the patient.

BEHAVIORAL MANIFESTATIONS OF SWALLOWING DIFFICULTIES

The neuroscience nurse charged with overseeing patient care may observe several behaviors that suggest the need for a swallowing evaluation protocol (Table 22–4). The nurse might observe the patient choking on food, or the patient may do better (or worse) with liquid consistencies than with a regular diet that includes solid foods. The patient might not swallow food when it is placed in the mouth or may appear to lack enough attention to follow through in the feeding process. This could be an associated characteristic of a cognitive disorder. Excessive drooling, especially unilaterally, might be observed. Several

TABLE 22–4 • COMMON PREDICTORS OF SWALLOWING PROBLEMS

- Inability to voluntarily produce effective cough
- Frequent coughing during or after drinking liquids
- Regurgitation of liquid or food particles through the nose or the tracheostomy
- Inability to effectively manage saliva or other oral secretions

hours after mealtime, the nursing assistant performing routine oral hygiene may find food pocketed on one side of the patient's mouth.

A patient who is being tube-fed may appear to be swallowing his or her own secretions, which might suggest adequate oral manipulation and thus feeding potential. Questionable secretions resembling thick liquid (such as milk shakes) on the patient's tray may have been expelled from a tracheostomy tube. The patient might complain of a sensation of food becoming stuck in the throat. Any of these observations suggests referral to the facility's dysphagia team. If there is no such team, the speech-language pathologist can evaluate the patient or make appropriate recommendations concerning swallowing assessments and treatment guidelines.

Assessment

A nurse's concern about the patient's ability to swallow food warrants referral to specific individuals on the dysphagia team. An orthodontist or dentist may be asked to evaluate the patient's teeth or dentures to determine the best possible oral structure for chewing food. If laryngeal aspiration is suspected, referrals for cineradiography or videofluoroscopy can be made to the otolaryngologist. It might be beneficial to evaluate the actual swallowing process from both a radiographic and a behavioral standpoint. Information obtained from these evaluations is used to establish therapeutic goals. Information from the radiographic studies will include comments on bolus propulsion and bolus transfer in the pharyngeal area and around the epiglottis to the cricoesophageal sphincter and into the stomach. Radiographic studies can be replayed frame by frame to outline the sequence of swallowing and to delineate any difficulties, peculiar findings, or significant problems, such as laryngeal penetration, laryngeal aspiration, and regurgitation from the esophagus or into the nasal passageway. The behavioral assessment by the speech-language pathologist begins with a focus on comments from the patient's history. Respiratory status, head-trunk control, and dental considerations are evaluated and commented on. A comprehensive oral mechanism evaluation of the structure and function of various components of the oral cavity, including both sensation and motor functions, is completed. The patient's ability to communicate basic needs and to follow commands is assessed.

The speech-language pathologist conducts a complete swallowing examination to evaluate swallowing of various consistencies, textures, and temperatures of food. The patient's responses, including comments about oral preparation, bolus, manipulation, swallowing, and laryngeal excursion, are recorded and analyzed. Cervical auscultation, a protocol that calls for the stethoscope to be placed at the level of the larynx where two distinct sounds of anatomic structures moving can be heard, helps to further determine the patient's performance. Cervical auscultation can assist the clinician in assessing the presence of residuals or pharyngeal pooling, warning signs that the swallow may not have been completed. A comprehensive review of behavioral assessment procedures has been outlined by Schwartz-Cowley and Gruen (1986) that includes special areas of interest and clinical considerations for each evaluative component.

Many swallowing centers use evaluative procedures similar to those used at the Montebello Rehabilitation Hospital of the Maryland Institute for Emergency Medical Services Systems in Baltimore, Maryland. The Diagnostic Summary of Swallowing Functions form currently in use at the R Adams Cowley Shock Trauma Center is found in Figure 22–1.

Various types of swallowing disorders can be identified through comprehensive formalized bedside and radiographic evaluations of the swallowing mechanism and process. Rubin, Battle, Snape, and Cohen (1989) presented a review of medical management for patients with swallowing problems but emphasized the absolute need for clear differential diagnosis and fact-finding.

A brief notation of disorders associated with the oral preparatory, pharyngeal, and esophageal phases of swallowing is warranted. Oral phase difficulties can arise from the presence of structural abnormalities that arise from developmental disorders, trauma-induced injuries, or surgical removal. Patients may not be able to close their lips completely or to use tongue movements effectively because of inflammation, weakness, or paralysis of muscles. Incoordination of oral movements results in leakage of the bolus out of the oral cavity. Lack of selective attention, perceptual deficits, confusion, and errors in judgment and insight result in possible functional disturbances in oral preparation.

Many problems are noted during the pharyngeal phase of swallowing. These might include delayed or absent swallowing reflexes, structural abnormalities, interference with normal swallowing as a result of inflammation or accessory sphincter action (although this may help in certain situations), or inadequate, weak pharyngeal peristalsis. Patients who have poor control of velopharyngeal closure, such as that induced by progressive neurologic disease processes, may demonstrate nasal regurgitation. Lazarus (1991) discussed several potential problem behaviors associated with the pharyngeal stage of swallowing, including pharyngeal swallow delay, reduced pharyngeal peristalsis, reduced laryngeal elevation, reduced laryngeal closure, and cricopharyngeal dysfunction.

Although many swallowing teams do not evaluate or monitor esophageal problems, a radiographic assessment can identify esophageal spasms, immobility, or structural abnormalities. Disorders in coordination of bolus movement through the cricopharyngeal and gastroesophageal segments can pose problems in effective transfer and may predispose the patient to episodes of regurgitation. Radiographic studies are essential for objective determination of esophageal disorders.

Results of the swallowing evaluation are discussed with the patient, family, physician, therapy team, and neuroscience nurse. Recommendations about diet consistency, problem foods, supervision of feeding, assistive devices for feeding, effects of fatigue, and times for best swallowing activity are provided. For some patients, oral intake of food may not be recommended because of significant physical risks posed by limited structural, physiologic, or mental abilities. Because the neuroscience nurse becomes a key individual in the pa-

Text continued on page 524

Diagnostic Summary of Swallowing Functions

Date of examination: _______________________

Examiner: _______________________

I. **IDENTIFYING INFORMATION**

Date of birth: _______________________   Date of onset: _______________________

Referring physician: _______________________   Date of admission: _______________________

II. **MEDICAL INFORMATION**

Primary diagnosis: _______________________

____

Reason for referral (Include subjective complaint if applicable): _______________________

____

____

Current diet order/method of intake: _______________________

____

Respiratory status: ______ normal   ______ impaired

______ on ventilator   comment: _______________________

______ tracheostomy tube: type _______________________

______ cuffed   ______ uncuffed   ______ fenestrated   ______ unfenestrated

If fenestrated, ______ plugged   ______ unplugged; duration plugging tolerated: _______________________

Duration of oral intubation (if applicable): _______________________

Ability to manage secretions: _______________________

____

III. **BODY POSTURE**

Head/trunk control: ______ normal   ______ impaired

Comment: _______________________

	Right	**Left**	Head/neck extended: ______ yes ______ no
Hemiparesis	______	______	Head/neck contracted: ______ yes ______ no
Flaccid	______	______	
Spastic	______	______	

IV. **COGNITIVE-LINGUISTIC COMMUNICATIVE STATUS**

Rancho level (if applicable): _______________________

Attending behaviors: _______________________

Follows motor commands: ______ consistently ______ inconsistently ______ absent

oral commands: ______ consistently ______ inconsistently ______ absent

Comment: _______________________

Expression of wants/needs: ______ functional   ______ nonfunctional

Modality of expression: ______ verbal ______ written ______ gestures ______ augmentative

system: _______________________

____

Speech articulation: ______ precise   ______ imprecise

Comment: _______________________

Vocal quality: _______________________

V. **ORAL MECHANISM EXAMINATION**

A. Sensation: (Mark boxes with: + = deficit, − = no deficit, 0 = could not assess)

Indicate R (right) or L (left) for unilateral deficits

FIGURE 22–1 • Speech–Communication Disorders Program. Ant, anterior; LOS, length of stay; PO, per os (orally); post, posterior; R/O, rule out; TMJ, temporomandibular joint. (This evaluation is used by the Montebello Rehabilitation Hospital of the Maryland Institute for Emergency Medical Services Systems in Baltimore, MD.)

Illustration continued on following page

| | Temperature | | Touch | | Taste | | | |
Structure	Hot	Cold	Light	Increased pressure	Sweet	Sour	Bitter	Other
Lips								
Tongue ant ⅓								
post ⅔								
Buccal cavity								
Palate								
Velum								

B. Motor (structure/function): Indicate N (normal), A (absent), or I (impaired) for each movement on each side; make reference to range, strength, speed, and coordination of movements under comments, as needed.

Lips: Right   Left
At rest   _____   _____
Pursing   _____   _____
Retraction   _____   _____
Strength (tight closure)   _____   _____
Drooling: _____ yes   _____ no
Rapid movements: _____ adequate
                 _____ decreased
Comments: ___________________________
____
____

Jaw: Right   Left
At rest   _____   _____
Closure   _____   _____
Depression   _____   _____
Lateralization   _____   _____
TMJ noises: _____ yes   _____ no
Comments: ___________________________
____
____

Tongue: Right   Left
At rest   _____   _____
Protrusion   _____   _____
Retraction   _____   _____
Lateralization   _____   _____
Elevation   _____   _____
Depression   _____   _____
Strength   _____   _____
Rapid movements: _____ adequate
                 _____ decreased
Tongue thrust: _____ yes   _____ no
Comments: ___________________________
____
____

Hard palate: Right   Left
At rest   _____   _____
Comments: ___________________________

Velum:
At rest   _____   _____
Elevation
  Reflexive (Gag)   _____   _____
  Gag: _____ hyperactive   _____ hypoactive
       _____ intact
  Volitional ("ah"):   _____   _____
  duration in seconds _____
Comments: ___________________________
____
____

Larynx:
  Prolong "ah" vocal quality: _____ hoarse _____ breathy _____ harsh other: ___________________
  Intermittent phonation (ah-ah-ah): ____
  Volitional cough/throat clearing (check all that apply):
    _____ normal   _____ weak   _____ delayed   _____ absent
  Reflexive cough/throat clearing:
    _____ normal   _____ weak   _____ delayed   _____ absent/not observed
  Ability to vary pitch: _____ adequate   _____ limited   _____ N/A
  Ability to vary loudness: _____ adequate   _____ limited   _____ N/A
  Ability to impound air: _____ adequate   _____ limited   _____ absent

FIGURE 22–1 *Continued*

Dentition: Indicate presence/absence and/or normal dentition and adequacy of alignment: _______________
____

Primitive reflexes (check all that apply):
______ bite reflex ______ sucking ______ rooting (______ L ______ R) ______ munching
Other: ____
Salivary function: ______ adequate ______ dry mouth ______ excess saliva

VI. **DEGLUTITION**
   A. Position of patient for evaluation:
      ______ bed ______ chair ______ Stryker frame ______ Clinitron bed ______ Other: _______________
      Degree of hip flexion: ______ 0° ______ 45° ______ 90° ______ Other: _______________
      Comments: ____
      ____

   B. Consistencies (check all that apply):
      1. Ice chips: Oral preparation: ______ adequate ______ impaired:
              Comment: ____
              Bolus manipulation: ______ adequate ______ impaired:
              Comment: ____
              Swallow: ______ complete ______ incomplete
                     ______ delayed (time: in seconds _______________) ______ Repetitive
                     ______ mouth emptied ______ food particles remain (location) _______________
              Laryngeal excursion: ______ adequate ______ limited ______ absent
                           ______ coughing ______ particles exiting trachea
              Cervical auscultation: postswallow ______ clear ______ wet
                            postcough: ______ clear ______ wet
              Not assessed _______________
      2. Pureed consistency—specify food, temperature:
              Oral preparation: ______ adequate ______ impaired:
              Comment: ____
              Bolus manipulation: ______ adequate ______ impaired:
              Comment: ____
              Swallow: ______ complete ______ incomplete
                       ______ delayed (time: in seconds _______________) ______ Repetitive
                     ______ mouth emptied ______ food particles remain (location) _______________
              Laryngeal excursion: ______ adequate ______ limited ______ absent
                           ______ coughing ______ particles exiting trachea
              Cervical auscultation: postswallow: ______ clear ______ wet
                            postcough: ______ clear ______ wet
              Not assessed _______________
      3. Soft food consistency—specify food, temperature:
              Oral preparation: ______ adequate ______ impaired:
              Comment: ____
              Bolus manipulation: ______ adequate ______ impaired:
              Comment: ____
              Swallow: ______ complete ______ incomplete
                       ______ delayed (time: in seconds _______________) ______ Repetitive
                     ______ mouth emptied ______ food particles remain (location) _______________
              Laryngeal excursion: ______ adequate ______ limited
                           ______ absent ______ coughing
                           ______ particles exiting trachea
              Cervical auscultation: postswallow: ______ clear ______ wet
                            postcough: ______ clear ______ wet
              Not assessed _______________
      4. Regular food consistency—specify food, temperature:
              Oral preparation: ______ adequate ______ impaired:
              Comment: ____

FIGURE 22–1 Continued

Illustration continued on following page

Bolus manipulation: _______ adequate _______ impaired:
Comment: ____
Swallow: _______ complete _______ incomplete
_______ delayed (time: in seconds ________________) _______ Repetitive
_______ mouth emptied _______ food particles remain (location) ________________
Laryngeal excursion: _______ adequate _______ limited
_______ absent _______ coughing
_______ particles exiting trachea
Cervical auscultation: postswallow: _______ clear _______ wet
postcough: _______ clear _______ wet
Not assessed ________________

5. Liquids
   a. Thick liquids—specify
      type, temperature:

Check all that apply:
_______ cup _______ straw
Lip protrusion: _______ adequate _______ limited _______ absent
Sucking: _______ adequate _______ decreased strength
_______ absent
Swallow: _______ complete _______ incomplete
_______ delayed (time: in seconds ________________)
_______ repetitive _______ mouth emptied
_______ particles remain (location): ________________
_______ liquid spills from mouth
Laryngeal excursion: _______ adequate _______ limited _______ absent
_______ coughing _______ particles exiting trachea
Cervical auscultation: postswallow: _______ clear _______ wet
postcough: _______ clear _______ wet
Not assessed ________________

   b. Thin liquids—specify
      type, temperature:

_______ cup _______ straw
Lip protrusion: _______ adequate _______ limited _______ absent
Sucking: _______ adequate _______ decreased strength
_______ absent
Swallow: _______ complete _______ incomplete
_______ delayed (time: in seconds ________________)
_______ repetitive _______ mouth emptied
_______ particles remain (location): ________________
_______ liquid spills from mouth
Laryngeal excursion: _______ adequate _______ limited _______ absent
_______ coughing _______ particles exiting trachea
Cervical auscultation: postswallow: _______ clear _______ wet
postcough: _______ clear _______ wet
Not assessed ________________

6. Postsuctioning Results: _______ clear _______ food particles
   _______ methylene blue _______ unable to suction

VII. **Impressions:**
A. Diagnosis: _______ Dysphagia _______ R/O Dysphagia
   Comment: ____
B. Severity: _______ mild _______ moderate _______ severe
C. Stages of deglutition affected: _______ oral _______ pharyngeal (_______ laryngeal) _______ esophageal
D. Consistencies affected: _______ pureed _______ ground _______ soft _______ regular _______ thick liquids
   _______ thin liquids
E. Comment: ____
____

F. Functional status:
   _______ Dependent: Requires enteral or parenteral techniques to maintain adequate nutrition.
   _______ Limited: Intake is primarily oral but requires constant supervision at meals to maintain
   nutrition and assure safety.
   _______ Assisted: Intake is primarily oral but requires some assistance for feeding or a specialized diet.
   _______ Independent: Requires no assistance and is able to tolerate safely most regular foods.

FIGURE 22–1 *Continued*

522

G. Prognosis: _______ good _______ fair _______ poor _______ guarded
H. Prognostic indicators: Favorable: _______ age _______ progress/recovery course thus far
_______ date of onset _______ severity _______ other: _______________
Unfavorable: _______ age _______ progress/recovery course
_______ date of onset _______ severity _______ other:_______________

VIII. **RECOMMENDATIONS**
A. Treatment: _______ no treatment at this time _______ treatment
_______ pending: ____
B. Estimated LOS: Individual therapy for _______ week(s) for _______ units (sessions)
C. Referrals: ____
____

D. Treatment goals:
Long-term goals/short-term goals
1. _________________________________   3. _________________________________
a. ______________________________   a. ______________________________
b. ______________________________   b. ______________________________
c. ______________________________   c. ______________________________

2. _________________________________
a. ______________________________
b. ______________________________
c. ______________________________

E. Ongoing patient/family education: _______________________________________
____

F. Suggestions to staff/family:
1. Optimal positioning for feeding: _______________________________________
____

2. Diet recommendations:
_______ PO intake
_______ PO intake *is not* appropriate
_______ To be fed only by speech pathologist at present time
Diet: ____
____

Foods to be omitted: ____
____
____

3. Supervision required: ____
____

4. Instructions to give patient: _______________________________________
____
____

5. Others: ____
____
____

The above was discussed with the patient and/or family.

____
Speech-Language Pathologist

____

If cineradiography study was completed, see following page for results.

Radiographic Dysphagia Assessment

☐ Supplemental assessment:

_______ cineradiography   _______ videofluoroscopy

FIGURE 22–1 *Continued*

Illustration continued on following page

☐ Summary of results:

I. **Oral Stage:** _______ normal _______ impaired. If impaired,
   A. Check consistencies affected: _______ thick barium _______ thin barium
       _______ barium/cookie mixture _______ other: _______________
   B. View difficulty noted: _______ lateral: R L (circle), _______ posterior/anterior
   C. Positioning affected: _______ supine _______ standing _______ sitting other: _____________________
   D. Specific difficulty: ____

II. **Pharyngeal Stage:** _______ normal _______ impaired. If impaired,
   A. Check consistencies affected: _______ thick barium _______ thin barium
       _______ barium/cookie mixture _______ other: _______________
   B. View difficulty noted: _______ lateral: R L (circle), _______ posterior/anterior
   C. Positioning affected: _______ supine _______ standing _______ sitting other: _____________________
   D. Specific difficulty: ____

III. **Esophageal Stage:** _______ normal _______ impaired. If impaired,
   A. Check consistencies affected: _______ thick barium _______ thin barium
       _______ barium/cookie mixture _______ other: _______________
   B. View difficulty noted: _______ lateral: R L (circle), _______ posterior/anterior
   C. Positioning affected: _______ supine _______ standing _______ sitting other: _____________________
   D. Specific difficulty: ____

☐ **Recommendations (See evaluation in part VIII of diagnostic Summary of Swallowing Functions.):**

FIGURE 22–1 *Continued*

tient's successful oral intake of food, it is imperative for nurses to understand basic treatment goals, environmental modifications, and feeding procedures.

Treatment Guidelines

Schwartz-Cowley and Gruen (1986) described the Swallowing Impairment Index, which quantifies risks associated with swallowing disorders by judging patient behaviors, including presence of swallowing reflex, consistencies affected, oral intake potential, and supervision required for safe swallowing. Use of this tool assists neuroscience nurses and other team members in determining the feasibility of an effective and fruitful swallowing treatment program for the individual patient.

Manipulating various components of the environment can greatly influence the success of the swallowing procedure for patients with swallowing difficulties who are candidates for oral feeding. The atmosphere should be calm, quiet, and free from distractions. Other patients, staff members, and visitors should be asked to leave or to remain quiet during the feeding process so that the patient can direct his or her complete attention to the chewing and swallowing process.

Food selection and presentation should be as inviting and pleasant as possible. This can be a monumental challenge when allowable safe consistencies are limited. Using patient preferences may enhance the potential of a successful feeding program.

Although the patient should be as comfortable as possible, proper positioning is extremely important and should not be compromised for the sake of comfort. Alexander (1987) emphasized the need for clinicians to determine the most appropriate position to facilitate as normal a tone as possible and to inhibit abnormal reflexes such as tonic jaw jerk, jaw opening, and bite reflexes. Table 22–5 displays basic considerations of positioning that can increase the potential for a successful feeding. It should be noted, however, that Lazarus (1991) presented convincing arguments for alteration in positioning, such as lying the patient down when residual food particles are aspirated after a swallow or tilting the patient's head back for increased propulsion speed in patients with demonstrated problems in transfer of the bolus to the pharyngeal area.

If the patient is receiving nourishment through tube-feeding, the doctor may order cessation of tube-feeding for 1 to 2 hours before oral feeding to help stimulate an appetite. The nurse should clean or freshen the patient's mouth to maximize the taste of the foods presented. Dentures or partial plates should be clean and used if they fit properly. However, neurologic events often induce physiologic and structural changes that make dentures fit improperly, especially after a prolonged illness. In these instances, it is often preferable to complete the feeding process with dentures or partial plates removed and to introduce foods that are easily palatable.

Several assistive feeding devices are available to help the patient with oral dysphagia. Patients may present with visual or physical limitations that necessitate the need for special, highly visual and functional, adaptive feeding products. These may include a push spoon, a vacuum mug, a universal cuff, weighted or angled utensils, one-way straws and straw holders (Miller, 1986), a nose-cut glass, and Styrofoam cups. Occupational therapists can offer other helpful suggestions specific to the patient's needs.

Many specialized pediatric assistive feeding devices are very successful with children. Such devices include weighted trainer cups designed to prevent

TABLE 22–5 • POSITIONING GUIDELINES TO FACILITATE EFFECTIVE SWALLOWING

- Have the patient sit in an upright position in a chair or bed for 10–15 min before eating.
- If the patient is bed bound, raise the back of the bed as far as is comfortable or place the patient in the reverse Trendelenburg position.
- Ensure comfort and safety of the patient in all sitting positions. Prop the patient with pillows or other positioning devices.
- Encourage the patient to flex the head and trunk slightly forward, if possible.
- The patient should remain at 45 degrees for approximately 30 min following completion of the meal.

spills; rolled-edge plates and bowls; flat utensils; and "doidy cups," which have a unique angle that reduces the need for the patient to tilt his or her head when drinking (North Coast Medical, 1993).

Care should be taken not to mix consistencies of food in early feeding trials. The swallowing evaluation will demonstrate the consistency best tolerated by the patient. Food consistencies that present the lowest risk for aspiration and the greatest potential for safe and effective delivery to the pharyngeal area should be used.

Although most foods prepared for any particular meal represent a variety of textures and temperatures, it is best not to mix different temperatures and textures in the same mouthful. Alternating cold and warm and smooth and coarse foods tends to enhance swallowing efficiency. Be certain not to mix liquids with solid foods in the same mouthful because of the significantly increased potential for aspiration of the liquid into the laryngeal area.

The patient should be instructed to move the food around the oral cavity with the tongue if he or she is physically capable of performing the activity. Initially, only small amounts of food (generally one-quarter to one-half teaspoon) should be given. Swallow retraining has the initial goal of the patient learning the process, not of maintaining patient nutrition. Augmentative feedings, such as nasogastric or gastric tube-feeding, should be continued until the patient can demonstrate the ability to take enough food orally to sustain nutritional requirements.

When feeding the patient, place the bolus on the stronger side of the mouth or on the opposite side from where weakness, drooping, or paralysis is noted. Additionally, have the patient tilt his or her head slightly in the direction of the stronger side to facilitate propulsion of the bolus to the back of the mouth. Logemann, Xahrilas, Robara, and Vakil (1989) reported success with this type of procedure. The caregiver may have to manually perform this function for the patient with dysphagia.

When feeding, allow the patient to close his or her lips around the spoon, and press slightly on the tongue when removing the spoon or other device. Gentle pressure on the upper lip may be needed to facilitate closure if the lips or the lower facial muscles are particularly weak.

Care needs to be taken with impulsive patients. The caregiver should always control the amount, consistency, and rate of intake of the bolus. This is particularly necessary with cognitively impaired patients, such as those with diagnoses of traumatic brain injury or progressive dementia, and with children.

The patient should be given ample time for the eating process. It is important to check for a complete swallow after each bolus presentation. Caregivers may want to look for laryngeal elevation as a predictor of swallow, although this should not be considered a fail-safe procedure. Family members are encouraged to aid the nurses in the time-consuming feeding process. Such family involvement also helps clarify teaching plans and provides a more natural social environment for eating.

As a final step in the oral feeding process, care should be taken to inspect the oral cavity to ensure that no residual food particles have been left in the mouth (pocketing). This is often found with patients who have decreased sensation or motor function unilaterally; also, cognitively impaired patients may forget that part of the meal is still in their mouth. In either case, the risk for aspiration at a later time is significantly increased.

The speech-language pathologist or other member of the swallowing team may attempt a variety of clinical procedures designed to increase swallowing proficiency. These may include selective icing, thermal stimulation, biofeedback, muscle reeducation, supraglottic swallow, and the Mendelsohn maneuver. Lazarus (1991) discussed a variety of specialized training procedures that facilitate the goal of improved swallowing in individuals with brain injury. Presented in Table 22–6, these procedures may have some beneficial effects in children and adults who present with other neurologic diagnoses. The speech-language pathologist should be consulted for more direct advice regarding the potential benefits of these procedures.

In patients with chronic alterations in mobility, the goal for those with inadequate nutritional status is to provide caloric intake that will meet the needs for growth, daily energy expenditure, and weight gain. The goal for the overweight patient is to structure the caloric requirements to meet growth and energy needs but to provide an organized pattern of weight loss in the context of the patient's exercise ability.

Interventions include planning meals that coincide with chewing and swallowing capabilities and reflect appropriate caloric requirements. Patients taking medication that facilitates swallowing (levodopa, anticholinesterases) should schedule meals for 1 hour after medication to coincide with the drug's peak effectiveness. The patient may want to avoid talking before or during meals.

TABLE 22–6 • POTENTIAL PROCEDURAL COMPONENTS IN DYSPHAGIA REHABILITATION

1. Reduce hypertonicity, hyperreflexia, and hypersensitivity.
2. Improve hypotonicity, hyporeflexia, and hyposensitivity.
3. Improve the oral and preparatory stages of swallowing as follows:
   Improve lip closure.
   Increase lip strength.
   Improve buccal tone.
   Redirect bolus flow.
   Improve range of motion of the tongue.
   Improve lingual control.
   Increase lingual strength.
4. Improve the pharyngeal stage of swallowing as follows:
   Enhance trigger of swallow reflex through thermal stimulation and suck-swallow maneuvers.
   Clear residue with liquid washes.
   Vary food consistencies.
   Employ postural maneuvers.
   Improve laryngeal adduction.
   Increase laryngeal elevation.

Data from Lazarus, C. (1991). Diagnosis and management of swallowing disorders in traumatic brain injury. In D. Beukelman & R. Yorkston (Eds.), *Communication disorders following traumatic brain injury: Management of cognitive, language, and motor impairments.* Austin, TX: Pro-Ed.

Many of the same muscles used for speaking are used in the swallowing process, and the muscles are likely to tire with repeated activity in patients with fatiguing muscle weakness, such as myasthenia gravis or multiple sclerosis (Kess, 1984). For the person with a movement disorder, performing two tasks at once interferes with the smooth accomplishment of either. In a patient with severe swallowing difficulty, high-caloric snacks such as puddings, eggnogs, and milk shakes may be used as supplements. A prospective study of weight loss in patients with Huntington's disease revealed that female patients who have diets high in fat lose proportionately less weight than their male counterparts (Shoulson et al., 1984). The overweight patient must be careful not to increase the total caloric intake with such supplements.

• C A S E   S T U D Y

Dale, a 23-year-old man, was admitted to a regional trauma center with a diagnosis of severe closed head trauma. The initial Glasgow Coma Scale score was 4/15. Predominant computed tomographic findings included significant diffuse cerebral edema and an acute left temporal-parietal epidural hematoma, which was removed quickly. Because of the low level of response, a tracheostomy with moist room air was completed 4 days after injury. A nasogastric tube was inserted, and the patient received 50% to 75% strength tube-feeding on a continuous basis. Behavioral rating was completed 7 days after onset. A Rancho Los Amigos Levels of Cognitive Functioning Scale was used to determine level III behaviors.

Characteristics included inconsistent reactions to stimulation provided by the examiner. The patient inconsistently followed simple commands such as "Point to the floor." Responses were delayed (5 to 10 seconds). Dale was unable to communicate his basic needs to the nursing staff. Responses were more consistent and exemplified higher levels of response when his girlfriend of 5 years gave the commands.

A referral to the speech-language pathologist for a swallowing evaluation was initiated. The patient appeared able to manage his secretions well without drooling. The bedside evaluation indicated impaired head and neck control, necessitating propping pillows and Posey restraints to position him in a gerichair. Cognitive-linguistic deficits included short selective attention span, inconsistent axial commands, remarkable decrease in gestural expression of personal needs, and nonverbal communication because of tracheostomy.

The oral mechanism examination was not reliable because of inconsistent patient response levels. The patient did, however, arouse when cold stimulation was provided to the teeth and the buccal cavities. Dale demonstrated tongue and jaw movements spontaneously. The cuffed tracheostomy tube was deflated. Saliva secretions were swallowed without coughing. Results of cervical auscultation were unremarkable before and after testing. Ice chips, soft potatoes, and a Popsicle were used to determine Dale's ability to swallow specific food textures and consistencies.

Results of oral feeding trials included successful oral manipulation through reflexive swallowing. No particles remained in the oral cavity. Breath sounds were normal to cervical auscultation, and an increase in overall awareness and cognitive-linguistic performance was noted. Recommendations were to decrease tube-feedings by 50% and to start supervised oral feeds while the patient was in the gerichair at 90 degrees. A soft diet without thin liquids was ordered. Suggestions about environmental distractions, positioning, and supervised feeding were provided to the primary nurse.

Dale's speech-language pathologist monitored swallowing functions in addition to implementing the cognitive-linguistic remediation program. Twenty-one days after onset, the tracheostomy tube was removed. The patient proceeded to a regular diet with liquids and tolerated oral feeding well. A significant positive change in overall cognitive-linguistic performance was also noted.

Nursing Diagnoses

POTENTIAL FOR ALTERATION IN NUTRITION—LESS THAN BODY REQUIREMENTS

Swallowing dysfunctions can considerably reduce the patient's nutritional intake (Carpenito, 1999). Adequate nutritional intake is critical to the healing process. The inability to meet metabolic requirements results in a loss of weight as well as a decreased ability of the body to grow and repair itself. Assessment of the patient's swallowing ability is the important first step in designing an appropriate nutritional plan for the patient.

Specific interventions include reducing causative and contributing factors, if possible. Before beginning a feeding, the nurse must assess that the patient is alert and responsive and has a good cough reflex. Suction equipment should be available. The patient should be positioned appropriately, and food must be given in small amounts and must be of the proper consistency. Following the plan outlined by the speech-language pathologist will ensure consistency of feeding. The use of a calorie count with supplemental intravenous or nasogastric nutritonal intake can ensure an adequate intake.

The expected outcomes for the patient are that he or she will experience an increase in the amount and type of nutrients ingested and will describe the rationale for the treatment plan initiated.

INSUFFICIENT AIRWAY CLEARANCE

The patient experiencing a swallowing disorder has great potential for aspiration, which could lead to upper and lower airway problems. Assessment of the cough and gag reflex is critical in every patient to prevent a possible catastrophe. Collaborating with the speech-language pathologist for guidelines on the best way to feed the patient also contributes to safeguarding the patient.

Specific interventions include the following:

1. Positioning the patient to facilitate swallowing by elevating the head of the bed to a 60- to 90-degree position. Avoiding a position that causes the patient to flex the neck or slouch can facilitate swallowing.

2. Allowing the patient adequate time to chew and swallow. Initially, patients undergoing swallowing therapy should be assessed on the quality of swallowing procedure rather than on the quantity consumed.

3. Avoiding patient fatigue and drowsiness. This is necessary because such conditions can increase the risk of aspiration during eating. Rest periods before eating allow the patient to be alert and responsive during the meal. Using assistive cough techniques and other pulmonary hygiene measures ensures clearing of the airway.

Expected outcomes are that the patient will have clear upper and lower airway on auscultation, have a decreased risk of aspiration, and demonstrate effective coughing techniques. The family can demonstrate the Heimlich maneuver in chronic care.

Although the ideal situation is to have all patients feeding either independently or with assistance, the realistic neuroscience nurse will realize that enteral or parenteral means will be required to maintain nutrition for some patients. Oral gastric and nasogastric tubes are frequently used for short-term swallowing problems. Gastrostomy or jejunostomy may be required for long-term nutritional management. Referrals to the gastroenterologist, internist, or surgeon are made when management issues are considered.

SUMMARY

Knowledge of the functional framework of the swallowing process, indications for assessment protocols, and therapeutic management options for the child or adult with swallowing difficulties aids the neuroscience nurse in developing an effective and appropriate nutrition and feeding program.

References

Alexander, R. (1987). Oral-motor treatment for infants and young with cerebral palsy. *Seminars in Speech and Language, 8,* 87–100.

American Speech-Language-Hearing Association (1992). *ASHA preferred practice patterns.* Rockville, MD: Author.

Blonsky, E., Logemann, J., Bosches, B., & Fisher, H. (1975). Comparison of speech and swallow function in patients with tremor disorders and in normal geriatric patients: A cinefluorographic study. *Journal of Gerontology, 30,* 299.

Carpenito, L. (1999). Nursing diagnosis application to clinical practice. In *Handbook of nursing diagnosis* (pp. 212–220). Philadelphia: J.B. Lippincott.

Donner, M. W., Bosma, J. F., & Robertson, D. L. (1985). Anatomy and physiology of the pharynx. *Gastrointestinal Radiology, 10*(3), 196–212.

Kess, R. (1984). Suddenly in crisis: Unpredictable myasthenia. *American Journal of Nursing, 84*(8), 994–998.

Lazarus, C. (1991). Diagnosis and management of swallowing disorders in traumatic brain injury. In D. Beukelman & R. Yorkston (Eds.), *Communication disorders following traumatic brain injury: Management of cognitive, language, and motor impairments* (pp. 325–338). Austin, TX: Pro-Ed.

Leopold, N. A., & Kagel, M. C. (1983). Swallowing, ingestion and dysphagia: A reappraisal. *Archives of Physical Medicine and Rehabilitation, 64*(8), 371–373.

Logemann, J. (1983). *Evaluation and treatment of swallowing disorders.* San Diego, CA: College Hill Press.

Logemann, J., Xahrilas, P., Robara, M., & Vakil, N. (1989). The benefit of head rotation on pharyngo-esophageal dysphagia. *Archives of Physical Medicine and Rehabilitation, 70,* 767–771.

Mandelstam, P., & Leiber, A. (1970). Cineradiographic evaluation of the esophagus in normal adults. *Gastroenterology, 58,* 32.

Miller, A. (1986). Neurophysiologic basis of swallowing. *Dysphagia, 1,* 91–100.

North Coast Medical (1993). *ADL: Products for the activities of daily living.* San Diego, CA: Author.

Roueche, J. (1980). *Dysphagia: An assessment and management program for the adult.* Minneapolis, MN: Sister Renny Institute.

Rubin, M., Battle, W., Snape, W., & Cohen, S. (1989). Managing the patient with dysphagia. *Hospital Medicine, 12,* 70–87.

Schwartz-Cowley, R., & Gruen, A. (1986). Rehabilitation assessment of communicative, cognitive-linguistic, and swallowing functions. *Trauma Quarterly, 3*(1), 63–75.

Shoulson, I., Miller, C., Welle, S., Panzik, J., Lipinski, B., Plumb, S., & Forbes, C. (1984). Huntington's disease: Body weight and metabolic indices [Abstract]. *Annals of Neurology, 16*(1), 126.

Zimmerman, J. E., & Oder, L. A. (1981). Swallowing dysfunction in acutely ill patients. *Physical Therapy, 61*(12), 1755–1763.

SENSATION PHENOMENA

23 | Sensation: An Overview

RUTH A. MULNARD

Sensation is an extremely personal concept, influenced by cultural, environmental, and psychologic factors. One might say that significant function and pure survival rely on the ability of the individual to receive, process, and take action on various forms of stimuli—external, from environmental influences, and internal, from within the individual.

From minute to minute, we experience situations within our environments and changes within our bodies by way of specialized sensory systems: hearing, vision, touch, taste, and smell. Each sensory system is architecturally specialized so that it reacts to a particular range of environmental influences. Sensation may be provocatively pleasant, irritating, or tearfully painful. It may be accentuated, altered, diminished, or even absent. There may be variety in intensity with no direct correlation to the stimulus, especially when the stimulus is of pathologic origin (Purchese, 1977).

Sensation may be viewed with respect to the implications it has for the person, family, and society. Many neurologic conditions alter sensory input, processing, or perception and thereby impose severe restrictions on the individual and the way he or she relates to family and society. In understanding the impact of lost sensation, several questions come to mind: How do normal sensations influence, enhance, or interfere with everyday life? How does an alteration in sensation affect daily living? Can one measure the devastation that is created when one of the senses has been impaired? Why do some people adapt to the effects of sensory loss better than others do? Is it their support systems, professional interest, culture, or life experiences? Should we even try to make a judgment about this, or should we instead heighten our awareness of the fact that alterations in sensory experiences are individual and may have profound implications for the person, family, and society?

This chapter discusses the anatomy, physiology, and assessment parameters for the various components of the sensory system, including the special senses. Disease states with primary pathology are reviewed.

PERIPHERAL SOMESTHETIC SENSORY SYSTEM

The pathway by which sensory information enters the central nervous system is variable in length and complexity. The general segments of the peripheral somesthetic system are addressed in this section, including levels of sensory receptors, sensory fibers, dermatomal distribution, and spinal cord tracts.

Sensory Receptors

The skin is considered the major source of sensory input to the nervous system and contains a variety of sensory receptors that relay information about the internal and external environments. The sensory receptors are specialized for converting various forms of energy in the environment into action potentials in the neurons (Ganong, 1987). The forms of energy converted by the receptors include mechanical (touch, pressure), thermal (degrees of warmth), electromagnetic (light), and chemical (odor, taste, carbon dioxide content of the blood). Because sensory receptors are highly specialized to respond to one particular form of stimulus, there must be many different types of receptors. The receptors pertinent to this chapter include mechanoreceptors, thermoreceptors, and nociceptors.

MECHANORECEPTORS

Mechanoreceptors facilitate the relative determination of positions and rates of movement of the different parts of the body. They are sensitive to touch, pressure, vibration, tickle, and position. There are six types of mechanoreceptors, as shown in Table 23–1.

THERMORECEPTORS

Thermoreceptors detect changes in temperature. There are various thermoreceptors throughout the body that function to inform the hypothalamic heat-regulating center of environmental temperature. That information plus the information from central temperature receptors normally stimulates the hypothalamus to activate either heat-gaining or heat-losing mechanisms; for example, when the body attempts to generate heat through shivering or when the body strives for heat containment by peripheral vasoconstriction.

Sensory information on the continuum of burning hot to freezing cold and degrees of temperature difference are discriminated by at least three types of peripheral sensory receptors: cold receptors, warmth receptors, and pain receptors. Central receptors are specialized neurons in the anterior hypothalamus (Table 23–2).

TABLE 23–1 • TYPES OF MECHANORECEPTORS

Type	Purpose	Location
Free nerve endings	Detect touch and pressure	Everywhere in the skin
Meissner's corpuscles	Discern spatial characteristics of touch sensation	Glabrous, nonhairy skin, especially fingertips and lips
Expanded-tip tactile receptors	Provide a continuous signal that gives the ability to determine continuous touch of objects against the skin	Skin
Hair and organs	Detect mainly movement of objects over the surface of the body as a result of stimulation of nerve fibers that entwine the base of the hair	Skin
Ruffini's end organs	Detect heavy continuous touch and pressure signals	Deep tissues and deeper layers of skin
Pacinian corpuscles	Detect tissue vibration; stimulated only by rapid movement	Beneath the skin, deep in the tissues of the body

NOCICEPTORS

Nociceptors are pain receptors that detect tissue damage of either physical or chemical origin.

Sensory Fibers

Sensory nerve fibers transmit impulses from the periphery to specific cortical or subcortical areas. Three types of fibers have been described according to

TABLE 23–2 • TYPES OF THERMORECEPTORS

Type	Purpose	Location
Cold receptors	Discriminate degrees of temperature difference, cold	Under the skin (there are three to four times as many cold receptors as heat receptors)
Heat receptors	Discriminate degrees of temperature difference, warmth	Under the skin
Pain receptors Warmth pain receptors Cold pain receptors	Pain receptors in combination with cold and warmth receptors are responsive to freezing cold and burning hot sensations (Guyton, 1987)	Under the skin
Central receptors	Monitor temperature of blood (core temperature)	Anterior hypothalamus

fiber diameter, conduction velocity, and physiologic characteristics. Generally, the greater the diameter of the nerve fiber, the greater its speed of conduction. The large fibers are concerned with proprioceptive sensation, whereas the smaller fibers are concerned with pain sensation (Ganong, 1987). The fibers are as follows:

Large Myelinated A Beta Fibers. These fibers transmit impulses generated via mechanical stimuli such as touch and pressure.

Small Myelinated A Beta Fibers. These fibers serve two functions. First, some fibers transmit impulses from nociceptors and mediate fast pain, such as removing a hand from a hot burner. Second, some fibers transmit impulses from mechanoreceptors. These are the fibers that carry temperature, crude touch, and prickling pain sensation.

C Fibers. These fibers are small, unmyelinated fibers with slow transmission velocity and are concerned basically with pain, temperature, itch, and crude touch sensation. A few C fibers also transmit impulses from mechanoreceptors. More than two thirds of all nerve fibers in peripheral nerves are C fibers. The large numbers of C fibers facilitate the transmission of tremendous amounts of information from the surface of the body, even though the velocity of transmission is slow.

Dermatomes

A dermatome is the cutaneous sensation of a specific area of skin supplied by the fibers of any one dorsal root. The cell bodies of the afferent fibers involved are located in the dorsal spinal nerve root ganglia and in the ganglia of the fifth, seventh, ninth, and tenth cranial nerves. Sensory stimuli travel toward the cell body from the periphery and continue to the spinal cord. The anatomic distribution represented by the dermatome correlates with a respective spinal cord segment and can be mapped out schematically. Using astute, accurate assessment of the cutaneous distribution of various nerve roots, it is possible to localize the site and the level of pathologic disturbance.

Spinal Cord

The spinal cord is a cylindrical, flexible structure that is the caudal continuation of the medulla oblongata. In the adult, it extends distally from the medulla, ending at the level of the first or second lumbar vertebra. The spinal cord travels through the hollow canal in the center of the vertebral column and serves as a communication cable carrying motor information from the brain to the peripheral nervous system and carrying sensory information from the peripheral nervous system back to the brain.

The spinal cord, approximately 45 cm long in the male and 42 cm long in the female, is divided into cervical (C), thoracic (T), lumbar (L), and sacral (S) segments. Two enlargements are present, one in the cervical region from C3 to T2, and the other in the lumbar region, corresponding to vertebrae T10 to T12. These enlargements receive additional nerves from the upper and lower extremities.

SPINAL NERVES

The spinal nerve roots are bundled together to form the 31 pairs of spinal nerves that originate from the spinal cord. Each nerve has an anterior or ventral root and a posterior or dorsal root (Fig. 23–1). The anterior or ventral nerve roots consist of efferent motor fibers originating in the ventral and lateral gray columns, with attachments to the front portion of the spinal cord. They carry motor information from the brain to various body parts.

The posterior or dorsal nerve roots contain afferent sensory fibers from the nerve cells in the spinal or dorsal root ganglion; ganglia are enlargements containing cells in the dorsal root of each nerve. The dorsal nerve roots have their attachment to the back portion of the cord and carry incoming sensory information to the cord, where it is then transmitted to the brain.

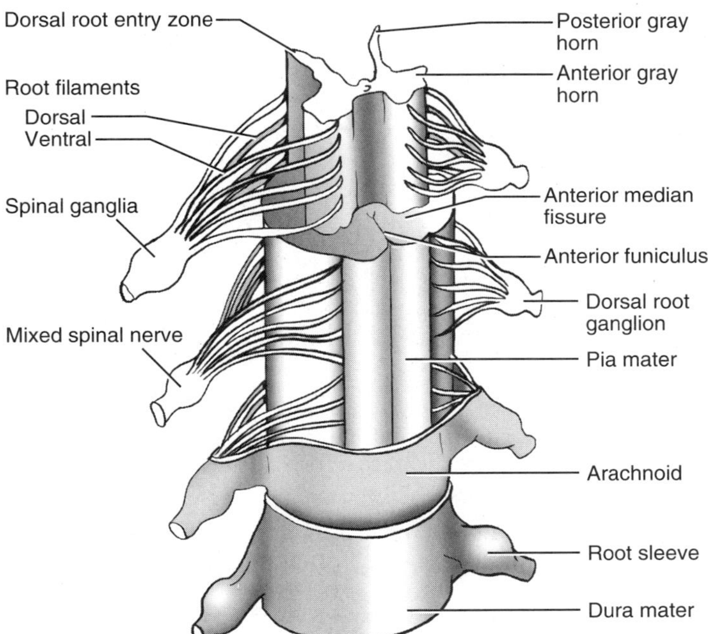

FIGURE 23–1 • Spinal cord and meninges.

The groups of spinal nerves are divided into 8 cervical, 12 thoracic, 5 lumbar, 5 sacral, and 1 coccygeal nerve. The lumbosacral nerve roots are collectively called the cauda equina because of their resemblance to the tail of a horse.

GRAY MATTER

The gray matter within the spinal cord is composed of cell bodies clustered in the central area, in the shape of a butterfly or an H (Fig. 23–2). White matter is composed of myelinated nerve fibers and surrounds the gray matter. The

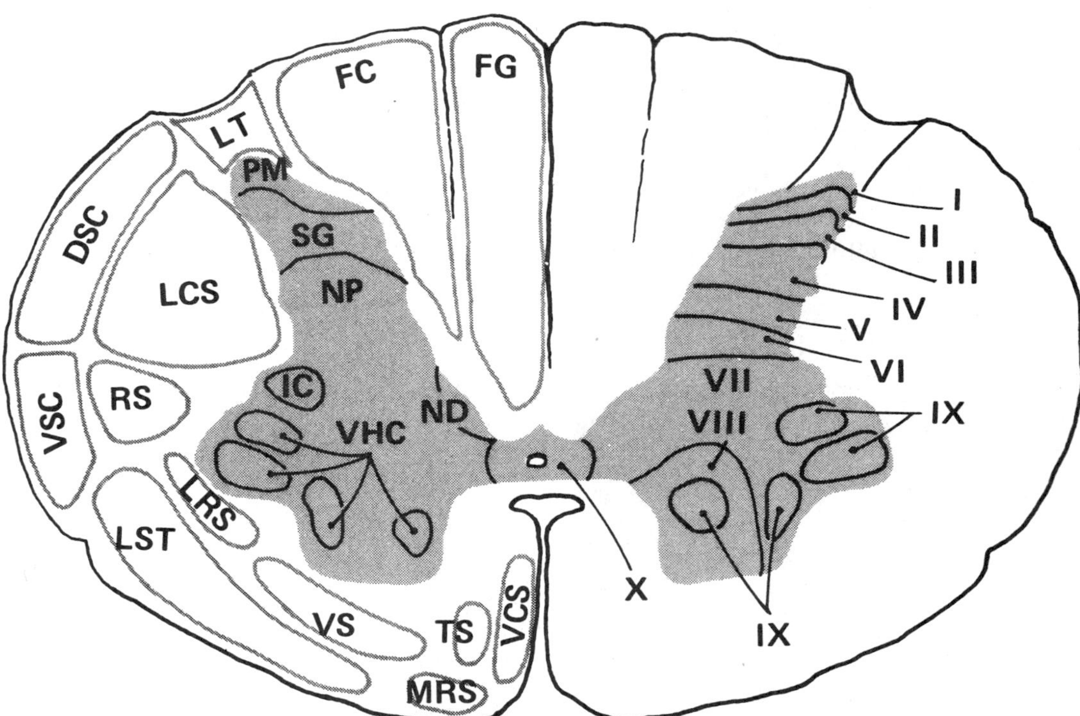

FIGURE 23–2 • Cross-section of the spinal cord at approximately the C-8–T-1 segmental level. Tracts and nuclei of the cord are illustrated on the left; Rexed's laminar organization of the gray matter is illustrated on the right. DSC, dorsal spinocerebellar tract; FC, fasciculus cuneatus; FG, fasciculus gracilis; IC, intermediolateral cell column; LCS, lateral corticospinal tract; LRS, lateral reticulospinal tract; LST, lateral spinothalamic tract; LT, Lissauer's tract; MRS, medial reticulospinal tract; ND, nucleus dorsalis; NP, nucleus proprius; PM, posteromarginal nucleus; RS, rubrospinal tract; SG, substantia gelatinosa; TS, tectospinal tract; VCS, ventral corticospinal tract; VHC, ventral horn cell columns; VS, vestibulospinal tract; VSC, ventral spinocerebellar tract. (From Gilman, S., & Winans, S. S. [1990]. *Manter & Gatz's essentials of clinical neuroanatomy and neurophysiology* [7th ed.]. Philadelphia: F.A. Davis.)

gray matter has three columns, the anterior, posterior, and lateral columns. The *anterior column (anterior horn)* is composed of cell bodies of motor neurons that relay motor information from the brain out through the anterior roots. The *posterior column (dorsal horn)* contains sensory relay cells that transmit incoming information received through the posterior root from the body to the brain. The *lateral column (lateral horn),* also called the *intermediolateral cell column,* extends from T1 through L2 or L3. This column consists of small motor-type cells and gives rise to preganglionic sympathetic fibers.

The gray matter is divided into 10 layers, or laminae, on the basis of cytoarchitecture and organization of neurons (see Fig. 23–2). Lamina I is in the most dorsal section of the dorsal horn, and lamina IX is in the most ventral section of the ventral horn. Each lamina extends the full length of the spinal cord. Laminae I to VI are located in the dorsal horns, with lamina I the most superficial and lamina VI the most deep. These laminae are primarily concerned with afferent sensory input to the spinal cord. Specifically, laminae II and III correspond to the substantia gelatinosa, which receives information from pain and temperature afferents. Lamina VII is located in the intermediate gray area and extends into the anterior horn, containing the nucleus dorsalis and the intermediolateral gray column. The anterior horn also contains lamina VIII, which has neurons that send commissural axons to the opposite side of the cord. Lamina IX is contained within the ventral horn and has motor neurons that send axons into the ventral roots of the spinal nerves and innervate the skeletal muscles. Lamina X surrounds the central column.

WHITE MATTER

The white matter in the spinal cord is composed chiefly of myelinated nerve fibers, although there are some unmyelinated fibers as well. The purpose of the white matter is to link different segments of the spinal cord and connect the spinal cord with the brain. The white matter is organized around longitudinal columns, also known as the anterior, posterior, and lateral funiculi (see Fig. 23–2). Each column consists of fiber tracts, some ascending (sensory) and others descending (motor).

For the purposes of this chapter, only major ascending tracts are discussed. The *lateral spinothalamic tract* is the main pathway for conveying impulses of pain and temperature, and the *anterior spinothalamic tract* is the pathway for simple touch and pressure. Recent evidence indicates that both the lateral spinothalamic tract and the anterior spinothalamic tract are capable of mediating nociceptive and tactile sensation. The *posterior* or *dorsal column tract* includes the fasciculus gracilis fibers from the leg and the fasciculus cuneatus fibers from the arm. These pathways are responsible for sensations of motion, movement, touch, and pressure. The *ventral spinocerebellar tract* relays information from pain, tactile, and pressure receptors in an extremity, and the *dorsal spinocerebellar tract* transmits information from individual muscles and joints. Both the ventral and the dorsal spinocerebellar tracts are concerned mainly with the lower extremities and provide predominantly proprioceptive information to the cerebellum. The name of each tract is descriptive of the column (funiculus) in which it travels, the location of its cells of origin, and the location of its axon termination.

There are two major ascending systems responsible for conveying somatosensory information to the cerebral cortex. Current literature divides them into the dorsal column, or lemniscal system, which mediates fine tactile and kinesthetic sensation, and the anterolateral system, which conducts impulses for pain, temperature, touch, and deep pressure.

Dorsal Column System. In general, fine touch, pressure, and proprioceptive fibers ascend on the ipsilateral side in the dorsal columns to the medulla, where they synapse in the gracile and cuneate nuclei. The second-order neurons from the gracile and cuneate nuclei cross the midline and ascend in the medial lemniscus to end in the specific sensory relay nuclei of the thalamus, which projects neurons to the somatosensory regions of the cerebral cortex. Dorsal columns transmit messages exclusively from mechanoreceptors, whereas information from the anterolateral system comes from mechanoreceptors, thermoreceptors, and nociceptors. Dorsal column lesions produce ipsilateral impairment of sensations.

Anterolateral System. The fibers mediating temperature and pain, as well as some touch fibers, synapse on the neurons in the dorsal horn. The axons from these neurons cross the midline and ascend on the contralateral side in the anterolateral quadrant of the spinal cord. This pathway ends in the reticular formation of the brain stem and in the thalamus. Anterolateral lesions produce sensory impairment on the contralateral side (Schmidt, 1978).

Fibers from within both the dorsal column (lemniscal system) and the anterolateral system are joined in the brain stem by fibers mediating sensation from the head.

CENTRAL SOMESTHETIC SENSORY SYSTEM

The body has two major sensory systems that influence and organize sensation. Neither is mutually exclusive, and they depend on each other's normal function and relay of impulses for the total delivery of the sensory experience. The first sensory system, the peripheral somesthetic system, has been discussed. The central somesthetic sensory system includes the fiber connections between the peripheral somesthetic sensory system, which communicates with the brain stem (reticular activating system), as well as the thalamus, hypothalamus, and parietal lobes (Schmidt, 1978).

Brain Stem Reticular Activating System

The reticular activating system (RAS) receives information from all the afferent cranial nerves and is thought to participate in a number of sensory influences. Schmidt (1978, p. 57) lists these as the following:

1. Influence the RAS has on control of consciousness by influence on the activity of cortical neurons
2. Mediation of the affective (emotional) effects of sensory stimuli—for example, the transmission of afferent pain information to the limbic system
3. Vegetative regulatory functions with vital reflexes (cardiovascular, respiratory, swallowing, coughing, and sneezing reflexes) in which many afferent and efferent systems must be coordinated
4. Participation in the motor mechanisms for body support and directed movement

Thalamus

The thalamus has many subdivisions and is a very important sensory center. The thalamus receives afferent communication from the periphery and from all other sensory modalities, with the exception of the olfactory impulses. Some of the fibers that terminate in the thalamus are those of the lateral spinothalamic tract, which carry sensations of pain and temperature, as well as those from the anterior spinothalamic tract, which are responsible for carrying sensations of light touch and pressure. In his work, Peele (1977, p. 311) stated that ''thalamic nuclei may serve as simple relays, as integrative centers for conscious recognition of certain impulses and as integrative and elaborative centers which project the product of their elaboration to the cerebral cortex.''

The thalamus serves to integrate sensory impulses, as in the recognition of pain or in the spectrum of temperature or touch variations. The thalamus also makes it possible for a person to realize the degree of contraction in muscles and around joints, allowing for a sense of movement or position. The ability to recognize size, shape, and quality of objects that have contact with touch receptors and to identify a particular point of stimulation are cortical functions that are possible only if thalamic relay functions are intact.

Hypothalamus

The hypothalamus is directly responsible for a variety of vital regulatory functions of the body and is involved with many aspects of emotion and behavior. With the limbic structures, the hypothalamus seems to be responsible for the interpretive nature of sensory sensation, whether pleasant or painful. Communicating pathways exist with all levels of the limbic system. Stimulation of various regions of the hypothalamus can create an increase in activity that can create the emotions of fear and rage and increased sexual drive.

Parietal Lobe

Adams and Victor (1985, p. 338) stated, ''The greater part of the parietal lobe functions as a center for integrating somatic sensory with visual and auditory information in constructing an awareness of the body and of its relation to extrapersonal space. Through frontal connections, proprioception and vision are combined for the movement of the body and manipulation of objects and for certain constructional activities, and impairment of these functions implicates the parietal lobe, especially the right."

The somesthetic area, the primary sensory projection area, is responsible for the reception of general sensation and is located in the parietal lobe. It receives fibers from thalamic radiations conveying skin, muscle, joint, and tendon sense from the opposite side of the body. The primary sensory areas are arranged topographically on the cerebral cortex to mirror image the primary motor area; this is called the *sensory homunculus.*

Conditions That May Alter Somatic Sensation

Many neurologic conditions may have alteration in sensation as a common symptom. Only those with an actual or potential marked sensory alteration are discussed.

COMPLETE SPINAL CORD INJURY

When there is a sudden transverse lesion to the spinal cord, all sensory and motor function is lost immediately below the level of the lesion; these functions do not return. Generally, there may be a hyperesthetic area near the upper margin of anesthesia, and loss of pain, temperature, and touch sensation may begin one or two segments below the level of the lesion.

INCOMPLETE SPINAL CORD INJURY SYNDROME

The most commonly seen incomplete spinal cord injuries are Brown-Sequard syndrome and central cord syndrome. *Brown-Sequard syndrome* is caused by hemisection of the spinal cord, resulting most commonly from bullet or stab wounds. This syndrome results in ipsilateral motor paralysis; ipsilateral loss of touch, pressure, vibration, and proprioceptive sensation; and contralateral loss of superficial pain and thermal sensation, usually beginning one or two segments below the lesion. *Central cord syndrome* occurs when damage is located specifically in the area of the central spinal cord. Motor ability of the upper extremities is more severely affected than is that of the lower extremities, and sensory loss is variable.

SYRINGOMYELIA

Syringomyelia (from the Greek *syrinx,* "pipe" or "tube") is a chronic progressive syndrome of the spinal cord associated with an enlarging accumulation of fluid in the spinal cord. Usually, the central canal of the spinal cord enlarges, or tubelike cavities open in the central region of the gray matter. As a result, there is destruction of the gray and white matter that lies adjacent to the central canal. Because pain fibers that cross anterior to the central canal may be interrupted or destroyed, the first symptom is often loss of pain and temperature sensation in the involved dermatomes. Pain may be a symptom, however, and if so, it is usually unilateral, of a burning, aching quality, and located in the region of sensory impairment. The cavitation, or syrinx, may extend into the anterior horn, destroying motor neurons and resulting in atrophy and weakness of the segments involved.

TRIGEMINAL NEURALGIA

Trigeminal neuralgia (*tic douloureux*) may result from the degeneration or compression of one or all branches of the fifth central nerve. It is characterized by mild to excruciating facial pain, described by many as the worst possible pain a person could ever suffer. The pain frequently occurs as severe, lightninglike, electric stabs or searing pain and may be accompanied by twitching of the facial muscles. The duration is usually short, lasting from a few seconds to minutes, but frequently pains occur in succession so that the pain seems endless. At times, the pain may be provoked by a slight breeze, brushing of the teeth, or washing of the face. The most common trigger points include the nostril, medial cheek, or lip.

THALAMIC LESIONS

Thalamic lesions involving the nucleus ventralis posterolateralis of the thalamus can create a decrease in or loss of sensation on the contralateral side of the body. The origin of this thalamic lesion is usually a vascular insult or a tumor. The sensory function most commonly involved is position sense, and deep sensory loss is usually but not always more profound than cutaneous loss. There may be spontaneous and extremely irritating pain on the affected side that may linger and be extremely unpleasant.

LESIONS OF THE PARIETAL LOBE

The best known anterior parietal lobe syndrome is described by Adams and Victor (1985) as Veger-DeJerine syndrome. It is characterized by disturbances of the discriminative sensory abilities on the contralateral side, especially of the face, arm, and leg. Impaired localization of touch and pain stimuli, loss of position sense, elevation of two-point threshold, astereognosis, and tactile agnosia (if the lesion is in the dominant hemisphere) are the most prominent findings. Seen frequently with lesions involving the parietal lobe is a sensory inattention or neglect response of body parts on the affected side. Stroke, head injury, and tumors may cause parietal lobe lesions.

HERPES ZOSTER

Herpes zoster (shingles) is a viral infection of primary sensory neurons. Generally, symptoms of fever and malaise precede the pain, and vesicles form over the segmental distribution of the involved roots. Itching, tingling, or burning sensations of the dermatomes often precede the vesicular eruption.

Any dermatome may be involved, but T5 to T10 dermatomes appear to be the most common, followed by the craniocervical regions. The pain and dysesthesia frequently linger for weeks, months, or, in some cases, years, creating difficult problems with pain management.

CAUSALGIA

Causalgia is a condition of constant burning pain, most commonly along the distribution of the median or tibial nerves. Causalgia usually follows traumatic lesions of the peripheral nerves. Symptoms may begin the first few days after injury and may involve trophic changes on the skin, sweating in the affected extremity, and changes in the hair and nails.

MULTIPLE SCLEROSIS

Multiple sclerosis is one of the most common neurologic diseases in the United States. It is chronic, often progressive, and characterized by destruction of multiple areas of central nervous system myelin. Sensory disturbances are common and depend on the area of sclerotic patch formation in the central nervous system. Sensory disturbance may be symmetrical or asymmetrical and involves the trunk and lower extremities more frequently than it involves the upper extremities. Lhermitte's sign is perhaps one of the most common sensory symptoms noted and is frequently described as a lightninglike sensation that radiates down the neck after neck flexion. Other forms of sensory changes experienced include loss of vibratory sense in the distal lower extremities; bandlike sensations about the trunk; tingling paresthesias, or numbness, of the face in the distribution of the fifth nerve; and pain that is individualized.

DIABETES MELLITUS

Diabetes mellitus, a disorder of abnormal glucose metabolism, is known to cause progressive destruction of the peripheral nerves, causing a neuropathy. Protracted elevations of the serum glucose as a result of lack of insulin have long-term detrimental effects on the end organs of sensory information as well, particularly on the eye.

BRAIN AGING

There appears to be a decrease in the efficiency of neurochemical activity as the brain ages, as a result of a decline in the production of some of the neurotransmitters, and also an increase in the activity of the enzymes responsible for neurotransmitter degradation (Havener, Saunders, Keith, & Prescott, 1974). These age-related changes, in combination with changes specific to the organs in the body, create an overall decrease in the functioning of the sensory nervous system. Age-related changes occur at different rates in each individual and are often complicated by a variety of situational, disease-related, and therapeutic aspects, such as nutrition, hypertension, hyperlipidemia, diabetes mellitus, and drugs. It is, therefore, important for the nurse to assess the elderly person's sensory functioning thoroughly and to determine the impact the changes have on the ability to perceive and respond to the environment.

SPECIAL SENSES

The special senses are complex neurologic systems consisting of hearing, vision, taste, and smell. Specific dysfunctions may occur in each system.

Hearing

In the United States, hearing loss is one of the most frequent forms of physical disability, affecting 10 to 20 million Americans. The potential for suboptimal educational, economic, and psychosocial advantage is a real concern to both individuals and society. Alterations in hearing affect each person and family unit differently. The meaning this disability has is a uniquely personal experience. Hearing levels adequate for one person, situation, or occupation vary. The effect of hearing loss might be different for a carpenter or a photographer than it would be for a musician (Meyerhoff, Liston, & Anderson, 1984).

There are both peripheral and central components to the sensation of hearing (Fig. 23–3). The *peripheral components* include the outer, middle, and inner ear as well as the auditory peripheral nerve (eighth cranial nerve). The *central auditory system* includes the brain stem cochlear nuclei, superior olive, lateral lemniscus, inferior colliculus, and medial geniculate body. Auditory representation on the cerebral cortex includes a diversity of connections and pathways. The brain stem assumes some responsibility for sound awareness, and the temporal lobe is responsible for the appreciation of sound, pitch, intensity, and discrimination.

A sound stimulus may be created by a moving body in some medium—for example, water or air—or it may be the sound, sensation, or sensory experience

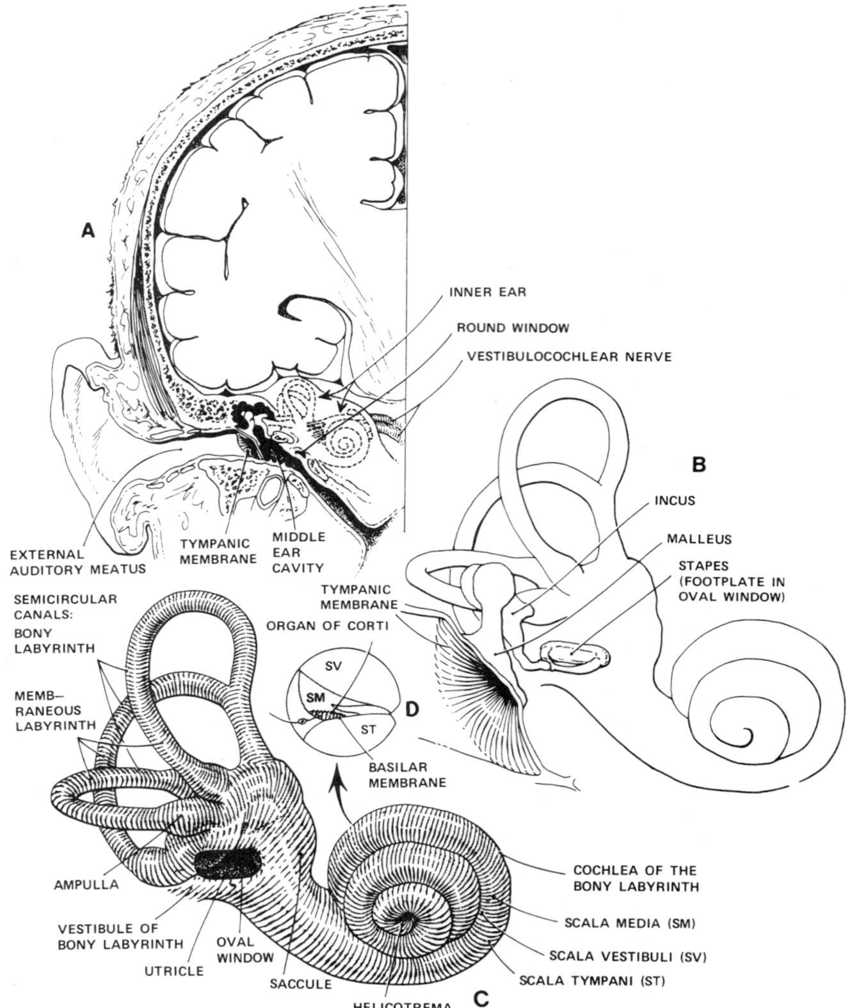

FIGURE 23–3 • The ear. *A,* The location of the three parts of the ear (external, middle, and inner) in relation to the skull and the brain. *B,* The relationship of the ear drum (tympanic membrane) and three bones (ossicles) in the middle ear that connect it to the inner ear. *C,* The bony labyrinth and the membranous labyrinth within it, forming the inner ear. *D,* A cross-section through the bony and membranous labyrinths of the cochlea to show the location of the organ of Corti within the membranous labyrinth. (From Gilman, S., & Winans, S. S. [1990]. *Manter & Gatz's essentials of clinical neuroanatomy and neurophysiology* [7th ed.]. Philadelphia: F.A. Davis.)

known only to the mind of the listener as it relates to our physical and emotional lives. Sound is interpreted by the brain as music, information, or noise. We can discriminate between sounds, such as footsteps versus horse's hooves, and even tell the direction of movement based on noise. Sound begins from a mechanical disturbance, such as that caused by the slamming of a door or the striking of the keys on a piano. The sound vibrations cause the formation of waves that radiate in all directions. The moving waves are heard as sound.

Sound waves are collected by the auricle of the outer ear and pass along the auditory canal to the tympanic membrane. The tympanic membrane vibrates in response to sound waves; these vibrations are then conducted through the malleus and incus to the stapes. The stapes footplate articulates with the oval window, and beneath it lie the utricle and saccule, surrounded by perilymph. Movement of the stapes footplate causes sound waves to be conducted through the oval window to move the endolymph. This movement stimulates the delicate hair cells of the cochlea, and from these cells impulses pass along fibers of the auditory nerve to reach the auditory cortex in the superior temporal gyrus on both sides of the brain (Pracy, Sieglar, & Stell, 1974, p. 35).

The auditory pathway contains a series of neurons that make synapses at each station of the ascending pathway and may be described as follows. Acoustic stimulation excites fibers of the cochlear nerve that terminate in the cochlear nucleus. The fibers leave the cochlear nucleus via three main tracts, one of which connects with the superior olivary complex. Fibers continue to ascend in the contralateral lemniscus to the inferior colliculus, which sits on the roof of the midbrain. The inferior colliculus gives rise to fiber tracts that terminate in the medial geniculate body, which is in the posterior portion of the thalamus. From here, fibers form the thalamic auditory relay, which connects to the auditory cortex (Bradford & Hardy, 1979; Karmody, 1983).

When hearing loss is assessed, hearing specialists attempt to determine the site of damage within the auditory system. Hearing loss is, therefore, generally broken down into three categories that relate to the anatomic areas of involvement. The first is a *conductive hearing loss,* in which there is damage involving the external auditory canal, eardrum, middle ear, or eustachian tube. The second is a *sensorineural hearing loss,* in which there is involvement of the inner ear, the auditory nerve, or both. The third is *central hearing loss,* in which damage to the auditory system lies in the central nervous system between a structure in the medulla oblongata, the auditory nucleus, and the cortex (Sataloff, Sataloff, & Vassallo, 1980).

Some nongenetic causes of sensorineural hearing loss in the neurologic realm include (1) trauma resulting from noise, penetrating injuries, or temporal bone fracture; (2) sudden pressure changes resulting from cerebrospinal fluid or barometric pressure changes, such as flying, diving, coughing, or sneezing; (3) metabolic disturbances resulting from hypothyroidism or adrenopituitary disorders; (4) toxic substances, such as heavy metals, antibiotics (especially the aminoglycosides, which are capable of destroying the hair cells and stria vascularis of the inner ear), and salicylates; (5) space-occupying lesions in the cerebellopontine angle, such as acoustic neuromas and meningiomas; and (6) inflammatory disease, either viral (herpes, cytomegalovirus, or adenovirus

III, which may create labyrinthitis, neuronitis, or vasculitis) or bacterial (meningococcal meningitis, which may involve the inner ear) (Meyerhoff et al., 1984).

Vision

Vision is an extremely complex and still not completely understood sensory modality. We begin by discussing the structure and composition of the eye. The *cornea* forms the anterior one sixth of the eyeball and is responsible for focusing and transmitting light to the interior of the eye. The *sclera* is white, opaque, and tough and is directly continuous with the edge of the cornea. It encircles the eye completely, except where it joins the emerging optic nerve. The donut-shaped structure that gives the eye its color is the iris. It surrounds the pupil, which is essentially a hole in the center of the iris. The two muscles in the iris are responsible for changing pupillary size (Havener et al., 1974). The *ciliary body* is in direct continuity with the iris and is adherent to the sclera. The ciliary muscle directly controls the focusing ability of the eye by controlling the size and shape of the lens. The richly vascular layer, the choroid, supplies nutrition to the outer half of the retina. The retina receives light and is the innermost layer of the eye. Each retina contains more than 125 million nerve cells able to respond to light, and many more millions of nerve cells to coordinate and transmit the impulses from the visual cells to the optic nerve. The two types of visual cells are called *rods* and *cones* and are the light-sensitive part of the retina. The rods are used for vision in dim light; the cones are used for daylight color and vision. The rods and cones are located in the deepest layer of the retina. The retina develops from the central nervous system and, in its component layers of nerve cells and fibers, resembles the architecture of the cerebral cortex (Havener et al., 1974).

The lens is just behind the iris and functions to focus light on the retina. The space behind the lens is the *vitreous body*. It is filled with fluid resembling gelatin and occupies two thirds of the volume of the eye. The *anterior chamber* is the space between the iris and cornea, which is filled with a crystal-clear fluid called *aqueous humor*, formed by the ciliary body. The posterior chamber is located between the iris and the lens and is also filled with aqueous humor.

OPTIC NERVE

The optic nerve emerges from the back of the globe to enter the cranial cavity via the optic canal. Intracranially, the two optic nerves join to form the optic chiasm (Fig. 23–4). Each optic nerve is covered by the meninges. The total length of the optic nerve is approximately 4 to 5 cm (Peele, 1977). Because the general cranial subarachnoid space is continuous with that surrounding the optic nerve, an increase in intracranial pressure is transmitted through the spinal fluid to the optic subarachnoid space, creating swelling of the optic

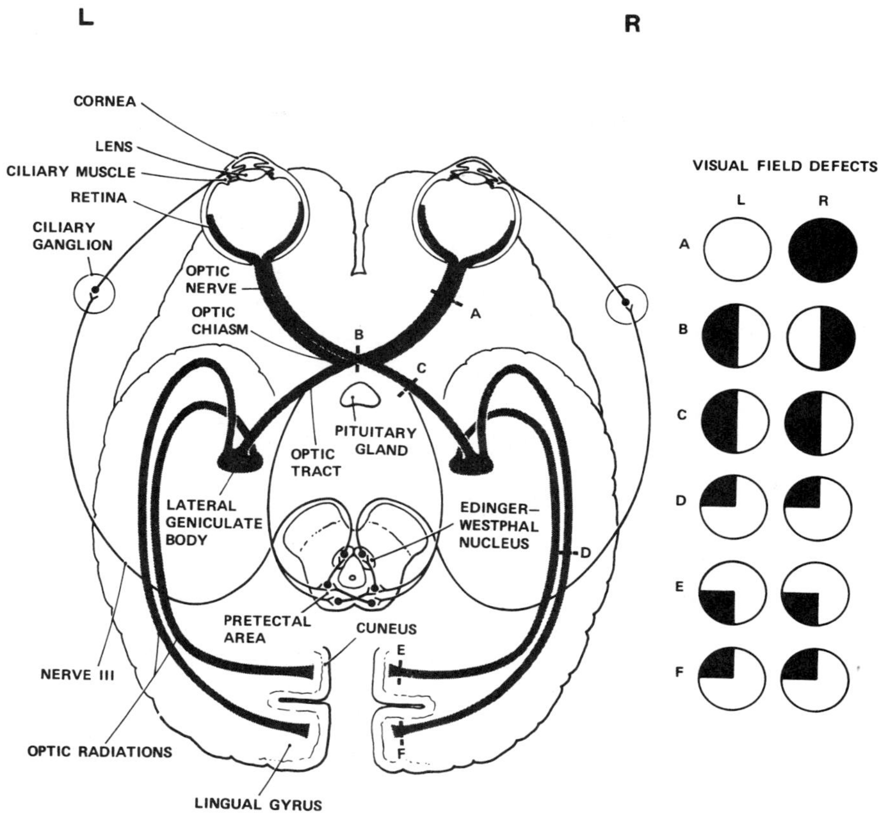

FIGURE 23–4 • The visual pathways. Lesions along the pathway from the eye to the visual cortex (lesions A through F) result in deficits in the visual fields, which are shown as black areas on the corresponding visual field diagrams. The pathway through the pretectum and nerve III, which mediates reflex constriction of the pupil in response to light, is also shown. (From Gilman, S., & Winans, S. S. [1990]. *Manter & Gatz's essentials of clinical neuroanatomy and neurophysiology* [7th ed.]. Philadelphia: F.A. Davis.)

papilla. This is known as *papilledema* and can be visualized on funduscopic examination of the eye.

EXTRAOCULAR MUSCLES

There are six extraocular eye muscles in each eye that are responsible for moving the ocular globe. These 12 must work in harmony all the time; they are amazingly coordinated and automatically aim the two eyes at exactly the same point in space. The innervation for these muscles is from the third, fourth, and sixth cranial nerves. Dysfunction of ocular movement is described in Chapters 19 and 21.

VISUAL PATHWAY

As the fibers leave the optic canal, approximately half of them cross to the opposite side at the optic chiasm (see Fig. 23–4). Once past the optic chiasm, these crossed fibers, which originated from the nasal half of each eye, intermingle with the fibers originating from the temporal half of the retina of the opposite eye. These intermingled fibers form the optic tracts.

Fibers from the optic tracts enter a relay station, the *lateral geniculate body.* From here, the fibers disseminate in a fan shape and traverse parts of the temporal and parietal lobes en route to the occipital cortex, the *striate area.* The area from which the retinas receive light impulses is the *visual field.* Mapping of the visual field provides information about the functioning of the retina and the visual pathways.

DISORDERS OF VISION

The eyes are in close concert with the brain and often supply much diagnostic information that may assist in the localization and diagnosis of central nervous system disorders. When there is abnormal function of the anatomic structures that are in close proximity to the eyes and optic pathways, such as those around the optic chiasm, third ventricle and pituitary gland, or internal carotid artery and optic nerve, there will be dysfunction of ocular movement and visual disturbance.

Optic neuritis is a sudden decrease in vision, often accompanied by central visual field defects. Optic neuritis may be attributed to a wide variety of causes, but sudden central monocular visual loss with pain on ocular movement is usually due to demyelinization of optic nerves. Multiple sclerosis appears to be one of the most common causes. *Pituitary tumors* have such a close proximity to the optic chiasm that the visual finding is commonly bitemporal hemianopsia. *Pupillary abnormalities* occur in Horner's syndrome, in which the affected pupil is small, regular, and associated with a mild ptosis and loss of sweating of the forehead. Horner's syndrome is usually associated with damage to or interruption of the sympathetic nerve supply, usually in the neck. *Argyll-Robertson pupils* are small, irregular pupils, usually occurring bilaterally, with a poor or absent reaction to light but appropriate response to accommodation. This condition is usually associated with neurosyphilis.

Taste

The sense of taste allows one to discriminate and recognize the salt of a potato chip, the bitterness of lemon, the sweet taste of sugar, and the sour taste of acid. The sense of taste, however, must usually depend on the sense of smell to appreciate the complete array of food flavors, such as fruit, meat, and coffee.

The sense of taste arises from the dorsal surface of the tongue, the epiglottis, and at times the mucous membranes of the cheeks, lips, and larynx. For taste discrimination, the tongue is divided into the following:

- Middorsal surface, which is insensitive to taste
- Tip, which senses sweet and salt but responds to all taste
- Borders of the tongue, which are most sensitive to sour tastes
- Base of the tongue, which is most sensitive to bitter tastes

Taste buds that recognize these flavors are present on the surface of the tongue and number approximately 100,000 in the human adult (Peele, 1977).

There are both peripheral and central taste pathways. The *peripheral pathways* are from the seventh, ninth, and tenth cranial nerves. The geniculate ganglion of the seventh cranial nerve, the superior petrosal ganglion of the ninth cranial nerve, and the nodose ganglion of the tenth cranial nerve pass centrally into the medulla, join the tractus solitarius, and synapse in the nucleus solitarius. The central pathways seem to be the secondary solitariothalamic fibers, which travel in company with the medial lemniscus fibers and synapse within the medial portion of the posteromedial ventral thalamic nucleus.

The tongue must be moist enough to allow for solution to stimulate the taste buds. If the tongue is very dry, the sense of taste is thus dramatically reduced. The number of taste buds decreases with age, thus creating a loss of full appreciation of flavor. Bell's palsy may create a loss of taste on one side that is annoying but tolerable. Stimulation of Brodmann's area 50 has elicited taste sensations. Taste may be altered by local disturbance of the mouth, and alterations in taste do not always indicate pathology of the taste pathways.

Smell

The airway of the nostril provides access to the sensitive nerve endings that are all but hidden high in a compartment at the top of the nasal cavity. This compartment, the olfactory cleft, occupies an area about 2.5 cm within each nostril. The nasal septum separates the two clefts. Most inspired air passes directly to the pharynx and lungs, bypassing the cleft. Some odor particles escape the air and find their way to the cleft. The nasal chamber of the nostril has an average volume of 17.1 mL. When one chews food, the movement of the palate and throat create small air movements that project odorous material up to the cleft via the nasopharynx, where it can stimulate the sensitive receptors. The surface of the olfactory cleft, the olfactory mucosa, is composed of millions of tiny endings of the first cranial nerve and an even larger number of supporting cells. The true endings of the olfactory nerve fibers or rods project through the supporting cells to the surface. Tiny cilia arise from the tip of each rod and project into the mucous layer, which bathes the entire surface of the olfactory epithelium (Geldard, 1972).

An altered sense of smell is very common. There are three major causes. Trauma to the head or neck seems to affect the olfactory tract by tearing or shearing of the tiny olfactory nerves, or by avulsion of the olfactory tract secondary to a basilar skull fracture in the anterior fossae. Compression of delicate olfactory tracts after trauma may result from cerebral edema or intracranial blood clots. Tumors, especially meningiomas of the olfactory groove, may alter smell. Frontal or temporal lobe tumors, or any swelling in the vicinity of the olfactory nerve, may impair sense of smell. Seizures, in particular partial sensory seizures, may be characterized by unpleasant olfactory sensations. The seizure focus may be located in an area responsible for normal olfactory perception, such as the olfactory bulb and receptor cells or the limbic system (Douck, 1974). The olfactory sensation may also represent an aura for another type of seizure. Smokers or persons who use the nares for drug abuse also have limited sense of smell.

Alzheimer's disease (AD) has been shown to be associated with impaired olfactory function, which can be detected early in the course of the disease. Deficits include impaired odor recognition, identification, and memory (Doty, Reyes, & Gregor, 1987; Moberg et al., 1987; Rezek, 1987). Interestingly, the hallmark signs of AD, namely, the senile plaques and neurofibrillary tangles, are increased in the central olfactory anatomy (cortical regions, anterior olfactory nuclei, and olfactory tract) in comparison to the peripheral regions of the olfactory apparatus (olfactory bulb, primary sensory neurons). This finding argues against the origin of AD via the olfactory pathway. In other words, the olfactory impairment in AD seems to be a consequence of the disease, not a causative factor or pathway for disease pathogens (Davies, Brooks, & Lewis, 1993).

ASSESSMENT OF THE SOMATIC AND SPECIAL SENSES

Somatic Sensation

When evaluating sensation, it is most important to have the full cooperation of the person being examined; otherwise, the findings will be inaccurate. In order to enhance the assessment, the person should be instructed about what to expect. The face, trunk, arms, and legs are most commonly tested. The examiner systematically tests the right and left sides and evaluates the dermatomes, working upward on the body from the impaired area to the normal area.

LIGHT TOUCH

Light touch may be tested with a wisp of cotton, first familiarizing the person with the stimulus by applying it to a normal body part. The person can be asked to say "yes" every time it is felt. When an area of impairment is discovered, the stimulus should be moved from the point of impairment outward until normal areas are found to map the boundaries of impairment.

PAIN

Pain may be tested with the sharp point of a pin. The person should be asked to indicate the degree of sharpness in addition to the feeling of contact or pressure. As in testing for light touch, the examiner should work upward, beginning with the areas of impaired sensation. The skin may be tested using both sharp and dull ends of the pin to have the person differentiate sharp from dull. Both right and left sides of the body should be tested.

TEMPERATURE

The perception of temperature at times is difficult to assess accurately. It depends on the temperature of the test object, the duration of the stimulus, and the area over which it is applied. The test object should be large; a flask of hot or cold water or a metal tuning fork may be used. The test object should be tested over a normal area, and the person should then be asked if the thermal sensation is less hot or less cold on the impaired area in comparison with the sensation in the normal part.

POSITION SENSE—PASSIVE MOVEMENT

To test for position sense, the examiner asks the person to close his or her eyes while the examiner moves the person's extremity and has the person describe the position of that extremity. The person may also be asked to hold the arms up and attempt to touch the nose with the index finger. Passive movement may be tested by the examiner's holding one of the fingers or toes firmly and moving it rapidly up or down. The person should be asked to report each movement as being up or down.

VIBRATION SENSE

Vibration and position sense are often lost together. Vibration sense is evaluated by placing a tuning fork over the sternum, fingers, elbow, iliac crest, ankles, and toes. The examiner must be careful that the person is responding to the vibration and not to the pressure of the tuning fork. When the person no longer feels the vibration, the fork is moved quickly to the same point on the corresponding limb. Perceived vibration at this point indicates an abnormality (Adams & Victor, 1985).

HIGHER CORTICAL SENSORY FUNCTION

Lesions in the sensory cortex or thalamocortical projections may leave touch, pain, temperature, and vibration sense intact but interfere with higher integrated sensation, such as form, discrimination, and shape. The following tests are higher-level tests of discriminating function.

Two-point discrimination is the ability to distinguish two points from one. The two points must be applied simultaneously and without pain. *Number writing* or *graphesthesia* can be tested by tracing a number or letter larger than 4 cm on the person's skin and asking him or her to identify it. *Stereognosis,* or ability to detect shape, is tested by placing an object in the patient's hand and asking him or her to identify the object without looking at it.

Special Senses

HEARING

Hearing can be evaluated by determining the person's perception of the whispered or spoken word. The ear not being tested should be blocked when performing this test. The patient is positioned 20 ft away, and a few words are whispered. This provides a quick, rough estimate of hearing loss. If a problem is detected, further evaluation is essential.

Weber's test assesses bone conduction. The base of the vibrating tuning fork is placed on the forehead or top of the skull, and the patient is asked if the sound is heard better in one ear or the other. *Rinne's test* involves placing the vibrating tuning fork on the mastoid process until the vibrations are no longer heard, then immediately moving the fork to the external ear canal to determine if sound is still present. Normally, sound should be heard longer by air conduction than by bone conduction.

VISION

Tests for vision include pupillary reaction, visual acuity, visual fields, and extraocular movement. Pupils are examined for size, shape, equality, and reaction to light, as well as for accommodation and consensual light reaction.

Visual acuity is best tested with Snellen's eye chart. The person is placed 20 ft from the chart and asked to read the lines of progressively smaller letters until they can no longer be read. Each eye is tested individually. Test line 8 is what the normal eye should be able to read at 20 ft, and such vision is described as 20/20. This indicates that what the person has read from a distance of 20 ft is what a normal eye should be able to read at 20 ft.

Visual fields are tested by comparing the patient's peripheral vision with that of the examiner by determining when both patient and examiner can see the object. The examiner stands in front of the person and assesses one eye at a time by having the person close one eye while the examiner closes the opposite eye. The examiner asks that the person fix on a point in the midline and brings his or her finger toward the midline in all four planes of vision. The patient indicates when the object comes into vision. Examination of *extraocular movement* is described in Chapter 19.

SMELL

With the eyes closed, the patient should be able to identify such common substances as chocolate, cinnamon, and tobacco. A well-known test for olfactory function is the University of Pennsylvania Smell Identification Test (UPSIT, sold commercially as the Smell Identification Test, or SIT), which consists of 40 self-administered odor patches that release a distinct odor when scratched.

Gross olfactory assessment can be approached in children of various ages who may not be able to identify specific smells. In these instances, very pleasant versus unpleasant odors may be used to elicit, at a minimum, the child's response to noxious stimuli to the olfactory pathway.

TASTE

Taste is tested by placing a few salt crystals or sugar crystals on the tongue. The person being tested must describe the taste. Perception of taste and smell diminishes with age.

SUMMARY

There are many conditions with a wide range of varying degrees of sensory alteration. The impact of these dysfunctions is addressed in Chapters 24 through 26.

References

Adams, R., & Victor, M. (1995). *Principles of neurology* (6th ed.). New York: McGraw-Hill.

Bradford, L., & Hardy, W. (1979). *Hearing and hearing impairment.* Philadelphia: Grune & Stratton.

Davies, D.C., Brooks, J.W., & Lewis, D.A. (1993). Axonal loss from the olfactory tracts in Alzheimer's disease. *Neurobiology of Aging, 14*(4), 353–357.

Doty, R.L., Reyes, P.F., & Gregor, T.P. (1987). Presence of both odor idenfication and detection deficits in Alzheimer's disease. *Brain Research Bulletin, 18*(5), 587–600.

Douck, E. (1974). *The sense of smell and its abnormalities.* New York: Churchill-Livingstone.

Ganong, W. (1987). *Review of medical physiology* (13th ed.). Stamford, CT: Appleton & Lange.

Geldard, F. (1972). *The human senses* (2nd ed.). New York: John Wiley & Sons.

Guyton, A. (1987). *Basic neuroscience: Anatomy and physiology.* Philadelphia: W.B. Saunders.

Havener, W., Saunders, W., Keith, C., & Prescott, A. (1974). *Nursing care in eye, ear, nose, and throat disorders.* St. Louis: C.V. Mosby.

Karmody, C. (1983). *Textbook of otolaryngology.* Malvern, PA: Lea & Febiger.

Meyerhoff, W., Liston, S., & Anderson, R. (1984). *Diagnosis and management of hearing loss.* Philadelphia: W.B. Saunders.

Moberg, P.J., Pearlson, G.D., Speedie, L.J., Lipsey, J.R., Strauss, M.E., & Folstein, S.E. (1987). Olfactory recognition: Differential impairments in early and late Huntington's and Alzheimer's diseases. *Journal of Clinical and Experimental Neuropsychology, 9*(6), 650–664.

Peele, T. (1977). *The neuroanatomic basis for clinical neurology* (3rd ed.). New York: McGraw-Hill.

Pracy, R., Sieglar, J., & Stell, P. (1974). *Ear, nose and throat.* London: English Universities Press.

Purchese, G. (1977). *Neuromedical and neurosurgical nursing.* Suffolk, U.K.: Bailliere Tindall.

Rezek, D.L. (1987). Olfactory deficits as a neurologic sign in dementia of the Alzheimer type. *Archives of Neurology, 44*(10), 1030–1032.

Sataloff, J., Sataloff, R., & Vassallo, L. (1980). *Hearing loss.* Philadelphia: J.B. Lippincott.

Schmidt, R. (1978). *Fundamentals of sensory physiology.* New York: Springer-Verlag.

Bibliography

Carpenter, M. (1985). *Core text of neuroanatomy* (3rd ed.). Baltimore: Williams & Wilkins.

Chusid, J. (1985). *Correlative and functional neuroanatomy* (19th ed.). Stamford, CT: Appleton & Lange.

Creutzfeldt, O., Schmidt, R., & Willis, W. (1984). *Sensory-motor integration in the nervous system.* New York: Springer-Verlag.

Dusenbery, D.B. (1992). *Sensory ecology: How organisms acquire and respond to information.* New York: W.H. Freeman.

Fisher, A.G., Murray, F.A., & Bundy, A.C. (1991). *Sensory integration: Theory and practice.* Philadelphia: F.A. Davis.

Gonzalez-Crussi, F. (1989). *The five senses.* San Diego, CA: Harcourt Brace Jovanovich.

Mitchell, P., Ozuna, J., Cammermeyer, M., & Woods, N. (1984). *Neurological assessment for nursing practice.* Paramus, NJ: Reston.

24   Alterations in the Special Senses

RUTH A. MULNARD

As an open system, each person is in constant interaction with the environment, exchanging matter, energy, and information. "The constant interchange of matter and energy between man and environment is at the basis of man's becoming. It is this interchange that portends the creativity of life" (Rogers, 1970, p. 54). Information from the environment is perceived by five senses—sight, hearing, smell, taste, and touch—which are important mechanisms for data collection vital to an individual's very existence in an ever-changing, complex environment. A person receives, processes, interprets, and responds to information perceived by the senses in a unique way as an individual.

Perception of the information received from the environment forms the basis for a response. Through experience, a degree of stability and predictability is established in this communication pattern. A deficit in one or more of the senses disrupts the individual's sense of predictability and can often bring chaos to the biopsychosocial functioning of that individual.

The impact of an alteration in one of the special senses is profound and dramatic, for it changes the way an individual has previously perceived and responded to the environment. A person's preference for environmental perception can often be inferred by the response to daily environmental input: "I hear you," "I see what you mean," "That feels right to me." The loss of a preferred sense may have greater impact on an individual's ability to interact constructively with the environment than will the loss of another modality. Neurologic disease processes are often responsible for creating alterations in the senses. Neuroscience nurses work daily with people who have sudden or progressive alteration in one or more of the special senses.

Research has shown that sensory impairment influences the perception of quality of life in older individuals residing at home. Single sensory impairments involving hearing or vision loss were associated with increased risk for depression and decreased self-sufficiency in activities of daily living. Visual dysfunction alone was also correlated with fewer social relationships (Carabellese et al., 1993).

The neuroscience nurse cares for, supports, and teaches the individual and the family to adapt and to repattern their communication with each other and their environment. The goals of the neuroscience nurse are to assess the individual's physical, emotional, and behavioral responses to a sensory deficit; to formulate nursing diagnoses; and to plan interventions with the patient and the family directed toward achieving independence and optimal health within the constraints of the illness.

The generalist focuses on the individual, the family, and the health care team while implementing nursing plans and coordinating overall care. The specialist, whose roles include education, clinical practice, consultation, and research, uses expertise in neurologic and neurosurgical clinical practice to serve as a resource to the generalist; intervenes as a change agent; and actively participates in the community to facilitate maximal attainment of skills and capabilities of neurologic patients and their families (Davis, 1985). The ability to cope with and adapt to changes in sight, smell, hearing, taste, and touch can be facilitated by the nurse's interventions with the individual, the family, and the community.

This chapter discusses the changes in the special senses that occur in the normal aging process and the impact of these changes on the nurse's interventions with the elderly person. Conditions and diseases that result in alterations in the special senses are reviewed briefly, and human responses are illustrated using a case-study format.

AGE-RELATED CHANGES IN SENSORY COMPONENTS OF THE NERVOUS SYSTEM

Infants and Children

The subject of pain in the late-term fetus and in the newborn infant has long been debated. Medical opinion has drawn attention to the ethical considerations of performing pain-producing procedures on individuals assumed to be immature and less mentally evolved who, in fact, display complex behavior patterns, such as altered sleep-wake cycles, irritability, abnormal eye movements during sleep, grimacing, and crying, and physiologic manifestations of pain common to all age groups, such as sweaty palms, elevations in blood pressure, increased pulse rate, and release of hormones linked to stress (Anand & Hickey, 1987). The consensus is that infants and children do experience pain and must have their pain treated.

Elderly Persons

Signs and symptoms of neurologic dysfunction are common in the elderly. According to Drachman and Long (1981), neurologic deterioration in the elderly person is the result of a cumulative summation of four factors:

1. Normal neuronal attrition (involution over time)
2. Previous neural damage

3. Decline in neural reserve or plasticity

4. Specific diseases of the nervous system present at the time of evaluation

Both structural and functional changes to the nervous system occur as it ages. Structurally, the brain loses weight and, therefore, volume within the fixed cavity of the cranium, giving it a shrunken appearance. Loss of both gray and white matter occurs (Kemper, 1984). The extracellular compartment volume and cerebral blood flow decrease, thereby providing fewer nutrients to the neurons and decreasing the efficiency of the cell functioning (Meyer & Shaw, 1981). Intracellularly, neurofibrillary tangles or intraneuronal fibrillary material in the cytoplasm develops, which is thought to decrease intracellular transport and thus cause a permanent decline in neuronal functioning (Kemper, 1984). There appears to be a decrease in the efficiency of neurochemical activity in the elderly person as a result of a decline in the production of some of the neurotransmitters and also an increase in the activity of the enzymes responsible for neurotransmitter degradation (Solkoe & Kosik, 1984). These age-related changes, in combination with changes specific to the organs in the body, create an overall decrease in the functioning of the sensory nervous system. Age-related changes occur at different rates in each individual and are often complicated by a variety of situational, disease-related, and therapeutic aspects, such as nutrition, hypertension, hyperlipidemia, diabetes mellitus, and drug usage. It is, therefore, important for the nurse to thoroughly assess the elderly person's sensory functioning and to determine the impact that changes have on the ability to perceive and respond to the environment. Table 24–1 describes changes in the sensory functions, commonly experienced symptoms, and some general nursing considerations when working with the elderly person.

CONDITIONS THAT MAY CAUSE ALTERATIONS IN SENSORY FUNCTIONS

Seeing

Visual anatomy is described in Chapter 23. Neurologic disorders that can impair vision along the visual pathway include degeneration of the receptor cells of the retina; lesions of the macula, retina, or optic nerve; pituitary tumors; temporal or occipital lobe lesions; and disruption of blood supply to the structures along the visual pathway.

Specialized diagnostic techniques that may be helpful in determining the type and location of these disorders include magnetic resonance imaging (MRI) and pattern-shift visual evoked responses (Adams & Victor, 1985). Medical management is specific to the disorder and may include control of intracranial pressure, surgical removal of tumors or other lesions, and revascularization procedures.

TABLE 24–1 • AGE-RELATED CHANGES IN SENSORY FUNCTIONING

Sensory Function	Vision Function	Hearing Function	Combined Vestibular, Visual, and Proprioception Functions
Functional changes	Decreased visual acuity, visual fields, color receptivity, pupil size, reactivity to light; opacification of lens	Stiffening and degeneration of auditory ossicles; altered auditory examination results	Decreased balance, coordination, and equilibrium
Common symptoms	Myopia, hyperopia, tunnel vision, decreased color discrimination, impaired vision in dim light or glare	Decreased ability to detect pitch (high frequencies, initially) and to understand spoken words, nonverbal sounds, and music	Vertigo; disturbances in gait; falls; difficulty walking and turning on uneven surface
Nursing considerations	Orient to environment; consistently locate furniture and personal objects; position objects within field of vision; provide adequate illumination and side lighting; ensure annual eye examination.	Face client when speaking; speak clearly and distinctly without artificial mouth configurations; keep pitch low in louder tones; use short sentences; request one response at a time; consider use of hearing aids; ensure annual auditory examination.	Encourage awareness of balance; turning slowly; rising gradually from sitting or lying; sitting to put on pants, socks, and shoes; using bathtub and stair rails.

Hearing and Balance

The ear is a complicated structure concerned not only with sensation of hearing but also with balance. Dysfunctions that can occur along the complicated neural pathways of the auditory system are varied, such as damage from excessive noise, ototoxic drugs, and a variety of neurologic disorders: acoustic neuroma, auditory cortex infarct, pontine lesion, chronic meningitis, or demyelinating plaque (Adams & Victor, 1985). In addition to the physical assessment findings, specialized hearing testing using audiograms and brain stem auditory evoked responses can be helpful in identifying the location and nature of hearing deficits (Weldon, Murray, & Ouine, 1983).

Prevention is the best intervention for limiting impairment from ototoxic drugs. Routine assessment of hearing for patients taking ototoxic drugs can provide early indication of this side effect, at which time the drug can be discontinued or the dosage adjusted if the side effect is dose related.

Conductive hearing loss may be improved by use of hearing aids or by surgical replacement of one or more of the auditory ossicles. Sensorineural hearing loss is difficult to treat because it is usually permanent, and the source of the dysfunction is the focus of therapy, such as surgical removal of tumors, revascularization, or antibiotic therapy for infections.

The endolymph in the semicircular canals of the vestibular labyrinth moves in response to changes in motion and position of the head. This neurologic information, in conjunction with visual input and impulses from the proprioceptors of the joints and muscles, is integrated to maintain equilibrium, balance, and orientation in space. Dysfunctions of the vestibular system, such as Meniere's disease, trauma, vertebrobasilar ischemia, and vestibular neuronitis can cause symptoms of vertigo, nystagmus, and unsteadiness. The goal of medical therapy is to treat the underlying disorder or the symptoms of the disorder. Examples of therapy include surgery, antihistaminic agents, rest, and mild sedatives (Adams & Victor, 1985).

Smell

The receptor cells of the olfactory sense are bipolar neurons found in the mucous membranes of the upper and posterior parts of the nasal cavity. Olfaction can be diminished (hyposmia) or lost (anosmia) by such common causes as allergies or rhinitis, in which swelling or congestion of the nasal mucosa occurs (Adams & Victor, 1985). The sense of smell is dependent on moistened, volatile air particles reaching the receptor cells and can therefore be impaired by inability to breathe in deeply through the nose or by inadequate moisture of the nasal mucosa (Brown, 1985). Damage resulting from head injury to the receptor cells as the cells converge and pass through the cribriform plate of the ethmoid bone can be severe, particularly with fractures of the ethmoid bone (Adams & Victor, 1985).

The central processes of the olfactory receptors of the first cranial nerve and their connections in the brain are complex; therefore, the influences of smell on the biopsychosocial behaviors of an individual are broad. Brown (1985) offered an overview of the anatomic structures and the interrelationships between the olfactory neuronal connections and the other structures and functions of the brain. Other etiologies that may affect the olfactory sense along its neural connections include tumors, multiple sclerosis, Parkinson's disease, and trauma (Adams & Victor, 1985). Olfactory hallucinations or an unpleasant smell (cacosmia) can occur as an aura in uncinate seizures. Again, medical therapy is aimed at treating the underlying causative factors, if possible.

Taste

The sensory receptors for taste are distributed over the surface of the tongue, with a smaller number over the palate, pharynx, and larynx. The taste receptors perceive only salty, sweet, bitter, and sour sensations. More complex tastes are the combined sensations of taste and smell (Adams & Victor, 1985).

Decreased sense of taste (hypogeusia) or loss of taste (ageusia) may be caused by extreme dryness of the oral mucosa or by lesions of the medulla oblongata or may follow influenza-like illnesses. Unilateral lesions of the thalamic region or the parietal lobe have been characterized by contralateral impairment of taste. Taste distortions can occur with some medications, such as antithyroid drugs, chlorambucil, colestyramine, and some anticancer drugs

(Adams & Victor, 1985). Treatment of the underlying cause is the basis of medical management.

Touch

Deficits in touch perception can occur as a result of damage to the many structures in the sensory nervous system. Review of the entire sensory nervous system is beyond the scope of this chapter, but deficits can result from pathologies occurring as distal as the sensory nerve receptor or the dorsal nerve root and ganglion. Altered touch can occur as a result of spinal cord disorders in which the anterolateral spinothalamic tract or the posterior columns are damaged, or with insult to the thalamus. Increased intracranial pressure or lesions affecting the parietal lobe can cause deficits characteristic of damage to the postcentral gyrus. In addition to a thorough history and physical assessment, computed tomography, MRI, and short-latency somatosensory evoked potentials can assist the physician in differential diagnosis of disturbances of touch in the sensory nervous system (Adams & Victor, 1985). Table 24–2 provides an overview of the anatomic structures involved in alterations in touch sensation, examples of causative neurologic disorders, and options for medical management.

TABLE 24–2 • UNCOMPENSATED DEFICITS IN TOUCH

Categories of Disorders	Examples of Disorders	Medical Management Options
Anatomic structure: peripheral nervous system		
Peripheral Neuropathies		
Chronic	Carcinoma and myeloma, amyloidosis	Removing or controlling tumor growth
Acute	Idiopathic polyneuritis, Landry's syndrome, Guillain-Barré syndrome	Corticosteroid therapy, physiotherapy to prevent pressure palsies
Subacute (symmetrical)	Nutritional deficiency states, uremia, drug intoxications	Nutritional supplementation, dialysis in renal failure, discontinuing or decreasing dosage of drugs
Subacute (asymmetrical)	Diabetes mellitus, polyarteritis nodosa	Control of blood sugar level, corticosteroid therapy
Other	Genetically determined disorder, trauma, entrapment neuropathies	Immobilization, physical therapy, surgery
Anatomic structure: central nervous system		
Cord (complete. posterior column. partial. thalamus. parietal lobe. postcentral gyrus.)		
Specific	Brown-Séquard syndrome of the partial cord	See below
Overall	Complications of surgery, trauma, lesions from tumors, infarcts, hemorrhages, or myelitis (as in demyelinative myelitis)	Therapy to treat underlying cause of symptomatology: surgery, immobilization, corticosteroids

HUMAN RESPONSES TO ALTERATIONS IN SPECIAL SENSES

The neuroscience nurse, in collaboration with the individual and the family, develops a realistic, individualized plan for assisting the patient in regaining and maintaining functions of daily living as safely and as independently as possible. In the following clinical case, a nursing care plan is developed for individuals with uncompensated sensory deficits and their families.

• C A S E   S T U D Y

Stroke

Mr. F, a 68-year-old man, was hospitalized with an admitting diagnosis of septal and posterior wall myocardial infarction. His recuperation was complicated by severe episodes of congestive heart failure, for which he was treated with diuretics. Three days after admission, Mr. F developed atrial fibrillation that was unresponsive to drug therapy. Because the dysrhythmia had a significant impact on his hemodynamic status, it was imperative that he undergo cardioversion, to which he agreed. Twenty-four hours after successful cardioversion, Mr. F suffered a cerebral embolus.

His patient profile and social history described Mr. F as a right-handed, 5 ft 11 in, 260-lb Caucasian male from South Carolina. He was married and had four children, all living away from home. His wife, a 58-year-old woman, was healthy and a homemaker with no work experience outside the home. Mr. F was a machine mechanic employed by a local garage. He and his family were Baptist and attended church regularly. Mr. F had no hobbies and often spent his leisure time at the local pool hall with his friends from town. Mr. F had been looking forward to retiring in a few months and had a modest savings account.

His past medical history revealed the usual childhood diseases: measles and chickenpox, with no history of rheumatic fever. He had a history of several broken bones, which were job-related and without complications. Mr. F stated that he had been put on a "water pill" and a "heart pill" about 12 years ago after several months of headaches, when he was diagnosed with hypertension. Mr. F stated that he sometimes forgot to take his medication and did not seek out medical attention often, "unless it's something I can't fix myself." He stated that he had had several episodes of "indigestion" over the last 3 or 4 months. The present episode "didn't go away, and it was more crushing than the other ones," which was why he agreed to let his wife bring him to the hospital. Mr. F stated that he had noticed a bilateral decrease in his hearing over the last few years, commenting, "My wife keeps saying I'm just ignoring her." Mr. F's medications before admission were furosemide (Lasix), methyldopa (Aldomet), and potassium chloride.

The day Mr. F sustained a cerebral embolus, he experienced a sudden onset of agitation, restlessness, and severe sensorimotor deficit of the right side. Athough he did not lose consciousness, Mr. F had decreased orientation to time and place and decreased awareness. He was initially aphasic and did not follow movements when they occurred in his right field of vision. Mr. F was incontinent of stool and urine at this time.

Three weeks after the cerebral embolus, Mr. F showed stable cardiac condition and improvement in motor function of his right leg but minimal improvement in his right arm and face movement. He continued to exhibit impairment of sensory function on his right leg, arm, and face to light touch, vibration, position, discrimination, and tactile localization. He understood written and spoken words and showed some improvement in speech. His inability to communicate with the health care staff, complicated by his sensorineural hearing loss, was extremely frustrating to Mr. F, and he often turned his head away when staff entered the room. Mr. F's physical therapy program continued to provide improvement in motor function, particularly in walking and gross motor movement in the right leg and arm. Mrs. F's visits had decreased in length and frequency, and often when she visited she spoke to Mr. F infrequently and tears welled up in her eyes. She mentioned to the staff that she realized that Mr. F wanted to come home soon, but "I just don't know how I can handle it all."

Nursing Diagnoses

PARTIAL SELF-CARE DEFICIT: FEEDING, DRESSING, AND BATHING, RELATED TO SENSORY DEFICITS

Decreased vision makes it difficult for an individual to locate self-care items as well as to perform self-care functions. Defining characteristics of decreased visual acuity include myopia, hyperopia, blurring, glare, visual loss, and clouding of the lens. Visual field defects, such as homonymous hemianopsia, bitemporal hemianopsia, quadrantanopsia, scotoma, and central field defects, make it difficult for the individual to locate items in the environment. Additional uncompensated sensory deficits that hinder self-care abilities include impaired depth perception, impaired temperature discrimination, impaired ability to determine objects by touch, and impaired ability to determine position of body parts.

The success of the individual in accomplishing self-care activities can be enhanced by both the nurse and the family encouraging the individual's independence in self-care activities as much as possible while providing adequate time for each activity. Praise and positive reinforcement of the individual's efforts and accomplishments encourage motivation and enhance the individual's self-esteem. As part of nursing interventions, the nurse and the family should consistently place items of self-care, such as water, soap, towels, or clothing, in designated locations while verbally identifying the location of objects to the individual. They can assist the individual in finding objects by creating cues, such as a brightly colored sign over bathing utensils. When meals are served, the family should identify the location of food and liquids on the meal tray or table by clock placement, such as, "The coffee is at 2 o'clock, and the fork is at 3 o'clock."

Depending on the functional limitations of the sensory deficit, the individual may need assistance with cutting food and pouring hot liquids. The individual can be instructed to fill cups and glasses only halfway to prevent spilling. If the meal tray has disposable containers, the nurse can open the lids only halfway to prevent spilling.

Emphasis on using intact senses for identifying objects can facilitate self-care efforts. The nurse can teach the individual to hold a knife and fork in the European style while the patient is learning to identify foods by how they feel through the knife and fork. Foods can be differentiated by an intact sense of smell. Using condiments, such as salt, pepper, catsup, mustard, lemon juice, and mayonnaise can also enhance food identification by smell or appearance. Amounts of salt, pepper, or sugar can be estimated by pouring them over the fingertips that have intact sensation.

The nurse can teach patients with peripheral or central visual field defects to scan the environment visually to locate self-care items and food on a tray or table. Self-care articles and food should be placed on the unaffected side of the patient's vision.

Individuals with disturbances in touch should be encouraged to use the unaffected side to determine the temperature of food, liquids, and bath water. These patients should also be encouraged to use the unaffected side to identify the location and texture of objects, such as towels or clothes. Individuals with loss of touch need to examine their skin daily for bruises, cuts, burns, and pressure areas; they should be taught to monitor the position of body parts while bathing, sitting, lying, or altering their position.

As the nurse works with the individual and the family, she can teach the family the extent of the individual's physical limitations, the compensatory techniques that facilitate self-care, and the activities that require assistance. Collaboration with other members of the health care team in teaching and reinforcing the use of compensatory techniques in the hospital and in the home is essential to promoting the individual's self-care independence.

The expected outcomes are that the individual will use compensatory techniques for maximizing functional abilities in performing self-care and will attain an acceptable level of self-care within the functional limitations, requiring minimal or moderate assistance. The family will assist the individual in those self-care efforts he or she is unable to perform.

With Mr. F's improved cardiac status and motor ability, the nurses were successful in encouraging him to perform more and more of his self-care. It was apparent to the nursing staff, though, that as Mr. F assumed more independence, he also increased his risk of accidents and falls.

POTENTIAL FOR INJURY RELATED TO IMPAIRED VISION AND HEARING

Impaired vision and impaired hearing can make it difficult for the individual to receive input from the environment, putting him at risk for falls, accidents from moving objects, or things as simple as not hearing a smoke detector alarm in a house fire. Impaired tactile sense also creates risk of injury from falls, burns, cold, and pressure areas. Additional defining characteristics that indicate potential for injury include impaired motor ability, history of falls or injuries, and lack of knowledge of necessary safety precautions.

To prevent injury, the individual with sensory deficits must reestablish familiarity with the environment. Some general environmental principles include orienting the individual to the environment, such as the location of furniture, lights, and light switches; keeping objects in consistent locations; and informing the individual of changes if objects are moved. People with sensory deficits should always be approached on the side of intact senses to reduce the startle effect. It is important for the nurse to instruct the family about the impact of the individual's physical deficits, the environmental hazards, and the safety precautions, including eliminating throw rugs, toys on the floor, and furniture that is situated away from room walls. While the patient is in the hospital, his or her bed should always be kept in the lowest position.

Specific nursing interventions for safety of individuals with impaired vision include the following procedures. To optimize visual capabilities, the nurse should encourage the use of adequate lighting, including night-lights. Incandescent light offers less glare than fluorescent light. Providing side lighting, or lighting in front of objects rather than behind them, can also help to reduce glare. Encouraging the individual to avoid looking directly at bright lights, such as headlights, while driving, and to wear sunglasses while outside on bright days can help diminish the blinding effects of glare. The use of color contrast can greatly enhance the visual discrimination of objects for individuals with impaired vision. The family can help alter the home environment to improve safety, using some of the following suggestions: place color strips on the edges of steps; avoid white on walls, countertops, and any working surface; paint door frames and doorknobs in bright colors; and use contrasting colors for light switches and electric outlet plates. If the individual has visual field defects, it is important to teach him or her to scan the environment to compensate for and identify safety hazards, such as door frames, furniture, and stairs inside the home or moving vehicles outside the home.

Specific safety interventions for individuals with impaired tactile sense include the following. To prevent burns, a common injury resulting from this impairment, the individual or the family can set the thermostat on the hot-water heater to provide warm but not extremely hot or scalding water. The individual can be taught to assess the temperature of the bath water with the unaffected extremity or with a bath thermometer. The individual should use thermal insulated mitts when handling pots and pans from the stove or oven and should avoid the use of hot-water bottles and heating pads. Skin injury can occur without the person realizing the injury; therefore, people with tactile deficits should inspect the skin daily for burns, scratches, bruises, cuts, or pressure areas. A common site of undetected injury is the feet; individuals should wear well-fitting, low-heeled, soft shoes. Monitoring the position of body parts during activities can help minimize the risk of injury from uncompensated tactile deficits.

As safety interventions for individuals with impaired hearing, the individual and family should be encouraged to have visual signals installed on smoke detectors, phones, and doorbells. Outside the home, scanning the environment can be helpful for those with this sensory deficit.

The expected outcomes for this diagnosis are that the individual will not sustain injury from falls, burns, wounds, or pressure sources and that the individual and the family will use safety precautions in the home environment.

Difficulty with communicating became frustrating for both the nurses and Mr. F. Implementation of the nursing care plan was hindered by the nurses' attempts to communicate through the normal visual and verbal signals. It became evident that alternative mechanisms for communication had to be developed to facilitate Mr. F's interactions with his environment.

ALTERATION IN VERBAL COMMUNICATION RELATED TO HEARING COMPOUNDED BY APHASIA

In an increasingly complex age of information, the mechanisms by which people exchange information with their environment have also become more varied and complex. In addition to face-to-face verbal exchange, radio, television, telephones, newspapers, magazines, letters, and computers are routine means of communication. Impaired hearing is the most common cause of communication difficulties. When it is accompanied by impaired vision, an individual's inability to receive information is compounded by the difficulty experienced in reading and observing lip movement during verbal exchanges.

Neurologic disorders can cause impairments that further inhibit an individual's ability to interact in the environment, such as motor or expressive aphasia, sensory or receptive aphasia, total or global aphasia, auditory language agnosia, visual language agnosia, and agraphia.

Establishment of a calm, unhurried environment is a key factor in establishing effective communication with an individual with uncompensated sensory deficit. Active and careful listening is essential to understanding the communication efforts of the individual while expressing positive regard for him or her. Approaching the individual with sensory deficits on the side of intact senses is an important principle in facilitating communication. In the hospital setting, this includes situating the patient's bed in the room with the side of intact senses facing the door. The nurse must initially determine with the patient an effective alternative form of communication. Some alternative interventions include using hand signals, pointing to letters on an alphabet board, or using a magic slate. The effectiveness of these methods of communication depends on the form of uncompensated sensory deficit as well as on the dexterity of the patient.

To facilitate communication, it is important to stand facing the individual when speaking. Speaking clearly in low-pitched tones can help the individual with hearing impairment understand spoken words. If it is appropriate, address verbal communication to the individual's normal or better ear.

To maximize the individual's sensory abilities, annual professional vision and hearing examinations should be performed. Visual aids, such as glasses, magnifying glasses, and hearing aids may be useful in improving vision and hearing.

With the individual and the family, the nurse can determine the need for various resources, such as speech therapists, large-print materials, and "talking books," available through the Library of Congress, closed-captioned television services, and the Commission for the Blind and Visually Handicapped.

The expected outcomes are that the individual will be able to communicate effectively within physical limitations and that the individual and the family will use compensatory techniques to enhance communication.

CONSEQUENCES OF SENSORY ALTERATION

Consequences for the Individual

Uncompensated sensory deficits severely alter the individual's established pattern of interaction with people and objects in the environment. Inability to receive stimuli from the environment can elicit fear, anger, anxiety, and frustration. Until an effective alternative method of receiving information is established, the individual may be unable to carry out activities of daily living, as well as normal role responsibilities.

Frustration and fear underlie the individual's desire to limit interaction with people. If alternative forms of communication are not established, social isolation can result. Nursing interventions can assist the individual in emphasizing intact senses for receiving environmental input. Collaboration with the individual and the family is essential in evaluating the effectiveness of compensatory techniques.

Consequences for the Family

Often it is the family who must assume the responsibilities of an individual with uncompensated sensory deficit. Breadwinner, parent, and homemaker are difficult roles for family members to assume. If the individual is unable to carry out activities of daily living, he or she may assume a childlike role, requiring assistance in eating, dressing, and bathing. The profound changes in family structure and functioning may stimulate feelings of anger, resentment, and frustration. It is extremely important that the family participate in the planning and implementation of the nursing actions so they may learn the necessary techniques for compensation of sensory deficits and subsequently encourage the individual to use them.

Consequences for the Community

Alterations in the senses of vision, hearing, or touch may mean that the individual is no longer capable of performing work responsibilities. New jobs may have to be learned whose responsibilities require use of intact senses. The financial impact and loss of work contributions resulting from uncompensated sensory loss can be significant unless effective rehabilitation is achieved.

UNCOMPENSATED SENSORY DEFICITS: IMPAIRED SMELL AND IMPAIRED TASTE

Deficits in smell and taste are discussed together because they are clinically interdependent and have similar impact on the individual's response to the environment. Two characteristics unique to the sense organs of smell and taste are that their receptor sites are chemoreceptors and that the receptor cells are constantly dying and being replaced; these are "the only examples of neuronal regeneration in humans" (Adams & Victor, 1985, p. 197).

Compared with the vast amounts of research and literature available about deficits in the other special senses, there is a scarcity of information about the impact of impaired smell and taste on an individual's interaction with the environment. The recognized impact that impairment of these two senses has on the individual is the lack of interest in or enjoyment of food. Just as the elderly person who has decreased functioning of these sensory receptors complains, individuals with impaired taste or smell often note that everything "tastes the same." This may leave the individual with a poor appetite and subsequent weight loss.

Nursing Diagnosis

ALTERATION IN NUTRITION: LESS THAN BODY REQUIREMENTS RELATED TO ALTERED TASTE AND SMELL

An interview with the individual with impaired smell and taste may reveal the defining characteristics of lack of interest in or enjoyment of food, often with a subsequent decrease in food intake. There may also be a verbalized decrease in appetite. The individual with impairment in these two senses usually does not seek medical care for this condition as a primary problem, but the medical history would likely indicate weight loss without other medical cause.

As an initial intervention, the nurse can discuss the specific foods that the individual avoids, likes, or dislikes. This will provide a basis for determining a diet plan that will be agreeable to the individual and, therefore, have greater chance of success.

Small, frequent, visually appealing meals may be more enticing to the individual and should be provided in a quiet, nondistracting environment. Adequate time must be made available for eating. Liquid supplements, provided in acceptable flavors, can supply the needed calories between meals. Thorough oral hygiene before and after meals may be helpful in improving the flavor of the food.

The individual and the family should be informed about the basic food groups and the recommended daily allowances to meet the individual's needs. Teaching the meal preparer of the family and the individual some simple, yet effective, methods of enhancing the enjoyment of food can improve the appetite of the individual with altered taste and smell. Some examples of these methods include varying the textures in food selections; using spices and seasonings, such as mint, cloves, thyme, or lemon juice, to enhance the aroma of foods; and adding supplements to routine food preparation to increase the nutritional quality of the meal—for example, adding powdered milk or eggs to sauces, gravies, puddings, or casseroles or adding raisins and nuts to cereals.

The individual can monitor the success of these efforts by maintaining a dietary log with calorie count to demonstrate adequate intake and by monitoring weight gain or loss once a week. Expected outcomes for this diagnosis are that the individual will increase the quantity and quality of nutritional intake necessary to meet metabolic needs and that the family will support the individual in meeting dietary requirements.

SUMMARY

The neurologic deficits that can impair an individual's ability to perceive input from the environment through the special senses are complex and varied. An impairment in the senses can have a major impact on the individual's ability to function and communicate with people and objects in the environment. The neuroscience nurse can assist the individual and the family within the community setting in maximizing independent, safe, and satisfying functioning within the constraints of the illness.

References

Adams, R., & Victor, M. (1985). *Principles of neurology* (3rd ed.). New York: McGraw-Hill.

Anand, K. J. S., & Hickey, P. R. (1987). Pain and its effects in the human neonate and fetus. *New England Journal of Medicine, 317*(21), 1321–1329.

Brown, I. A. (1985). The widespread influence of olfaction. *Journal of Neurosurgical Nursing, 17*(5), 273–279.

Carabellese, C., Appollonio, I., Rozzini, R., Bianchetti, A., Firsoni, G. B., Frattola, L., & Trabucchi, M. (1993). Sensory impairment and quality of life in a community elderly population. *Journal of the American Geriatrics Society, 41*, 401–407.

Davis, A. K. (1985). Focus on rehabilitation in the acute care setting: The role of the neuroclinical nurse specialist. *Journal of Neurosurgical Nursing, 17*(4), 244–246.

Dekosky, S. T., & Palmer, A. M. (1994). Neurochemistry of aging. In M. L. Albert (Ed.), *Clinical neurology of aging* (pp. 79–101). New York: Oxford University Press.

Drachman, D. A., & Long, R. R. (1994). Neurological evaluation of the elderly patient. In M. L. Albert (Ed.), *Clinical neurology of aging* (pp. 159–180). New York: Oxford University Press.

Kemper, T. (1994). Neuroanatomical and neuropathological changes during aging and dementia. In M. L. Albert (Ed.), *Clinical neurology of aging* (pp. 3–67). New York: Oxford University Press.

Meyer, J. S., Kawamura, J., & Terayama, Y. (1994). Cerebral blood flow and metabolism with normal and abnormal aging. In M. L. Albert (Ed.), *Clinical neurology of aging* (pp. 214–234). New York: Oxford University Press.

Rogers, M. E. (1970). *An introduction to the theoretical basis of nursing.* Philadelphia: F.A. Davis.

Weldon, P. R., Murray, T. J., & Ouine, D. B. (1983). Hearing changes in multiple sclerosis. *Journal of Neurosurgical Nursing, 15*(2), 98–103.

Bibliography

Carpenito, L. (1983). *Nursing diagnosis: Application to clinical practice.* Philadelphia: J.B. Lippincott.

Creutzfeldt, O., Schmidt, R., & Willis, W. (1984). *Sensory-motor integration in the nervous system.* New York: Springer-Verlag.

Dusenbery, D. B. (1992). *Sensory ecology: How organisms acquire and respond to information.* New York: W.H. Freeman.

Fisher, A. G., Murray, E. A., & Bundy, A. C. (1991). *Sensory integration: Theory and practice.* Philadelphia: F.A. Davis.

Freimer, M. L., & Cornblath, D. R. (1994). Peripheral neuropathy in the elderly. In M. L. Albert (Ed.), *Clinical neurology of aging* (pp. 521–536). New York: Oxford University Press.

Gonzalez-Crussi, F. (1989). *The five senses.* New York: Harcourt Brace Jovanovich.

Kopac, C. (1983). Sensory loss in the aged: The role of the nurse and the family. *Nursing Clinics of North America, 18*, 373–387.

Mitchell, P., Ozuna, J., Cammermeyer, M., & Woods, N. (1984). *Neurological assessment for nursing practice.* Paramus, NJ: Reston.

Singh, R. N., & Strausfeld, N. J. (1988). *Neurobiology of sensory systems.* Reading, MA: Plenum Press.

Smith, J. F., & Nachazel, D. P. (1980). *Ophthalmologic nursing.* Boston: Little, Brown.

Souder, E., & Yoder, L. (1992). Olfaction: The neglected sense. *Journal of Neuroscience Nursing, 24*(5), 273–280.

Stein, B. E., & Meredith, M. A. (1993). *The merging of the senses.* Cambridge, MA: MIT Press.

Stewart, C. M. (1982). Age-related changes in the nervous system. *Journal of Neurosurgical Nursing, 14*(2), 69–73.

Wallace, E., Hayes, D., & Jerger, J. (1994). Neurology of aging: The auditory system. In M. L. Albert (Ed.), *Clinical neurology of aging* (pp. 448–464). New York: Oxford University Press.

Weinberger, M., & Radelet, M. L. (1983). Differential adaptive capacity to hearing impairment. *Journal of Rehabilitation, 49*(4), 64–69.

Pain: Acute and Chronic

NORMA D. MCNAIR

Pain is one of the symptoms most often managed by health professionals. Common factors influence an individual's responses to pain, but the responses to and the treatment of acute and chronic pain differ. The purpose of this chapter is to delineate these differences and guide the practitioner in effective nursing management of both acute and chronic pain.

NEUROPHYSIOLOGY OF PAIN

Pain is regarded as a primary sensation, with nociceptor stimuli from the periphery transmitted to the central nervous system. This neurophysiologic approach to pain adequately explains acute pain with known pathology but excludes much of chronic pain, where the organic basis and the sensory receptor stimulus are unknown or absent. In the instance of chronic pain, the phenomenon is better described as the subjective interpretation of perceived nociceptive input. Several authors have argued that pain is a perceptual rather than a sensory experience (Chapman, 1978; Fordyce, 1978). Perception, in this context, is defined as "the awareness of a noxious sensation, appreciation of negative emotion, and attribution of meaning to the experience" (Chapman & Bonica, 1983, p. 7). This definition eliminates the need for sensory input in the pain experience.

Nociception is defined as a neural event and reflex response produced by a noxious stimulus. Pain is defined as an unpleasant sensory and emotional experience associated with actual or potential tissue injury. The nociceptor is a responder to noxious stimulation. Sensation is transmitted to the spinal cord, and autonomic and nociceptive reflexes are activated and perceived in the brain. The autonomic reflex is a protective reflex that causes an increase in heart rate, blood pressure, and respiratory rate (Cleland & Gebhart, 1997).

There are four stages of nociception. These stages are transduction, central processing and abstraction, modulation, and development and plasticity. In transduction, neural activity travels along a primary afferent neuron or specialized receptor that transduces somatic and visceral stimuli. The axon enters the spinal cord, cranial nerve nuclei, or cell body located in the ganglion of the nerve. Transduction may occur with unimodal or polymodal receptors. Central processing and abstraction allow for the processing of nociceptive neural signals to extract relevant information. Modulation is the adaptation of nociceptive activity to changes in the environment and the needs of the individual. Development and plasticity indicate that permanent changes in the neural mechanisms that mediate nociception have occurred in response to development, experience, and injury (Cleland & Gebhart, 1997).

The anatomy that relates to pain perception and transmission involves the dorsal root ganglion, the spinal cord, and the brain. Cell bodies of nociceptors are found in the dorsal root ganglia. Of the two axons in the ganglia, one axon goes to the periphery to transmit sensory information, and the other terminates in the cord and synapses to the brain. The spinal cord gray matter consists of three regions related to pain. The posterior horn processes sensory information. The intermediate region integrates sensorimotor information, and the anterior horn provides motor commands for spinal reflexes. The spinal cord is divided into 10 laminae. Laminae I through VI are in the posterior horn, VII and X are in the intermediate region, and VIII and IX are in the anterior horn (see Fig. 23–2). The synapses for nociceptive stimuli are in laminae I, II, V, and VI (Cleland & Gebhart, 1997).

The periaqueductal and periventricular gray matter is the nodal point of the endogenous pain modulation system. Exogenous opioids and endogenous released opioid peptides activate inhibitory influences that descend the cord. These synapses occur between the midbrain and the spinal cord in the medulla. The neurotransmitters that mediate descending inhibition are serotonin and norepinephrine. Drugs that mimic the action of serotonin and norepinephrine are analgesic when given into the spinal epidural or intrathecal space. Stress, fear, and pain can activate the descending systems that inhibit pain. Anxiety and apprehension can lead to enhancement of pain. Descending facilitation of pain may play a role in unusual chronic pain states (Cleland & Gebhart, 1997). Although the term pain generally describes a somatic or body experience, the work of Melzack et al. (Melzack, 1975; Melzack & Casey, 1968; Melzack & Torgerson, 1971; Melzack & Wall, 1965, 1970, 1982) indicates that pain includes sensory, affective, and cognitive dimensions. The most useful clinical definition is a verbal report from the person experiencing the pain (McCaffery, 1979; Zborowski, 1969).

PAIN THEORIES

Current thinking about the psychophysiologic basis of pain was introduced in the gate control theory proposed by Melzack and Wall in 1965. The theory was updated in 1968 and 1982 (Melzack & Wall, 1982). This theory proposes that both peripheral and central nervous systems influence pain. The primary processing area, or gate, is composed of cells in the substantia gelatinosa (SG), located in the posterior horn of the spinal cord. From the periphery, the balance of large-diameter and small-diameter fibers regulate ascending nociceptive input through the gate. Descending input to the SG originates centrally, from the cerebral cortex, midbrain, and lower brain stem. Reticular projections to the dorsal horn have an inhibitory effect on cells in the SG. The presence of opiate receptors and the high concentration of enkephalins and other neurotransmitters in areas of the thalamus, midbrain, and posterior horn provide possible mechanisms for descending control of pain.

Three types of endogenous opioid are now known: enkephalins, dynorphins, and beta endorphins. Enkephalins are widely distributed through the central nervous system. They are primarily found in the dorsal horn, periaqueductal gray matter (PAG), raphe magnus, and globus pallidus. Dynorphins are found in the hypothalamus, PAG, mesencephalic reticular formation, and spinal and medullary posterior horn. Beta endorphins are found throughout the nervous system. In addition to these endogenous opioids, there are opiate receptors that have been isolated in the PAG, the nucleus raphe magnus, and the medial thalamus. Opiate agonists and antagonists compete for the same receptor sites, and the antagonists displace the opiate agonist from the receptor site (Bonica, 1990a; Greer & Hoyt, 1990). The gate opens, and nociception is facilitated by the activity in small-diameter afferent fibers. The gate is closed by activity in large diameter myelinated nonnociceptive afferent fibers (Cleland & Gebhart, 1997).

The multiple ascending and descending projections are shown in Figure 25–1. Nociceptive input ascends the cord via the neospinothalamic (rapid transmission) and paleospinothalamic (slow transmission) tracts. The neospinothalamic tract carries sensory and discriminative information to the thalamus and cerebral cortex. This tract also processes sensory information regarding location, intensity, and duration of pain (Bonica, 1990a). Multiple synapses of the paleospinothalamic tract in the reticular formation and limbic system relate to the affective and motivational dimensions of pain. The motivational dimension assists the individual into action in order to deal with the painful stimulus (Bonica, 1990a). Communication via neurotransmitters from the periaqueductal gray area to the SG is linked to descending modulation (Pert, 1982). Cortical projections may also exert descending control indirectly via the reticular projections and directly via the pyramidal tract. Despite lack of current knowledge about mechanisms, it is apparent from clinical observation that both affective and cognitive factors greatly influence pain and responses to it.

Persistent pain in the absence of peripheral stimulation is explained by the gate control theory. Degeneration of nerves produces abnormal, high-frequency firing and bursting activity analogous to the neural activity found in epilepsy (Crue, Kenton, & Carregal, 1979). This neural activity occurs without nociception and, in some cases, without peripheral stimulation at all. Continued pain may be caused by (1) overwhelming input from bursting activity into the SG, (2) a lack of or reduced effect of the descending inhibitory system, and (3) memory patterns developed by prolonged, intense nociception (Melzack & Wall, 1982).

Loeser's (1986) model of pain defines nociception as the transmission of a painful impulse from where it begins to perception in the brain. The interaction

Pain Pathways

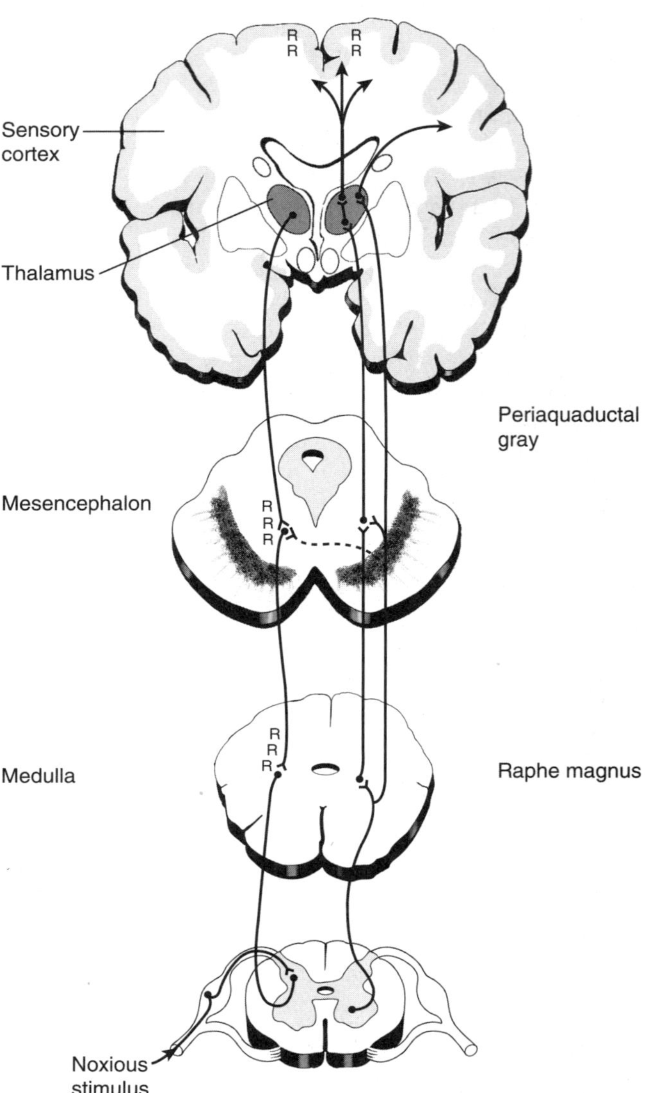

FIGURE 25–1 • Ascending and descending pain pathways. R, opiate receptor site.

of impulses in the midbrain, pons, and medulla and the impact on ascending and descending tracts in the spinal cord result in a modulated pain experience. The depletion of serotonin decreases the analgesic effects of opiates. The release of epinephrine during the sympathetic response sensitizes the nociceptive nerve endings and exacerbates pain transmission.

Other models of pain include the sensory-discriminative and motivational-affective models. The sensory-discriminative model describes pain as a physical sensation. A noxious stimulus activates nociceptors and initiates a series of neural events that are transmitted to the brain. These events include the location, intensity, and duration of the stimulus (Cleland & Gebhart, 1997). The motivational-affective theory states that the nature and intensity of emotional responses is what makes the pain personal and unique. There are older, relatively indirect neural pathways, and cognitive contributions can significantly modulate the response and reaction to a painful stimulus (Cleland & Gebhart, 1997).

DIFFERENTIATION BETWEEN ACUTE AND CHRONIC PAIN

Recognizing the differences between acute pain and chronic pain is important in providing effective pain management. Acute pain "consists of a complex constellation of unpleasant sensory, perceptual and emotional experiences and certain associated autonomic, psychologic, emotional and behavioral responses" (Bonica, 1990c, p. 180). The International Association for the Study of Pain (IASP) defines pain as an unpleasant sensory and emotional experience associated with actual or potential tissue damage or described in terms of such damage (Merskey, 1986). The National Institutes of Health Consensus Development Conference (1987) defined three categories of pain based on cause: pain following acute injury, disease, or some type of surgery (acute pain); pain associated with cancer or other progressive disorders (chronic malignant pain); and pain in persons whose tissue injury is nonprogressive or healed (chronic, nonmalignant pain). The most consistent differentiator of acute or chronic pain is time. According to Bonica (1990b), chronic pain persists for a month beyond the usual course of acute disease or the reasonable time for an injury to heal. Some clinicians use 6 months to designate the pain as chronic. This definition of chronic pain could make the difference between potential for healing an injury and causing it to become irreversible. The IASP defines chronic pain as that which persists beyond the normal time of healing. In practice, this may be less than 1 month or more than 6 months. Three months is the most convenient division between acute and chronic pain (Bonica, 1990b).

Both acute and chronic pain may begin with organic pathology, in which pain is a symptom that warns of impending or actual tissue damage. Acute pain is self-limiting; as healing occurs, the pain resolves. Once pain has persisted past the healing phase, it no longer functions as a warning signal. The individual begins to question whether there will be an end to the pain. As the individual moves from the acute to the chronic state, pain becomes a syndrome rather than a symptom.

Common pain syndromes include tension, migraine, and cluster headache; trigeminal neuralgia; temporal-mandibular joint syndrome; and low back pain. Neuropathic pain can occur from dorsal root avulsion, postherpetic neuralgia, diabetic neuropathy, and phantom limb pain. Musculoskeletal syndromes include fibromyalgia and myofascial pain syndrome. In addition, cancer can cause pain syndromes from bone metastasis, neuritis, plexus or epidural invasion, and bone marrow transplantation (Byas-Smith, 1997).

Types of pain include somatic, visceral, and vascular. The skin is densely innervated, and this allows for pain to be accurately localized. Noxious stimulation causes a protective withdrawal reflex. This is somatic pain. Visceral pain is diffuse and often difficult to localize. The pain is referred from the deep, internal structures of the body to the skin. Examples of visceral pain are angina and the pain of cholecystitis. Veins have nociceptors, and vascular pain is also often diffuse and difficult to localize, as it may be referred to other structures such as the eyes, teeth, or head or neck muscles (Cleland & Gebhart, 1997).

Acute Pain Response

The most common sources of acute pain are trauma, planned surgery, and childbirth. Cancer pain is considered a special subset of chronic pain (Grichnik & Ferrante, 1991). The observable responses to acute pain include physiologic, behavioral, and affective behaviors.

PHYSIOLOGIC RESPONSES

Acute, rapid-onset pain produces sympathetic arousal, the "fight or flight" response that is mediated by the reticular formation. Sympathetic stimulation that is often observed includes tachycardia, hypertension, tachypnea, sweating, and pallor. Patients may also have an increase in cardiac output, decreased gastric motility, and vasoconstriction. This response is to facilitate escape from the cause of injury or to assist with coping with the injury (Grichnik & Ferrante, 1991). Typically, the sympathetic nervous system adapts rapidly, making it difficult to rely on these observations to indicate the presence of pain.

BEHAVIORAL RESPONSES

There is a set of reflexive responses that follows the onset of nociception. The sequence of events includes sudden withdrawal of the injured part, turning of the head to examine the injury, vocalization, and muscle splinting to protect the injured part (Melzack & Wall, 1970). The usual response to acute pain is anxiety. Anxiety becomes modified by an individual's preparation for pain and the etiolgy and anticipated duration of pain (Grichnik & Ferrante, 1991).

Operant learning leads to behavioral manifestations of acute pain such as withdrawal, avoidance of activity that exacerbates the pain, and attempts to escape from noxious sensations. Acute pain behaviors can be controlled by external reinforcement. The patient is not aware of behaviors and is not consciously motivated to obtain positive reinforcement. Treatment focuses on elimination of pain behaviors by withdrawal of attention and increasing well behavior through positive reinforcement. The flaws with operant learning are that there is (1) narrow focus on motor pain behaviors, (2) failure to consider emotional and cognitive aspects of pain, and (3) failure to treat the subjective experience of pain. There is an emphasis on overt behaviors and the use of them as the basis for understanding pain, distress, and suffering (Beutler et al., 1986; Blumer & Heilbronn, 1982; Edwards, Zeichner, Kuczmierczyk, & Boczkowski, 1985).

With respondent learning, chronic or recurrent acute pain is initiated and maintained by classical or respondent conditioning. If a painful stimulus is paired with a neutral stimulus, there is a pain response. Patients may have learned to associate increases in pain with all types of stimuli. In addition, social learning and cognitive factors play a role in pain response. Acquisition of pain behavior can occur from observation and modeling of others. Behavior and emotions can be influenced by interpretation of events (Beutler et al., 1986; Blumer & Heilbronn, 1982; Edwards et al., 1985).

The description of the pain-prone personality (Beutler et al., 1986; Blumer & Heilbronn, 1982; Edwards et al., 1985) and caregivers' experiences with patients in pain may make it difficult to be objective in the management of pain. The pain-prone personality is described as that of a person who may deny emotion and interpersonal problems; be unable to deal with anger and hostility while craving affection and dependency; have a family history of depression, alcohol abuse, and chronic pain; and have difficulty expressing anger and intense emotions. These may be predisposing factors that link chronic pain to depression (Beutler et al., 1986; Blumer & Heilbronn, 1982; Edwards et al., 1985). It is also thought that some individuals with pain have a motivational view of their pain. They are thought to be motivated by financial gain. In this situation, pain is often unsubstantiated by observed physical pathology. There may be an expression of symptom exaggeration or malingering. No studies have demonstrated a dramatic improvement in pain reports after receiving disability awards, however (Beutler et al., 1986; Blumer & Heilbronn, 1982; Edwards et al., 1985).

AFFECTIVE RESPONSES

Anxiety, like pain, is subjective experience that produces nonspecific sympathetic arousal. Sources of anxiety with acute pain are identified easily: Why does it hurt? Will I have more pain than I can bear? Will this pain affect my future (immediate or long term)? Acute pain is associated with a transient situational state of anxiety that motivates the individual to cope with acute pain. Keefe, Brown, Scott, & Ziesat (1982) described three important coping behaviors: reducing activity until healing begins, using medications to relieve pain, and seeking medical assistance. At this time, the person relies on medical professionals to diagnose and cure the source of pain. An active cognitive coping style is prevalent (Keefe et al., 1982), using such techniques as distraction and future-oriented planning. Unrelieved pain can lead to distress, suffering, and sleep deprivation. There is extensive evidence that a variety of social factors influence the experience of pain as well as pain-related cognition and behavior. These include mood, personality, attention, perceptual processes, expectations, social factors, perceived control of pain stimulus, and anxiety. The most frequently noted psychologic consequence of pain is anxiety (Justins & Richardson, 1991).

Other psychologic aspects of pain include the fact that persistent pain can lead to uncertainty in the diagnosis. One conceptualization of pain is the unidimensional sensory model (Turk, 1997). This model states that the amount of pain that is experienced is a direct result of the amount, degree, or nature of sensory input or physical damage. Pain is explained in terms of specific physiologic mechanisms, and the report of pain will be directly proportional to the amount of pathology. Assessment should focus on identifying the cause of the pain, and treatment should focus on removal of the cause or blocking of the pain pathway (Turk, 1997). Factors that are not taken into consideration with this model are that patients with equivalent degrees or types of pathology vary widely in the report of pain severity. In addition, surgical procedures to cut pain pathways may not alleviate pain. Finally, patients respond differently to therapeutic intervention even if it is exactly the same (Turk, 1997). These responses—physiologic, behavioral, and affective—reflect observations of acute pain but bear little resemblance to the responses of the individual who is experiencing chronic pain.

Chronic Pain Response

There are many disease states labeled as chronic pain. Arthritis and migraine headaches, which are characterized by periods of pain with intervals of no pain, are considered recurrent chronic pain. Syndromes with more constant pain, such as postherpetic neuralgia and low back pain, are termed chronic nonmalignant pain, which is defined as pain of unknown origin that is not life threatening. Chronic pain is caused by pathologic process in the somatic structures or viscera or by prolonged and sometimes permanent dysfunction of the central or peripheral nervous systems. It can also be caused by psychologic mechanisms or environmental factors. Therapy for chronic pain is often more difficult than for acute pain (Bonica, 1990c). The intensity of the pain complaint cannot be explained by the pathology. In the intractable syndrome, the pain is refractory to medical treatment. In contrast to the variable nature of acute pain, clients with chronic pain report a constant and high-intensity pain (Keefe et al., 1982).

The behaviors developed during the acute pain stage continue to be used to manage chronic pain. Unfortunately, they are no longer appropriate in coping with persistent pain. Activity has been limited over a period of time (usually longer than 3 months), leading to deconditioning of the skeletal muscles, heart, and lungs. The person has not worked or has done so in a limited capacity since the onset of pain. Reliance on pain medications may lead to narcotic and nonnarcotic dependence. The client may continue to look for the medical cure, which can lead to doctor shopping and other behaviors such as obtaining multiple prescriptions for medication (Sternbach, 1982).

PHYSIOLOGIC RESPONSES

Patients with chronic pain syndromes who experience continuous or near-continuous pain do not experience the same response to pain as do those in acute pain. Habituation of the sympathetic response may occur, and patients usually remain physiologically stable for a long period of time. Muscle hyperactivity may be a direct or indirect source of persistent pain, whereas muscle hypoactivity may be a result of decreased activity. In both cases, muscle tone is abnormal and requires intervention. Eventually, patients may experience sleep disturbances, lack of appetite, constipation, increased irritability, decreased interest in sexual activity, and lowered pain tolerance (Bonica, 1990c).

BEHAVIORAL RESPONSES

From a learning framework, the duration of chronic pain allows changes in behavior patterns to occur in both the client and the family. These patterns evolve as the environment provides rewards for behavior or avoidance of negative consequences. Fordyce (1978) has labeled these behaviors, which are determined by environmental consequences, operants. The operant nature of behavioral responses has been termed pain behavior, defined by Block (1982, p. 51) as "overt indices of putatively painful condition—all of which are influenced by a number of nonpathologic variables." Some pain behavior seeks to communicate pain; facial expressions, posture, vocalization, and guarding alert others to the suffering experienced. Fordyce (1978) included inappropriate coping behaviors as well. The benefits of having pain behavior include spouse and family attention, spouse and family control, avoidance of social (home and work) responsibilities, and financial gain. Sleep disturbances are the most common complaint. Clients have difficulty falling asleep because of discomfort. Patients state that they feel exhausted and drained of energy because of lack of sleep and because the continuous pain wears them down (Bonica, 1990c).

AFFECTIVE RESPONSES

Many studies have investigated the psychologic profile of clients with chronic pain (Capka, Griffin, Harris, & Pinsky, 1979; Gentry, Shows, & Thomas, 1974). Agreement has been found on a pattern of affective responses, based on the Minnesota Multiphasic Personality Inventory (MMPI), consisting of increased scores on measures of hypochondriasis, depression, and hysteria. It has been suggested that people who develop chronic pain have difficulty expressing emotions. Somatic preoccupation (hypochondriasis) and hysterical denial allow the person to repress unpleasant affect (depression) (Sternbach, 1982), leading to anxiety (Capka et al., 1979). Although people with chronic pain often have multiple personal and interpersonal problems, they commonly insist that with alleviation of their pain all their problems will be solved (Pilowsky, 1978). Clients may develop "abnormal illness behavior" that consists of increased preoccupation with their pain. Their anxiety about their health is severe and may be accompanied by a persistent conviction that they have serious pathology (Bonica, 1990c).

Depression is the affective state most closely related to chronic pain. This reactive or neurotic depression is related to conflict or loss (Pinsky, 1979). It is easy to understand how feelings of sadness, hopelessness, and helplessness arise after long-term persistent pain. Losses as a result of pain may be great—loss of function, support systems, and job. Many depressive symptoms are indicative of chronic pain. These include decreased mobility, productive activity, and appetite; loss of libido; change in sleep pattern; and withdrawal from social activity (Fordyce, 1978; Keefe et al., 1982; Melzack & Wall, 1982; Sternbach, 1982). The chronic pain client's approach to interpersonal relations has been described as hostile and manipulative (Violon & Giurgea, 1994). Additional vegetative signs are also found frequently in chronic pain; these manifestations often overlap with the adverse effects of narcotics. As with anxiety and acute pain, the behavioral responses to chronic pain are closely related to those of depression. Chronic anxiety, which is almost as prevalent in chronic pain as in depression, may also produce some of these vegetative symptoms (Sternbach, 1982).

Chronic pain has the potential to disrupt all aspects of life: physical, psychologic, and social. This disruption affects not only the individual suffering from chronic pain but the individual's family as well.

SOCIOLOGIC EFFECTS

Clients with chronic pain often develop problems within the family and with friends. There may be a decrease in social interaction. Some clients are unable to work, others may be on Worker's Compensation, and others lose their jobs because of absenteeism. Those that are on disability usually receive less income than they received previously, which may add an additional strain on the family. Other role changes within the family can change relationships and decrease self-esteem (Bonica, 1990c).

Influencing Factors

In all pain states, there are many factors that influence perception of and response to pain. Factors that influence pain involve the cognitive-evaluative and affective-motivational aspects of pain, which explain the highly variable and individual responses to pain. The sensory-discriminative aspect of pain is relatively stable across individuals with normal sensory capabilities (Melzack & Wall, 1982). Individual factors that influence the severity of pain include meaning attached to pain, familial model, culture, personality, and socioeconomic characteristics. Attention has long been one of the manipulable factors of pain perception. Attention focused on pain increases the perception of pain. Applying the gate control theory, attention activates descending control mechanisms that either open or close the gate in the SG.

The response to pain attributed to "heartburn" differs from that of "heart attack," although the location and quality may be similar. This exemplifies the effect that meaning of pain has on response to pain. The meaning of pain may be influenced by familial models and by culture. The influence of familial models on pain experience arises from social learning theory. Behavior patterns may be learned by observation. The rewards and punishments for pain behavior are observed easily in the family setting. In some studies, the influence of family modeling significantly affected complaints of pain in a general population (Cleland & Gebhart, 1997) and was significantly related to chronic pain (Yarton, 1979). Craig (1978) suggested that modeling begins in the family context and may be the underlying mechanism for observed cultural differences.

The classic study of cultural differences by Zborowski (1969) suggested that culture influences the expression of pain rather than any physiologic or sensory factors. He found that people from Mediterranean areas (Italians and Jews) were more expressive of pain, whereas Anglo-Saxons (Irish and Old Americans) were more stoic. Some of the findings from this study are accepted as generalizations but may not be observed in our culturally mixed American society. The sources of cultural differences in response to pain are not clear, but a learned rather than an innate source is suggested (Craig, 1978; Stimmel, 1985; Zborowski, 1969).

It is important to recognize that health care providers also carry cultural biases, again based on learning of past familial models. The American medical system operates on an Anglo-Saxon model of illness behavior (Zborowski, 1969). Adhering to this model means that clients control their expression of pain and submit to necessary painful procedures without complaint. In the past, health care professionals rewarded clients who responded in the appropriate manner by giving more credence to their pain complaints (Zborowski, 1969) and, it is presumed, by providing faster and more adequate pain relief (McCaffery, 1979). Now, institutions and physicians recognize that procedures and activities in the hospital cause pain. In most institutions, protocols have been developed to provide conscious sedation or an additional dose of pain medication to patients for painful procedures such as insertion of chest tubes.

Research and clinical observation have identified several personality characteristics that influence pain responses. Neuroticism, of which the largest component is anxiety, is related to higher levels of reported pain (i.e., lower pain tolerance) in both acute and chronic pain states. Introversion-extroversion, in contrast, is related to willingness to express pain (Sternbach, 1982). This characteristic may also be related to culture (Zborowski, 1969) and social learning.

Socioeconomic factors influence pain responses. Sternbach, Wolf, Murphy, and Akeson (1973) described the chronic pain patient as a member of the working class, engaging in physical labor, with a high school education. Physical labor increases the possibility of being injured at work, a common location of initial injury. The medical compensation system, particulary in the United States, gives greater support for physical than for psychologic disabilities and treatment (Carron, DeGood, & Tait, 1985).

Involvement in litigation may be a strong influence on pain, because receiving money for disability can be a potent secondary gain. Timmermans and Sternbach (1974) found the MMPI scores for hypochondriasis, depression, and hysteria to be greater in clients involved in litigation than in those who were not. Carron et al. (1985), in a comparison of low back pain in the United States and New Zealand, found that although clients entered with similar pain intensity and frequency, subjects in the United States had more emotional and behavioral disruptions. These authors proposed that the emotional distress was related to the cumbersome compensation system in the United States.

It has long been thought that newborns or premature infants do not feel pain and consequently have not been medicated for pain for various procedures that are performed. For younger children, fear of the risks of narcotics has meant that they have received little or no pain relief. Many institutions have now developed interdisciplinary pain management teams with a focus on the pediatric population. Interventions include using other family members for assistance and psychologic intervention and changing the way pain medications are administered. The physiologic response to pain of children is similar to that of adults and includes increased heart rate and blood pressure, impaired sleep, altered eating pattern, and decreased immune function (Agency for Health Care Policy and Research, 1992).

Elderly patients have multiple medical needs and frequently experience pain. More than 80% of elderly persons suffer from arthritis, which may be accompanied by acute pain. Elderly clients are more likely to have emergency surgery or to have pain related to cancer. Pain may be reported differently by the elderly. Assessment is often difficult because of cognitive impairment, delirium, or dementia. The use of visual analog scales, descriptor scales, or numerical scales has not been fully studied in this population. Because the elderly often have visual, auditory, or motor impairment, such scales may not be useful. Finally, the elderly are at risk for under- or overmedication. There are negative consequences to unrelieved or unmanaged pain in the elderly. Some physiologic consequences include increased stress, increased metabolic rate, increased blood clotting, water retention, delayed healing, decreased gastrointestinal motility, decreased mobility and ambulation, interference with sleep and appetite, impaired immune function, and unnecessary suffering. Key principles in pain management in the elderly include believing the report of pain. Assessment should be ongoing and comprehensive and should include the use of a pain scale for those who can use it. The goal is to prevent pain rather than treat it, and interventions should be individualized (Dellasega & Keiser, 1997). Few studies are available that look at optimum medication dosing in the elderly, and further work is needed (Agency for Health Care Policy and Research, 1992).

HUMAN RESPONSES IN ACUTE PAIN

Acute Pain

The defining characteristics of acute pain are primarily behavioral responses. Behavioral signs, such as verbalization, restlessness or agitation, guarding, avoidance of activity, and physiologic evidence of increased muscle tension indicate the presence of pain. Of these manifestations, verbal report of pain may be the only sign present. Nevertheless, in clients who conform to the stoic model of expression, pain may be denied despite other clinical signs.

Assessment of pain is organized according to the sensory-discriminative, affective, and cognitive dimensions. Responses and influencing factors are initially assessed; ongoing assessment of relevant factors is derived from the initial contact with the patient.

The client's self-report of pain is important in obtaining information to evaluate nursing care and in communicating to the client that his or her pain is believed. Several tools are available to assess clinical pain. The PPQRST (Provocation, Palliation, Quality, Radiation, Severity, Temporal), a simple, non–research-oriented interview guide, is summarized in Table 25–1. The PPQRST provides comprehensive data on the sensory and cognitive dimensions but lacks complete affective information. It is, therefore, necessary to assess affect through observation of behavior and client self-report.

The McGill Pain Questionnaire (MPQ) and Pain Rating Scale (PRS) are two instruments developed for research purposes that may be helpful in clinical assessment. The MPQ is conceptually congruent with the gate control theory and includes rank ordered verbal descriptors of the three dimensions of pain (Melzack, 1975; Melzack & Casey, 1968; Melzack & Torgerson, 1971). In addition, location, influencing factors, and palliative measures are assessed with this instrument. The PRS, developed by Johnson (1972), is useful because it measures the sensory and affective dimensions of pain. It is composed of two 10-cm lines and uses numerical descriptors (0 to 10), verbal descriptors (none,

TABLE 25–1 • PPQRST ASSESSMENT OF PAIN

Provocation	Is there an identifiable incident related to the initial onset of pain?	Cognitive
	What provokes the pain (including activity, affect, environmental stress)?	Affective
Palliation	What reduces or relieves the pain (activity changes, analgesics, assistive devices, medical assistance)?	Cognitive
	Is there exposure to alternative methods (relaxation, imagery, hypnosis)?	Sensory
Quality	What words are used to describe the pain?	Sensory
Radiation	Where is the location of pain? Is the pain localized or generalized? Does it radiate, and if so, where?	Sensory
Severity	What is the intensity of pain (on a scale of 0 [no pain] to 10 [worst cognitive pain imaginable] using the descriptors none, mild, moderate, severe)?	Cognitive Evaluative
Temporal	Is there a pattern to the pain? Is the pain constant or intermittent?	Sensory

PPQRST, Provocation, Palliation, Quality, Radiation, Severity, Temporal.

mild, moderate, severe), or both. One line assesses intensity of pain sensation (sensory dimension), and the other assesses distress (affective dimension) caused by these sensations. Whereas the MPQ is a multifaceted, comprehensive instrument, the PRS is simple to use and therefore more appropriate for serial measures. The PRS may be more useful in a critical care setting where the patient can point to a descriptor. The PRS is easy to use even for an intubated patient. In addition, patients who are non–English-speaking are still able to use the PRS or a Visual Analogue Scale (VAS) to communicate the extent of their pain.

Acute pain typically has an organic basis. Peripheral free nerve endings respond to thermal and mechanical stimuli, and these compose the initial stimulus for acute pain. Etiology may be organized by the anatomic structures affected by the pathologic changes. Medical management, which is directed at the source as well as the palliation of pain, is summarized according to anatomic structure in Table 25–2.

Nursing intervention involves application of the nursing process to both the individual and the family. Interventions specific to pain and its effects are organized as peripheral and central, following the gate control theory. Peripheral techniques alter receptor input entering the SG, whereas central techniques

TABLE 25–2 • MANAGEMENT OF PAIN SYNDROMES

Type of Pain	Origin	Medical Management
Myofascial	Muscle and fascia	Activity: mobilization Procedure: local nerve block Pharmacology: muscle relaxants, nonsteroidal anti-inflammatory drugs (NSAIDs) Surgery: none Other: stress management, counterirritation
Rheumatic	Bone, joint, ligament	Activity: mobilization Procedure: deep heat Pharmacology: NSAIDs, corticosteroids Surgery: joint replacement
Neuralgia	Peripheral	Activity: mobilization for peripheral, immobilization for dorsal root (e.g., intervertebral disk, dorsal root) Procedure: local nerve block Surgery: nerve release from entrapment (e.g., diskectomy) Pharmacology: analgesics
Trigeminal neuralgia	Central neuron	Activity: mobilization Procedure: none Pharmacology: antiepileptic (phenytoin, carbamazepine) Surgery: fifth cranial nerve root decompression
Causalgia	Sympathetic nervous system	Activity: mobilization Procedure: ganglion block Pharmacology: alpha blockers Surgery: sympathectomy
Vascular	Vascular	Pharmacology: vasodilators Surgery: specific to site (e.g., bypass surgeries)

alter the affective and cognitive dimensions, thus exerting descending control from the supraspinal structures.

Radwin (1987) identified several research-based nursing interventions for acute pain that can be performed autonomously. Interventions include relaxation techniques and patient teaching. Other studies (Diers, Schmidt, McBride, & Davis, 1972; McBride, 1967) determined that relaxation decreased the sensation of pain in patients with acute pain. Patient teaching can assist the patient through painful procedures. Radwin (1987) suggested that a holistic approach to the patient and allowing the patient to choose among methods of pain relief is helpful in relieving the patient's pain. The Agency for Health Care Policy and Research (1992) has also determined that a transcutaneous electrical nerve stimulation (TENS) unit may assist in nonpharmacologic pain relief.

• C A S E   S T U D Y   1

Grace is a 51-year-old woman with pain of 2 months' duration. The pathologic source of pain is an invasive pelvic tumor. Grace is admitted for pain control. On admission, she displays a tense facial expression, a slightly flexed posture (guarding), and slow, rigid movements. She reports pain in the low back and pelvis only when asked. She denies any familial pain models and, in fact, finds it difficult to remember either of her parents expressing pain. To Grace, the pain indicates that the tumor is growing and, hence, is anxiety producing.

In assessing the primary complaint, Grace notes that the pain worsens with vigorous activity (e.g., a half-day shopping trip) and when she is tired. Emotions seem to play a part; when she is feeling low, the pain is at its worst. Rest and the analgesics ordered by her physician (650 mg acetaminophen and 60 mg codeine) reduce her pain from 6 to 7 on a scale of 0 to 10 to 4 to 5 on a scale of 0 to 10. She used imagery during chemotherapy but is not using it to control pain. The pain is usually located in her low back, pelvis, and perineum and occasionally radiates to the lower extremities. She rates her present pain at 6 and her distress at 8 on a scale of 0 to 10.

A general systems review reveals an adequately nourished woman with lower abdominal and pelvic tenderness. Trunk mobility is decreased; range of motion in extremities is within normal limits. The client reports a recent decrease in appetite and constipation, which she attributes to the pain and the analgesics ordered.

Nursing Diagnoses in Acute Pain

ALTERATION IN COMFORT—ACUTE PAIN

Client involvement in the planning and use of selected interventions increases the likelihood that the techniques will be effective (Moss & Meyer, 1966; Regan, 1984). If the client has used methods of pain relief, they become the basis for instruction in additional techniques. The rationale for newly introduced techniques should be explained in understandable terms and in a way that is congruent with the client's pain model (Meichenbaum & Turk, 1976).

Pain relief is related to the expectation for success of treatment that the client has. As an intervention for the nurse generalist, approaching the client with a positive suggestions, such as, "I think this will relieve your pain," may increase the likelihood that the treatment will work. Giving false reassurances, such as, "After this analgesic you shouldn't feel any pain," may be counterproductive because the client may stop trusting the nurse if pain is still felt.

Massage is a common nursing intervention for immobility. The effects include muscle relaxation and, potentially, sedation, both of which provide comfort. Massage may close the gate to nociception because of large-diameter fiber stimulation. It may also reduce a source of nociception by promoting muscle relaxation.

Assessing the client's knowledge and use of imagery provides a basis for instruction as intervention for the nurse specialist. Imagery is the use of cognitive activity to produce a therapeutic goal (McCaffery, 1979), in this case, pain reduction. As Grace had used, for example, diversional, pleasant imagery to cope with the adverse effects of chemotherapy, it would have been appropriate to begin with this technique. Relaxation typically precedes imagery. Images to promote muscle relaxation may reduce muscle tension as well as anxiety. Imagery may also be used to transform sensations (sensory transformation) and context and produce disassociation (Wolff, 1985). Postimagery suggestion, which is similar to posthypnotic suggestion (McCaffery, 1979) may prolong the analgesic effects of the imagery. Imagery is considered a benign therapy but should be used with caution in patients with depression and not used in those patients with psychotic disorders.

Outcomes

Desired outcomes are that the client will (1) participate in the planning and evaluation of therapeutic modalities used, (2) report increased comfort and decreased pain, (3) report an increased sense of well-being, and (4) use imagery as a self-initiated pain relief measure (Regan, 1984).

Because of the severity of Grace's pain and the etiology, 8 mg morphine intramuscularly every 4 hours as required is ordered. The use of narcotic analgesia requires selecting the drug and route of administration and determining suitable initial dose, frequency of administration, optimal doses of nonopioid analgesics, adverse effects, and the setting in which the drug is to be administered. Titration to maintain a desired effect should also occur (Agency for Health Care Policy and Research, 1992). Parenteral morphine is indicated for pain of moderate to severe intensity, which Grace experiences (i.e., pain of 5 to 8 on a scale of 0 to 10). From observation, it is apparent that Grace continues to experience pain with activity. A review of analgesic administration reveals that she is receiving 8 mg morphine at variable intervals ranging from 4 to 8 hours (Fig. 25–2).

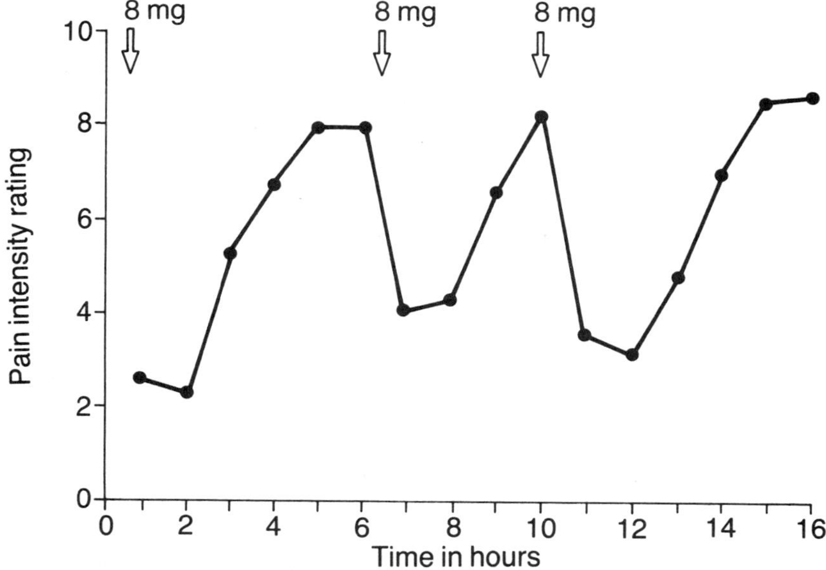

FIGURE 25–2 • Report of pain intensity with variable administration of morphine 8 mg.

It is apparent that Grace is not requesting analgesics to prevent severe pain or that the nursing staff is not offering it on a regular basis. Because of this, the dosage is not sufficient to relieve severe pain. After talking with Grace, the nurse finds that fear of addiction and of losing control are preventing her from requesting medications to prevent pain.

INEFFECTIVE COPING WITH ACUTE PAIN RELATED TO LACK OF KNOWLEDGE

Fear of addiction is a common reason for undertreatment of pain with narcotics. McCaffery (1979) stated that tolerance (decreased effectiveness of a drug after repeated administration) and physical dependence (development of withdrawal symptoms when a repeatedly administered narcotic is abruptly stopped) are involuntary physiologic effects of narcotic administration. In contrast, addiction and drug abuse are voluntary behavior patterns that result in psychologic and social disruption for the individual.

The incidence of addiction is less than 1% in clients with acute pain requiring narcotics. According to Porter and Jick (1980), physical dependence is unusual in the patient with short-term narcotic use (Ready, Murphy, Loeser, & Fordyce, 1980). In addition, it is unlikely that patients will develop psychologic dependence or addiction if they have no history of drug abuse. In clients such as Grace, comfort is the first priority. Because of the limited nature of pain, addiction should not be an issue. If pain has not been adequately relieved, clients may behave like an addict—that is, crave narcotics; in fact, what they crave is pain relief (McCaffery, 1979). Once the pain has been relieved, the addictive behavior disappears.

The goal of treatment for acute pain is pain prevention. If pain is prevented or kept at a manageable level, anxiety is reduced, which, in turn, reduces the amount of analgesic required. The common practice of pro re nata (prn, as needed) administration of analgesics has been criticized because the variable intervals between administration produce wide swings in pain intensity that require variable doses of analgesic. Morphine, the most frequently ordered narcotic, is typically prescribed for 4-hour intervals, although its mean duration of effectiveness is 3 hours and the client may require higher doses for pain relief (Agency for Health Care Policy and Research, 1992).

Respiratory depression is the most dangerous adverse effect of narcotics. To prevent respiratory depression, assessment of respiratory rate, depth, and character is necessary before administration and at the onset of the first two doses of a narcotic (McCaffery, 1979). Opioids should be withheld if the patient is sedated or whenever there is respiratory depression (less than 10 breaths per minute) (Agency for Health Care Policy and Research, 1992). Additional adverse effects and potential nursing diagnoses are summarized in Table 25–3.

After discussing with Grace the issue of addiction and the need to "keep on top" of the pain, a mutually agreed-upon plan of interventions by the nurse generalist is determined. Morphine is administered on a regular schedule, every 4 hours, and effectiveness and adverse effects are evaluated over the next several days. Figure 25–2 displays the peaks and valleys of pain intensity that occur with this type of medication schedule.

Evaluation of regular administration reveals that the interval of doses is too long (i.e., pain returns to its initial level before the next dose is due). The interval of morphine is reduced to every 3 hours, which flattens out the pain intensity curve (Fig. 25–3) and is more appropriate for the action of the drug. Because of the moderate pain intensity, the dosage of morphine may be reduced.

TABLE 25–3 • ADVERSE EFFECT OF NARCOTICS

Adverse Effect	Mechanism of Action	Nursing Diagnoses
Respiratory depression	Reduced responsiveness of respiratory center to CO_2 levels	Potential for inadequate ventilation
Nausea and vomiting	Stimulation of chemoreceptor trigger zone depresses medullary vomiting center	Potential for fluid and electrolyte imbalance
Orthostatic hypotension	Local effect of peripheral vasodilation	Potential for unsafe ambulation (falling)
Increased intracranial pressure	Cerebral vasodilation	Potential for altered level of consciousness
Constipation	Increased smooth muscle tone and decreased motility	Potential for constipation

CO_2, carbon dioxide.

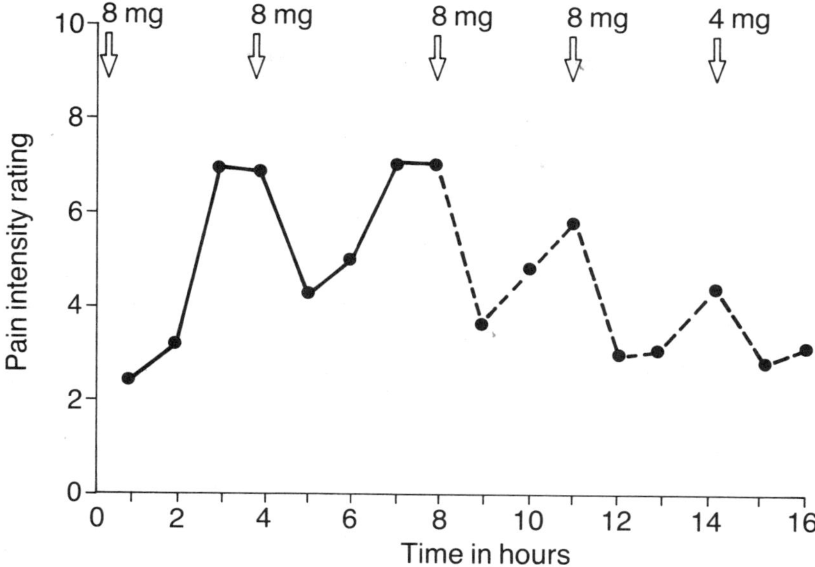

FIGURE 25–3 • Report of pain intensity with regular administration of morphine 4 to 8 mg.

The use of meperidine for pain management has decreased over the last few years because of some of its side effects. Meperidine metabolizes to normeperidine, which is excreted through the kidneys. Normeperidine is a cerebral irritant that can cause dysphoria, irritable mood, or seizures. This can occur in any patient if high doses of meperidine are given. Other opioids should be considered before use of meperidine. Meperidine should be used for short-term pain relief only, if at all (Agency for Health Care Policy and Research, 1992).

Regular administration of analgesics seeks to eliminate blood level variability and to provide more adequate relief. It also eliminates the need for the client to prove he or she has pain and, therefore, reduces the risk of receiving reinforcement for pain behavior. Although regular administration provides excellent pain control, it allows little control for the individual suffering from pain.

On-demand or self-administered analgesic systems have been developed to allow the individual control over pain management. Systems developed for self-control include intravenous, intramuscular, and epidural administration of various narcotics. Research suggests that client-controlled administration decreases the amount of narcotic used and increases alertness (Turk, Meichenbaum, & Genest, 1983). These benefits are a result of reduced anxiety from anticipation of pain and enhanced feelings of self-control. The pain intensity curve is relatively flat, which eliminates the need for narcotic adjustment because of variable pain intensities. Tolerance will occur with long-term administration, but because tolerance develops to both the analgesic and the adverse effects of narcotics, increasing the dosages of narcotics does not pose any greater danger.

The only adverse effect Grace notes is mild sedation. Grace finds this bothersome, in that it limits the amount and type of activity in which she can engage. Most narcotics have similar actions and adverse effects at equianalgesic doses; however, an individual may receive a better response and fewer adverse effects from one drug than from another. One action, therefore, is to discuss with the physician a change in narcotic. Because the client is concerned about losing control, a better alternative is to institute an adjunctive self-management technique, such as analgesic imagery, and to reduce the dose of morphine or change the route of administration.

Imagery is used as an intervention by the nurse specialist. Grace is instructed to imagine the girdle area as numb or warm rather than painful. After achieving this sensory transformation, the nurse suggests that this sensation will remain on termination of the imagery session. In planning, the nurse may suggest the use of imagery either on a regular basis—for example, 2 hours after analgesic administration—or as required. It is important to discuss the preventive use of imagery because it is more effective if used for pain of moderate intensity (Melzack & Wall, 1982). The goals of imagery or other cognitive-behavioral therapies are to change patient perception of pain, alter pain behavior, and provide patients with a greater sense of control over their pain. Nonpharmacologic interventions are intended to supplement, not replace, pharmacologic interventions.

Several palliative medical therapies are available to manage Grace's pain. Injectable narcotics, although effective, may be replaced by an oral, patch, or epidural route of administration for home use. In clients with a limited life expectancy, neurolytic blocks or cordotomies may be effective means of pain control. In both procedures, the success rate is approximately 50%, and the pain tends to recur 6 to 12 months after the procedure.

After discussion with Grace and her family, the decision is made to continue to use narcotics to manage her pain. Oral methadone is tried, but the adverse effects of nausea and sedation are distressing to Grace. The next step is to insert a temporary epidural catheter for self-administration. Grace is scheduled for this procedure, to be performed under local anesthesia.

ANXIETY RELATED TO PAINFUL PROCEDURES

Preparatory information alters responses to the distressful aspects of pain during anxiety-producing procedures. Preparatory information includes temporal, sensory, and coping skill information. Providing the sequence of events and describing some of the equipment, environment, and personnel involved composes temporal information. Sensory information includes the sensations that are typically experienced during a procedure. Sensory information reduces the affective dimension of pain, with little effect on the sensory experience (Agency for Health Care Policy and Research, 1992; Hartfield, Cason, & Cason, 1982; Johnson & Levanthal, 1974; Padilla et al., 1981; Regan, 1984), by providing accurate expectations of the sensations experienced (Levanthal & Johnson, 1983).

Coping skills information instructs the client in activities that will reduce pain or distress during the procedure (e.g., deep breathing and swallowing during nasogastric intubation) or after the procedure to prevent complications and hasten recovery (e.g., turning, deep breathing, and coughing after general anesthesia). There is an additive effect when sensory information and coping skills are combined (Johnson, Rice, Fuller, & Endress, 1978).

Although responses are influenced by individual differences, such as preference for control (Padilla et al., 1981) and level of preoperative fear (Klos, Cummings, Joyce, Graichen, & Quigley, 1980), there are no contraindications to providing preparatory information. The intervention is most effective if the level of knowledge is initially assessed, the level of understanding is frequently checked, and the information is tailored to the client's needs and anxiety level. Methods of pain management are included to reassure the client that he or she will not suffer severe pain and to inform the client of expected behavior.

Providing temporal and sensory information is an intervention for the nurse generalist. A description of the sequence of events before epidural insertion and the sensations that may be experienced are provided the evening before the procedure (Regan, 1984).

Specific coping skills, such as deep breathing and distraction, can be taught, because they require little concentration and can be reinforced during the procedure with short commands. Deep breathing is a component of relaxation, because taking deep breaths counteracts the shallow, rapid respirations associated with sympathetic arousal. Deep breathing has a calming effect that may help the client gain control over his or her responses to pain and reduce anxiety. There are many types of deep breathing exercises that act as distractors—for example, "he-who" breathing and counting and breathing (McCaffery, 1979). Distraction redirects attention or awareness from the pain to other environmental stimuli, thus providing a sensory shield (Fordyce, 1978; McCaffery, 1979). Many activities, such as counting, singing, listening to music, describing pictures, or engaging in conversation are distractors that can be used during stressful procedures. Grace is asked to describe several complicated pictures during the procedure.

The administration of epidural morphine is successful in controlling Grace's pain with minimal adverse effects. Several days later, she undergoes permanent placement of the catheter, with the end extending through a fistula in the abdomen. This surgical procedure is performed under general anesthesia. Preparatory information, including postoperative coping skills of deep breathing, coughing, and turning, are used to reduce presurgical anxiety and promote postoperative recovery (Agency for Health Care Policy and Research, 1992). Grace and her husband are instructed in self-administration and in care of the catheter (Sternbach, 1974).

CONSEQUENCES OF ACUTE PAIN

Consequences for the Individual

Acute pain produces many responses, but the most significant to the individual is suffering. Suffering is defined as "negative affective response generated in higher nervous centers by pain and other emotional situations, such as loss of loved objects, stress, anxiety or depression" (Loeser, 1986). The individual may be asking such questions as, "Why is this happening to me? What does it mean? Will I be able to cope?" Seeking medical attention is an appropriate response to acute pain because medical therapies may treat the source of pain and thus eradicate it. Nursing interventions assist the client in controlling the perception of pain through knowledge of pharmacologic and self-initiated techniques. Collaboration with the client is essential in effective management of acute pain.

If pain limits the individual's ability to engage in daily activities, there will be a temporary change in role function and responsibilities. Hospitalization is the most obvious situation in which this occurs; a functioning adult who enters the hospital forfeits most responsibilities to become a patient. This may be a welcome rest for some, but the majority of patients have some difficulty giving up control and fitting into the hospital's structured routine. The client may be unable to meet family responsibilities, which places an added burden on family members. Assessment of the patient with pain should include a history of the pain and a medication history. In addition, health patterns, relationships and goals, pain behaviors, a summary of pain status, and the treatment recommended should be included. This information provides the foundation for discussion of the plan with the patient and the family (Simon, 1996).

Consequences for the Family

The family is typically concerned about the client's suffering, related again to the meaning of pain and the diagnostic and therapeutic procedures necessary to relieve it. Inability of the client to fulfill his or her family role responsibilities means that the remaining members must do so. Preoccupation with pain and related anxiety may make the client irritable with those closest to him or her, possibly leading to confusion or anger in family members. This, in turn, may produce guilt: "How can I be angry when my family member is experiencing such pain?" Both the person in pain and the family need to adapt to the temporary changes brought about by pain.

Consequences for the Community

The person with acute pain may be temporarily unable to fulfill work responsibilities. The incidence and impact of acute pain on the community has not been investigated. However, because pain is one of the most prevalent symptoms that motivates people to seek medical care, the overall consequences for the community are presumably significant.

HUMAN RESPONSES TO CHRONIC PAIN

Nursing Diagnoses in Chronic Pain

INEFFECTIVE COPING WITH CHRONIC PAIN

The defining characteristics of ineffective coping with chronic pain are behaviors learned during the acute phase of the process. Activity reduction is related to exercise avoidance, work avoidance, and minimal social participation. There is a continued reliance on medications, leading to overuse of addictive and nonaddictive drugs. This overuse leads to mental cloudiness, disorientation, memory loss, and demands for more medications (Snyder, 1984). Repeated contact with and failure of the health care system to alleviate pain result in manipulative and alienating behavior toward caregivers that carries over to all interpersonal relationships. Depression, and the vegetative signs associated with it, also assists in diagnosing ineffective coping with chronic pain. The result of these behaviors is an inability to meet role demands and responsibilities.

The assessment of chronic pain includes the areas identified under acute pain: the primary complaint and its sensory, affective, and cognitive dimensions. The manifestations of anxiety may be coupled with depressive symptoms. The client may focus totally on physical problems experienced (hypochondriasis) and deny any other affective or interpersonal difficulties (hysterical denial). Because of the dysfunctional nature of the pain problem, more data are gathered on daily activity, medication use, family relations, social participation, and employment status. Other evaluations that may assist the family with coping with the patient's pain include discussion of the meaning of the pain to the client; evaluation of the physical, emotional, cognitive, and behavioral responses to the pain; evaluation of the impact of the pain on all aspects of life; and responses of the significant others to the pain. In addition, discussion of coping strategies for the patient and family should be included (Simon, 1996).

The etiologies of ineffective coping with chronic pain fall into three categories: personal, psychodynamic, and environmental. Personal etiologies include failure to relate the pain to psychologic as well as physical factors and lack of knowledge of pain management techniques based on psychology. Psychodynamic etiologies include an inability to express feelings and resolve conflicts. Continued pain meets the need for dependency and conflict avoidance. Inability to cope with life stressors is one environmental etiology. Reinforcement of pain behavior is another environmental etiology. Pathology may be included as a contributing factor in chronic pain, although not as an etiology of ineffective coping. The philosophy held about the etiology of chronic pain guides the approach to treatment.

The most effective treatment of chronic pain is in multidisciplinary pain programs, which have multiplied rapidly since the 1980s. The objective of most pain programs is to assist the client in developing effective coping mechanisms. If, in the process, pain is alleviated, the client has received a bonus. The emphasis of each program is unique and in part dependent on the philosophical and etiologic orientation of the multidisciplinary team. For example, programs with a pathologic (peripheral) focus would result in the use of techniques that interrupt nociception before it reaches the SG. In contrast, a psychodynamic (central) focus would place more emphasis on altering the affective and cognitive responses to pain. Regardless of the focus, all programs combine, to some degree, both peripheral and central approaches.

The physician may orchestrate the therapeutic program, but multiple disciplines are involved. The goals of most pain programs include increasing functional status, reducing pain-related medication use, and increasing use of effective coping mechanisms. These goals, if attained, will produce a better quality of life for the client with chronic pain.

• C A S E   S T U D Y   2

Paul, a 32-year-old man, is admitted to an inpatient pain treatment program with a diagnosis of low back pain of myofascial origin. Paul has a tense facial grimace, algetic (painful) gait, and difficulty sitting for more than 5 minutes. His affect is withdrawn, his speech is slow and hesitant, and he avoids eye contact. He becomes more animated when discussing his pain and the poor treatment received from health care professionals.

The injury to his low back occurred on a construction site 2 years previously. The initial pain was severe, leading him to seek medical treatment. He underwent many diagnostic tests, which revealed evidence of a herniated disk. A diskectomy of L4 through L5 was performed, which provided relief for 2 months. With the return of pain, Paul began searching for another physician to "do the surgery right." A second back surgery to remove scar tissue provided little relief of his pain. Assistive devices were then tried with little relief.

On admission, Paul uses a back brace and cane as required. He describes the pain as continuous and severe (8 to 9 on a scale of 0 to 10). Distress is rated at 6 on a scale of 0 to 10. The location includes the lumbar area, with dull aching pain radiating down both legs to the knee. He obviously experiences pain when changing position but can stay in one position for only 5 to 10 minutes. He s taking multiple medications, none of which really relieves his pain. The only palliative measure he uses is distraction with television. Paul reports that his wife used some type of relaxation with childbirth, but he never paid much attention to it. He has not worked since the original injury 2 years ago.

Paul is married, with two school-age children. He expresses guilt about his behavior toward his family, about the fact that his wife had to take a full-time job to help with the expenses, and about his inability to be a real father for his two sons. Paul attributes these difficulties to his pain and believes things would return to normal if the pain could be relieved. He reports a familial model for pain behavior in that his mother suffered from severe migraines that frequently disrupted family life.

On examination, Paul is nourished but pale and reports a 10-lb weight loss over the past year. He complains of a poor appetite and frequent constipation. Difficulty with sleep onset and frequent awakenings are also problems. Physical examination of the back and the lower extremities is difficult because of his anticipatory responses (i.e., increased pain behavior) to pain.

ALTERED MUSCLE TENSION IN LUMBAR AREA RELATED TO GUARDING AND ANXIETY

Muscular hyperactivity is commonly the only physiologic defining characteristic noted in clients with chronic pain. It may be directly related to the etiology, as in Paul's case with myofascial pain, or it may indirectly increase another source of pain through reflex muscle contraction. There is typically a trigger point, which is a small, tender nodule found in the muscle belly. The primary interventions aim at reducing muscle tension, either peripherally with heat, cold, or TENS, or centrally with somatic relaxation (Agency for Health Care Policy and Research, 1992).

Application of heat is an intervention for the nurse generalist. Heat produces several physiologic changes: increased pain threshold, muscle relaxation, and increased blood flow, all of which may influence pain perception. Heat may be dry (heating pads and hot water bottles) or moist (Hydrocollator packs and warm soaks). Trapping the body's own heat with unbreathable materials—for example, plastic—may reduce joint stiffness and pain (Carpenito, 1983; McCaffery, 1979). All applications of heat should be wrapped adequately to prevent burning of the skin. Heat should be applied with caution to clients with altered sensation (peripheral vascular disease, paresthesias) and altered ability to communicate (poststroke, coma, vegetative state). Because of the increased blood flow produced by heat, it is contraindicated in clients with malignancies or potential for hemorrhage (McCaffery, 1979).

Cold application decreases nerve conduction velocity and, therefore, increases pain threshold. In addition to promoting muscle relaxation, cold application is particularly useful in pain of inflammatory origin, because it decreases blood flow and edema, thus reducing the inflammatory process. Cold may be dry (ice bag or gel pack) or moist (ice-soaked towels). Cold application is indicated for pain of musculoskeletal origin—for example, muscle sprains or strains. Although heat is more commonly used for stiff arthritic joints, cold may be helpful in reducing inflammation and pain and improving function. Cold can also burn the skin; therefore, the cold pack should be well covered to prevent injury. Cold is contraindicated in patients with altered sensation, altered ability to communicate, and sensitivity to cold (Raynaud's disease).

Electrical stimulation using TENS or mechanical stimulation using a vibrator are two methods of counterirritation that the nurse specialist uses as interventions. Following the gate control theory, it is hypothesized that counterirritation closes the gate peripherally by stimulating large-diameter fibers. Because the analgesic effects long outlast the treatment, it is believed to act centrally as well by stimulating descending inhibitory mechanisms. The most effective electrode placement, pulse wave intensity, and frequency are identified by trial and error. An intact nerve supply is needed in the area of electrode placement.

Counterirritation may be applied for 10 to 60 minutes at regular intervals but can be used for up to 24 hours a day. Counterirritation increases muscle relaxation and blood flow (McCaffery, 1979) and, therefore, has added effects in pain accompanied by muscle tension. TENS has been used primarily in the treatment of chronic pain, providing relief in 20% to 30% of clients (North, 1989). The use of TENS is contraindicated in patients with pacemakers and cardiac arrhythmias because of the electrical activity of the TENS and the potential interference with the pacemaker. Instruction in the use of counterirritation is imperative if the client is to increase self-control of pain.

Spinal cord stimulation devices are also helpful in the long-term management of chronic pain. These devices have been used since the 1960s for intractable pain. Stimulation of the large-diameter fibers in the peripheral nerves or the posterior columns could block central transmission of pain. This has been a successful mode of treatment for pain. Criteria for implanting a spinal cord stimulator include the following: objective pain complaint exists; alternative therapies are exhausted, psychiatric clearance is obtained, and underlying pathology is amenable to stimulation. Specific indications include chronic arachnoiditis, spinal cord lesions, phantom limb pain, peripheral neuropathy, peripheral vascular disease, and reflex sympathetic dystrophy. The benefits usually last about 6 to 12 months (Abram, 1993; North, 1989), but prolonged pain control has been reported.

Spinal and epidural narcotic use is also helpful in chronic pain, but its overall long-term success has not been as high as initially anticipated. There is a problem with dose escalation over time, which seems to be increased in patients with intermittent bolusing as compared with those with continuous infusion. Pain occurring with activity seems to be more difficult to control, and patients with noncancer pain seem to be more resistant to management with spinal or epidural narcotics (Abram, 1993). In addition, a variety of neurotransmitter receptor systems have been identified in the posterior horn that are not related to opiate receptors. Limited clinical application of nonnarcotic agents is under study and includes clonidine, baclofen, somatostatin, and N-methyl-D-aspartate receptor agonists (Abram, 1993).

Relaxation techniques are most appropriate for clients with muscular hyperactivity. Because of the negative influence of anxiety and the prevalence of anxiety in chronic pain, relaxation may be beneficial for any type of chronic pain state. Relaxation increases susceptibility to the suggestions of comfort (McCaffery, 1979), which is why hypnosis and imagery are commonly preceded by a short relaxation technique.

Relaxation is a common technique used in multifaceted pain programs because it enhances the effects of other pain management techniques and places increased responsibility for pain management on the client. The suggested use of relaxation is 20 to 30 minutes twice a day (Benson, 1975). If used more frequently, withdrawal and psychotic manifestations may occur. Consequently, relaxation is contraindicated in clients who have a history of psychosis and should be used with caution in clients who are depressed (McCaffery, 1979; Sternbach, 1978). In clients with cardiovascular disease, tight muscle contraction used in progressive relaxation should be avoided (Sternbach, 1978).

Although relaxation is considered a relatively benign procedure, some adverse effects have been noted. Muscle cramps, feelings of suffocation, and increased awareness of pain are effects that may be reduced by altering the technique. Intrusive thoughts, either anxiety producing or sexually arousing, may occur early in therapy (Bernstein & Borkovec, 1973). The nurse may be aware of these difficulties and openly discuss them with the client. In clients who keep tight control over their feelings, the open awareness suggested may increase feelings of fear, anxiety, or sadness. In this case, the nurse should terminate the exercise and therapeutically listen to the individual.

Paul learns a progressive relaxation technique (Bernstein & Borkovec, 1973), and, to provide structure to the program, Hydrocollator packs are available every 4 hours and are applied for 20 minutes. Because Paul has some difficulty with back and leg muscle relaxation, a collaborative decision is made to apply the hot pack for 20 minutes before relaxation. The use of heat is effective, and Paul begins to fall asleep during the relaxation exercise. Because Paul has difficulty with sleep onset, he decides to use the relaxation technique in the early afternoon in a sitting position to prevent sleep and while recumbent at bedtime to promote sleep.

PAIN PREOCCUPATION RELATED TO NARROWED FOCUS OF ATTENTION

Preoccupation with pain is a manifestation of somatization (hypochondriasis), which may be inadvertently reinforced by staff members. The approach to chronic pain management is focusing on wellness. Therefore, the emphasis and reinforcement are placed on well behaviors, one of which is non–pain-related interpersonal interactions. It is important to initially assess the client's pain and convey that the pain is believed. Once this attitude is communicated, the general nursing intervention related to chronic pain is selective nonintervention (Zborowski, 1969). Ignoring pain behavior and reinforcing well behavior will alter the client's behavior but will not alleviate the pain. This presents a double-edged sword, because nursing responsibility includes early detection of non–pain-related problems, of which pain may be an early symptom.

Pain behavior, which includes verbalization of pain complaints, algetic gait, facial grimaces, and moaning or sighing, is acknowledged but not acted on in nursing intervention. Nurse-client interactions are initiated surrounding well behaviors, such as increased activity and the use of alternate self-management techniques. The structure of a pain program and the milieu provide opportunities for the client to engage in these well behaviors. Program structure is important in setting consistent limits on client behavior, thus avoiding manipulation of staff. Structure may reduce anxiety as it identifies expected client behaviors.

Milieu therapy is defined in the context rather than the content of therapy (Radwin, 1987). Exposure to pain peers may reduce the feelings of isolation and assist individuals in identifying and owning up to dysfunctional or maladaptive behaviors. The health team members function as part of the milieu. Their responsibilities include assisting clients in developing awareness and insight into their responses and working through alternative modes of behavior and showing role model responses to emotions such as anger, joy, and adaptive interpersonal exchanges.

Paul responds to the milieu by taking an active role in the group. As he gains insight into other client behaviors, he is able to apply these ideas to his own behavior. Paul accepts responsibility for planning and implementing extracurricular activities for the peer group.

The three most dysfunctional pain responses are activity reduction, drug abuse, and continued reliance on medical therapies to eliminate pain. Paul completed the Daily Activity Diary (DAD) (Fordyce, 1976), which identifies on an hourly basis the number of minutes spent standing, sitting, and reclining during the week before admission. Paul's activity tolerance is assessed in preparation for physical and occupational therapy. His tolerance for sitting is 10 minutes, for standing, 25 minutes, and according to the diary, he spends as much as 18 hours a day reclining. The DAD also includes medication use, and the following pattern of medication use is identified: 650 mg acetaminophen with 60 mg codeine, two tablets four to five times daily; 5 mg diazepam three times daily; 250 mg methocarbamol two times daily; and 50 mg diphenhydramine at bedtime.

To provide effective treatment, nursing works interdependently to support and reinforce treatment programs designed to increase activity, reduce medication use, and increase self-management of pain. Table 25–4 presents multidisciplinary management of chronic pain, and Table 25–5 shows specific nursing diagnoses and interventions.

Paul begins an activity program designed by the physical therapy department, and his tolerance for activity increases as he is weaned from the back brace and cane. Paul successfully completes detoxification with only mild withdrawal symptoms. Because he is skilled in relaxation by the time detoxification begins, Paul is able to control his withdrawal symptoms with relaxation. This success increases his ability to cope with pain.

INEFFECTIVE FAMILY COPING RELATED TO LACK OF KNOWLEDGE

Assessment of the interaction between spouse and client yields information about the possible rewards gained from pain behavior. The spouse may provide rewards for pain behavior that make it difficult for the client to give up his or her symptom. Spouse support may, in contrast, be an important variable in pain reduction and positive mood elevation (Kerns & Turk, 1984). The shift in family roles and the added burden on the spouse may be important in explaining their interactions. The previous (prepain) pattern of function will indicate the adaptation that has taken place. Flor and Turk (1985) suggested that the development of chronic pain may be a reflection of family function and may, in fact, be a stabilizing force.

The perception of marital satisfaction may significantly differ between client and spouse, with the client denying difficulties that the spouse reports

TABLE 25–4 • MULTIDISCIPLINARY MANAGEMENT OF CHRONIC PAIN

Management Plan	For Client Activity Reduction	For Client Dependence on Addictive Medications	For Client Reliance on Health Professionals for Pain Management
Goals	Restore muscle tone, strength, and flexibility to increase activity tolerance. Decrease or eliminate assistive devices.	Eliminate use of medications with minimal withdrawal symptoms. Reduce use of nonaddictive medications.	Promote self-management of pain.
Methods	Replace pain contingent with time or activity quotas. Increase by 10% each week (Fordyce, 1978; Sternbach, 1982). Increase functional activity. Perform physical education: anatomy and physiology, body mechanics.	Plan time-contingent medication schedule. Reduce active analgesic by 10% each day (Fordyce, 1978; Sternbach, 1982). Use sedatives and tranquilizers to manage withdrawal symptoms. Perform drug education.	Set small, mutually agreed-upon goals to increase belief in self-efficacy (Turk et al., 1983). Review progress frequently and concretely (e.g., using flow charts). Explore relationship between thoughts, emotions, and behavior (Turk et al., 1983). Identify maladaptive patterns and plan adaptive alternatives. Promote problem-solving education.

TABLE 25–5 • NURSING DIAGNOSES AND RELATED INTERVENTIONS FOR THE MANAGEMENT OF CHRONIC PAIN

Diagnosis	Specific Interventions	Outcome Criteria
Reduced activity related to pain	Monitor activity and rest. Mutually plan activity-rest periods, increasing activity weekly. Reinforce functional activity.	Client will Participate in planning activity. Demonstrate increased tolerance for activity.
Use of addictive medications related to pain and physical dependence	Assess medication use in preparation for detoxification. Evaluate effects of detoxification. Instruct in use of self-management techniques to reduce withdrawal symptoms.	Client will Be drug free. Demonstrate effective use of self-management techniques.
Reliance on health professionals to manage pain related to lack of knowledge	Assess need for sedative or tranquilizer. Assess beliefs in self-efficacy, ability to cope with pain. Instruct in self-management techniques. Reinforce self-initiated pain management.	Client will Verbalize positive expectations for self-management of pain. Use selected pain relief modalities.

(Maruta, Osborne, Swanson, & Hallnig, 1981). A high incidence of sexual dysfunction in clients with chronic pain has also been reported (Maruta & Osborne, 1978; Maruta et al., 1981). Marital adjustment and sexual satisfaction should be discussed with the spouse and client individually.

Because effective self-management is a goal of treatment for the client, nurse specialist interventions involve the spouse as well. If the chronic pain is indicative of family dysfunction, self-management techniques may assist in the development of more effective family coping mechanisms. Counseling is recommended as well. Both client and spouse should be instructed in promoting well behaviors, and spouse involvement in techniques to manage pain may be one aspect of this.

If the spouse is providing reinforcement for pain behavior, operant techniques to develop his or her awareness of this process are necessary. This may be done with the use of videotapes of family interaction, diaries, or evaluation in a family or group setting. Working with the family members to change their pattern of behavior is imperative if the client's behavior is to change.

Paul and his wife meet with the social worker regularly during his hospitalization. In planning for discharge, family counseling and vocational retraining are recommended on an outpatient basis.

Desired outcome criteria are that the client will participate in the development and implementation of a pain management program, report an improved sense of well-being, use selected pain relief modalities effectively, and engage in non–pain-related social interactions. The family members of the client will assist the client in effective coping with chronic pain.

CONSEQUENCES OF CHRONIC PAIN

Consequences for the Individual

The suffering of chronic pain is obvious, and the use of ineffective coping behaviors only compounds this. Irritability and withdrawal alienate others and serve only to further isolate the client with his or her suffering. This puts the client in the difficult position of being dependent on the spouse and family members to meet role responsibilites previously assumed. If the family situation deteriorates and spouse support decreases, the client will become more manipulative to meet dependency needs.

Treatment of ineffective coping with chronic pain involves a multidisciplinary and multitherapeutic approach. The blending of operant principles and psychodynamic therapy aimed at developing awareness of ineffective behaviors shows promise in assisting the client to cope effectively with chronic pain. The goal is to restore the client to wellness (Fordyce, 1978) and thus provide a better quality of life.

Consequences for the Family

As pain becomes more of a focus for the client and maladaptive behavior increases, disruption of family function and role responsibilities occurs. Adaptation to altered role function occurs over time, but the family members may become frustrated, angry, and depressed. Because the client is so obviously suffering, the family members may hesitate to express these feelings. A successful treatment program requires involvement of both the identified client and his or her family. The ineffective coping behaviors may be an indication of maladaptive family function, in which case family therapy is a crucial element in restoration of wellness. Family members may need support in coping with their own feelings about the member with chronic pain and will need assistance in dealing with ongoing therapies when the client has returned home.

Consequences for the Community

Chronic pain presents a problem for the community. Bonica (1980) reported that over one third of the U.S. population, more than 50 million people, experience chronic or recurrent pain requiring medical therapy. The financial burden to the community includes extensive medical costs, compensation for work time lost, and liability. The human suffering of the individual with chronic pain and the family cannot be calculated (Chapman & Bonica, 1983).

SUMMARY

Acute and chronic pain present two distinct clinical pictures. The pathology and influencing factors are shared, but the individual's physiologic, affective, and cognitive responses differ markedly. Because of the behavioral differences and the potential treatment outcomes, goals of therapy differ as well. The goal of medical therapy in acute pain is to identify and treat the pathologic condition causing the pain. Rest, gradual mobilization, and pharmacologic agents are helpful in palliative treatment. The goal of nursing therapy is to prevent severe pain and promote a feeling of well-being. The duration, persistence, and refractory nature of intractable chronic pain make it highly doubtful that a cure will be found. Multidisciplinary treatment for chronic pain includes the involvement of nurses, occupational therapists, physicians, physical therapists, psychologists, social workers, and vocational counselors. The goal of therapy is improving quality of life by providing more effective or adaptive coping mechanisms. Nursing diagnoses for clients with chronic pain relate to the effects of ineffective coping patterns.

References

Abram, S. E. (1993). Advances in chronic pain management since gate control. *Regional Anesthesia, 18*, 66–81.

Agency for Health Care Policy and Research (1992). *Acute pain management: Operative or medical procedures and trauma* (Clinical Practice Guideline). Rockville, MD: U.S. Department of Health and Human Services.

Benson, H. (1975). *The relaxation response.* New York: William Morrow.

Bernstein, D. A., Borkovec, T. D. (1973). *Progressive relaxation training.* Champaign, IL: Research Press.

Beutler L. E., Engle, D., Oro-Beutler, M. E., Daldrup, R., & Meredith, K. (1986). Inability to express intense affect: A common link between depression and pain. *Journal of Consulting and Clinical Psychiatry, 54,* 752–759.

Block, A. R. (1982). Multidisciplinary treatment of chronic low back pain: A review. *Rehabilitative Psychology, 27,* 51–58.

Blumer, D., & Heilbronn, M. (1982). Chronic pain as a variant of depressive disease: The pain-prone disorder. *Journal of Nervous and Mental Disease, 170,* 381–406.

Bonica, J. J. (1980). Pain research and therapy: Pain and current status and future needs. In L. K. V. Ng & J. J. Bonica (Eds.), *Pain, discomfort, and humanitarian care* (p. 1). New York: Elsevier.

Bonica, J. J. (1990a). History of pain concepts and therapies. In *The management of pain* (2nd ed., pp. 2–17). Malvern, PA: Lea and Febiger.

Bonica, J. J. (1990b). Definition and taxonomy of pain. In *The management of pain* (2nd ed., pp. 18–27). Malvern, PA: Lea and Febiger.

Bonica, J. J. (1990c). General considerations of chronic pain. In *The management of pain* (2nd ed., pp. 180–196). Malvern, PA: Lea and Febiger.

Byas-Smith, M. G. (1997). Common pain syndromes. In *Expert pain management* (pp. 87–123). Springhouse, PA: Springhouse.

Capka, D., Griffin, S., Harris, G., & Pinsky, J. J. (1979). Selected psychometric evaluations before and after treatment on a pain unit. In *Chronic pain* (p. 373). New York: SP Medical and Scientific Books.

Carpenito, L. J. (1983). *Nursing diagnosis: Application to clinical practice.* Philadelphia: J. B. Lippincott.

Carron, H., DeGood, D. E., & Tait, R. (1985). A comparison of low back pain patients in the United States and New Zealand: Psychosocial and economic factors affecting severity of disability. *Pain, 21,* 77–84.

Chapman, C. R. (1978). The perception of noxious events. In R. Sternback (Ed.), *The psychology of pain* (pp. 169–173). Lancaster, CA: Raven.

Chapman, C. R., & Bonica, J. J. (1983). *Current topics: Acute pain.* Kalamazoo, MI: Upjohn.

Cleland, G. L., & Gebhart, G. F. (1997). Principles of nociception and pain. In *Expert pain management* (pp. 1–30). Springhouse, PA: Springhouse.

Craig, K. (1978). Social modeling influences on pain. In R. Sternbach (Ed.), *The psychology of pain* (pp. 73–96). Lancaster, CA: Raven.

Crue, B. L., Kenton, B., & Carregal, E. J. A. (1979). Neurophysiology of pain: Peripheral aspects. In B. L. Crue (Ed.), *Chronic pain* (p. 59). New York: SP Medical and Scientific Books.

Davis, A. E. (1996). Primary care management of chronic musculoskeletal pain. *Nurse Practitioner, 21*(8), 72–82.

Dellasega, C., & Keiser, C. L. (1997). Pharmacologic approaches to chronic pain in the older adult. *Nurse Practitioner, 22*(5): 20–35.

Diers, D., Schmidt, R. L., McBride, M. A. B., & Davis, B. L. (1972). The effect of nursing interaction on patients in pain. *Nursing Research, 21,* 419–423.

Edwards, P. W., Zeichner, A., Kuczmierczyk, A. R., & Boczkowski, J. (1985). Familial pain model: The relationship between family history of pain and current pain experience. *Pain, 21,* 379–382.

Engle, G. L. (1959). Psychogenic pain and the pain-prone patient. *American Journal of Medicine, 26,* 899–918.

Flor, H., & Turk, D. C. (1985). Chronic illness in an adult family member: Pain as a prototype. In D. C. Turk & R. D. Kerns (Eds.), *Health, illness and families* (p. 255). New York: John Wiley & Sons.

Fordyce, W. E. (1976). *Behavioral methods in chronic pain and illness.* Philadelphia: C.V. Mosby.

Fordyce, W. E. (1978). The learning process in pain. In R. Sternbach (Ed.), *The psychology of pain* (p. 49). Lancaster, CA: Raven.

Gentry, W. D., Shows, W. D., & Thomas, M. (1974). Chronic low back pain: A psychological profile. *Psychosomatics 15,* 174–179.

Greer, K. R., & Hoyt, J. W. (1990). Pain: Theory, anatomy and physiology. *Critical Care Clinics, 6*(2), 227–234.

Grichnik, K. P., & Ferrante, F. M. (1991). The difference between acute and chronic pain. *Mount Sinai Journal of Medicine, 58*(3), 217–220.

Hartfield, M. T., Cason, C. L., & Cason, G. J. (1982). Effects of information about a threatening procedure on patients' expectations and emotional distress. *Nursing Research, 31,* 202–207.

Johnson, J. E. (1972). Effects of restructuring patients' expectations on their reactions to threatening events. *Nursing Research, 21,* 499–502.

Johnson, J. E., & Levanthal, H. (1974). Effects of accurate expectations and behavioral instructions on reactions during a noxious medical examination. *Journal of Personality and Social Psychology, 29,* 710–713.

Johnson, J. E., Rice, V. H., Fuller, S. S., & Endress, M. P. (1978). Sensory information, instruction in a coping strategy, and recovery from surgery. *Research in Nursing and Health, 1,* 4–7.

Jones, S. L. (1997). Pharmacology of pain management. In *Expert pain management* (pp. 31–64). Springhouse, PA: Springhouse.

Justins, D. M., & Richardson, P. H. (1991). Clinical management of acute pain. *British Medical Bulletin, 47*(3), 561–583.

Keefe, F. J., Brown, C. J., Scott, D. S., & Ziesat, H. (1982). Behavioral assessment of chronic pain. In F. J. Keefe & J. Blumenthal (Eds.), *Assessment strategies in behavioral medicine* (p. 321). Philadelphia: Grune and Stratton.

Kerns, R. D., & Turk, D. C. (1984). Depression and chronic pain: The mediating role of the spouse. *Journal of Marriage and Family, 46,* 845–851.

Klos, D., Cummings, K. M., Joyce, J., Graichen, J., & Quigley, A. (1980). A comparison of two methods of delivering presurgical instruction. *Patient Counseling and Health Education, 2,* 6–12.

Levanthal, H., & Johnson, J. E. (1983). Laboratory and field experimentation: Development of a theory of self-regulation. In P. J. Wooldridge, M. H. Schmitt, J. K., Skipper, & R. C. Leonard (Eds.), *Behavioral science and nursing theory* (pp. 189–197). St. Louis: C. V. Mosby.

Loeser J. D. (1980). A definition of pain. *U W Med, 7*(1): 3–6.

Loeser, J. D. (1986). Pain and its management: An overview—NIH Consensus Development. In *National Institutes of Health, The integrated approach to the management of pain* (pp. 1–8). Bethesda, MD: National Institutes of Health.

Marks, R. M., & Sachar, E. J. (1973). Undertreatment of medical inpatients with narcotic analgesics. *Annals of Internal Medicine, 78,* 173–175.

Maruta, T., & Osborne, D. (1978). Sexual activity in chronic pain patients. *Psychosomatics, 19,* 531–534.

Maruta, T., Osborne, D., Swanson, D. W., & Hallnig, J. M. (1981). Chronic pain patients and spouses: Marital and sexual adjustment. *Mayo Clinic Proceedings, 56,* 307–311.

McBride, M. A. B. (1967). Nursing approach, pain and relief: An exploratory experiment. *Nursing Research, 16,* 337–342.

McCaffery, M. (1979). *Nursing management of patients in pain* (2nd ed.). Philadelphia: J. B. Lippincott.

Meichenbaum, D., & Turk, D. (1976). The cognitive behavioral management of anxiety, anger, and pain. In P. O. Davidson (Ed.), *Behavioral management of anxiety, depression and pain* (pp. 1–27). Philadelphia: Brunner Mazel.

Melzack, R. (1975). The McGill pain questionnaire: Major properties and scoring methods. *Pain, 1,* 277–283.

Melzack, R., & Casey, K. L. (1968). Sensory, motivational, and central control determinants of pain: A new conceptual model. In D. Kenshalo (Ed.), *The skin senses* (p. 423). Westport, CT: Thomas.

Melzack, R., & Torgerson, W. S. (1971). On the language of pain. *Anesthesiology, 34,* 50–54.

Melzack, R., & Wall, P. D. (1965). Pain mechanisms: A new theory. *Science, 150,* 971–975.

Melzack, R., & Wall, P. D. (1970). Psychophysiology of pain. *International Anesthesiology Clinics, 8*(1), 3–11.

Melzack, R., & Wall, P. D. (1982). *The challenge of pain.* New York: Penguin.

Merskey, H. (1986). International association for the study of pain. Pain terms: A current list with definitions and notes on usage. *Pain, 3*(Suppl), S1–S225.

Moss, F. T., & Meyer, B. (1966). The effects of nursing interaction upon pain relief in patients. *Nursing Research, 15,* 303–307.

National Institutes of Health Consensus Development Conference. (1987). The integrated approach to the management of pain. *Journal of Pain and Symptom Management, 2,* 35–44.

North, R. B. (1989). Spinal cord stimulation for intractable pain: Indications and technique. In D. M. Long (Ed.), *Current therapy in neurological surgery 2* (pp. 297–301). Hamilton, ON: BC Decker.

Padilla, G. V., Grant, M. M., Rains, B. L., Hansen, B. C., Bergstrom, N., Wong, H. L., Hanson, R., & Kubo, W. (1981). Distress reduction and the effects of preparatory teaching films and patient control. *Research in Nursing and Health, 4,* 375–381.

Pert, A. (1982). Mechanisms of opiate analgesia and the role of endorphins in pain suppression. *Advances in Neurology, 33,* 107–120.

Pilowsky, I. (1978). Psychodynamic aspects of the pain experience. In R. Sternbach (Ed.), *The psychology of pain* (pp. 203–209). Lancaster, CA: Raven.

Pinsky, J. J. (1979). Aspects of the psychology of pain. In B. L. Crue (Ed.), *Chronic pain* (pp. 301–311). New York: SP Medical and Scientific Books.

Pinsky, J. J., & Malyon, A. K. (1979). The eclectic nature of psychotherapy in the treatment of chronic pain syndromes. In B. L. Crue (Ed.), *Chronic pain* (pp. 321–329). New York: SP Medical and Scientific Books.

Porter, J., & Jick, H. (1980). Addiction rare in patients treated with narcotics (letter). *New England Journal of Medicine, 302,* 123.

Radwin, L. E. (1987). Autonomous nursing interventions for treating the patient in acute pain: A standard. *Heart and Lung, 16*(3), 258–266.

Ready, B., Murphy, T. M., Loeser, J. D., & Fordyce, W. E. (1980). The management of chronic pain. *University of Wisconsin Medicine, 7*(1), 13–17.

Regan, P. (1984). *Teaching guides for patients with neurological disorders.* Paramus, NJ: Reston.

Simon, J. M. (1996). Chronic pain syndrome: Nursing assessment and intervention. *Rehabilitation Nursing, 21*(1), 13–19.

Simon, J. M., & McTier, C. L. (1996). Development of a chronic pain assessment tool. *Rehabilitation Nursing, 21*(1), 20–24.

Snyder, M. (1984). Progressive relaxation as a nursing intervention. *Advances in Nursing Science, 6*(3), 47–54.

Sternbach, R. A. (1974). *Pain patients: Traits and treatments.* McLean, VA: Academic Press.

Sternbach, R. A. (1978). *The psychology of pain.* Lancaster, CA: Raven.

Sternbach, R. A. (1982). The psychologist's role in the diagnosis and treatment of pain patients. In J. Barber & C. Adrian (Eds.), *Psychological approaches to the management of pain* (pp. 3–12). Philadelphia: Brunner Mazel.

Sternbach, R. A., Wolf, S. R., Murphy, R. W., & Akeson, W. H. (1973). Traits of pain patients: The low back "loser." *Psychomatics, 14,* 226–229.

Stimmel, B. (1985). Pain, analgesia, and addiction: An approach to the pharmacological management of pain. *Clinical Journal of Pain, 1*(1), 14–18.

Timmermans, G., & Sternbach, R. A. (1974). Factors of human chronic pain: An analysis of personality and pain reaction variables. *Science, 184,* 806–808.

Turk, D. C. (1997). Psychological aspects of pain. In *Expert pain management* (pp. 124–178). Springhouse, PA: Springhouse.

Turk, D. C., Meichenbaum, D. H., & Genest, M. (1983). *Pain and behavioral medicine: A cognitive behavioral perspective.* New York: Guilford Press.

Upton, R. N., Semple, T. J., & Macintyre, P. E. (1997). Pharmacokinetic optimisation of opioid treatment in acute pain therapy. *Clinical Pharmacokinetics, 33*(3), 225–244.

Violon, A., & Giurgea, D. (1994). Familial models for chronic pain. *Pain, 18,* 199–202.

Wolff, B. B. (1985). Ethnocultural factors influencing pain and illness behavior. *Clinical Journal of Pain, 1*(1), 23–29.

Yarton, P. (1979). The role of the nurse on the pain unit. In B. L. Crue (Ed.), *Chronic pain* (pp. 413–432). New York: SP Medical and Scientific Books.

Zborowski, M. (1969). *People in pain.* San Francisco, CA: Jossey-Bass.

ELIMINATION PHENOMENA

26 | Elimination: An Overview

ROSE ROSSI SCHWARTZ

The elimination of stored waste products in the form of urine and feces is essential to maintaining health. The content of the waste products varies with the quantity and quality of food and fluids ingested. Elimination during health is affected by physical activity, maintenance of body temperature within 1°F above or below the average, and amount of usual life stress experienced. More importantly, equilibrium between the central nervous system and the urinary and gastrointestinal systems is essential for elimination.

Bladder elimination, or micturition, involves the kidneys, which create the urine; the bladder, which stores the urine; the bladder neck, through which the urine flows after voluntary relaxation; and the urethra, which carries the urine out of the body. Disruption of bladder elimination can occur when disease processes invade the structures themselves, when neurogenic pathways are interrupted, or when cortical control centers are affected.

Bowel elimination in the form of bowel movements or evacuation of stool involves ingestion and digestion of food and fluids and activities of the small and large intestines, the anal canal, and the rectum. Voluntary relaxation of the external anal sphincter is under cortical control. The neural pathways include the sacral spinal cord, the ascending and descending spinal cord tracts, and the spinal nerves. Several key reflexes, such as the gastrocolic reflex, play an important role in defecation. As with bladder elimination, bowel elimination can be disrupted when disease processes invade the structures involved with digestion and storage, when neural pathways are interrupted, or when cortical control centers are involved.

BLADDER ELIMINATION

Voiding is primarily a spinal reflex facilitated and inhibited by higher voluntary centers in the brain (Ganong, 1987). The formation of urine is the response of the body in regulating the internal environment in relation to volume, osmolality, and acid-base balance (Duling, 1988). The organs that make up the urinary system are the kidneys, ureters, bladder, and urethra. Other than the kidneys, which produce urine, these structures are primarily involved in transportation, storage, and elimination.

Anatomy of the Urinary System

The kidneys are approximately 11.25 cm in length, 5 to 7.5 cm wide, and 2.5 cm thick. They lie retroperitoneally anterior and lateral to the twelfth thoracic vertebra. The major structures of the kidneys are the pelvis, the medulla, and the cortex. The renal pelvis is the expanded upper end of the ureter and lies within the renal sinus. The medulla is made up of a varying number of renal pyramids. The cortex forms the peripheral layer under the fibrous capsule covering the kidney. The major functions of the kidneys are filtration, reabsorption, and secretion.

The ureters are approximately 28 to 35 cm long, arising from the pelvis on the medial sides of the kidneys and extending to the base of the bladder, and are composed of smooth muscle. The ureters fan out at the ureteral orifice and extend into the trigonal region (Elbadawi, 1991). They travel under the bladder epithelium for several centimeters before opening into the bladder (Guyton, 1987). The mechanism of the ureterovesical junction allows free efflux but prevents any reflux of urine (Tanagho, 1992).

The bladder is a hollow muscular organ composed of (1) the body, which is primarily detrusor muscle; (2) the trigone, a small area through which the ureters and urethra pass; and (3) the bladder neck or posterior urethra. The detrusor, posterior urethra, and trigone are smooth muscle.

The urethra extends from the bladder to the surface of the body. In females, the urethra is approximately 4 cm long. Striated (voluntary) circular muscle, which is under voluntary control, forms the external sphincter of the bladder, where the urethra passes through the urogenital diaphragm. The male urethra is approximately 20 cm long and is divided into three parts: prostatic, membranous, and cavernous (Kabalin, 1992). The prostatic urethra extends from the bladder for approximately 3 cm and passes through the prostate to the pelvic floor. The ejaculatory ducts empty into the urethra on the posterior wall of the prostatic urethra. The membranous urethra is approximately 1 to 2 cm long and passes through the external sphincter to form the cavernous urethra for its remaining length.

Neural Regulation

The neurologic control of micturition involves the micturition reflex, the sympathetic and parasympathetic nerve supply, and the cerebral centers involved in voiding (Fig. 26–1).

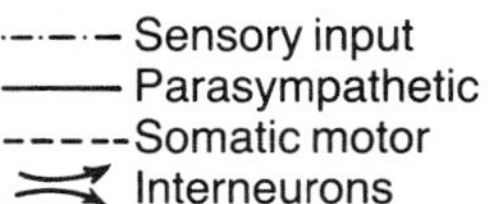

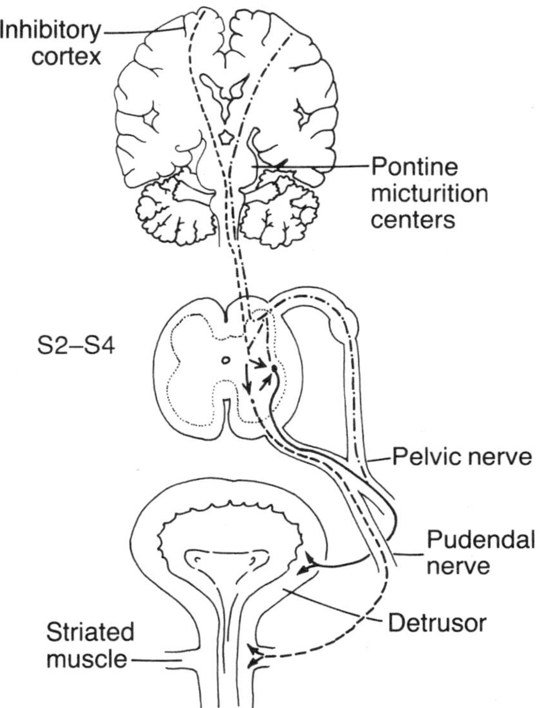

FIGURE 26–1 • Neural regulation of micturition at three levels: cortex, spinal cord, and end organ. (Modified from Mitchell, P. H., Cammermeyer, M., Ozuna, J., & Woods, N. F. [1984]. *Neurological assessment for nursing practice.* Reston, VA: Reston Publishing Co.)

PROCESS OF MICTURITION

The bladder fills at an average rate of 1 mL/min. As it fills, intravesical pressure rises. The micturition reflex is stimulated at a threshold pressure, accompanied by a conscious desire to void. Voiding will occur if there is no voluntary inhibition. In adults, the desire to void is usually felt when the bladder contains 300 to 400 mL of urine. Cystometrographic studies of the bladder demonstrate that as the bladder fills, there is a gradual rise in intravesical pressure from approximately 0 cm water when the bladder is empty to 5 to 10 cm water with 100 mL of urine. This pressure does not change dramatically until approximately 400 mL of urine is collected. The pressure can then rise to more than 400 cm water because of reflex contractions of the detrusor (Guyton, 1987).

As the bladder fills to 300 to 400 mL of urine, stretch receptors in the bladder wall send sensory impulses through the pelvic nerves to the sacral spinal cord segments. Impulses from the spinal segments return to the bladder through parasympathetic fibers in the pelvic nerves. This initiates reflex contractions of the detrusor, which are self-regenerating; each contraction activates further afferent impulses from the bladder. These bladder contractions send sensory input to the micturition center in the brain, which responds with inhibitory signals to the bladder (Perkash, 1990). As the bladder fills, the external sphincter remains contracted. Perkash (1990) described this as the holding reflex. The voiding process begins with inhibition of the holding reflex and is followed by relaxation of the bladder neck. The opening of the bladder neck is accomplished by immediate contraction of the detrusor, which allows urine to flow from the bladder through the open bladder neck and urethra. The flow of urine usually continues until the bladder is empty, but it can be stopped voluntarily.

CENTRAL INNERVATION

Both voluntary control and involuntary control over the micturition reflex are represented in specific anatomic areas of the brain. The pons contains centers that both facilitate and inhibit the micturition reflex. In addition, centers in the medial cerebral cortex serve voluntary inhibition of the reflex (Guyton, 1987). Afferent impulses that trigger the sensation to void travel on the pudendal or pelvic nerve to the S2–S4 spinal cord segments to the pons and cortex via the spinothalamic tracts (Elbadawi, 1991).

PARASYMPATHETIC NERVE SUPPLY

The detrusor muscle is supplied by parasympathetic fibers that originate in the S2–S4 segments of the spinal cord and pass through the pelvic splanchnic nerves. Postganglionic fibers travel to the detrusor, and sustaining bladder contractions during micturition are under parasympathetic control (Perkash, 1990).

SYMPATHETIC NERVE SUPPLY

The sympathetic nerve supply originates in the T11 and L2 segments of the spinal cord. In the male, it serves to prevent semen from entering the bladder during ejaculation. Sympathetic stimulation functionally closes the bladder neck by stimulating relaxation of the detrusor muscle (Perkash, 1990).

Factors Affecting Micturition

Many variables can affect bladder elimination, such as injury, infection, and disease. These factors can affect the normal structures of the genitourinary system, the afferent or efferent neural pathways, and the cortical control centers. Abnormal bladder function as a result of interruption of the neural pathways is termed neurogenic bladder. Several forms of neurogenic bladder are sources of alterations in bladder elimination. These are discussed in Chapter 27.

BOWEL ELIMINATION

Patterns of elimination of stool vary from individual to individual, from once to twice daily to once every 3 days. A neurogenic bowel may result when there is a disruption of signals among the brain, the spinal cord, the spinal nerves, and the gastrointestinal tract (Banwell, Creasey, Aggarwal, & Mortimer, 1993).

Anatomy of the Defecation System

Food enters the alimentary canal through the mouth and undergoes a series of changes in the process of digestion, absorption of nutrients, and elimination of waste products. Enzymes and digestive juices assist with the process in the stomach to break down food substances. In the small intestine, complete digestion occurs with the aid of additional enzymes, and it is here that the absorption of nutrients occurs. Chyme enters the large intestine, where the absorption of water and electrolytes takes place primarily in the proximal half; the distal half of the colon is concerned with the storage of stool.

The content of stool is inorganic material, undigested plant fibers, bacteria, and water. Variations in diet do not affect stool content greatly because the largest percentage of stool content is nondietary in origin. Even with prolonged starvation, feces will continue to be passed because of its nondietary component. The transit time varies in individuals, but it usually takes 8 to 9 hours for a meal to reach the colon. In 72 hours, approximately 70% of the meal has been evacuated from the colon, and the remaining 30% may take as long as a week to be passed (Ganong, 1987).

The four major parts of the colon are the ascending, transverse, descending, and sigmoid colons. The hepatic flexure is formed as the ascending colon turns abruptly forward and to the left. The transverse colon turns downward to become the descending colon at the splenic flexure. The descending colon is the narrowest part of the large intestine; it swings into an S curve to midline, forming the sigmoid colon, which gives way to the anal canal and the rectum, which terminates with the internal and external anal sphincters. The internal anal sphincter is composed of circular smooth muscle, and the external anal sphincter is composed of striated (voluntary) muscle. The mucosa of the rectum and the anal canal is thick and highly vascular (Banwell et al., 1993). The angulation of the rectum and the spiral folds, or Houston's valve, serves to maintain continence.

Neural Regulation of Digestion and Defecation

Neural control of digestion and defecation occurs at several levels of the nervous system, similar to the levels of control described in bladder elimination. The defecation reflex involves central voluntary control as well as spinal cord and autonomic reflex control. Several reflexes play a key role in defecation. The gastrocolic reflex is initiated by distention of the stomach after a meal. The distention stimulus sends signals to higher centers in the brain that are sensed as the urge to defecate (Banwell et al., 1993). Giant contractions are initiated in the colon to bring about mass movements to propel fecal material. These occur three or four times in 24 hours and are often initiated when some part of the colon becomes overfilled (Banwell et al., 1993).

The defecation reflex produces reflex relaxation of the internal anal sphincter and contraction of the gut wall in response to fecal material in the rectum. The bowel empties if the external anal sphincter is also relaxed. This reflex subsides after several moments and usually will not return for several hours, but it can be initiated by straining (Banwell et al., 1993).

PROCESS OF DEFECATION

When stool enters the rectum, the stretch response initiates signals that spread through the myenteric plexus. This response initiates reflex peristaltic waves in the descending and sigmoid colons. These waves move toward the anus, causing relaxation of the internal anal sphincter. Stimulation of the rectum initiates afferent signals, which are transmitted to the S2, S3, and S4 segments of the spinal cord. Impulses travel to the descending colon, sigmoid colon, rectum, and anus along parasympathetic nerve fibers, intensifying peristalsis. Stretch receptor impulses also travel from the sacral segments to the brain, where the desire to defecate is perceived.

The spinal cord reflex initiates contraction of the abdominal muscles, inhalation of a deep breath, and closure of the glottis, as well as contraction of the pelvic floor musculature. If the external anal sphincter is voluntarily relaxed, defecation will occur. Defecation can be prevented if the timing is not appropriate by maintaining the normal tonic contraction of the sphincter until an more propitious time. These pathways are shown in Figure 26–2 and described in detail below.

The intramural plexus of the intestine is composed of two layers of neurons and connecting fibers: the outer is the myenteric plexus or Auerbach's plexus, and the inner is the submucosal or Meissner's plexus. These plexi begin at the esophagus and end at the anus. The primary effects of stimulation of the intramural plexus are increased tone of the gut wall, increased intensity and rate of rhythmic contractions, and increased velocity of conduction of excitatory waves along the gut wall. Coordination of peristalsis is also controlled by this plexus.

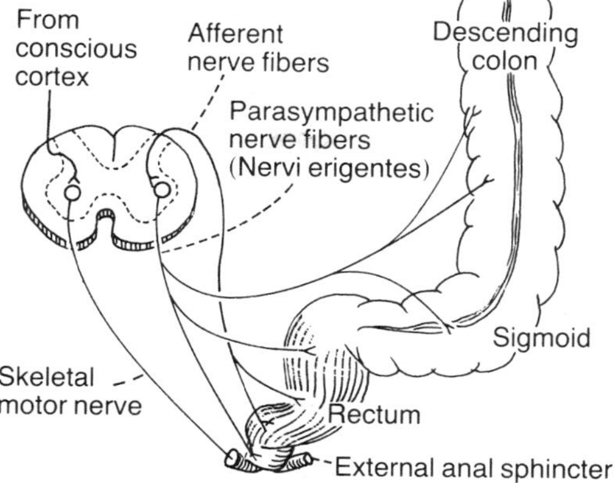

FIGURE 26–2 • Neural regulation of defecation reflex. (Redrawn from Guyton, A. C. [1981]. *Textbook of medical physiology* [6th ed.]. Philadelphia: W.B. Saunders.)

PARASYMPATHETIC INNERVATION

The vagus nerves innervate the esophagus, stomach, pancreas, part of the small intestine, gallbladder, and first half of the colon. The sacral parasympathetic supply originates from the S2, S3, and S4 segments of the spinal cord and passes through the nervi erigentes to the distal half of the large intestine, the sigmoid colon, and the rectum.

Stimulation of the parasympathetic nervous system increases activity of the intramural plexus, which, in turn, excites the reflexes of the gastrointestinal tract.

SYMPATHETIC INNERVATION

Sympathetic fibers involved in digestion and defecation originate in the spinal cord between T8 and L3. Postganglionic fibers spread to all parts of the gut. The overall effect of sympathetic nervous system stimulation is inhibitory, except when sympathetic stimulation excites contraction of the ileocecal sphincter, the internal anal sphincter, and the muscularis mucosae throughout the entire gastrointestinal tract.

CENTRAL INNERVATION

Afferent impulses travel by way of the spinothalamic tracts to the brain from S2–S4 segments of the spinal cord, which provide the sensation underlying the desire to defecate. The pudendal nerve innervates the striated muscle of the external anal sphincter (Ganong, 1987).

Factors Affecting Bowel Elimination

Diet is an important variable in the process of elimination. Certain foods add bulk to the stool, which is needed to provide the stimulus for bowel reflexes to occur. Inadequate fluid intake promotes constipation or infrequent, hard stools. Medication can often cause constipation or diarrhea and needs to be considered when bowel problems are being assessed. Activity and exercise enhance digestion and bowel motility as well as the strength of Valsalva's maneuver, which is necessary to initiate defecation (Pires & Kelly-Hayes, 1990). As Staas and DeNault (1973) noted, it is difficult to defecate without the ability to sit for any length of time. Severe emotional stress can cause excessive parasympathetic stimulation, with resultant overproduction of mucus in the colon. Increased mucosal secretions lead to decreased absorption and can contribute to diarrhea (Doughty & Jackson, 1993). Disease or injury causing neurogenic effects to the bowel are discussed in Chapter 28.

ASSESSMENT OF ELIMINATION

Assessment of the type and extent of voiding or defecating dysfunction is mandatory as the initial step of the nursing process. Baseline and ongoing assessment direct the nurse in planning individualized programs and preventing complications that could compromise renal or intestinal functions. The following assessment areas can be evaluated simultaneously in a given individual but are separated into bladder and bowel assessments for clarity.

Neurologic Assessment

Many patients with neurologic disorders may present initially with bladder or bowel dysfunction. An in-depth neurologic assessment can detect an underlying disease process, as well as explain the cause of the presenting problem. A comprehensive neurologic examination can be divided into five main parts: (1) mental status, (2) cranial nerve function, (3) motor system, (4) reflexes, and (5) sensory function (Siroky & Krane, 1991). For the purposes of this chapter, we will concentrate on the areas important to neurologic bladder and bowel dysfunction.

Mental status is determined by assessing the patient's memory, cognition, orientation, speech, and comprehension. Cerebral awareness is an essential part of maintaining continence. Disorders of mentation that may produce complications of elimination include dementia, brain tumors, cerebrovascular disorders, Parkinson's disease, and multiple sclerosis.

An examination of the motor system may determine the level of a neurologic lesion (Siroky & Krane, 1991). The location of the lesion plays a role in the type of dysfunction present. Assessment should include evaluation of strength and coordination. Common causes of motor disturbance include spinal cord injury, congenital malformations of the spinal cord and spinal column, Parkinson's disease, multiple sclerosis, and cerebrovascular disorders. "Normal" aging changes producing lumbar and cervical stenosis, as well as myelopathy, may also produce motor, reflex, and sensory changes.

Evaluation of the deep tendon reflexes indicates segmental spinal cord function and suprasegmental function (Siroky & Krane, 1991). Assessment of deep tendon reflexes and superficial abdominal reflexes may relay information about the corticospinal tract. The superficial abdominal reflex, however, may be absent because of obesity, abdominal surgery, or tension.

Assessing the external anal sphincter provides details on pelvic floor innervation. The tone of the sphincter and the patient's ability to produce a voluntary contraction are assessed digitally.

The bulbocavernous reflex is used to test the perineal striated muscle. It can be elicited by squeezing the glans penis or glans clitoris and monitoring the external anal sphincter (Siroky & Krane, 1991). The anal reflex or "anal wink" is relayed through somatic pudendal nerves. This reflex consists of a visible contraction of the external anal sphincter in response to a pinprick to the adjacent perianal skin.

Sensory function is associated with anatomic correlates. The patient's extremities should be assessed for deep and light touch, deep and light pain, vibration, and proprioception. Patients should be assessed for the ability to discern bladder or bowel fullness, sensation during elimination, or feeling of wetness after elimination. Saddle sensation is a perianal sensation elicited by response to pinprick or light touch. Disorders such as diabetes mellitus, alcoholism, spinal cord lesion, or cerebral lesion may produce diminished or absent sensation.

Urologic Assessment

HISTORY

A history of the patient's voiding patterns should be obtained. Any past problems such as enuresis, urinary tract infection, kidney stones, and sexual dysfunction should be noted. Present history should include questions concerning nocturia, frequency, urgency, burning, hesitation, retention, force and flow of stream, incontinence, sensation changes, pain, and sexual dysfunction.

ASSESSMENT

Urinary assessment should begin at the abdomen. Inspect the abdomen for asymmetry, swelling, or bulging. The bladder is located in the lower abdomen. Observe the lower abdomen for bladder distention. Palpate the lower abdomen starting at the umbilicus and moving toward the symphysis pubis (Stark, 1988). Assess for bladder distention, tone, and urinary retention. To palpate the kidney, position your hand on the patient's flank and ask the person to take a deep breath. Flank pain from kidney inflammation can be assessed by placing one hand over the 12th rib at the costovertebral angle on the back. Thump that hand with the edge of your other fist. Note any discomfort during this procedure.

Next, inspect the perineum and genital area for any evidence of bruising, bleeding, swelling, skin breakdown, or urethral discharge. For the male patient, the penis and scrotum are examined, and it is noted whether he is circumcised, because this may influence the type of urinary management if an external collection device is used.

The prostate should be assessed digitally in males. With females, the labia and the location of the urethral meatus are examined, and a menstrual history and the date of the last menstrual period are obtained.

Two final general assessment areas are the patient's physical abilities and the potential for cooperation. Evaluation of self-care skills for bladder management must begin early. Physical assessment of upper extremity strength and hand function and any limitations in mobility are necessary before program planning can begin. The ability of the patient to cooperate fully in the bladder management program is crucial to the outcome. Communication problems and decreased mentation, motivation, and receptiveness to learning can all have a negative impact on the goals and success of the program.

DIAGNOSTIC STUDIES

In conjunction with data gathering from the general urologic assessment, the nurse must incorporate findings from medical diagnostic tests describing the functional state of the external urinary sphincter, bladder, ureters, and kidneys. Evaluation and knowledge of laboratory, radiologic, and urodynamic studies will assist in these determinations. The data collected are essential in formulating an accurate nursing diagnosis and establishing appropriate nursing interventions.

Laboratory tests detailing composition and physical properties of the urine include (1) urinalysis, (2) urine culture, and (3) urine and serum creatinine clearance. In a urinalysis, evaluation of certain properties can signal subtle changes occurring in urologic function. The specific gravity (1.010 to 1.025) is an indicator of urinary concentration, and a low reading can herald the development of early loss of tubular reabsorption. Urine pH is determined by its hydrogen ion concentration. Normal urine is usually slightly acidic (4.5 to 7.5), and infection can flourish if the urine is alkaline. Maintaining urine pH levels below 6 may be indicated in patients with neurogenic bladders to prevent urinary infection and calculi formation. Evidence of microscopic hematuria could be indicative of trauma, stones, tumor, or acute cystitis. Pyuria greater than five white blood cells per high-powered field signifies an inflammatory response, with probable bacteriuria, and urinary casts indicate an inflammatory or renal parenchymal disease.

Urine cultures are necessary to monitor the incidence of bacteriuria, which is a constant threat in patients with urologic dysfunction. The urine culture should be obtained through a clean-catch voiding technique. If the patient is unable to obtain a clean-catch sample, catheterization may be necessary. A colony count greater than 10^5 per milliliter of urine, along with pyuria, represents signficant bacteriuria and usually requires antibiotic treatment (Perkash, 1990). It is important to remember that some patients with neurogenic bladders may not exhibit the classic symptoms of a urinary tract infection because of their neurologic deficit. Therefore, observing the patient for subtle changes—for example, dysreflexia symptoms, increased cloudiness or odor to the urine, general malaise, temperature elevation, or a spastic bladder with increased incontinence—can provide clues to the presence of bacteriuria.

Both urine and serum creatinine clearance tests are used to determine the glomerular filtration rate. Serum and 24-hour urine creatinine clearance tests are run simultaneously. Creatinine blood levels are normally 0.6 to 1.2 mg/dL and are generally constant unless renal failure has begun. The 24-hour urine measurement gives the amount of creatinine that can be cleared by the kidney in 1 minute. The normal value is 100 mL/min.

Initial radiologic studies, such as intravenous pyelography and voiding cystourethrogram, assess the anatomic structure of the upper and lower genitourinary tract and delineate any abnormalities. Abnormalities that can be visualized include (1) calculi, (2) hydronephrosis or chronic pyelonephritis indicating parenchymal damage, and (3) vesicoureteral reflux. Renal scintiradiography with ^{131}I hippuran has become an important diagnostic tool for assessing actual renal function through calculations of effective renal plasma flow (Tempkin, Sullivan, Paldi, & Perkash, 1985).

To definitively diagnose the functional state of the bladder, urodynamic evaluation is mandatory. In general, urodynamic testing encompasses simultaneous measurement of (1) bladder pressure during filling and voiding, (2) urine flow rate during voiding, and (3) urethral pressure and electromyography of the periurethral striated sphincter (Hinman, 1991). These measurements assist in identifying (1) sensation of normal bladder filling, (2) bladder pressure response to increased volume, (3) urethral pressure to assess urinary continence and detrusor sphincter muscle contraction, and (4) pelvic floor and external sphincter muscle activity.

Gastrointestinal Assessment

Bowel habits are unique and specific to the individual. The presence of a neurogenic disorder complicates the individual's pre-disability bowel regimen. A comprehensive assessment of bowel function must be instituted before an effective approach can be planned or a bowel management program can be implemented. Often, bowel programs are instituted without adequate assessment and planning in regard to the unique needs of the individual. A program based on trial and error is discouraging for the individual as well as for the nurse or care provider and is doomed to fail. Successful bowel management programs are based on careful evaluation.

HISTORY

Concomitant medical history, age, nutrition history, bowel history, and medication history are all important in determining factors influencing elimination. The presence of concurrent or previous medical conditions, such as diverticular disease, bowel surgery, anal fissure or abscess, hemorrhoids, ulcerative colitis, cancer, diabetes, psychiatric disorder, or depression must be assessed for any relationship to the current elimination problem.

Diet assessment includes meal patterns and routines and food preferences, with consideration of cultural influences on diet, fluid intake, and type of food that has caused an alteration in normal bowel patterns, as well as types of food accessible based on the patient's socioeconomic status. Foods that previously promoted regular evacuation or upset the individual's bowel routine will likely have similar effects after the onset of neurologic dysfunction. In addition, mechanical problems, such as teeth in poor repair or ill-fitting dentures, may cause mastication problems and the avoidance of foods that would otherwise be encouraged to promote an adequate bowel regimen. A bowel program may also be disrupted by the presence of gas in the gastrointestinal tract. Sensory awareness of rectal distention normally occurs with as little as 15 mL of gas (Doughty & Jackson, 1993). Large volumes of gas formation may lead to abdominal distention and cramping, causing decreased gastric motility.

In the pediatric population, congenital defects such as myelomeningocele, meningocele, scoliosis, and tethered cord may all affect bowel elimination to varying degrees. The "normal" effects of aging must also be evaluated. Altered or impaired activity from lumbar or cervical stenosis or degenerative joint disease may affect the success of a bowel program.

Neurologic deficits that affect facial and tongue sensation or interfere with the swallowing process may compromise an adequate diet. Roughage may be particularly deficient in the diet, causing further digestion and evacuation problems. Tube-feeding may increase the frequency of evacuations or cause stools of loose consistency, further complicating a regular bowel routine. Disorders that create dependence on others for feeding may interfere with food and fluid intake. Functional limitations of the upper extremities and positional restrictions may decrease food and fluid intake.

The examiner must assess the fluid intake to determine if it is adequate to prevent constipation. Water is reabsorbed into the systemic circulation from the stool in the proximal colon. If fluid intake is inadequate, hard, dry stool will result. A fluid intake of 2000 to 3000 mL/day is recommended to maintain a stool of soft yet formed consistency. One must also consider the type of bladder management program the individual is on. Fluids may be restricted during an intermittent catheterization program, and planning for the bowel program must take this into account.

Previous bowel habits, including the history of any gastrointestinal disorders, must be reviewed with the patient. Other areas explored include pre-onset evacuation time, frequency of bowel movements, methods used to stimulate defecation, pre-onset stool consistency, pre-onset incontinence, laxative or enema use, past medication use, obstetric history, and prior abdominal or gastrointestinal surgical history. Bowel habits that were previously healthful and workable should be continued as much as possible.

Present history should include questions concerning stool consistency, frequency of bowel movements, occurrence of incontinence, consistency of content lost, sensation at time of defecation, sensation before defecation, ability to differentiate expelled contents, and associated pain (Marcio, Jorge, & Wexner, 1993).

Medications that affect elimination may cause either constipation or diarrhea. Anticholinergics, antihypertensive agents, analgesics, tranquilizers, anticonvulsants, and certain antacids containing calcium or aluminum may have a constipating effect. Antibiotics may deplete the bowel of normal flora and can contribute to diarrhea. Habitual use of laxatives or enemas can cause atony of the rectal musculature, which results in decreased awareness of rectal sensation. Decreased appreciation of the urge to defecate can cause further constipation.

ASSESSMENT

Gastrointestinal assessment entails evaluation of the nervous system and of functional status as well as an abdominal assessment.

Assessment of the abdomen assists in evaluation of elimination dysfunction, particularly in regard to constipation, diarrhea, and paralytic ileus. With the patient in a supine position, inspect the entire abdomen for contour, symmetry, masses, peristalsis, and pulsation. Auscultation is performed in all four quadrants, noting the frequency and character of bowel sounds. Bowel sounds may be increased with diarrhea or early intestinal obstruction and are absent in the presence of paralytic ileus. Percussion is useful for identification of air in the stomach or bowel. A tympanic percussion note may be associated with gaseous distention. If distention is suspected, the abdominal girth at the level of the umbilicus should be measured and serial comparisons should be made daily, with the examiner being alert for the absence of bowel sounds. A dull sound of the descending colon may be due to accumulation of fecal material. Palpation is required to delineate abdominal organs and masses, to elicit areas of tenderness, and to evaluate hypotonic abdominal muscles or reduced contractility (Doughty & Jackson, 1993).

Physical activity and exercise generally promote peristalsis and bowel activity. If an individual is immobilized because of bedrest, functional limitations, or neurologic or orthopedic instability, bowel motility is slowed and constipation results. Functional ability and muscle strength must be assessed to determine (1) use of accessory muscles in exerting Valsalva's maneuver, (2) sitting tolerance, (3) trunk balance, and (4) ability to transfer to a commode chair or toilet. Hand function must also be considered when planning for the level of self-care ability to carry out a bowel program.

DIAGNOSTIC STUDIES

In the presence of abdominal tenderness, distention, or increased or absent bowel sounds, an abdominal x-ray will help rule out bowel obstruction. The condition of the intestinal pathways and the extent and location of intestinal distention can be determined.

Barium enema and proctosigmoidoscopy are performed when an acute change in bowel habits has occurred unrelated to the neurologic dysfunction. The purpose of these tests is to help rule out other organic disorders, such as cancer of the colon, ulcerative colitis, or diverticulitis.

The most frequently used tests to diagnose the functional state of bowel elimination are anal manometry, cinedfecography, and electromyography. Anal manometry measures the pressure generated by the anal sphincter. A microtransducer pressure catheter is placed in the anal canal to measure the pressure. Cinedfecography is a radiologic study of rectal emptying. A barium paste is placed in the rectum, and the patient is asked to squeeze the sphincter and to evacuate while fluoroscopic images are recorded. Electromyography is useful to evaluate the integrity of external anal sphincter innervation. Either concentric needles or single fiber electrodes are placed in the anal sphincter, and electrical impulses are measured (Madoff, Williams, & Caushaj, 1992).

Chemical and microscopic examination will determine the presence of occult blood or the actual composition of the stool. If diarrhea persists and cannot be explained as a result of antibiotic therapy, fecal impaction, or dietary factors, Gram's stain, stool culture, or testing for ova and parasites is useful to determine the source of an intestinal infection.

References

Banwell, J. G., Creasey, G. H., Aggarwal, A. M., & Mortimer, T. (1993). Management of the neurogenic bowel in patients with spinal cord injury. *Urologic Clinics of North America, 20*(3), 517–525.

Doughty, D. B., & Jackson, D. B. (1993). Interference with fecal elimination. In D. B. Doughty (Ed.), *Gastrointestinal disorders* (pp. 254–283). St. Louis: Mosby–Year Book.

Duling, B. (1988). Regulation of the composition of extracellular fluid. In R. M. Berne & M. N. Levy (Eds.), *Physiology* (pp. 794–816). St. Louis: Mosby–Year Book.

Elbadawi, A. (1991). Anatomy and innervation of the vesicourethral muscular unit of micturition. In R. J. Krane & M. B. Siroky (Eds.), *Clinical neurourology* (pp. 5–23). Boston: Little, Brown.

Ganong, W. F. (1987). *Review of medical physiology.* Stamford, CT: Appleton & Lange.

Guyton, A. C. (1987). *Basic neuroscience: Anatomy and physiology.* Philadelphia: W.B. Saunders.

Hinman, F. (1991). Critique of urodynamics. In R. J. Krane & M. B. Siroky (Eds.), *Clinical neurourology* (pp. 161–162). Boston: Little, Brown.

Kabalin, J. N. (1992). Anatomy of the retroperitoneum and kidney. In P. C. Walsh, A. B. Retik, T. A. Stamey, & E. D. Vaughan (Eds.), *Campbell's urology* (p. 340). Philadelphia: W.B. Saunders.

Madoff, R. D., Williams, J. G., & Caushaj, P. F. (1992). Fecal incontinence. *New England Journal of Medicine, 326*(15), 1002–1007.

Marcio, J., Jorge, N., & Wexner, S. D. (1993). Etiology and management of fecal incontinence. *Diseases of the Colon and Rectum, 36*, 70–97.

Perkash, L. (1990). Management of neurogenic dysfunction of the bladder and bowel. In F. J. Kottke & J. F. Lehmann (Eds.), *Krusen's handbook of physical medicine and rehabilitation* (pp. 810–832). Philadelphia: W.B. Saunders.

Pires, M., & Kelly-Hayes, M. (1990). Collaborative nursing therapies for clients with neurological dysfunction. In D. A. Umphred (Ed.), *Neurological rehabilitation* (pp. 791–810). St. Louis: Mosby–Year Book.

Siroky, M. B., & Krane, R. J. (1991). The history and examination in neuro-urology. In R. J. Krane & M. B. Siroky (Eds.), *Clinical neurourology* (pp. 275–284). Boston: Little, Brown.

Staas, W. E., & DeNault, P. M. (1973). Bowel control. *American Family Physician, 7*(1), 126–128.

Stark, J. L. (1988). A quick guide to urinary tract assessment. *Nursing88, 18*(7), 57–58.

Tanagho, E. A. (1992). The anatomy of the lower urinary tract. In P. C. Walsh, A. B. Retik, T. A. Stamey, & E. D. Vaughan (Eds.), *Campbell's urology* (pp. 40–67). Philadelphia: W.B. Saunders.

Tempkin, A., Sullivan, G., Paldi, J., & Perkash, F. (1985). Radioisotope renography in spinal cord injury. *Journal of Urology, 133*(2), 228–230.

Alterations in Bladder Elimination

ROSE ROSSI SCHWARTZ

The central and peripheral nervous systems are intricate components of the urinary system (see Chapter 26). As a result, a variety of lesions and neurologic states affect the neural control of the bladder and associated structures. A disruption at any segment of the micturition reflex center leads to impaired urinary elimination. The most common neuro-urinary symptoms are storage problems, emptying problems, or a combination of the two. The problems that may ensue are ones of varying degrees and intensities. Variability in symptomatology creates a challenge for the nurse. Nursing care should help the individual return to as independent a life as possible. The integral component of effective nursing care is an in-depth knowledge state of the urinary tract and the neurologic influence that oversees the system.

CLASSIFICATION OF NEURO-UROLOGIC DISORDERS

Neuro-urologic dysfunction has been classified by location of lesion or response of the bladder. Previous classifications may have represented an oversimplification of the anatomy involved. Lapides (1970) developed a taxonomy focusing on the response of the bladder. It consists of five categories of bladder dysfunction. The classification is lacking in that it does not consider the action of the urethral or smooth muscle sphincter in relation to the bladder. Krane and Siroky (1979) proposed an innovative classification system with a focus on function and therapy. This system places neuro-urologic dysfunctions into two major categories, detrusor hyperreflexia and detrusor areflexia. Each division is subdivided on the basis of the action of the sphincters. Table 27–1 contrasts the pathophysiology and symptom categories of Lapides (1970) and Krane and Siroky (1979). General assessment techniques are discussed in Chapter 26. This chapter discusses the urologic complications of neurologic disorders. For each dysfunction, the nursing process is applied. Appropriate pharmacologic and nonpharmacologic management strategies are discussed as indicated.

TABLE 27–1 • TYPES OF NEUROGENIC BLADDERS AS DELINEATED BY LAPIDES, ADAPTED FROM GIROUX, AND TYPES OF NEURO-UROLOGIC COMPLICATIONS AS DELINEATED BY KRANE AND SIROKY

Pathophysiology	Symptoms
Uninhibited neurogenic bladder 　　Defect in corticoregulatory pathways	Urinary frequency and urgency; uninhibited contractions
Reflex neurogenic bladder 　　Lesions above S2–S4 segments	Involuntary reflex voiding
Autonomic neurogenic bladder 　　Lesions involving S2–S4 segments	Varies from constant urinary dribbling to overflow incontinence
Motor paralytic neurogenic bladder 　　Lesions involving the anterior horn cells and anterior roots of segments S2–S4	Ability to perceive bladder fullness but inability to initiate voiding; possible straining to void
Sensory paralytic neurogenic bladder 　　Lesions involving the dorsal horn cells or dorsal roots of S2–S4 segments	Inability to perceive bladder fullness but ability to initiate voiding; possible overflow incontinence
Detrusor Hyperreflexia 1. Coordinated urethral sphincters Lesion of suprasacral cord and higher centers	Urgency; urge incontinence
2. Dyssynergia of the external urethral sphincter Suprasacral cord lesions	Outflow obstruction; increased postvoid residual urine volume; incontinence
3. Dyssynergia at proximal smooth muscle sphincter Spinal cord lesions (T6–T12) and associated with autonomic dysreflexia	Decreased urinary flow rate
Detrusor Areflexia 1. Coordinated urethral sphincters Sacral cord lesions or peripheral nerves	Difficulty emptying bladder; increased postvoid residual volume
2. Nonrelaxing striated sphincter Sacral cord lesions or peripheral nerves	Inability to empty bladder; increased postvoid residual volume
3. External urethral sphincter Denervation lesions involving parasympathetic and pudendal outflows	Incontinence with residual urine volume
4. Nonrelaxation of smooth muscle sphincter Lesions involving parasympathetic outflow	Decreased urinary outflow rate; increased residual volume

Data from Giroux (1988). Alterations in bladder elimination. In *AANN's neuroscience nursing* (pp. 431–440). Norwalk, CT: Appleton & Lange. Krane, R. J., & Siroky, M. B. (1979). Classification of neuro-urologic disorders. In *Clinical neuro-urology* (pp. 143–158). Boston: Little, Brown. Lapides, J. (1970). Neuromuscular vesical and ureteral dysfunction. In M. F. Campbell & J. H. Harrison (Eds.), *Urology* (p. 1343). Philadelphia: W.B. Saunders.

Nursing Diagnoses

URINARY FREQUENCY, URGENCY, OR INCONTINENCE RELATED TO DETRUSOR HYPERREFLEXIA WITH COORDINATED URETHRAL SPHINCTERS

Detrusor hyperreflexia is typified as an involuntary contraction of the detrusor muscle during bladder filling. This has been referred to by other names, including motor unstable bladder, autonomic bladder, cord bladder, reflex neurogenic bladder, and uninhibited neurogenic bladder (Lapides, 1970). The cause of this pathologic process is poorly understood. Detrusor hyperreflexia appears to stem from a new micturitional reflex center located in the sacral cord after it has been disconnected from the pontine reticular formation (Krane & Siroky, 1979). The separation may be the result of lesion or trauma. The combination of detrusor hyperreflexia with an intact urethral sphincter is most commonly seen with lesions of the cerebrum or basal ganglia and with incomplete supraspinal cord lesions. Related factors associated with detrusor hyperreflexia with an intact urethral sphincter include multiple sclerosis (MS), dementia, stroke, and Parkinson's disease. Most often, patients with this disorder display urgency and urge incontinence.

Defining characteristics consist of intact bladder sensation and normal bulbocavernous reflex. Urodynamic evaluation shows involuntary detrusor contraction, decreased bladder capacity, and intact external urethral sphincter.

The goal of the treatment plan is to decrease or eliminate episodes of incontinence. This can be accomplished through nonpharmacologic or pharmacologic methods. Nonpharmacologic therapies are appealing because of their high yield, low cost, and minimal side effects (Weiss, 1991). Nonpharmacologic therapies (Table 27–2) recommended for detrusor hyperreflexia include scheduling regimens and biofeedback.

There are several interventions for the patient with detrusor hyperreflexia. These interventions include behavioral therapy, biofeedback, and pharmacologic therapy. Behavioral therapies used in bladder scheduling regimens are based on the concept of timed voiding. Frequent timed toileting maintains low intravesical volume and reduces bladder hyperactivity. Clinical trials have found that bladder training is an effective alternative to drug therapy (Weiss, 1991). Environmental factors that facilitate continence should also be considered (Table 27–3).

Biofeedback uses physiologic responses converted to electrical signals and routed back to the patient. For detrusor hyperreflexia, electrodes are placed on the abdominal wall and external sphincter. Signals are sent to a biofeedback unit and displayed visually. Techniques to assist visually, cognitively, or auditorily impaired patients are also available (O'Donnell & Doyle, 1991).

The objective of drug therapy is to decrease the hyperreflexic state of the detrusor muscle. The pharmacologic categories (Table 27–4) most effective are anticholinergic agents such as propantheline and direct smooth muscle relax-

TABLE 27–2 • NONPHARMACOLOGIC MODALITIES

Modality	Indication
Conditioning	
Trigger voiding	Hyperreflexic bladder; incomplete bladder emptying
Credé's maneuver	Areflexic bladder; incomplete bladder emptying
Kegel exercises	Improved functioning of the pubococcygeus muscle; urge incontinence in women
External collection devices	
Condom catheter (male)	Detrusor hyperreflexia; incontinence
Urinary pouch (female)	Detrusor hyperreflexia; incontinence
Biofeedback	Detrusor hyperreflexia; urge incontinence; stress incontinence
Catheterization	
Intermittent	Incomplete bladder emptying; total retention; incontinence
Indwelling	Above reasons; intermittent catheterization not feasible
Anesthetic technique	
Sacral nerve root block	Detrusor hyperreflexia with or without external sphincter spasm; increased bladder capacity; assessment of benefit of sacral neurectomy or sacral nerve sectioning
Pudendal nerve block	Relaxed spastic striated external sphincter and pelvic floor muscle; incomplete bladder emptying; assessment of benefit of pudendal neurectomy
Surgical techniques	
Transurethral external sphincterotomy	Outflow resistance from vesicosphincter dyssynergia
Pudendal neurectomy	Resistance of external urethral sphincter
Transurethral resection of the bladder neck	Hyperreflexic bladder
Enterocystoplasty	Increased bladder capacity
Rhizotomy sacral nerve root	Hyperreflexic and contracted bladder
Urinary diversion	
Suprapubic cystostomy	Incontinence when catheterization is not indicated
Cutaneous vesicostomy	
Continent vesicostomy	
Urinary diversion ileal loop	Long-term hydronephrosis
Artificial urinary sphincter	Weak external urethral sphincter
Sacral nerve electrodes	Hyperreflexic bladder with weak external urethral sphincter
Vesicoureteroplasty	Irreversible vesicoureteral reflux

Data from Hackler, R. (1979). Surgical treatment of the adult neurogenic bladder dysfunction. In R. J. Krane & M. B. Siroky (Eds.), *Clinical neuro-urology* (pp. 197–212). Boston: Little, Brown. Khanna, O. P. (1979). Nonsurgical therapeutic modalities. In R. J. Krane & M. B. Siroky (Eds.), *Clinical neuro-urology* (pp. 159–196). Boston: Little, Brown. Henderson, J. S. (1988). A pubococcygeal exercise program for simple urinary stress incontinence: Applicability to the female client with multiple sclerosis. *Journal of Neuroscience Nursing, 20*(3), 185–188.

TABLE 27-3 • ENVIRONMENTAL FACTORS THAT FACILITATE CONTINENCE

Environmental Factors	Modifications
Bed	A low position facilitates getting in and out of bed.
Chair	Arms should extend to the front of the chair, and seat should be 16–18 in from the floor.
Bathroom	Bathroom should accommodate assistive devices (e.g., wheelchair, walker) and have grab bars, toilet seat arms, raised toilet seat, well-marked door, and well-lighted path.
Toilet substitutes (commode)	These should be of proper size and in an accessible location.
Clothing	Wrap-around skirts, clothing with Velcro fasteners, elastic waistbands, and footwear with traction.

Adapted from Morishita, L. (1988). Evaluation and treatment of incontinent geriatric outpatients. *Nursing Clinics of North America, 23*(1), 200.

ants such as oxybutynin, dicyclomine, and flavoxate (Khanna, 1979). Contraindications include glaucoma, obstruction of the gastrointestinal tract, paralytic ileus, and myasthenia gravis. Urinary retention may result from the use of this therapy. In the elderly person, assess for changes in mental status, vision changes, dysphagia, and constipation (Peggs, 1992).

•C A S E   S T U D Y   1

Ms. B was a 49-year-old woman with a 5-year history of MS. Ms. B had been experiencing increased episodes of urinary frequency and urgency with incontinence. Urinalysis and urine culture and sensitivity testing were normal. Laboratory data, including complete blood count (CBC) with differential, blood urea nitrogen (BUN), and creatinine test results, were also within normal limits, suggesting that the upper urinary tract was intact. The cystometrogram showed involuntary detrusor contractions at 100 mL. External sphincter electromyogram demonstrated relaxation during the involuntary detrusor contractions. On examination, Ms. B had a normal bulbocavernous reflex and intact bladder sensation.

Nursing interventions included a planned toileting schedule based on Ms. B's bladder capacity. For Ms. B to achieve an effective voiding technique, stimulation of the trigger areas to induce reflex voiding was begun. Trigger voiding measures for patients include pulling of the pubic hairs, stroking of the glans penis, rubbing of the thighs, and anal dilatation. For Ms. B, manual tapping of the suprapubic region in conjunction with Valsalva's maneuver facilitated maximum voiding. An every-3-hours voiding schedule was necessary to avoid incontinence.

To further improve Ms. B's bladder capacity, oxybutynin chloride was added to decrease detrusor contractions and increase bladder capacity. Ms. B was instructed on (1) her bladder dysfunction, (2) the potential side effects of oxybutynin, (3) adherence to the timed voiding schedule, and (4) signs and symptoms of a urinary tract infection.

TABLE 27–4 • USE OF MEDICATIONS IN NEURO-UROLOGICAL DYSFUNCTION

Drug	Lass	Dosage	Indication
Cholinergic agents			
Bethanechol (Urecholine)	Muscarinic	40–150 mg per day/divided doses	Functional urinary retention; detrusor atony
Carbachol	Muscarinic	6–12 mg per day/divided doses	Functional urinary retention; detrusor atony
Anticholinergic agents			
Propantheline bromide (Pro-Banthine)	Antimuscarinic/ ganglionic blocking	30–120 mg per day/divided doses	Detrusor spasticity
Adrenergic agents			
Ephedrine sulfate	Alpha/beta sympathomimetic	75–100 mg per day/divided doses	Stress urinary incontinence; urethral sphincter atony
Phenylephrine (Neo-Synephrine)	Alpha sympathomimetic	75–100 mg per day/divided doses	Stress urinary incontinence; urethral sphincter atony
Ornade Spansules (50 mg phenylpropanolamine, 2.5 mg isopropamide, 8 mg chlorpheniramine)	Sympathomimetic, antimuscarinic, and antihistaminic	1 caps every 12–34 hr	Urethral atony; detrusor hyperreflexia
Imipramine (Tofranil)	Alpha/beta sympathomimetic	100–200 mg per day/divided doses	Decreased bladder capacity; urethral sphincter atony
Dibenzyline	Alpha blocking agent	10–60 mg per day	Increased urethral tone
Adrenergic blocking agents			
Phentolamine (Regitine)	Alpha-adrenergic blocking agent	100 mg per day/ divided doses	Increased urethral tone
Phenoxybenzamine hydrochloride	Alpha-adrenergic blocking agent	10–40 mg per day/ divided doses	Neurogenic obstruction of the bladder neck and urethral smooth muscle; urgency incontinence; detrusor areflexia, with or without functional outflow obstruction
Prazosin (Minipress)	Alpha-adrenergic blocking agent	3–20 mg per day/ divided doses	Bladder neck and sphincter spasticity
Propranolol (Inderal)	Beta-adrenergic receptor blocking agent	40–80 mg per day/ divided doses	Stress incontinence
Direct smooth muscle relaxants			
Flavoxate (Urispas)	Smooth muscle relaxant	300–800 mg per day/divided doses	Detrusor spasticity
Oxybutynin chloride (Ditropan)	Antimuscarinic/ antispasmodic	10–15 mg per day/ divided doses	Detrusor hyperreflexia with urgency incontinence
Terodiline	Antimuscarinic/calcium antagonist	12.5–25 mg/day	Detrusor instability
Dicyclomine hydrochloride	Anticholinergic	60–80 mg per day/ divided doses	Detrusor spasticity
Lisidonil (Hydramitrazine)	Inhibits polysynaptic reflexes	10 mg/kg body weight per day/ bladder	Hyperreflexic neurogenic bladder with or without spasticity of the external sphincter

TABLE 27–4 • USE OF MEDICATIONS IN NEURO-UROLOGICAL DYSFUNCTION *Continued*

Drug	Lass	Dosage	Indication
Baclofen (Lioresal)	Inhibits monosynaptic and polysynaptic reflexes	30–100 mg per day/divided doses	Spastic external sphincter
Diazepam (Valium)	Inhibits polysynaptic reflexes	15–40 mg per day/ divided doses	Spasm of the striated external sphincter
Skeletal muscle relaxants			
Dantrolene sodium (Dantrium)	Skeletal muscle relaxant	50–400 mg per day/divided doses	External sphincter spasm
Miscellaneous			
Conjugated estrogens (Premarin orally, Estrace, Premarin intravaginally)	Increases periurethral blood flow, strengthens periurethral tissue	0.625 mg daily or 2 times weekly	Stress incontinence associated with sphincter weakness

Data from Khanna, O. P. (1979). Nonsurgical therapeutic modalities. In R. J. Krane & M. B. Siroky (Eds.), *Clinical neuro-urology* (pp. 143–158). Boston: Little, Brown. Wiseman, et al. (1991). Terodiline with bladder retraining for treating detrusor instability in elderly people. *British Medical Journal, 302*(6783), 994–996.

INCOMPLETE INVOLUNTARY BLADDER EMPTYING AND INCONTINENCE RELATED TO DETRUSOR HYPERREFLEXIA AND DYSSYNERGIA OF THE EXTERNAL URETHRAL SPHINCTER

This pattern, also known as vesicosphincter dyssynergia, is usually seen in patients with suprasacral cord lesions (Krane & Siroky, 1979). It is believed that the detrusor muscle and the urethral sphincter are coordinated from the pons. Therefore, a lesion between the sacral cord and the pons results in detrusor hyperreflexia and also in urethral sphincter dyssynergia. The related factors associated with dyssynergia of the external sphincter include advanced MS of the spinal cord, spinal cord injury, spinal cord tumor, and transverse myelitis (Bradley, 1993). The combination of detrusor hyperreflexia and dyssynergia of the external sphincter can lead to autonomic dysreflexia.

Clinically, patients with vesicosphincter dyssynergia have outflow obstruction and postvoid residual urine volume. The difficulty lies in the short, ineffective detrusor contraction despite high intravesical pressures (Krane & Siroky, 1979). There is some degree of incontinence as well as upper urinary tract disorder. This state is due to the loss of the coordinating reflexes from the pontine reticular formation.

Defining characteristics include decreased or absent bladder sensation. The bulbocavernous reflex is hyperactive. The bladder does not empty easily with suprapubic tapping. Urodynamic studies show involuntary detrusor contractions on cystometrogram. External sphincter electromyogram displays bursts of electrical activity in the sphincter. Sphincter contractions usually occur at the time of detrusor contraction, causing high intravesical pressure and an outflow obstruction.

The desired outcome for a patient with vesicosphincter dyssynergia is to achieve a catheter-free, reflex voiding state with a urinary volume of less than 100 mL. Interventions for this disorder include catheterization, pharmacologic agents, surgery, and sacral nerve electrodes. Initially, the use of intermittent catheterization prevents damage to the upper urinary tract and also decreases the risk for urinary tract infection. It is important to remember that if resistance is met during catheterization, the patient may be experiencing bladder neck obstruction or reflex spasms. A Coudé catheter or lidocaine jelly may be necessary (Perkash, 1993). Once the initial shock stage has subsided, a bladder-retraining program should be initiated. Close monitoring of the patient's intake and output is necessary.

Pharmacologic agents are aimed at decreasing urethral resistance and detrusor contractions. However, drugs that relax smooth muscle, such as flavoxate, often cause bladder neck or urethral obstruction. Alpha-adrenergic blocking agents, such as prazosin or phenoxybenzamine, can reduce bladder neck and sphincter spasticity. Patients taking these medications should be assessed for cardiac or pulmonary disease, gastrointestinal obstruction, and glaucoma.

Surgical interventions are reserved for patients who are not successful with bladder retraining and medications. Transurethral sphincterotomy is indicated for vesicosphincter dyssynergia, bladder wall trabeculations, persistent high voiding pressure, autonomic dysreflexia, and vesicoureteral reflux (Perkash, 1993). This procedure surgically reduces the bladder neck and urethral resistance to allow more adequate emptying. In some cases, however, this may result in some degree of incontinence, loss of erectile ability, or retrograde ejaculation. If the patient has any functional use of the upper extremities, neurosurgery or medications may be used to convert a hyperreflexic bladder to an areflexic bladder. As a result, the external sphincter may become the mechanism of continence through intermittent self-catheterization (Krane & Siroky, 1979). This is not a realistic option for most quadriplegics.

Implanted sacral nerve electrodes have been tried for urinary incontinence associated with detrusor hyperreflexia and sphincter weakness. Neurostimulation of the S3 foramen produced an adequate sphincter closure (Schmidt, 1991). Involuntary voiding because of detrusor contractions was able to be suppressed. Patients retained voluntary bladder emptying. This may be an appropriate modality for incomplete, low spinal cord injuries; however, further research is needed to ascertain its long-term effectiveness.

Once a balanced bladder state and reflex voiding are achieved through bladder retraining, medication, surgery, or a combination of these, an external method of urinary collection is usually required. For the male patient, this does not usually present a problem because there are many types of external catheter devices from which to choose. For the female patient, however, the choice of external devices is limited. The Female Urinary Pouch by Hollister was tested in a nursing home and found to be an alternative. It was not as effective in maintaining dryness as a urethral catheter, but the incidence of bacteriuria was substantially lower (Johnson, Muncie, O'Reilly, & Warren, 1990). Because of this limited selection, sphincterotomy is not a viable choice for women. Remaining choices include intermittent catheterization, indwelling catheter, or incontinence pads. Generally, incontinence pads or garments should be used with discretion, especially in asensory patients, because of the potential risk of skin breakdown.

INCOMPLETE INVOLUNTARY BLADDER EMPTYING AND INCONTINENCE RELATED TO DETRUSOR HYPERREFLEXIA AND DYSSYNERGY AT THE LEVEL OF THE PROXIMAL SMOOTH MUSCLE SPHINCTER

A lesion above the thoracolumbar sympathetic outflow (T6–T12) results in detrusor hyperreflexia and loss of coordination between the detrusor and the smooth muscle sphincter. This may result in the loss of inhibition of sympathetic discharges to the smooth muscle (Krane & Siroky, 1979). This is believed to be one of the mechanisms of autonomic dysreflexia. Autonomic dysreflexia is a life-threatening condition associated with a sharp rise in blood pressure, bradycardia, and sweating and an increase in spasticity. The usual trigger is a distended bladder or a fecal impaction. Related factors associated with detrusor hyperreflexia and dyssynergia include spinal cord trauma, tumor, MS, and vascular disease.

Defining characteristics include outflow obstruction, postvoid residual volume, and bladder distention. The desire to void is absent. Urine outflow may occur in spurts or with interrupted voiding (Yalla & Bushra, 1991).

Cystometrograms are commonly performed to detect detrusor hyperreflexia. External sphincter electromyograms may also be used to discover dyssynergia at the external striated sphincter, but this method is less reliable. To diagnose dyssynergia of the proximal smooth muscle, phentolamine may be given and urinary flow rates or urethral pressures measured.

Interventions and outcomes are similar to those used in detrusor hyperreflexia with dyssynergia of the external sphincter. The most common pharmacologic therapy is oral phenoxybenzamine. If this is not effective, a transurethral sphincterotomy is indicated.

• C A S E   S T U D Y   2

Mr. M was a 20-year-old C6–C7 quadriplegic man who had been recently injured in a diving accident. On admission, he had an indwelling catheter for bladder management. An intermittent catheterization program every 4 hours was begun. Twenty-four–hour intake and output recordings were started, with fluid restricted to 100 mL/hr. After resolution of the spinal shock phase, some reflex bladder activity was observed. The nurse stimulated trigger voiding before each intermittent catheterization by suprapubic tapping. Because Mr. M's level of injury precluded fine hand movement, Mr. M was taught to use the ulnar surface of his hand to initiate suprapubic tapping when he was in an upright position. With increased spontaneous and stimulated voiding, Mr. M's catheterizations were reduced in frequency to every 6 hours and then to every 8 hours.

Residual urines, however, remained greater than 250 mL, and Mr. M occasionally displayed signs of autonomic dysreflexia. During an episode of dysreflexia, the nurse would elevate the head of Mr. M's bed, monitoring his blood pressure and pulse, and would check for the source of the stimuli. With urologic involvement, the bladder must be assessed for overdistention caused by kinked or plugged catheters, full drainage bags, or a full bladder. After manual stimulation did not produce bladder emptying, Mr. M was catheterized, with resolution of the dysreflexic symptoms. A trial of prazosin was begun. Mr. M's residual urines remained high, and occasional dysreflexic symptoms persisted. After weighing all the facts, Mr. M decided on a transurethral sphincterotomy. Postoperatively, Mr. M was instructed on the importance of regular, timed reflex bladder triggering. A self-adhesive external catheter was recommended to maximize Mr. M's self-care skills and increase his independence.

Additional areas of instruction should focus on (1) daily inspection of penile skin for cuts or abrasions, (2) daily perineal hygiene and condom change to reduce risks of bladder infection, (3) signs and symptoms of urinary infection, (4) importance of fluid intake of 2500 to 3000 mL/day including fluids that acidify the urine, and (5) daily cleaning of the urinary drainage bags with a disinfectant solution.

URINARY RETENTION AND OVERFLOW INCONTINENCE RELATED TO DETRUSOR AREFLEXIA ASSOCIATED WITH COORDINATED URETHRAL SPHINCTERS

Patients in this category have the absence of the detrusor reflex in the presence of high intravesical pressure. This disorder is usually the result of a lesion involving the sacral cord, cauda equina, or pelvic nerves. It is not associated with any obstruction at the level of the smooth muscle or striated muscle sphincter (Krane & Siroky, 1979). Related factors associated with detrusor areflexia with coordinated urethral sphincters are sacral cord MS and complications of pelvic surgery. Patients display the inability to voluntarily initiate voiding with associated urinary retention. Overflow incontinence may occur.

Defining characteristics demonstrate decreased or absent bladder sensation in light of high intravesical pressure. The bulbocavernous reflex is absent. Cystometrogram demonstrates an areflexic bladder. External sphincter electromyogram shows a decrease in electrical activity at the time of the attempted detrusor contraction.

Nursing interventions and outcomes should be directed toward preventing overdistention of the bladder by reducing residual urine and managing incontinence. Voiding can be accomplished with the use of Credé's and Valsalva's maneuvers. Credé's maneuver involves external manual pressure applied over the bladder to force the urine out. Valsalva's maneuver used together with Credé's maneuver increases intra-abdominal pressure, further emptying the bladder. If feasible, the patient should be taught abdominal strengthening exercises. Stimulation of the muscarinic cholinergic receptors with the use of medications, such as bethanechol, may be effective in increasing detrusor tone and decreasing bladder spasticity. Contraindications to this therapy include peptic ulcer disease, coronary artery disease, Parkinson's disease, and epilepsy.

Cholinergic agents may cause gastrointestinal or urinary obstructions. If incomplete voiding cannot be overcome with these methods, intermittent catheterization usually becomes the treatment of choice.

Mr. P was a 28-year-old man who had developed urinary retention and overflow incontinence as a result of spinal cord MS. Cystometrogram demonstrated detrusor areflexia at an intravesical volume of 500 mL. Postvoid residual volume was 250 mL. Stimulated voiding was taught to Mr. P using Credé's and Valsalva's maneuvers. Fluid intake was limited throughout the day. A voiding schedule was instituted. On reevaluation, Mr. P continued to have difficulty with postvoid residuals. Bethanechol was added with an improvement in residual urine volume. Mr. P. was instructed on (1) importance of maintaining his voiding schedule, (2) signs and symptoms of urinary infection, (3) importance of fluid intake of 2500 to 3000 mL/day including fluids that acidify the urine, and (4) potential side effects of bethanechol.

URINARY RETENTION: INABILITY TO INITIATE URINATION AND OVERFLOW INCONTINENCE RELATED TO DETRUSOR AREFLEXIA ASSOCIATED WITH NONRELAXING STRIATED SPHINCTER

Nonrelaxation of the striated sphincter in the face of detrusor areflexia is thought to be related to overdistention of the areflexic bladder with continued input to the spinal cord via the sympathetic pathways (Krane & Siroky, 1979). The result is contraction of the external sphincter during voiding attempts. As intra-abdominal pressure increases, so does sphincter contraction. This pattern of dysfunction is often related to lesions of the pudendal nucleus in the sacral cord or peripheral nerves. Patients are unable to voluntarily empty their bladders, with high residual urine volume.

Defining characteristics demonstrate absent bladder sensation. Bulbocavernous reflex is absent. Perineal sensation may also be decreased or absent. Urodynamic evaluation reveals detrusor areflexia. External urethral sphincter electromyogram displays increased electrical activity during a patient's attempt to void. This increase in activity causes a flow obstruction.

Nursing interventions and outcomes are limited in this population. Outcomes are to decrease urine volume and prevent chronic changes in the bladder resulting from overdistention. Interventions include pharmacologic agents and catheterization. Pharmacologic therapies to improve bladder tone are not usually effective and may increase the outflow obstruction. This group experiences the greatest results from intermittent self-catheterization. For discharge, patients should be taught clean intermittent catheterization techniques. As a result of the urethral sphincter contractions, patients are usually continent between catheterizations.

Ms. L was a 48-year-old woman who had developed urinary retention and overflow incontinence after an S4 spinal cord tumor. Urodynamic evaluation demonstrated detrusor areflexia with a residual urine volume of 350 mL. Contractions of the external urethral sphincter at attempts to void were also present. Laboratory study results, including those for CBC with differential, BUN, and creatinine, were within normal limits. Urinalysis and urine culture did not reveal any signs of infection. Stimulated voiding was initiated but resulted in high postvoid residuals. Intermittent self-catheterization was initiated every 4 hours to keep residuals below 400 mL. A fluid intake program was started to maintain low residuals. Ms. L could increase the length of time between catheterizations to every 6 hours. Any further increase in length of time between bladder emptyings might increase the risk of bacteriuria and urinary infection.

Additional education should focus on (1) attempting to void before catheterization, (2) importance of a clean environment during catheterizations, (3) care of catheters between catheterizations, (4) signs and symptoms of urinary infections, (5) signs of bladder distention, and (6) monitoring of fluid intake.

URINARY INCONTINENCE AND RETENTION RELATED TO DETRUSOR AREFLEXIA ASSOCIATED WITH URETHRAL SPHINCTER DENERVATION

The neurologic basis for detrusor areflexia with urethral sphincter denervation may be related to a lesion involving both the parasympathetic outflow and the pudendal outflow. Related factors for this disorder are often seen in severe cauda equina syndrome. Patients often experience overflow incontinence with increasing residual urine volume.

Defining characteristics include absent bladder sensation. Bulbocavernous reflex is either increased in latency or absent (Bradley, 1993). A diminished anal reflex is noted on neurologic examination. Cystometrogram shows detrusor areflexia. Sphincter activity is depressed or absent. Pudendal neuropathy is present.

Interventions for the incontinence associated with sphincter denervation are often limited and ineffective. Strategies such as medication, bladder training, or intermittent catheterization are frequently attempted. Medications such as bethanechol may decrease postvoid residual volume but do not affect incontinence. Indwelling catheterization is a viable alternative for maintaining continence. The outcome of treatment is to reduce postvoid residuals and eliminate incontinence.

Some patients with sphincter denervation may benefit from an artificial urinary sphincter. The device, which is most effective in this patient population, increases resistance at the bulbous urethra (Hackler, 1979). To be considered for this procedure, patients must have adequate bladder capacity and voiding pressures. This procedure together with intermittent catheterization may be effective in maintaining continence.

• C A S E   S T U D Y   5

Ms. R was a 32-year-old woman who developed cauda equina syndrome after the delivery of her third child. On examination, she had decreased perianal sensation. The anal sphincter and bulbocavernous reflex were diminished. She was incontinent, with a palpable bladder. Urologic evaluation demonstrated detrusor areflexia with sphincter denervation. Ms. R was placed on an intermittent catheterization schedule of every 4 hours with attempts at voiding using Credé's and Valsalva's maneuvers. Incontinence between catheterizations remained a problem. An indwelling catheter was instituted to decrease the risk of skin breakdown.

Discharge planning included instruction on the insertion and care of an indwelling catheter and on proper positioning and taping to promote urethral draining. Additional education focused on (1) daily perineal hygiene and drainage bag care, (2) signs and symptoms of urinary infections, (3) risk of catheter-associated ascending bacteriuria, (4) importance of fluid intake of 2500 to 3000 mL/day, and (5) catheter management during sexual activity.

URINARY RETENTION RELATED TO DETRUSOR AREFLEXIA WITH NONRELAXATION OF THE SMOOTH MUSCLE SPHINCTER

The relaxation of the smooth muscle at the time of detrusor contraction may be mediated peripherally through the neuroterminal plexus. A decrease in parasympathetic outflow from the sacral cord might result in detrusor areflexia and smooth muscle sphincter obstruction (Krane & Siroky, 1979). Related factors associated with this disorder include lesions affecting parasympathetic outflow, which create an inability for smooth muscle sphincter relaxation or cauda equina syndrome. Patients present with urinary retention.

Defining characteristics on urologic evaluation are detrusor areflexia on cystometrographic analysis with external sphincter relaxation during voiding attempts. Urinary flow rate is diminished in this population.

Interventions include catheterization and pharmacologic and surgical strategies. Intermittent catheterizations decrease the vesicle and prevent damage to the upper urinary tract and urinary tract infections. Pharmacologic therapy is aimed at detrusor tone as well as smooth muscle sphincter contractions. Drugs of choice include cholinergic agents (bethanechol) or alpha-adrenergic agents (phenoxybenzamine, phentolamine). This group of agents should be used with caution in patients with coronary artery disease, Parkinson's disease, and hypotension. They may cause loss of ejaculation in young men. Surgical interventions may include transurethral resection of the bladder neck (Krane & Siroky, 1979). The outcome is to decrease urinary retention.

NEURO-UROLOGIC DISORDERS IN CHILDREN

This section explores the neuro-urologic dysfunctions commonly seen in the pediatric population. The major neurologic causes of voiding dysfunction include myelodysplasia, spinal cord tumor, injury to spinal cord, or spinal cord malformation (Krane & Siroky, 1979). The functional and anatomic causes of voiding dysfunction are not discussed here.

Myelodysplasia is a cystic dilation of the meninges associated with dysplasia of the underlying spinal cord (McGuire, 1988). There is an absence of skin covering the meningomyelocele. The neurologic complications rise from damage to specific nerve root and from spinal cord injury. At birth, the child presents with an areflexic bladder and an open, nonfunctional vesical outlet. Upper urinary tract damage, such as ureteral dilatation, vesicoureteral reflux, hydroureteronephrosis, stone formation, and ultimately chronic renal failure, may occur (McGuire, 1988).

Loss of voluntary bladder control may be the result of an areflexic (60%) or hyperreflexic (25%) detrusor muscle (Bauer, 1979). Electromyogram of the striated urethral sphincter shows denervation. With increased intra-abdominal pressure, the sphincter fails to relax, producing an outlet obstruction. As a result, patients are incontinent with poor bladder emptying.

Continence may be obtained through alpha-adrenergic stimulating agents, such as ephedrine. Intermittent catheterizations may improve continence; however, this is dependent on urethral sphincter competence. Oxybutynin infused intravesically in combination with intermittent catheterization has been found to improve bladder capacity and decrease incontinence between intermittent catheterizations (Greenfield & Fera, 1991). An artificial sphincter or rectal fascia sling may also be useful in promoting continence (Belloli, Campobasso, & Mercurella, 1992; Herschorn & Radomski, 1992).

Strategic planning for this disorder requires input from the child, the parents, and the health care professional. Management is based on changing the child's voiding habit through education, behavioral therapy, and psychosocial support. Parents are encouraged to learn catheterization techniques along with the child. A schedule of frequent voiding or catheterization is created, along with administration of medications and behavioral therapy. For school-aged children, health care professionals and parents should discuss the child's problem with school administrators, teachers, and the school nurse. Supplies for catheterizations may be stored in the nurse's office during school hours. Children should be encouraged to have a change of clothing available at school should an accident occur.

Another congenital abnormality responsible for neuro-urologic dysfunction is sacral agenesis. This is a congenital abnormality of the vertebral column. One or more parts of the sacral segment are missing. Other abnormalities may be present from the cephalad to the sacral lesion.

Detrusor denervation may produce a hyperreflexic or areflexic bladder. Urethral sphincter electromyogram reveals denervation. Sacral sensation is present. Patients often present with urinary retention, abnormal voiding, or incontinence.

Treatment for sacral agenesis is similar to that for myelodysplasia. The plan focuses on bladder elimination and promotion of continence.

PSYCHOSOCIAL CONCERNS

Any source of altered urinary elimination is a natural cause of concern for an individual. It may signify a loss of control over a very private body function and may decrease self-esteem. Disruption of daily routine and lifestyle, as well as work and family dynamics, can occur. Coping with these alterations and achieving acceptable forms of bladder elimination are of prime importance to the patient. To attain success, a bladder reconditioning program must be individualized, taking into consideration the patient's psychosocial, vocational, and physical needs. Personal preference is a factor that cannot be overlooked.

The outcome of a bladder retraining program depends on a realistic plan and on maximizing involvement of the patient and the family. The nurse has a unique role in coordination of the patient's bladder rehabilitation program, incorporating essential components from all disciplines involved in the team. By assessing the patient's total needs and including clinical and diagnostic findings, the nurse is able to assist the patient in a healthy adaptation to the neuro-urologic disorder. Within the realm of the team's therapeutic program, the knowledgeable and skilled nurse can help the patient choose the type of urinary drainage most suitable and plan a mutually workable regimen. It is important to remember that these adjustments must be adaptable to the patient's home and community environments. Anticipating these changes benefits discharge planning and ensures a realistic management regimen for the patient.

References

Bauer, S. B. (1979). Pediatric neuro-urology. In R. J. Krane & M. B. Siroky (Eds.), *Clinical neurourology* (pp. 275–293). Boston: Little, Brown.

Belloli, G., Campobasso, P., & Mercurella, A. (1992). Neuropathic urinary incontinence in pediatric patients: Management with artificial sphincter. *Journal of Pediatric Surgery, 27*(11), 1461–1464.

Bradley, W. E. (1993). The diagnosis and treatment of patients with neurologic dysfunction of the urinary bladder. In P. A. Low (Ed.), *Clinical autonomic disorders* (pp. 573–588). Boston: Little, Brown.

Greenfield, S. P., & Fera, M. (1991). The use of intravesical oxybutynin chloride in children with neurogenic bladder. *Journal of Urology, 146*(8), 532–534.

Hackler, R. (1979). Surgical treatment of the adult neurogenic bladder dysfunction. In R. J. Krane & M. B. Siroky (Eds.), *Clinical neuro-urology* (pp. 197–212). Boston: Little, Brown.

Henderson, J. S. (1988). A pubococcygeal exercise program for simple urinary stress incontinence: Applicability to the female client with multiple sclerosis. *Journal of Neuroscience Nursing, 20*(3), 185–188.

Herschorn, S., & Radomski, S. B. (1992). Fascial slings and bladder neck tapering in the treatment of male neurogenic incontinence. *Journal of Urology, 147*(4), 1073–1075.

Johnson, D. E., Muncie, H. L., O'Reilly, J. L., & Warren, J. W. (1990). An external urine collection device for incontinent women. *Journal of the American Geriatrics Society, 38*(9), 1016–1022.

Khanna, O. P. (1979). Nonsurgical therapeutic modalities. In R. J. Krane & M. B. Siroky (Eds.), *Clinical neuro-urology* (pp. 159–196). Boston: Little, Brown.

Krane, R. J., & Siroky, M. B. (1979). Classification of neuro-urologic disorders. In R. J. Krane & M. B. Siroky (Eds.), *Clinical neuro-urology* (pp. 143–158). Boston: Little, Brown.

Lapides, J. (1970). Neuromuscular vesical and ureteral dysfunction. In M. F. Campbell & J. H. Harrison (Eds.), *Urology* (p. 1343). Philadelphia: W.B. Saunders.

McGuire, E. J. (1988). Myelodysplasia. *Seminars in Neurology, 8*(2), 145–149.

O'Donnell, P. D., & Doyle, R. (1991). Biofeedback therapy techniques for treatment of urinary incontinence. *Urology, 37*(5), 432–436.

Peggs, J. F. (1992). Urinary incontinence in the elderly: Pharmacologic therapies. *American Family Physician, 46*(6), 1763–1769.

Perkash, L. (1993). Long-term urologic management of the patient with spinal cord injury. *Urologic Clinics of North America, 20*(3), 423–434.

Schmidt, R. A. (1991). Treatment of unstable bladder. *Urology, 37*(1), 28–32.

Weiss, B. D. (1991). Nonpharmacologic treatment of urinary incontinence. *American Family Physician, 44*(2), 579–586.

Wiseman, P. A., Malone-Lee, J., & Rai, G. S. (1991). Terodiline with bladder retraining for treating detrusor instability in elderly people. *British Medical Journal, 302*(6783), 994–996.

Yalla, S. V., & Bushra, A. F. (1991). Spinal cord injury. In R. J. Krane & M. B. Siroky (Eds.), *Clinical neuro-urology* (2nd ed., pp. 319–331). Boston: Little, Brown.

Alterations in Bowel Elimination

ROSE ROSSI SCHWARTZ

Bowel elimination depends on several factors including cognition, stool volume and consistency, colonic transit, rectal distention, anal sphincter function, anorectal sensation, and anorectal reflexes (Madoff, Williams, & Caushaj, 1992). Abnormalities in any of these factors may lead to incontinence, constipation, or diarrhea. For the patient with a neurologic disorder, disruption of the balance between the nervous system and the gastrointestinal system may compromise bowel function or voluntary control of defecation (Table 28–1). Factors impeding bowel control include loss of cerebral awareness and ability to inhibit defecation, loss of anal sphincter sensation, and loss of anal sphincter control. The location and extent of a lesion determine what type of bowel dysfunction is present. Nursing care of the patient with alteration in bowel elimination is aimed at promoting continence, maintaining bowel function, and encouraging independence. Assessment of bowel function and of defecation patterns is presented in Chapter 26.

NEUROGENIC BOWEL DYSFUNCTIONS

Neurogenic bowel is defined as a bowel dysfunction that occurs because of an interruption of the neural pathways that supply the rectum, external sphincter, and accessory muscles that inhibit or initiate evacuation. The function of each part of the system is greatly dependent on the others. Five classifications of neurogenic bowel dysfunction, based on the location of a neural lesion, are discussed: uninhibited, reflex, autonomous, motor paralytic, and sensory paralytic. These categories and their neural correlates, related disease states, and associated signs and symptoms are shown in Table 28–2.

Urgency or Bowel Incontinence Related to Uninhibited Neurogenic Bowel

Supraspinal bowel dysfunctions are related to lesions above the level of the pons. Related factors associated with uninhibited neurogenic bowel include

TABLE 28–1 • CLASSIFICATION AND ETIOLOGY OF FECAL INCONTINENCE

I. Altered stool consistency
  A. Diarrhea
  B. Constipation

II. Inadequate rectal sensation
  A. Neurologic condition
    1. Dementia
    2. Stroke
    3. Tabes dorsalis
    4. Multiple sclerosis
    5. Injuries
      a. Brain
      b. Spinal cord
      c. Cauda equina
    6. Neoplasms
      a. Brain
      b. Spinal cord
      c. Cauda equina
    7. Sensory neuropathy
  B. Overflow incontinence
    1. Fecal impaction
    2. Encopresis
    3. Use of psychotropic drugs
    4. Use of antimotility drugs

III. Abnormal sphincter mechanism of pelvic floor
  A. Anatomic sphincter defect
    1. Traumatic
    2. Neoplastic
    3. Inflammatory
  B. Pelvic floor denervation
    1. Primary
      a. Pudendal neuropathy
      b. Chronic straining at stool
    2. Secondary
      a. Injuries to the spinal cord, cauda equina, or pelvic floor nerves
      b. Diabetic neuropathy
  C. Congenital abnormalities
    1. Spina bifida
    2. Myelomeningocele

Adapted from Marcio, J., Jorge, N., & Wexner, S. D. (1993). Etiology and management of fecal incontinence. *Diseases of the Colon and Rectum, 36*(1), 70–97.

stroke, multiple sclerosis (MS), head injury, Parkinson's disease, and brain tumor. Perception of the need to evacuate and also motor function to reach the bathroom and initiate the motor activity of evacuation are necessary for voluntary elimination (Liptak & Revell, 1992). Defining characteristics of uninhibited neurogenic bowel include delayed gastric emptying, constipation, and fecal incontinence (Caruana, Wald, Hinds, & Eidelman, 1991). In the elderly, incontinence is usually the result of abnormal sensation and decreased resting sphincter pressure (Madoff et al., 1992).

TABLE 28–2 • LEVELS OF NEURAXIAL DYSFUNCTION AFFECTING DEFECATION

Bowel Function	Level in Neuraxis	Possible Etiology	Upper Motor Neuron Lesion	Lower Motor Neuron Lesion	Sensory Loss	Saddle Sensation	Bulbocavernous Reflex	Fecal Incontinence
Uninhibited neurogenic	Cortical and subcortical	Stroke, MS, brain tumor, brain trauma	+	0	0	Normal	Normal or increased	Present—associated with sudden urge
Reflex neurogenic	Spinal cord above conus medullaris	Trauma, tumor, vascular disease, MS, syringomyelia, pernicious anemia	+	0	+	Diminished or absent	Increased	Present—occurs without warning or during mass reflex
Autonomous neurogenic	Conus medullaris or cauda equina	Spina bifida, trauma, tumor, intervertebral disk	0	+	+	Diminished or absent	0	Present—may be continuous or may occur during stress
Motor paralytic	Anterior horn cells or S2, S3, S4 roots (ventral)	Poliomyelitis, intervertebral disk, trauma, tumor	0	+	0	Normal	0	Rare, except in widespread disease
Sensory paralytic	S2, S3, S4 roots (dorsal), cells of origin or dorsal horns of spinal cord	Diabetes mellitus, tabes dorsalis	0	0	+	Diminished or absent	Normal, decreased, or absent	Rare, except in advanced stages

From Staas, W. E., & DeNault, P. M. (1973). Bowel control. *American Family Physician, 7*(1), 126–128.
Abbreviation: MS, multiple sclerosis.

The rectum does not have sensory receptors. The proprioceptors are situated in the levator muscles, puborectal muscle, and anal sphincter surrounding the rectum (Marcio, Jorge, & Wexner, 1993). In this disorder, the sacral reflex arc and perianal sensation are intact, but cerebral inhibitory or facilitory interpretation of the sensory impulses to defecate is interrupted. When a fecal bolus is in the rectum, a reflex relaxation of the anal sphincter occurs. A sense of urgency and involuntary elimination or incontinence occurs because the sacral reflex acts alone without inhibition from higher cerebral centers. Medications often used in the treatment of neurologic disorders, as well as resulting immobility, may also contribute to a decrease in the ability to evacuate effectively.

On examination, bowel and saddle sensations are intact. The bulbocavernous reflex is intact or increased. Fecal incontinence with urgency is present.

The outcomes of therapy are aimed at complete evacuation of stool and creation of a pattern of elimination. The individual with a cerebral lesion may have cognitive dysfunction in attention, concentration, judgment, and memory. These impairments may lead to difficulty with integration of stimuli and generalization of the bowel program to the home environment. Therefore, the program must be uncomplicated so that the individual can master it.

Nursing interventions include pharmacologic therapy, bowel training, biofeedback, and alternative therapies. Rectal suppositories have been a useful part of a bowel-training program. Suppositories increase rectal sensation and increase awareness of the urge to defecate. They are also an effective means of stimulating lubrication of the anal tract. For bowel training, suppositories are initially used to stimulate the anorectal reflex. This, combined with a management program including timing of evacuation and increased intake of fluid and dietary fiber, has been found to be effective (Venn, Taft, Carpentier, & Applebaugh, 1992). Once a routine is established, the suppositories should be discontinued.

Biofeedback has also been found effective in increasing rectal sensation. The treatment uses physiologic responses converted to electrical signals that are routed to the patient. For rectal sensation, a balloon is placed in the rectum to simulate the sensation of stool. This is coordinated with a contraction of the external sphincter (Madoff et al., 1992). These signals are sent to a biofeedback unit and displayed visually. Techniques are available to assist visually, cognitively, or auditorily impaired patients.

For the control of incontinence not managed by conservative means, one option may be an anal incontinence plug. The Conseal colostomy plug provides an alternative to surgical management of incontinence. It is not intended for permanent use but may be useful on occasions when fecal leakage may create social embarrassment (Christiansen & Roed-Peterson, 1993; Mortensten & Humphreys, 1991).

As with any treatment plan, planning bowel elimination requires assessment of the patient's preexisting bowel habits as well as his or her present needs (see Principles of Bowel Management). The goal for this patient is to be free from incontinence and constipation.

• C A S E   S T U D Y   1

Mrs. C, a 63-year-old right-handed woman, came to the emergency department with left-sided weakness and slurred speech. The symptoms had progressed since their onset the previous morning shortly after she arose from bed. Findings included left hemiparesis with diminished position sense and stereogenesis of the left hand, left homonymous hemianopsia, and Babinski's reflex on the left. A diagnosis of a stroke secondary to thrombosis of the right middle cerebral artery was made. Mrs. C had a history of untreated transient ischemic attacks persisting for the past 2 to 3 months. She had been treated for hypertension.

Mrs. C was admitted to the neurologic unit. Her nursing care plan, which focused on immediate as well as long-term physical, functional, and psychosocial needs, included the nursing diagnosis of potential constipation and fecal impaction: altered bowel elimination pattern exhibited by a person with a cerebral lesion. Expected outcomes included establishment of a habit pattern of elimination in which a persistent and consistent approach was used to encourage Mrs. C to focus attention on elimination.

During the acute recovery stages, Mrs. C's nursing care focused on maintenance of normal body functions. The bowel management program, in particular, was directed toward prevention of constipation and fecal impaction. A comprehensive nursing assessment included investigation of previous bowel habits, nutrition, and diet history. Mrs. C had been accustomed to a daily evacuation in the morning. Her present neurologic and physical status was reviewed. Saddle sensation and bulbocavernous reflex were intact. The gag reflex was intact. She was initially on bedrest. After 48 hours, it was determined that there was no further neurologic deficit, and nutrition was advanced from intravenous to regular diet as tolerated. The left-sided hemiparesis persisted. When solid foods were tolerated, Mrs. C was encouraged to feed herself while sitting in high Fowler's position. She was encouraged to place food in the right side of her mouth because of left lower facial muscle weakness.

At this point, Mrs. C's bowel program consisted of 30 mL of milk of magnesia at bedtime followed by a glycerine suppository in the morning after breakfast to coincide with the gastrocolic reflex and her previous elimination patterns. An elimination record was started. Her stool was soft and firm, negating the need for a stool softener. She had a sense of urgency just before defecation, resulting in incontinence. The occurrence of incontinence was embarrassing for Mrs. C and discouraging to her husband. Emotional support, understanding, and explanations were provided. Initially, bowel care was performed in bed in a side-lying position (see Principles of Bowel Management for positioning techniques and suppository administration procedure). Privacy was ensured, and a relaxed atmosphere was established. Mrs. C was instructed not to bear down during defecation.

Within the first week after the stroke, Mrs. C tolerated her diet well. Increased fiber was then added to her diet. She was taking fluids well without restriction. When bathroom privileges were allowed, toileting was done on a commode chair in the bathroom. Mrs. C required assistance with transfer activities, and a safety belt was used on the commode chair. Her feet were supported on a footstool to encourage a squatlike position. Abdominal massage was used to facilitate defecation.

Bowel management goals soon advanced to establishment of a planned "habit time" elimination routine. As Mrs. C's therapy program progressed, ambulation and functional abilities increased. The bowel record showed that Mrs. C was having daily adequate bowel movements after suppository administration without spontaneous stools between elimination times. Suppository use was discontinued, and Mrs. C started using the toilet for evacuation. A schedule of toileting immediately after breakfast was maintained. Milk of magnesia at bedtime was later replaced with prune juice. At the time of hospital discharge, a bowel care routine of prune juice at bedtime and toileting after breakfast had proved workable for Mrs. C. A habit of routine elimination had been attained.

Potential Fecal Impaction or Incontinence Related to Reflex Neurogenic Bowel

Reflex neurogenic bowel occurs with lesions between the pons and the sacral spinal cord (Liptak & Revell, 1992). Related factors of reflex neurogenic bowel include spinal cord trauma, spinal tumors, spinal vascular disorders of the cord, or disease processes such as MS or syringomyelia. The presence of a lesion at this level, especially above the S2, S3, and S4 spinal cord segments, causes an interruption of ascending sensory signals between the sacral reflex center (S2–S4) and the brain. This results in an inability to feel the urge to defecate. The most significant loss of bowel function presents as a loss of voluntary control over the external anal sphincter. The external sphincter remains in a contracted state because of parasympathetic innervation through the sacral segments of the spinal cord (Martin, Holt, & Hicks, 1981). Anal tone is also reduced because of decreased sympathetic outflow to the gastrointestinal tract (Sun, Read, & Donnelly, 1991). Because the lesion is above the conus medullaris, the S2, S3, and S4 nerve segments that govern defecation are intact.

Assessment of the patient with reflex neurogenic bowel demonstrates absent cerebral awareness and voluntary control. Saddle sensation is diminished or absent. The bulbocavernous reflex is hyperactive. Fecal incontinence may occur but is rare. Fecal impaction and retention are common.

The outcome goal of the treatment plan is to have planned, predictable eliminations. Management of this disorder focuses on stimulation of the intact sacral reflex arc. A structured bowel management program is developed to ensure adequate emptying and prevent incontinence.

During the acute stages after spinal cord injury, the focus of nursing interventions is on prevention of complications of spinal cord injury and on control of incontinence. Gastrointestinal complications include paralytic ileus and stress ulcers. Other complications may include autonomic dysreflexia.

Initially, following spinal cord injury, there is a state of spinal cord shock that may result in loss of gastrointestinal activity for as long as 2 to 3 days. This is the result of tonic paralysis of the intestines together with a flaccid anal sphincter. Lack of tone results in a loss of bowel sounds and abdominal distention. Progressive abdominal distention can cause vomiting, with possible aspiration, or may interfere with diaphragmatic excursion, resulting in respiratory distress. Intravenous fluids are usually ordered to replace oral intake until bowel sounds return. A rectal tube may be required to decompress the bowel. Rectal tubes should be used for short, intermittent periods because of the asensory state of the anorectal cavity. There is a danger of ischemia to the rectal mucosa from the constant pressure of the tube.

When bowel sounds return and flatus passes, the patient's diet should advance slowly from fluids to a full diet as tolerated. A manual rectal examination and evacuation of any stool are performed daily (Table 28–3).

During the acute period, the patient is prone to the development of gastric mucosal hemorrhages and stress ulcerations in the stomach or the duodenum. Stress ulcers generally occur within the first 4 weeks and can result in hemorrhage (Kewalramani, 1979). Stress ulcers are thought to be caused by increased levels of catecholamines and steroids after injury. Patients with a history of gastric or duodenal ulcerations are particularly susceptible to recurrence (Perkash, 1990). Drugs such as ranitidine or antacids are useful in the prevention of stress ulcers (Table 28–4). Emesis, gastric drainage, and stool should be tested for the presence of occult blood.

Autonomic dysreflexia is a life-threatening condition associated with a sharp rise in blood pressure, bradycardia, sweating, piloerection, blurred vision, nasal congestion, and increase in spasticity. This disorder may be the result of a hyperactive outflow of sympathetic signals at the interrupted level of the cord. Symptoms may be precipitated by many noxious stimuli, especially a

TABLE 28–3 • TECHNIQUES TO STIMULATE OR FACILITATE BOWEL EVACUATION

Digital Stimulation

Insert a gloved, lubricated finger into the rectum, pointed posteriorly, and use a gentle circular massage for 1–2 min. When the internal sphincter relaxes, stop the massage. Wait for 30 min for evacuation to occur.

Valsalva's Maneuver

Instruct patient to bear down and push. This requires the use of abdominal and pelvic muscles and is dependent on intact innervation of the lower thoracic cord. Similar activities include forward bends and pushups from the toilet seat. To accomplish this, patient should grasp the toilet seat on each side with his or her hands and lift his or her trunk off the toilet seat.

Abdominal Massage

Instruct patient to massage abdomen in a clockwise direction following the anatomic course of the colon.

Positioning

Patient should be sitting in a high Fowler's position. A squatting position with the knees higher than the hips is achieved by supporting the feet on a footstool. This position further increases intra-abdominal pressure.

Manual Evacuation

1. Should be performed with patient in a sitting position to increase intra-abdominal pressure on the bladder. The rectum is then digitally emptied of stool. Manual evacuation should be stopped at any signs of autonomic dysreflexia.
2. Flexion of hips and knees with feet supported on a stool assists patient in assuming a squatting position. Valsalva's maneuver, forward bends, and abdominal massage are also used.
3. A gloved, well-lubricated finger is inserted into the rectum in a posterior direction to avoid pressure.

TABLE 28–4 • PHARMACOLOGIC AGENTS

Drug	Indication	Dose	Mechanism of Action
Anti-ulcer			
Cimetidine (Tagamet)	Duodenal ulcer	800 mg daily in divided doses	Inhibits the action of histamine (H_2), decreasing gastric acid secretions
Famotidine (Pepcid)	Duodenal ulcer	40 mg daily in divided doses	Inhibits the action of histamine (H_2), decreasing gastric acid secretions
Nizatidine (Axid)	Duodenal ulcer	300 mg daily	Inhibits the action of histamine (H_2), decreasing gastric acid secretions
Omeprazole (Prilosec)	Esophagitis, gastroesophageal reflux	20 mg daily for 8 weeks	Inhibits the activity of the acid pump; blocks the formation of gastric acid
Ranitidine (Zantac)	Duodenal and gastric ulcers	300 mg daily in divided doses	Inhibits the action of histamine (H_2), decreasing gastric acid secretions
Sucralfate (Carafate)	Duodenal ulcer	4 g daily in divided doses	Adheres to and protects the ulcer surface by forming a barrier
Antacid			
Aluminum hydroxide (Amphojel)	Gastric upset	Depends on product chosen	Reduces total gastric load in the GI tract; strengthens gastric mucosal barrier
Aluminum hydroxide/ magnesium hydroxide (Maalox)			
Aluminum hydroxide/ magnesium hydroxide/ simethicone (Mylanta)			
Magaldrate/simethicone (Riopan)			
Antidiarrheal			
Diphenoxylate (Lomotil)	Diarrhea	10–20 mg daily in divided doses	Increases smooth muscle tone in the GI tract; inhibits motility and propulsion
Loperamide (Imodium)	Diarrhea	Maximum of 16 mg daily	Inhibits peristaltic activity, prolonging transit of intestinal contents
Laxatives and softeners			
Bisacodyl (Dulcolax)	Constipation	Up to 30 mg p.o. or 1–2 suppositories daily	Increases peristalsis by irritating the musculature or stimulating the colonic intramural plexus
Calcium polycarbophil (FiberCon)	Constipation	4 g daily in divided doses	Increases bulk and moisture content of the stool

TABLE 28–4 • PHARMACOLOGIC AGENTS *Continued*

Drug	Indication	Dose	Mechanism of Action
Docusate (Colace)	Stool softener	50–300 mg per day in divided doses	Reduces surface tension of interfacing liquid contents of the bowel
Lactulose (Chronulac)	Constipation	30–120 mL daily in divided doses	Produces an osmotic effect in the colon
Magnesium hydroxide (milk of magnesia)	Constipation	10–20 mL daily	Produces an osmotic effect in the small intestine
Methylcellulose (Citrucel)	Constipation	1 tsp t.i.d.	Increases bulk and moisture content of the stool
Psyllium (Metamucil)	Constipation	1 tsp t.i.d.	Increases bulk and moisture content of the stool
Senna (Senokot)	Constipation	1 to 8 tablets daily in divided doses	Increases peristalsis by irritating the musculature or stimulating the colonic intramural plexus

Abbreviations: GI, gastrointestinal; p.o., per os (by mouth); t.i.d., ter in die (three times a day).

distended bladder or fecal impaction (Ropper, 1993). It is commonly seen in reflex neurogenic bladder. If the precipitating factor can be identified and eliminated, this will usually result in resolution of the symptoms within 2 to 10 minutes.

Interventions to promote fecal continence and prevent retention are possible through a bowel-retraining program. This can be accomplished through timed bowel programs (Table 28–5), bowel stimulation techniques (see Table 28–3), biofeedback, a diet generous in high fiber foods (Table 28–6), and medication (see Table 28–4) if necessary. Frequent bowel care will prevent colonic

TABLE 28–5 • BOWEL RETRAINING PROGRAM

1. Check the rectum with a gloved, lubricated finger, and remove any stool that is present. Insert a suppository into the rectum so that it touches the wall of the rectum above the anal sphincter. Suppositories must be in contact with the rectal mucosa to be effective. If stool is present in the rectum, manually disimpact the patient and proceed in placing the suppository.
2. Patients should be encouraged to facilitate bowel elimination through Valsalva's maneuver (bearing down), forward bends, and abdominal massage in a clockwise direction.
3. On the next day and thereafter, give the patient an opportunity to defecate without external stimulation at the scheduled time. If no spontaneous bowel movement occurs within 4 hr, administer a suppository until a pattern of regular defecation occurs for five consecutive scheduled times.
4. Once the pattern has been established, attempts should be made to discontinue the suppository to determine if the patient can have a spontaneous bowel movement without external stimulation.
5. If the suppository is not effective in stimulating defecation, digital stimulation of the rectum should be performed if this procedure is not painful to the patient or contraindicated by the patient's condition.

Adapted from Sun, W. M., Read, N. W., & Donnelly, T. C. (1991). Anorectal function in incontinent patients with cerebrospinal disease. *Gastroenterology, 99*(5), 1372–1379.

TABLE 28–6 • HIGH-FIBER FOODS		
Vegetables	**Fruits**	**Whole-Grain Products**
Asparagus	Apples	Wheat bran
Baked beans	Apricots	Wheat germ
Broccoli	Cherries	Cracked wheat
Brussels sprouts	Figs	Whole wheat bread
Cabbage	Oranges	Pumpernickel bread
Carrots	Berries	Oatmeal
Cauliflower	Grapefruit	Bran
Celery	Peaches	Shredded wheat
Corn	Pears	Rye crisp
Eggplant	Plums	Wheat crisp
Green beans	Prunes	Brown bread
Lima beans	Dried fruits	Cornmeal
Onions		Brown rice
Peas (all varieties)		Nuts
Peppers		Sunflower seeds
Potato skins		Popcorn
Radishes		
Spinach		
Squash		
Tomatoes		
Turnips		

distention with stool and may enhance colonic transit by the anocolic reflex (Liptak & Revell, 1992).

The individual is encouraged to participate actively in the bowel program. Patients and families, as well as attendants if needed, must learn all aspects of bowel management. If the individual has adequate hand and finger function, he or she will assume the responsibility of independent bowel care before returning home. If hand functioning for glove and digital stimulation is lacking, a digital stimulator may be appropriate. For the high cervical level quadriplegic patient with very limited hand and finger ability, attendant care is necessary for elimination.

Constipation and Overflow Incontinence Related to Autonomous Neurogenic Bowel

Complete or partial injury to the cauda equina or sacral segments (S2–S4) results in loss of lower motor neuron function, causing an autonomous bowel (Banwell, Creasey, Aggarwal, & Mortimer, 1993). The presence of a spinal cord lesion at this level destroys the sacral reflex center. Related factors of autonomous neurogenic bowel include trauma, spina bifida, tumor, or intervertebral disk disease. Resulting complications include loss of effective propulsive stimulation of the colon, lack of rectal sensation, decreased intra-abdominal pressure, and decreased anal sphincter tone (Banwell et al., 1993). Defining characteristics of autonomous neurogenic bladder include lack of awareness of the urge to defecate and loss of voluntary control of the external anal sphincter.

Examination demonstrates decreased or absent rectal and saddle sensation. Bulbocavernous reflex is absent. Patients present with retention and oozing of stool through the relaxed anal sphincter.

Outcomes are aimed at keeping the rectum free of stool and preventing incontinence. Nursing interventions include dietary management, bowel training, and surgery. Stool consistency should be firm but not hard. This can be accomplished through the use of dietary fibers and fluid intake (see Table 28–6). Manual evacuation of stool may become necessary (see Table 28–3). Techniques used to trigger a stimulus-response reflex, such as digital stimulation or suppository administration, are not effective with areflexic bowel because of the absence of the sacral reflex arc. When diarrhea is present, fecal impaction must be ruled out. Loose stools that occur suddenly are generally characteristic of diarrhea; however, the frequent or continuous oozing of stool is usually indicative of inadequate bowel emptying or fecal impaction.

In patients who have failed all attempts to manage their bowel care, colostomy may provide relief. However, colostomy should be reserved for patients with severe long-term disability, weight loss, and exhaustion of all nonsurgical options. Transit time studies determine the length of colon to be removed (Liptak & Revell, 1992).

Constipation Related to Motor Paralytic Bowel

Disease of the anterior horn cells or S2, S3, and S4 ventral roots results in motor paralytic bowel. Factors related to motor paralytic bowel may be secondary to poliomyelitis, intervertebral disk disease, trauma, or tumor. Defining characteristics include constipation and, rarely, incontinence. Constipation usually occurs as a result of poor rectal compliance. Incontinence may also occur as a result of smaller volumes of feces leading to higher intraluminal pressure (Marcio et al., 1993).

On examination, sensation is intact. The bulbocavernous reflex is absent. An areflexic bowel is exhibited with sensory sparing. The patient faces constipation as a complication of this disorder.

The outcome goal of motor paralytic bowel is prevention of constipation. The individual has sensory awareness of rectal fullness but does not have the advantage of the sacral reflex arc to stimulate peristalsis. A sluggish bowel results.

Nursing interventions are similar to those used with other types of neurogenic bowel dysfunction in which constipation is a problem. Bowel training includes planning for a scheduled bowel routine. The plan should take advantage of the gastrocolic reflex. Dietary management includes consumption of high-fiber foods (see Table 28–6) and increased fluid intake. Physical activity and exercise are encouraged to promote peristalsis. Positioning and techniques to increase intra-abdominal pressure to aid in stool evacuation may also be helpful.

Constipation Related to Sensory Paralytic Bowel

Lesions that involve the sacral (S2, S3, S4) dorsal roots, cells of origin, or the dorsal horns of the spinal cord result in sensory paralysis with sparing of the upper and lower motor neurons. The pudendal nerve is affected, causing diminished or absent denervation of the external anal sphincter, levator ani muscle, and puborectal muscle (Marcio et al., 1993; Vernava, Longo, & Daniel, 1993). Factors related to sensory paralytic bowel are seen with diabetes, tabes dorsalis, and anal sphincter tears. Constipation usually occurs as a result of diminished sensory awareness of distended rectum and slowed colonic motility. Chronic constipation can lead to overdistention of the colon, with further loss of tone. The occurrence of megacolon must be avoided.

On examination, the patient displays diminished or absent saddle sensation. Bulbocavernous reflex may be normal, diminished, or absent. Patients present with constipation and increased rectal compliance.

The outcome goals of sensory paralytic bowel are directed toward prevention of constipation and overdistention of the bowel. Interventions include bowel retraining, diet, exercise, and surgery. The plan of care is based on assessment of nutrition and bowel habit history. A bowel-retraining program, in conjunction with diet and fluid intake modification, exercise, positioning, and use of medications as needed, is required to prevent constipation.

Patients suffering from pudendal neuropathy may benefit from stimulation of the pudendo-anal reflex. Electrodes are placed on the pelvic floor and the external sphincter. As a result of the stimulation, the pudendo-anal reflex is activated, causing contraction of the external sphincter and expulsion of stool (Binnie, Kawimbe, Papachrysostomou, & Smith, 1990). Further research is necessary to determine the long-term benefits of this therapy.

If constipation is unmanageable by conservative means, a surgical approach may be required. Sphincter repair is considered in patients with a defined muscular defect. This can be accomplished by reconstruction of the sphincter and the pelvic floor (Christiansen & Sparso, 1992). The procedure may be beneficial in neurogenic and idiopathic constipation, but the results have been suboptimal (Marcio et al., 1993). One development is an implantable artificial anal sphincter. This device contains an inflatable cuff that provides complete control over bowel function (Christiansen & Sparso, 1992; Madoff et al., 1992).

PEDIATRIC ISSUES

Children are also faced with the prospect of neuromuscular bowel dysfunction. Disorders, such as myelomeningocele, spina bifida, and spinal cord injury, may lead to fecal incontinence or retention. The ability to manage one's personal hygiene is a major milestone in the child's personal and social development (Lie et al., 1991).

Parents and children are often not provided with information on incontinence or how to deal with it. Options for this population had previously been limited to incontinence pads or colostomy, but bowel management programs have been successful in some cases. Other alternatives include medication or surgery. Blair et al. (1992) found the bowel management tube to be an effective alternative for controlling fecal incontinence. A small enema is administered through the tube and retained for 5 minutes with the use of a Silastic balloon. This system is not effective on children younger than 4 years. Also, leakage around the balloon during the enema may occur. The most serious risk is bacteremia (Lisenmeyer & Stone, 1993). Further research on the long-term effectiveness of this technique is still required.

Continence is an important objective in the development of independence in children and must be a goal for children with neuromuscular bowel dysfunction (Lisenmeyer & Stone, 1993). Little information addressing this issue is available to parents and children. Additional knowledge and research are needed in this area.

PRINCIPLES OF BOWEL MANAGEMENT

Goals of Bowel Management

Bowel management is a planned program that uses comprehensive and individualized approaches based on the nursing assessment and the specific bowel dysfunction present to predetermine the method and the timing of evacuation (Table 28–7). A well-planned, workable bowel program makes it possible for the individual to regain control over defecation when voluntary control is precluded because of motor or sensory dysfunction. The goals for an effective bowel care program are as follows:

1. The program focuses on establishing a regular, predictable, and reliable time for evacuation to prevent accidental or spontaneous bowel movements.

2. The program must be consistent and maintained, yet flexible enough to meet the needs of the individual's lifestyle. It must be convenient and practical to fit into her or his daily activities comfortably.

3. The program should ensure adequate elimination to maintain satisfactory bowel function and prevent complications.

Implementing a Bowel Management Program

In addition to determination of the type of bowel dysfunction exhibited and comprehensive assessment of preexisting conditions affecting bowel elimination, other factors must be considered in planning and implementing a bowel management program.

TABLE 28–7 • NEUROGENIC BOWEL DYSFUNCTION—NURSING MANAGEMENT

Level of Lesion	Dysfunction Classification	Potential Problems and Characteristics	Nursing Interventions	Potential Problems
Cortical and subcortical	Uninhibited	Sense of urgency, involuntary defecation that may be infrequent or frequent	Consistent habit time Physical exercise High fluid intake High-fiber foods Suppository as needed	Constipation Elimination record
Spinal cord above S2, S3, S4	Reflex, automatic	Infrequent, sudden, unexpected, occurs without warning	Stimulus response evacuation Suppository use Digital stimulation Consistent habit time with planned evacuation every 2–3 days Elimination record Physical exercise High fluid intake High-fiber foods Valsalva's maneuver Techniques to increase intra-abdominal pressure at evacuation	Fecal impaction Autonomic dysreflexia

Spinal cord at S2, S3, S4 or cauda equina	Areflexic-flaccid, autonomous	May be frequent if rectum not emptied of stool, induced by physical exertion	Manual evacuation Maintain firm stool Maintain empty rectum Consistent habit time with planned evacuation daily Elimination record Physical exercise High fluid intake High-fiber foods Valsalva's maneuver Techniques to increase intra-abdominal pressure at evacuation	Fecal retention with oozing of stool
Anterior horn cells or S2, S3, S4 ventral root	Motor paralytic	Infrequent	Consistent habit time Elimination record Physical exercise High fluid intake High-fiber foods Valsalva's maneuver Techniques to increase intra-abdominal pressure at evacuation	Constipation
S2, S3, S4 dorsal root, cells of origin, or dorsal horn	Sensory paralytic	Infrequent	Same as motor paralytic	Constipation Bowel overdistention

Adapted from Martin, N., Holt, N., & Hicks, D. (1981). *Comprehensive rehabilitation nursing.* New York: McGraw-Hill.

TIMING

Planning a consistent schedule for time of evacuation is of utmost importance in establishing a predictable and reliable bowel routine. In the acute care stages, a morning schedule may be most convenient. As activity and mobility increase, however, a program needs to be developed into which the patient's previous bowel habits and the routine the individual will follow after discharge are incorporated. A person's life should not be governed by a bowel routine. It may be necessary for the individual to change the time of bowel evacuation to accommodate such factors as work or school schedule or time of attendant care. Because it may take 1 to 2 weeks or longer to reestablish a bowel routine on a new schedule, frequent time changes are discouraged. If it is necessary to change the timing of bowel care, starting a day early at the new time and administering a mild laxative 8 hours previously will get the bowel started on the new schedule.

Evacuation should be scheduled for 15 to 30 minutes after a meal, generally in the morning or evening, taking advantage of the gastrocolic reflex action. Drinking a warm liquid before defecation may also assist in stimulating peristalsis. Frequency of evacuation is individualized to the type of bowel dysfunction present, the patient's pre-onset bowel habits, and the present lifestyle. A pattern of evacuation of soft, formed stools, without spontaneous accidental stools between planned bowel care intervals, is the goal. Maintaining a bowel record or a flow sheet will assist in evaluating the effectiveness of the routine. The longer that stool remains in the colon, the drier and harder it becomes, increasing the potential for constipation and fecal impaction. Generally, more than 3 days between evacuations is not advised.

Once a workable elimination schedule has been attained, it should be maintained. If the schedule is upset, it may take weeks to reestablish a reliable new schedule. It is, therefore, critical to encourage active patient participation in the planning stages so that the schedule is tailored to specific needs and lifestyle.

DIET

Frequency and consistency of stool are related to type and amount of food and fluid ingested. Beyond being well balanced, the diet must provide adequate fiber. Fiber increases the bulk of the feces by enhancing water absorption. A diet that has inadequate fiber will result in a hard, dry, constipating stool. High-fiber foods, including nuts; the bran of whole grain, rather than refined, breads and cereals; and the cellulose of fresh fruits and vegetables with skins and seeds should be incorporated into the diet (see Table 28–6).

EXERCISE

Physical activity and exercise aid in the digestive process, promote peristalsis, and aid in elimination. Elimination is dependent on the integration of smooth and skeletal muscular activity and visceral reflex patterns. Immobility may interfere with these mechanisms, resulting in constipation. The primary muscles involved in defecation—abdominal, diaphragm, and levator muscles—work simultaneously to increase intra-abdominal pressure and expel the fecal mass. Immobility contributes to muscular atrophy, loss of tone, and generalized weakness. As a result, the individual is unable to help with the defecation process, and retention or incomplete evacuation results. As the individual's activity level increases, so does the physiologic response of elimination.

When the individual's condition warrants, encouraging participation in the daily care regimen will increase general conditioning and also bowel function. Basic daily activities, such as bathing, dressing, and transfer activities, in addition to participation in therapies, will aid in the process. Active exercise, such as pelvic tilting, hiking of the hips off the bed, range-of-motion exercises, turning in bed, and wheelchair pushups, will promote intestinal motility, muscular strengthening, and elimination.

POSITIONING AND FACILITATORY TECHNIQUES

Bowel care may have to take place in bed immediately after the onset of disability. Bedpans should not be used for people with sensory impairment because of the risk of pressure sores; rather, incontinent pads should be used for bowel care in bed. Positioning can capitalize on the anatomic position of the descending and sigmoid colons. Positioning on the left side promotes absorption and increases effectiveness of suppositories or enemas by using gravity. After stimulation, positioning on the right side aids in stool expulsion.

As soon as the condition allows, a sitting position is recommended for bowel care. The sitting position facilitates the use of gravity and increases intra-abdominal pressure for ease in stool expulsion. Flexion of the hips and knees with feet supported on a stool assists the patient in assuming a squatting position. Valsalva's maneuver, forward bends, and abdominal massage are also used to further facilitate increased intra-abdominal pressure. Environmental factors, such as the type of commode chair or toilet seat used, must be considered in planning care for this population (Table 28–8).

MEDICATIONS

Bowel stimulants, including laxatives, stool softeners, and bulk-producing agents, are frequently abused or considered a cure-all for elimination problems. Because the planning and management of a bowel care program are generally nursing functions, nurses must be knowledgeable about the actions, effects, and consequences of long-term bowel medications for safe and appropriate use. Short-term, judicious use of medications may be indicated (Table 28–9).

TABLE 28–8 • ENVIRONMENTAL FACTORS THAT FACILITATE CONTINENCE

Environmental Factors	Modifications
Bed	A low position facilitates getting in and out of bed.
Chair	Chair arms should extend to the front of the chair, and the seat should be 16–18 in from the floor.
Bathroom	The bathroom should accommodate assistive devices (e.g., wheelchair, walker). Grab bars, toilet seat arms, a raised toilet seat, or a padded toilet may be used if there is sensory loss. A well-marked door and a well-lighted path should be used.
Toilet substitutes (commode)	These devices should be of the proper size and in an accessible location.
Clothing	Wraparound skirts, Velcro fasteners, elastic waistbands, and footwear with surface friction may be used.

Adapted from Lincoln R., & Roberts, R. (1989). Continence issues in acute care. *Nursing Clinics of North America, 24*(3), 741–754.

ENEMAS

Large-volume enemas are not used in routine bowel care programs. Persistent use of enemas can result in diminished bowel tone by overstretching the bowel and causing a loss of the colon's natural elasticity. The result is a bowel that is more sluggish and prone to further constipation.

During the administration of an enema, the neurogenic bowel can go into spasm and trap fluid in the bowel segment behind the spastic area. If the enema is of large volume, the pressure exerted on the intestinal walls could result in rupture. In a flaccid colon, the enema fluid can flow in without resistance, and the bowel may balloon to accommodate the volume and then rupture, because there is no muscle tone or contraction force to express the fluid. Perforation of the rectum can occur because of enema-tip trauma if the patient has rectal sensory loss.

TABLE 28–9 • PRINCIPLES OF MEDICATION USE IN BOWEL MANAGEMENT

- The effect and action time of drugs may be altered in the presence of a neurogenic bowel, which can take 24 hr longer to respond than a normal bowel takes. Usual suggested dosages may result in cumulative effects that are difficult to control. Begin with the minimum recommended dose, and increase the dose gradually until the effective dose is reached.
- Plan bowel evacuation to coincide with peak effectiveness of the oral medication.
- The use of bulk-forming medications requires adequate fluid intake to prevent constipation and obstruction.
- Should medications need adjusting, only one element of the bowel program should be changed at a time and sufficient time allowed to evaluate the results.
- Use of harsh laxatives is avoided.
- Enemas and laxatives ordered in preparation for diagnostic tests may upset an established, workable bowel routine. The routine may take several weeks to reestablish. A modified bowel preparation is generally indicated for the individual with neurogenic bowel.

PSYCHOSOCIAL IMPLICATIONS

Elimination is a basic physiologic need that is particularly significant to the person with neurogenic bowel dysfunction. Planning, initiating, and maintaining a successful bowel elimination program prevents the occurrence of physical complications. The physical complications in themselves do not have as great a significance for the individual as do the psychosocial ramifications of the complications. Bowel management must fit the individual's lifestyle. Problems associated with dysfunction should not be accepted as inevitable; they must be anticipated and prevented.

An alteration in bowel function affects the individual and his or her total environment. The individual is part of the environment from which he or she has come, including culture, family, job, and community. The nurse must explore and acquire an understanding of the environment from which the individual comes to plan future goals effectively. What do bowel dysfunction and its consequences mean to the individual?

In addition to the responsibility of educating the patient, the family, and the other care providers, the nurse has a supportive role. Understanding and encouragement are of utmost importance. Impaired bowel function itself has an emotional impact on the patient and her or his significant others. Although optimal independence within functional limitations is encouraged and strived for, total independence is not always possible. If functional limitations necessitate the physical assistance of another person for the performance of bowel care, the problem is amplified. Who will perform bowel care at home? This problem should be explored with the individual and his or her partner, if indicated. It may not be conducive to a sexual relationship for the partner to provide bowel care, and, if possible, alternative arrangements should be planned. The nurse must be sensitive to the myriad of emotions associated with altered bowel function.

References

Banwell, J. G., Creasey, G. H., Aggarwal, A. M., & Mortimer, J. T. (1993). Management of neurogenic bowel in patients with spinal cord injury. *Urology Clinics of North America, 20*(3), 517–524.

Binnie, N. R., Kawimbe, B. M., Papachrysostomou, M., & Smith, A. N. (1990). Use of the pudendo-anal reflex in the treatment of neurogenic faecal incontinence. *Gut, 31*(9), 1051–1055.

Blair, G. K., Djonlic, K., Fraser, G. C., Arnold, W. D., Murphy, J. J., & Irwin, B. (1992). The bowel management tube: An effective means for controlling fecal incontinence. *Journal of Pediatric Surgery, 27*(10), 1269–1272.

Caruana, B. J., Wald, A., Hinds, J. P., & Eidelman, B. H. (1991). Anorectal sensory and motor function in neurogenic fecal incontinence. *Gastroenterology, 100*(2), 465–470.

Christiansen, J., & Roed-Peterson, K. (1993). Clinical assessment of the anal incontinence plug. *Diseases of the Colon and Rectum, 36*(8), 740–742.

Christiansen, J., & Sparso, B. (1992). Treatment of anal incontinence by an implantable prosthetic sphincter. *Annals of Surgery, 215*(4), 383–386.

Kewalramani, L. S. (1979). Neurogenic gastroduodenal ulceration and bleeding associated with spinal cord injuries. *Journal of Trauma, 19*(4), 259–265.

Lie, H. R., Lagergren, J., Rasmussen, F., Lagerkvist, B., Hagelsteen, J., Borjeson, M. C., Muttilainen, M., & Taudorf, K. (1991). Bowel and bladder control of children with myelomeningocele: A Nordic study. *Developmental Medicine and Child Neurology, 33*(12), 1053–1061.

Lincoln, R., & Roberts, R. (1989). Continence issues in acute care. *Nursing Clinics of North America, 24*(3), 741–754.

Liptak, G. S., & Revell, G. M. (1992). Management of bowel dysfunction in children with spinal cord disease or injury by means of the enema continence catheter. *Journal of Pediatrics, 120*(2), 190–194.

Lisenmeyer, T. A., & Stone, J. M. (1993). Neurogenic bladder and bowel dysfunction. In J. A. DeLisa (Ed.), *Rehabilitation medicine: Principles and practice* (pp. 733–762). Philadelphia: J.B. Lippincott.

Madoff, R. D., Williams, J. G., & Caushaj, P. F. (1992). Fecal incontinence. *New England Journal of Medicine, 326*(15), 1002–1007.

Marcio, J., Jorge, N., & Wexner, S. D. (1993). Etiology and management of fecal incontinence. *Diseases of the Colon and Rectum, 36*(1), 70–97.

Martin, N., Holt, N., & Hicks, D. (1981). *Comprehensive rehabilitation nursing.* New York: McGraw-Hill.

Mortensten, N., & Humphreys, M. S. (1991). The anal incontinence plug: A disposable device for patients with anorectal incontinence. *Lancet, 338*(8762), 295–297.

Perkash, L. (1990). Management of neurogenic dysfunction of the bladder and bowel. In F. J. Kottke & J. F. Lehmann (Eds.), *Krusen's handbook of physical medicine and rehabilitation* (pp. 810–832). Philadelphia: W.B. Saunders.

Ropper, A. H. (1993). Acute autonomic emergencies and autonomic storm. In P. A. Low (Ed.), *Clinical autonomic disorders* (pp. 747–765). Boston: Little, Brown.

Staas, W. E., & DeNault, P. M. (1973). Bowel control. *American Family Physician, 7*(1), 126–128.

Sun, W. M., Read, N. W., & Donnelly, T. C. (1991). Anorectal function in incontinent patients with cerebrospinal disease. *Gastroenterology, 99*(5), 1372–1379.

Venn, M. R., Taft, L., Carpentier, B., & Applebaugh, G. (1992). The influence of timing and suppository use on efficiency and effectiveness of bowel training after stroke. *Rehabilitation Nursing, 17*(3), 116–120.

Vernava, A. M., Longo, W. E., & Daniel, G. L. (1993). Pudendal neuropathy and the importance of EMG evaluation of fecal incontinence. *Diseases of the Colon and Rectum, 36*(1), 23–7.

HUMAN SEXUALITY PHENOMENA

29 Human Sexuality: An Overview

DONALD D. KAUTZ

DIMENSIONS OF HUMAN SEXUALITY AND SEXUAL HEALTH

Human sexuality is a complex phenomenon. Our sexuality pervades our biologic being, our sense of ourselves, and the way we relate to other human beings. Human sexuality is a multidimensional construct, with sexual function, sexual self-concept, and sexual roles and relationships constituting important dimensions. Sexual function refers to the ability of the individual to give and receive sexual pleasure. Sexual self-concept refers to the image one has of oneself as a man or a woman and the evaluation of one's adequacy in that role. Sexual self-concept also includes body image, reflecting the abstract representation of one's body and the evaluation of that image against personal and cultural standards. Sexual relationships refer to interpersonal relationships through which our sexuality is expressed. These dimensions have important correlates in expression of sexual health and are mirrored in the World Health Organization's definition of sexual health as the "positive integration of the somatic, emotional, intellectual, and social aspects of sexual being in ways that are positively enriching and that enhance personality, communication, and love" (World Health Organization, 1975, p. 6). This chapter examines the complex of biologic function, self-concept, and roles and relationships as they develop throughout the life span.

HUMAN SEXUALITY AND HUMAN DEVELOPMENT

Beginnings

Humans are sexual beings from the moment of fertilization. Chromosomal sex establishes the first of a series of developmental influences on our sexuality.

The male's sperm contributes either an X or a Y chromosome, which combines with the female's X chromosome, resulting in the XX (female) or XY (male) combination (Fig. 29–1).

After fertilization, there are critical points in the evolution of gender identity: the point at which induction of development of internal and external genitalia occurs and the point at which the hypothalamus takes on a male or a female pattern. At about 5 to 6 weeks of fetal life, the XX or XY chromosomal combination determines whether undifferentiated fetal gonads will develop as ovaries or testes. Further differentiation occurs in response to secretion of fetal androgen in the male fetus. If androgens are not present at critical periods and in appropriate amounts, male structures will not develop from the wolffian ducts, and the fetus with XY chromosomes will develop female genitalia. Biologic sex is well established by the 12th week of fetal life. Although there does

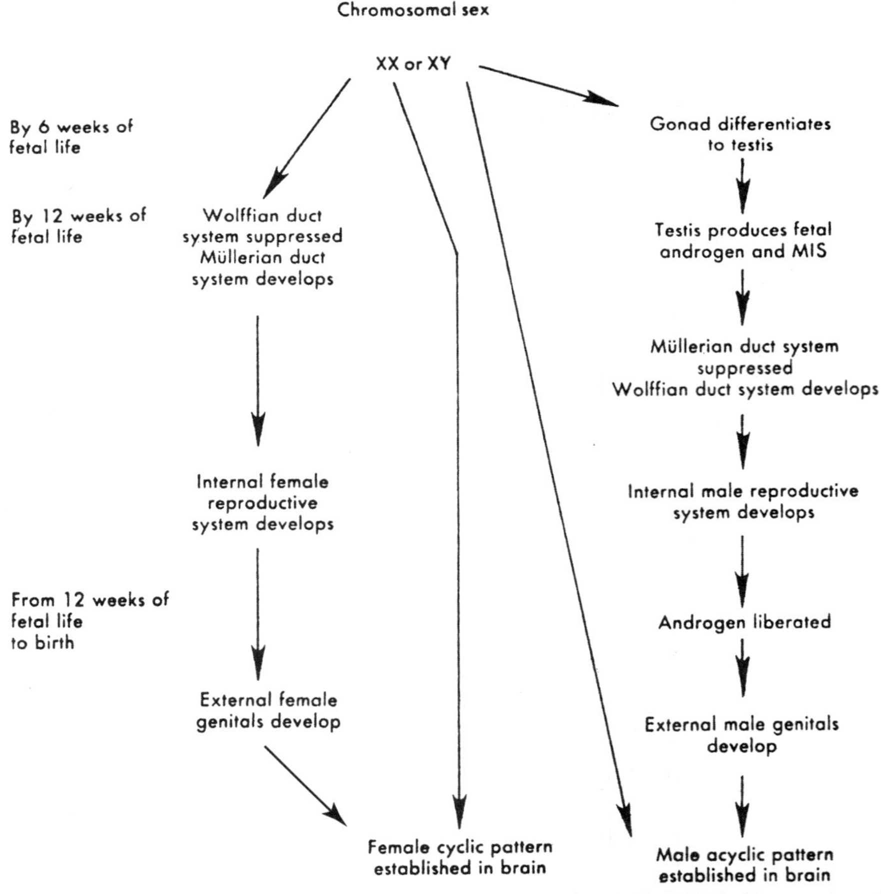

FIGURE 29–1 • Fetal sexual development. (From Woods, N. F. [1984]. *Human sexuality in health and illness* [3rd ed.]. St. Louis: C.V. Mosby.)

not appear to be a hormone necessary for induction of ovarian function in female fetuses, estrogen is necessary for full development of female genitalia (Money & Erhardt, 1972).

Another critical stage occurs around the time of birth, at which point another set of sexual controls is introduced. Testosterone is thought to influence the hypothalamus in such a way that it develops a male acyclic pattern for the release of pituitary gonadotropins. In the female, a cyclic pattern of gonadotropin release is established (Money & Erhardt, 1972).

Although the infant is born with an established chromosomal sex, gender identity and gender role are not yet established. Gender identity is the feeling that one is male, female, or ambivalent. Usually gender identity is solidified in children by the time they are 3 years old. Caregivers assign gender shortly after birth of the child, and their behavior confirms and reinforces the child's sense of maleness or femaleness. Children also respond to cues from their own bodies. For example, they respond to the appearance of their genitals and to verbal and nonverbal messages from caregivers in relation to their developing sense of self as female, male, or ambivalent. Gender role, the outward expression of one's gender, is learned early in life. Distinctions between appropriate masculine and feminine behaviors vary greatly among cultures. In Western cultures, these distinctions are becoming much less rigid, with the androgynous person (an individual who possesses both female and male characteristics) becoming synonymous with a healthy person.

Sexual development continues throughout the life span, with each component of sexuality being influenced by biologic development as well as sociocultural forces (Denney, 1992). Some of the significant developmental experiences related to sexual function, sexual self-concept, and sexual relationships are outlined in Table 29–1. A brief discussion of the sexual development of children is included below.

As children develop sexually, nurses can assist children and their caregivers by providing practical education to promote healthy, responsible behavior (Smith, 1993). Infant boys experience erections, and infant girls experience vaginal lubrication. These occurrences may be upsetting to some parents who do not realize that they are normal. After developing hand coordination, infants touch their own genitals during bathing and diaper changing. Caregiver acceptance is necessary as infants are not capable of comprehending their actions. As children learn the names of body parts, *penis* and *vagina* are better terms to teach children than are nicknames. Infants also learn how to show affection from those who provide their daily care. Toddlers are curious about their own bodies and learn through genital exploration that touching their own penis or vagina is pleasurable. Masturbation is normal; however, caregivers will need to set limits on when and where this behavior is acceptable. Setting limits on sexual exploration throughout childhood is best done matter-of-factly. By preschool age, children engage in sex play and exploration of playmates' bodies. Strict limits will need to be set to prevent trauma to the genitals or the rectum during sex play and to prevent children from shaming or sexually intimidating each other, but otherwise the limits on exploratory play can be modified depending on the values of the caregivers; opinions as to what is acceptable

TABLE 29–1 • SIGNIFICANT DEVELOPMENTS RELATED TO SEXUAL FUNCTION, SEXUAL SELF-CONCEPT, AND SEXUAL RELATIONSHIPS

Life Stage	Sexual Function	Sexual Self-Concept	Sexual Role and Relationship
Infancy	Orgasmic potential present; erectile function present	Gender identity reinforced; association of sexuality and good or bad; distinction between self and others	
Toddlerhood	Genital pleasuring and exploration; sensual activity (e.g., hugging)	Core gender identity solidified (by age 3 years)	Sex role differences learned; discrimination between male and female role models; sexual vocabulary learned
Preschool age	Sex play—exploration of own body and those of playmates; self-pleasuring (masturbation)		Sex roles learned; parental attachment and identification
School age		Curiosity about sex; sexual fears and fantasies; interest in aspects of sexual development; self-awareness as sexual being	Same-sex friends
Adolescence, prepubertal	Menarche; seminal emission	Concerns about body image; sexual thoughts, fantasies	Sexual experiences as part of friendships with same-sex friends
Early adolescence	Awkwardness in first sexual encounter (50% not sexually active)	Anxiety over inadequacy, lack of partner, virginity	Appropriate sex friendships; dating
Late adolescence	Masturbation, petting; may or may not be sexually active	Responsibility for sexual activity—sex role behaviors, lifestyles explored	Intimacy in relationships learned
Young adulthood	Experimentation with sexual positions, expression; exploration of techniques	Responsibility for sexual health (e.g., contraception, STD prevention); development of adult sexual value system, tolerance for others	Giving and receiving pleasure learned; long-term commitment to relationship developed
Middle adulthood	Adaptation to altered sexual function (e.g., vaginal dryness of menopause, slower erections)	Acceptance of body image changes related to aging	Adjustment of relationship as roles change
Late adulthood	More gradual sexual function	Acceptance of sexual response cycle without ending sexual aspects of relationship	New ways of sharing sexual pleasure and intimacy developed; adaptation to loss of partner or illness of partner

Abbreviation: STD, sexually transmitted disease.

vary greatly. For example, children who grow up in an environment where household nudity among family members is the norm learn that nudity within the household is acceptable. Children who grow up in a household where all family members make a point of not emerging from the bathroom or bedroom unless fully covered learn quickly that being clothed at home is proper behavior. Both extremes of households produce normally adjusted children, even though the children obviously emerge with differing values about nudity in the home.

During school years, children learn their own cultural expectations of sexual development, relationships, gender expectations, and role modeling (Smith, 1993). Many adults express a great deal of concern over the prominence of sexual content in the media, particularly on television shows and in videos. Even media that are not expressly sexual in nature are scrutinized for the sexual undertones portrayed. For example, the Disney movie *The Lion King*, released in 1994, was heralded by some as a wonderful return to traditional mother-father family values and as reinforcing the importance of father-son relationships and heterosexual relationships. Others criticized the movie for portraying chaos and destruction of society as the outcomes of challenging tradition and for suggesting that females need males to solve their problems. In our multicultural, multiethnic society, children are taught about sexuality from a multitude of caregivers, teachers, and media sources that portray multiple, conflicting points of view. Traditionally, parents, teachers, and other caregivers often ignore many sexual issues, which leaves sex education to the media and a child's peers. Those who wish to influence the sexual development of the children under their own care are encouraged to explore the many sources available, including schools, libraries, bookstores, churches, and health care providers such as nurses, physicians, and organizations like Planned Parenthood. Most agree that by the time boys and girls reach early adolescence, all should know strategies to protect themselves against rape, sexual abuse, and exploitation by adults and by other teens, as well as pregnancy, sexually transmitted diseases (STDs), and acquired immunodeficiency syndrome (AIDS).

Adolescence is a time of great sexual growth, both physically, because of the changes of puberty, and mentally, as the social pressures both to explore sexuality and to limit sexual exploration become dominant forces in a teenager's life (Smith, 1993). Nurses may be asked by both teenagers and their parents or caregivers to provide guidance on teen sexual development, realization of sexual orientation, and development of intimate relationships, as well as guidance on birth control and safe sex. Two articles illustrate how pediatric nurses have taken on these challenges, including making content relevant to African-American teenagers (Doswell, 2000; Jemmott, 2000).

Sexual development continues throughout adulthood. The rest of Chapter 29 as well as Chapter 30 expounds on sexual development as outlined in Table 29–1.

Human Sexual Responses

Human sexual response illustrates the interplay of biology, society, and culture with the individual's thoughts, feelings, and experiences. Masters and Johnson's pioneering work in the 1960s in the area of human sexual response contributed greatly to our understanding of the physiologic aspects of sexual function (Masters, Johnson, & Kolodny, 1998). Their laboratory studies revealed that the changes that accompany human sexual response result from two physiologic mechanisms: vasocongestion and myotonia. Vasocongestion is the primary response to sexual stimulation and refers to the engorgement of blood vessels with blood. Vasocongestion is responsible for swelling of vascular tissues in both women and men and for vaginal lubrication in women. Myotonia refers to muscle tension seen in the contraction of the woman's perivaginal muscles and the man's vas deferens and urethra during orgasm. Both vasocongestion and myotonia occur throughout the body with sexual response. Sexual response is thus best thought of as a total-body response rather than as only a genital response.

Masters and Johnson's original concept of the human sexual response cycle was revised in the work of Kaplan in the late 1970s (Kaplan, 1990). Kaplan later described human sexual response as consisting of three phases: desire, excitement, and orgasm (Kaplan, 1990). These phases are related components of sexual response but are governed by separate neurophysiologic systems. Kaplan's concept of sexual response is useful for understanding the physiology of sexual response, the consequences of pathophysiology, the etiology of sexual dysfunctions, and the appropriate therapies.

The desire phase of sexual response is the experience of sexual appetite or drive produced by the activation of neural systems in the brain. Sexual desire is experienced as sensations that move the person to seek out sexual activity. Although the precise neurons involved in sexual desire are unknown, it is believed to involve the limbic system and the preoptic nuclei of the hypothalamus. It is likely that the brain's sexual centers have either neural or chemical connection with the pleasure centers of the brain. The pleasure centers are stimulated during sexual activity, resulting in the pleasurable quality of sexual behavior. Some suggest that the pleasure centers are stimulated by release of endorphins with sexual behavior. Stimulation of the pain centers can inhibit sexual desire. If an object or situation evokes pain, it may cease to evoke desire.

Testosterone is important in mediating sexual desire in both men and women; low levels of testosterone are associated with low levels of sexual desire. Luteinizing hormone may also be important in mediating sexual desire. Two neurotransmitters, serotonin (5-hydroxytryptamine) and dopamine, are believed to be important in mediating sexual desire. Serotonin acts as an inhibitor and dopamine as a stimulant to the sexual centers of the brain.

Bonding with another person and love are both powerful stimuli to sexual desire. Many other stimuli are capable of evoking sexual desire, including sight, smell, and other sensory cues. Many of these stimuli are conditioned by culture. Fear and pain are the most potent inhibitors of sexual desire. Neural connections between the sexual centers and the other parts of the brain make it possible for people to turn off sexual desire when other stimuli are more important or when it is not adaptive to the individual to pursue sexual activity. These same connections also make it possible to enhance sexual desire.

During the excitement phase of sexual response, the level of sexual tension intensifies. Physiologic changes characteristic of the excitement phase—swelling of genitalia and vaginal lubrication—are produced by reflex vasodilation of the genital blood vessels. Two centers in the spinal cord (S2–S4 and T11–L2) cause the arterioles to dilate. This vasodilation causes the genitals to swell and changes their shape to adapt to their reproductive function. Vasocongestion is primarily a parasympathetically mediated response. Intense sympathetic response, such as that produced by fear and anxiety, can instantly lead to loss of erection. It is believed that erection is governed by two spinal reflex centers. The thoracolumbar center, the psychogenic area, appears to respond more to psychic stimuli, whereas the sacral center is stimulated by tactile input to the genitals. It is believed that the spinal reflex centers and the higher neural connections are analogous in males and females.

Orgasm refers to the peak and release of sexual tension. The orgasm phase of sexual response is characterized by a genital reflex governed by spinal neural centers and consists of reflex contractions of certain genital muscles. Sensory influences that trigger orgasm enter the cord via the pudendal nerve at the sacral level; the efferents are T11 and L2. Orgasmic sensations have been described in several ways, but women tend to note one or more of these forms: vulval, uterine, and blended. The vulval orgasm involves involuntary contractions of the orgasmic platform, the vascular tissues at the outer third of the woman's vagina, and the labia minora. The uterine orgasm depends on deep stimulation of the cervix that displaces the uterus, thus stimulating the peritoneum. Blended orgasms combine features of both vulval and uterine orgasms.

VARIATIONS IN SEXUAL EXPRESSION

Sexual pleasure may be experienced in a variety of ways. Culture influences the forms of sexual expression deemed acceptable and an individual's value system about sexual behavior. Indeed, culture plays an important role in defining what is normal. Contrary to what some espouse, there has never been consensus in our society about what sex acts are considered normal, moral, and healthy. There can be no "return to traditional sexual values and practices," as there was never a time in the United States when there was agreement over what constituted normal sexual expression. The difference between current sexual practices and those of earlier times is that variances in sexual expression are now discussed in public and portrayed in the media.

The search for a definition of "normal sex" has been pursued for centuries. Janus and Janus (1993) struggled to define what types of sexual acts could be classified as deviant when designing the questionnaire and interview guide for their broad-scale, scientific, nationwide survey. They found it much more useful to classify sexual acts as either harmful or harmless to the individual or the sex partner. Some sex acts are always harmful, wrong, criminal, and immoral, such as rape and sex between adults and children. Others that seem "kinky" to some but are probably not harmful unless pursued obsessively include cross-dressing, fetishes, and consensual dominance and bondage.

Sex on the Internet, or "cybersex," is another form of sexual variation. Sexual exploration "online" allows individuals to anonymously gain answers to sex questions that are too embarrassing to ask in person, learn to flirt, and practice or develop successful dating behaviors, as well as fulfill real-life sexual fantasies safely. Levine (1998) is an excellent resource for additional information.

Sexual Pleasuring

Each culture provides for a variety of erotic behaviors, but nearly all cultures are concerned with sexual modesty. Incest taboos are common to most societies, although the definition of incest varies from culture to culture. Each society has some form of legal system to regulate sexual behavior; for example, sexual intercourse may be restricted to marriage, or premarital sexual freedom may be encouraged.

The initiation of sexual activity and types of sexual acts vary greatly among individuals. Positions used for intercourse are highly variable, including female astride (on top), male astride, and side-to-side or squatting positions. In some relationships, women initiate sexual activity, but in others, only men do so. In some relationships, men are encouraged to ejaculate rapidly, whereas in others, the man's ability to prolong intromission is valued. Sexual stimulation is highly variable. Although kissing is nearly ubiquitous, by some it is regarded as unsanitary. Stimulation of the female breasts manually, orally, or with a man's penis is common. Manipulation of the female genitalia by the male is a common prelude to penile intromission. Oral stimulation of the woman's genitals (cunnilingus) is common in many relationships, and somewhat less common is oral stimulation of the male's genitals (fellatio). Painful stimulation is sometimes used to enhance arousal. Beliefs about sexual frequency also vary, as some believe intercourse should not occur during menses, lactation, or pregnancy, whereas others enjoy sex at these times.

Sexual Behavior

There are many variations in sexual behavior that involve variation in partners or goals. For example, heterosexuals choose partners of the opposite sex, whereas homosexuals seek partners of the same sex. Bisexuals choose both same-sex and opposite-sex partners at various times. Although heterosexuality is the most prevalent form of sexual expression in our society, it is certainly not the only type of sexual behavior in which people engage.

HOMOSEXUALITY

Because homosexuality is a very prevalent and poorly understood sexual variation, it is discussed here in more detail than are other variations. Two classic studies made a significant contribution to our knowledge of homosexuality. The Institute for Sex Research conducted a large study of homosexuals in the San Francisco Bay Area, and Masters and Johnson have published the results of their research (Bell & Weinberg, 1978; Masters & Johnson, 1979).

Bell and Weinberg (1978) studied 979 homosexual men and women and a comparison group of 477 heterosexual men and women from the San Francisco Bay Area. Through extensive interviews, these investigators determined that homosexuality involved much more than just sexual practices. Men and women in the homosexual sample varied in the degree to which they were involved in homosexual and heterosexual experiences, ranging along a continuum from those with exclusively homosexual feelings and behaviors to those with more heterosexual than homosexual feelings and behaviors. Homosexuals were predominantly covert about their homosexuality, although frequently their families were aware of their sexual preferences. Many common assumptions about homosexuality were not supported by this study. For example, homosexuals could not be typified as sexually hyperactive or hypoactive. The investigation made clear the uniqueness of homosexual lifestyles and the differences in lifestyles for men and women. For example, "cruising" (purposefully searching for a partner) was common among men but less common among women. Men tended to have more partners than women, but both men and women preferred a relatively steady relationship with a lover.

The homosexual men and women in this study used a variety of sexual techniques. Gay men most frequently used fellatio, hand-genital contact, and anal intercourse, and lesbian women most frequently participated in masturbation and cunnilingus with their partners. Sexual problems were more commonly reported by gay men than by lesbian women and included difficulty finding a partner and difficulty meeting the partner's sexual requests. Although STDs were a common health problem for gay men, this was not the case for lesbian women.

Bell and Weinberg (1978) found that the homosexual men and women they interviewed were involved in a variety of relationships, ranging from quasimarriages to having multiple short-term contacts. In contrast, some were not involved in a relationship, had little sexual interest, or regretted being homosexual.

When psychologic adjustment of the homosexual sample was compared with that of the heterosexual group, it was apparent that the homosexual persons who were in dysfunctional sexual relationships or who were asexual were less well adjusted than heterosexual persons. However, when the comparison was restricted to those who were functional (had little regret about homosexuality) or were in a coupled relationship, homosexuals were no more distressed than heterosexuals.

Masters and Johnson (1979) compared the physiology of sexual response in homosexual and heterosexual persons in the laboratory setting. They found no significant difference in homosexual and heterosexual subjects' facility for orgasm in response to masturbation, partner manipulation, fellatio, or cunnilingus. There were no demonstrable physiologic differences in the sexual response cycles of homosexual and heterosexual persons. Instead, lesbian women responded in the same manner as heterosexual women did, and similar results were obtained for men.

Both Masters and Johnson's and Bell and Weinberg's studies were conducted before the onset of the AIDS epidemic in the United States. AIDS was initially discovered in the United States among gay men, has been labeled as a gay disease, and is still thought by a good number of Americans to be primarily contracted by gay men through anal sex. However, worldwide, human immunodeficiency virus (HIV) is primarily contracted through heterosexual contact. Because of the AIDS epidemic, there is a great deal of postulation about the numbers and practices of gay men and lesbian women. Janus and Janus (1993) asked about sexual orientation in their survey. Of 1333 men, 91% identified themselves as heterosexual, 4% as homosexual, and 5% as bisexual. Of 1411 women, 95% identified themselves as heterosexual, 2% as homosexual, and 3% as bisexual. However, 22% of the men reported at least one sexual experience with a man, and 17% of the women reported at least one sexual experience with a woman. Janus and Janus (1993) also asked about multiple partners of all the male and female participants (lesbian, gay, heterosexual, and bisexual), who ranged in age from 18 years to older than 80 years, and found that of all the men, more than 70% had had sexual relations with more than 10 partners, and of all the women, 55% had had sex with more than 10 partners. More than 80% of the respondents were seriously concerned about STDs, but this concern did not necessary result in behavioral changes to prevent the spread of HIV and other STDs. Several respondents reported that of the people they knew who were sexually active with many partners, none had been infected with HIV. Some of these respondents had come to the conclusion that the risk of HIV infection was greatly exaggerated by both the media and the government. Overall, nurses are challenged to ensure that health needs of homosexuals are met, regardless of sexual behavior.

AGING AND HUMAN SEXUALITY

Research on sexuality and aging does not confirm the stereotypes of elderly people as either disinterested in sex or abnormally obsessed with it. For many aging persons, sexuality is an important dimension of living. Unfortunately, the sexual concerns of elderly people that arise from either aging or chronic illnesses are largely ignored by both physicians and nurses.

Although there is a decline in reports of sexual interest and activity with aging, there is no single point in the life cycle at which sexual activity ceases for all. Kaplan (1990) summarized work that has demonstrated that both sexual interest and sexual activity persist well into the seventh, eighth, and ninth decades of life. By analyzing multiple studies, Kaplan (1990) estimated that approximately 50% of healthy adults older than 50 years are sexually active.

Changes in sexual function occur gradually throughout the life span, and some may pass unnoticed. Processes essential for sexual response tend to occur more slowly with age, and the phase-specific changes may appear somewhat less intense. Nevertheless, the capacity for sexual pleasure persists among the elderly who are in reasonably good health.

As women age, there are gradual changes in their genitalia and breasts, reflecting the change in estrogen levels. Delay in the production of vaginal lubrication may occur in some women, and others notice that the vagina becomes smaller in both diameter and length. In general, vasocongestive responses are less pronounced. Some women may experience painful intercourse because of slow or absent vaginal lubrication and thinning of the vaginal walls. Using estrogen and water-soluble lubricant and having a sensitive, informed sexual partner are all helpful. Many texts recommend K-Y Jelly as a good water-soluble lubricant; however, it tends to become gummy quickly. Excellent vaginal lubricating agents include Replens, Lubrin, or Gyne-Mostrin, which can be obtained over the counter and are generally stocked with the feminine hygiene products. Sexual lubricants that are water soluble include Slippery Stuff and Astroglide, which may be available in drugstores or can be ordered through the Xandria Collection catalogue or the Sex Over 40 catalogue, both of which are listed in Table 30–5. Many older women also take estrogen on a daily basis as a treatment for vaginal dryness.

Age-related changes in men parallel those seen in women. As men age, the time necessary to experience an erection increases, and the erection is likely to be less full than it was earlier in life (Kaiser, 1991). Erectile dysfunction is one of the major health care problems of older adult men, and it is discussed further in Chapter 30. As with women, vasocongestive responses are less pronounced, and muscular contraction is less intense.

For many older people, absence of a sexual partner through death or illness means lack of sexual opportunity. Some find this frustrating, and others inhibit their sexual desire. Still others find new opportunities for sexual pleasure and explore alternative means of obtaining sexual pleasure, such as masturbation or partner stimulation. Usually, the most common reason given by both men and women for discontinuing sexual activity is the inability of the male partner to have an erection (Kaiser, 1991).

ASSESSING SEXUAL HEALTH

Assessment of sexual health begins with a sexual history and is supplemented by data about the person's general health, such as information obtained from the physical examination or the general health history (Mims & Swenson, 1980). A brief sexual assessment can be based on a few short questions that are integrated into the health history (Table 29–2). The approach described here deals with the person's role and relationships, sexual self-concept, and sexual function. Often, it is necessary to ask only the first or the second item on the questionnaire, and the client will volunteer data related to the other items. When a specific problem is identified that requires a referral to another clinician, or when more data are needed for planning an approach to a specific problem, a sexual problem history can be obtained.

When conducting a nursing assessment, screening for STDs can be done by asking the patient if he or she has either penile or vaginal discharge or open

TABLE 29–2 • BRIEF SEXUAL ASSESSMENT QUESTIONS

- Now I am going to ask a few questions about sexuality. Many patients with (back pain, spinal cord injury, head injury, stroke, multiple sclerosis, myasthenia gravis, etc.) have sexual concerns, and I may have some information that will help you.
- Has your (illness, hospitalization) interfered with your being (mother, father, wife, husband)? If so, how?
- (If the patient has acknowledged a sexual partner) Has your (stroke, head injury, multiple sclerosis, etc.) interfered with your relationship with your (spouse, sexual partner)? If so, how?
- Has your (spinal cord injury, Parkinson's disease, etc.) changed the way you see yourself as a (man, woman)? If so, how?
- Has your (disability, illness) changed your ability to function sexually (or your sex life)? If so, how?
- Have you noticed any open sores on your genitals (privates, penis, labia) or discharges from your (penis, vagina)?

lesions or sores on the genitals. These two questions will identify most patients with STDs.

Initially, a nurse may become anxious when asking these questions. With practice, the comfort level increases. Most nurses experience a great deal of anxiety when giving their first injection or starting their first intravenous line, yet no one believes that this fear is an acceptable reason for not learning the procedures. Unfortunately, a nurse's anxiety over asking about sexual concerns often means that the sexuality of many patients is ignored (Mims & Swenson, 1980).

Sexual Problem History

Although not absolutely necessary, a more in-depth history and assessment may be conducted to gain further insight into any problems the patient mentions in the brief assessment. Schover and Jensen (1988) offered interview guidelines on which the following recommendations are based.

The first component of the sexual problem history is a description, in the client's terms, of the current problem or concerns. Next, the onset and course of the problem are explored. The practitioner may wish to inquire about the client's age when the problem began, about whether the problem had an insidious onset or occurred suddenly, about whether the client can identify any precipitating events, and about whether there are other life events associated with the sexual problem. The course of the sexual problem can be described in terms of its fluctuations over time, such as with the changing intensity of a disease process, and in terms of its possible functional relationship to such phenomena as medication or alcohol use.

Of great importance is the client's concept of the cause and persistence of the problem. These data will enable the nurse to respond directly to the client's concerns rather than deal with them indirectly. Past attempts at treatment and their results may be explored, including evaluations by other health care practitioners, such as physicians; use of other professional help, such as professional counselors; and attempts that the client has made to cope with the problem.

The last component of the sexual problem history is an examination of the client's current expectations and the goals identified for treatment. A woman complaining of the inability to experience orgasm may have expectations of having orgasm with intercourse rather than by self-stimulation. If her expectations are not stated precisely, the practitioner may inappropriately treat her with the latter goal in mind or refer her to a practitioner whose approach to therapy would not be congruent with her goals.

Diagnosing sexual problems is frequently difficult. Often sexual problems are entangled in problems with relationships or with intrapersonal problems. As a consequence, the sexual problem may be a symptom of another problem, such as power struggle in a relationship or depression. Therefore, eliciting a careful description of the problem is essential.

Disorders at any level of the nervous system have the potential to influence some or all of the phases of sexual response. Cerebral lesions or strong emotions may inhibit the desire phase or the reflex responses of the excitement phase. Lesions of the brain stem and spinal cord may partially or completely interrupt the connections between cognitively mediated desire and the effector systems necessary to achieve intercourse. Neuropathies and spinal cord lesions that affect sensation in large parts of the body, particularly erotic areas, may decrease the sensory components of desire. Autonomic neuropathies, lesions of the sacral cord and cauda equina, and peripheral neuropathies may prevent any reflex activity in the excitement and orgasmic phases, while leaving desire intact.

Erectile dysfunction may also be the presenting sign of a chronic illness, particularly in older men (Kaiser, 1991). An otherwise-healthy older man who reports difficulty having an erection should have some basic diagnostic tests for diabetes, hypertension, and cardiac disease. Erectile dysfunction may also be the first sign of cognitive impairment as a result of dementia.

Preservation of reflex activity in the genital area makes physical intercourse potentially achievable for the person with spinal cord damage. Loss of such reflexes prevents intercourse but does not prevent sexual expression and is not necessarily damaging to sexual health. People with dysfunction of physical sexual response do not lose their sexuality and can achieve intimacy and affection with alternative forms of expression.

Physical Examination

Although most dimensions of sexual health are best assessed by means of a sexual history, physical assessment techniques provide useful data about potential changes in sexual function, particularly when the client has a health problem involving the nervous system, such as a spinal cord injury. Examination of sexual response is not necessary if there is no history of problems with sexual function or evidence of functional loss of lower extremity function. Sensation, volitional control, and reflex tone each provide important data about potential capacity for sexual response. Aspects of the neurologic examination of both men and women are directed toward determining the segmental level of injury (or peripheral level of injury, as in cauda equina lesions), as well as the completeness or incompleteness of spinal cord transections.

Rectal examination evaluates reflex motor function of the sacral cord segments S2–S4, important in reflex erection in men and sexual lubrication and swelling in women. Reflex control is assessed by inserting a gloved, lubricated finger into the rectum, noting the presence or absence of pressure from the contracting sphincter, and then asking the client to voluntarily contract the sphincter and noting the presence or absence of pressure on the gloved finger (Fig. 29–2). The bulbocavernosus reflex is another way to elicit the anal reflex. Squeezing the glans penis in the male or the glans clitoris in the female produces contraction of the anal sphincter if the reflex is present. Alternatively, one may elicit the anal reflex by stimulating the perianal skin lightly and observing for contraction of the sphincter. This response is often termed the anal wink (Mitchell et al., 1984).

If sensation is abnormal in the lower extremities and trunk, or if there is a history of injury involving the spinal cord, the sensory examination should include response to touch and pinprick over the genital and rectal areas (Fig. 29–3), as well as careful mapping of sensation over the trunk and lower extremities. Such findings help determine the potential for residual sexual response, as discussed in Chapter 30. Finally, reflex penile erection in men should be noted in response to sensory stimuli. Some men with complete spinal cord injuries may not be aware that they are having erections during catheterization or bathing. Nurses can tactfully acknowledge that the erection is occurring and offer the explanation that it is common in men with spinal cord injuries and is a reflex.

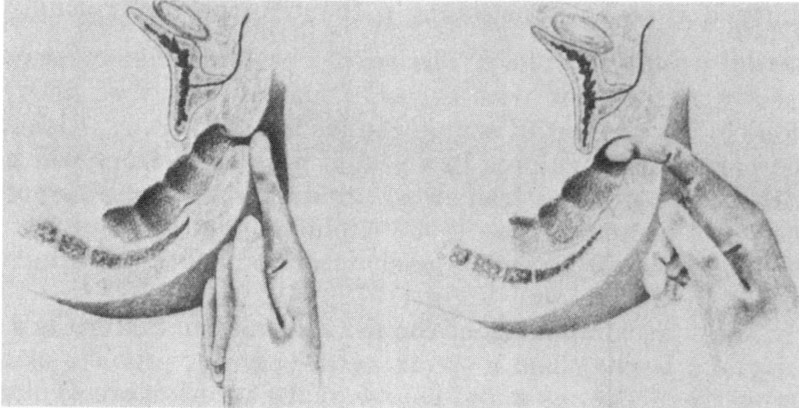

FIGURE 29–2 • Examining the anal sphincter reflex. (From Mitchell, P. H., Cammermeyer, M., Ozuna, J., & Woods, N. F. [1984]. *Neurological assessment for nursing practice.* Paramus, NJ: Reston.)

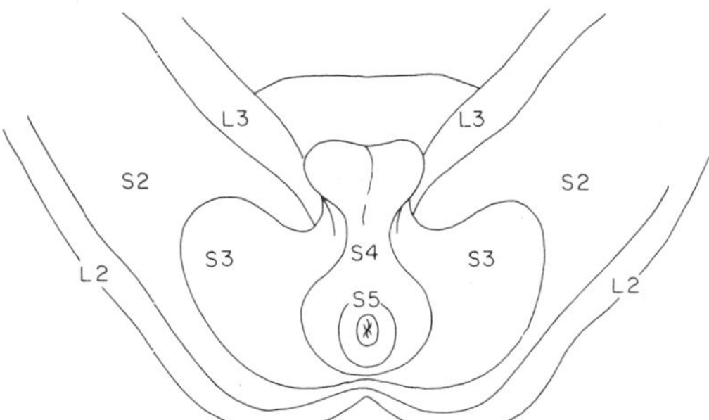

FIGURE 29–3 • Sensory mapping of genital and rectal areas. L2 and L3 indicate areas innervated by sensory roots entering the spinal column at the lumbar vertebrae. S2–S5 are areas sending sensory fibers to enter the spinal column at the sacral levels. (From Mitchell P. H., Cammermeyer, M., Ozuna, J., & Woods, N. F. [1984]. *Neurological assessment for nursing practice.* Paramus, NJ: Reston.)

SUMMARY

Human sexuality is a complex phenomenon consisting of the interrelated components of sexual function, sexual self-concept, and sexual relationships. Sexuality develops over the life span and may be affected by a variety of factors. Sexual health should be assessed and interventions developed accordingly; Chapter 30 deals with more detailed problem assessment and interventions.

References

Bell, A., & Weinberg, M. (1978). *Homosexualities.* New York: Simon & Schuster.

Doswell, W. M. (2000). Promotion of sexual health in the American cultural context: Implications for health promotion in school age African-American girls. *Journal of National Black Nurses Association, 11*(1), 51–57.

Janus, S. S., & Janus, C. L. (1993). *The Janus report on sexual behavior.* New York: John Wiley & Sons.

Jemmott, L. S. (2000). Saving our children: Strategies to empower African-American adolescents to reduce their risk for HIV infection. *Journal of National Black Nurses Association, 11*(1), 4–14.

Kaiser, P. E. (1991). Sexuality and impotence in the aging man. *Clinics of Geriatric Medicine, 7*(1), 63–72.

Kaplan, H. S. (1990). Sex, intimacy, and the aging process. *Journal of the American Academy of Psychoanalysis, 18*(2), 185–205.

Levine, D. (1998). *The joy of cybersex.* New York: Ballantine Books.

Masters, W. H., & Johnson, V. E. (1979). *Homosexuality in perspective.* Boston: Little, Brown.

Masters, W. H., Johnson, V. E., & Kolodny, R. C. (1998). *Heterosexuality.* New York: Grammery.

Mitchell, P. H., Cammermeyer, M., Ozuna, J., & Woods, N. F. (1984). *Neurological assessment for nursing practice.* Paramus, NJ: Reston.

Money, J., & Erhardt, A. (1972). *Man and woman, boy and girl.* Baltimore, MD: Johns Hopkins University Press.

Smith, M. (1993). Pediatric sexuality: Promoting normal sexual development in children. *Nurse Practitioner, 18*(8), 37–44.

World Health Organization. (1975). *Education and training of health professions in the treatment of human sexuality* (WHO Technical Report Series No. 572). Geneva, Switzerland: Author.

Alterations in Human Sexuality

DONALD D. KAUTZ

Alterations or changes in several aspects of human sexuality occur throughout the life span, frequently in response to illness. These sexual changes can be divided into four types: problems children experience, need to practice safe sex, fertility changes with illness, and sexual dysfunctions experienced by adults. The first part of this chapter explores sexual problems that children with nervous system trauma and disease may experience and how nurses can assist children, parents, and caregivers to overcome them. This is followed by discussions on safe sex and fertility changes with illness. Finally, sexual dysfunctions of adults are presented. Sexual dysfunctions may be categorized as sexual dysfunctions, alterations in sexual self-concept, and alterations in sexual relationships. Nursing diagnoses and management of alterations in each of these categories are presented, with special emphasis on problems that clients with nervous system problems are likely to experience.

SEXUAL DEVELOPMENT IN CHILDREN WITH NEUROLOGIC DISEASES AND DISABILITIES

Most insults to the nervous system in children have the potential to affect sexual development. The sexual needs of children with chronic neurologic illnesses and as survivors of neurologic trauma have largely been ignored. Nurses can take on the challenge of assisting children and their parents and caregivers in providing sexual education, preventing and reporting sexual abuse, preventing inappropriate sexual acting out, preventing shame, promoting the development of a healthy sexual self-concept, and assisting children to overcome sexual stereotypes about disabled people.

Sex Education for Children, Parents, and Caregivers

Sex education for children with disabilities or chronic illness should mirror that provided for healthy children and needs to be modified depending on the age group. Preschoolers can be taught about their own bodies, as well as about respect and the need for privacy concerning their own bodies and the bodies of others. Children from age 8 to 11 years can understand more about self-esteem and autonomy and that it is normal for them to be interested in same-sex friends. They will understand the concept of trust with adults. Children at this age can also be taught that sexual behavior is inappropriate for children of their age, even though they are curious. Questions about relationships and sexual expression can be answered matter-of-factly.

Adolescents and young adults who have neurologic impairments need specific information about the effects of their disability or chronic illness on sexuality and fertility. Selekman and McIlvain-Simpson (1991) recommended that these be done concretely, using dolls to demonstrate positions and scenes of sexual activity. Those with mobility impairments may need to modify positions for intercourse. All adolescents and young adults should be informed that manual stimulation of a partner's genitals and oral-genital sex are normal activities. A number of books have been written that nurses can use to illustrate these options and recommend for adolescents and young adults to purchase on their own. In addition, several written resources on sexuality have been published specifically for people with neurologic impairments and are included in Table 30–1. All include stories of people growing up with impairments who have experienced sexual problems and have overcome them. Although the books are generally written for adult audiences, older adolescents may find them to be very useful.

Adolescents and young adults with disabilities also need information on developing into sexual adults with a positive body image and appropriate social, dating, and intimacy skills. Those with neurogenic bowel and bladder problems who are not totally continent or who have ostomies will need to learn to use powders or deodorants to counteract offensive odors. Assisting them to choose clothes, hairstyles, and makeup and ensuring that their teeth, body, and hair are clean will enhance their self-image and improve the likelihood of social interactions in spite of severe disability. Encourage them to think of activities they can participate in for dating. Discussion groups or role-playing can be used to help them think through how they can express intimacy with others in ways other than sexual intercourse, including hugging, back rubs, or other nonsexual touching. Finally, adolescents and young adults need to have a clear idea of methods of sexual expression open to them in spite of their disability. In order to achieve penile-vaginal intercourse, they may need to use side-lying positions or semi-sitting positions using their wheelchair. In order to meet their own and their partner's needs, they may need to adopt many different methods of genital stimulation, including masturbation, manual stimulation of their partner, and oral sex. The references in Table 30–1 will help them anticipate their needs in advance so they can talk this through with potential sexual partners. There is a great deal of societal concern over teaching adolescents methods of sexual expression, even though there is no evidence that teaching about sex encourages teenage sexual activity.

Unfortunately, a disabled teenager may lose a potential lifelong partner if he or she cannot knowledgeably discuss what a lifelong sexual relationship

TABLE 30–1 • SEXUALITY RESOURCES

Books

- Kroll, K., & Klein, E.L. (1992). *Enabling romance: A guide to love, sex, and relationships for the disabled (and the people who care about them)*. Bethesda, MD: Woodbine House.
- Boston Women's Health Book Collective (1998). *Our bodies, ourselves for the new century: A book by and for women*. New York: Simon & Schuster.
- Corbet, B., Dobbs, J., & Brown, B. (1998). *Spinal network* (3rd ed.). Boulder, CO: Spinal Network. (Includes a comprehensive listing of both national and state organizations for people with neurologic diseases and disabilities. To order, call 1-800-543-4116).
- Griffith, E.R., & Lemberg, S. (1993). *Sexuality and the person with traumatic brain injury: A guide for families*. Philadelphia: F.A. Davis.
- Cole, S.S. (1993). *Reproductive issues for persons with physical disabilities*. Baltimore: Brooks Publishing.
- Levine, D. (1998). *The joy of cybersex*. New York: Ballantine Books.
- Ducharme, S.H. & Gill, K.M. (1997). *Sexuality after spinal cord injury*. Baltimore, MD: Brookes Publishing.
- Block, J.D. (1999). *Sex over 50*. Paramus, NJ: Reward Books.

Videotape

- Alexander, C., & Sipski, M. (Producers). (1993). *Sexuality reborn* [videotape]. West Orange, NJ: Kessler Institute for Rehabilitation.

Pamphlets

- Multiple Sclerosis Society. *Sexuality and MS.*
- American Heart Association. *Sexuality after Stroke.*

Mail Order

- Xandria Collection/Lawrence Research Group, P.O. Box 319005, San Francisco, CA 94131 (1-800-242-2823). Sexual aids, including lubricants, educational videos, books, and sex toys. Special edition of their catalog available for the disabled.
- Sex over Forty, P.O. Box 1600, Chapel Hill, NC 27515 (1-800-285-0444). Monthly newsletter available covering topics specific to older adults including health problem effects on sexuality. Educational videos and books, lubricants, and sexual aids also available.

will be like in spite of the disability. Limiting sexual information to disabled teens may very well prevent them from achieving a lifelong, mutually monogamous relationship, the goal supported by those who most ardently oppose sex education for teenagers.

Preventing and Reporting Sexual Abuse in Children

Neuroscience nurses may come in contact with children who have been sexually abused. In a case reported by Moglia (1993), Susan, born with cerebral palsy, began to be sexually abused by her stepfather when she was 10 years old. He would turn her so she was lying on her back so that she couldn't move and force her to engage in oral sex, anal sex, and coitus with him. The abuse heightened over the next few years as her stepfather and mother would bring men over to have sex with her. Moglia reported (1993) one estimate that 99% of disabled children experience at least one incident of incest, fondling, exposure, rape, physical injury, or financial harm by the time the child reaches 18 years. Nurses need to be alert for signs of physical trauma or a child's becoming anxious or afraid around certain adults. One of the factors that facilitates the abuse of disabled children is that a child may feel that he or she has no place to go or that the abuse is expected because of the disability. To prevent abuse, nurses who provide care to children with disabilities can include strategies to prevent victimization as a part of routine sex education. If sexual abuse is suspected, nurses can assist in referring the child to the social worker or psychologist in their own work setting to intervene.

Preventing Inappropriate Sexual Acting Out by Children

Inappropriate sexual behavior may occur in children in the neuroscience setting. Children with and without disabilities learn at an early age that sexual comments, exposure of genitals, and touching other people's genitals are sure ways to get a reaction out of adults. These behaviors in disabled and chronically ill children may indicate a form of protest and independence, may be a sign of sexual abuse at home, or may suggest a need for sexual education. Rather than looking at these behaviors as a need for help, nurses may react to the behavior by avoiding the child, instituting punishment or restrictions, becoming overprotective, or showing disgust. All these reactions are inappropriate because they do not extinguish the behavior or meet the child's need for intervention. Intervening is necessary to help the child grow up to be a sexually appropriate adult. Unfortunately, there is little agreement as to the best behavioral strategies to extinguish acting out behaviors and at the same time reward appropriate behavior. Although education is always a good first step, other measures will often need to be instituted. Devising a system of rewards (stickers or video game or television privileges) for times when acting out does not occur may work with some children. Others may benefit from role-playing of appropriate behavior. Others may need "time out." For more information, see Carrey and Adams (1992).

Because of the lack of privacy in most health care and educational settings, nurses may discover a child masturbating. Masturbation can be performed with only minimal hand function and requires little cognitive function yet is likely to be one of the most enjoyable, self-pleasuring activities a disabled child can engage in. Unfortunately, nurses may believe, as many other adults do, that masturbation is—at worst—harmful or immoral or—at best—a poor use of time and energy. Nurses can reassure parents and children that masturbation has been intensively studied and that it has no harmful effects and is completely normal when performed in private. Helping the child and her or his caregivers or parents to identify appropriate places for masturbation will convey that masturbation is appropriate at some times but not others. If nursing staff and caregivers consistently knock and wait a few seconds before entering a child's room, the number of times children are discovered masturbating will decrease dramatically.

Nurses may be required to perform bathing, bowel programs, catheterization, and dressing of children. Requiring assistance may lead to embarrassment or shame in boys and girls, especially those experiencing pubertal changes. When confronted with an embarrassing situation, children may use strategies such as pretending or joking during the embarrassing activity or may try to avoid the embarrassing situation altogether to prevent shame (Flaming & Morse, 1991).

Nurses may interpret these behaviors as noncompliance or wanting to avoid treatment, when the behaviors are more likely a protective measure for the child. Teaching independence will help limit the number of embarrassing episodes. However, the teaching itself may be too embarrassing for the child to tolerate. Approaches nurses can use to reduce embarrassment and shame include verbally recognizing the embarrassment, providing for as much privacy as possible, and treating the child as a developing sexual adult. Poking fun at the child's anxiety or making comments like, "You don't have anything I haven't seen before," belittle the child's sense of autonomy and heighten his or her anxiety and shame.

Promoting the Development of a Healthy Sexual Self-Concept

Nurses can aid in promoting the development of a healthy sexual self-concept. In some rehabilitation settings that serve head-injured adolescents and young adults, recreation therapists, nursing staff members, and therapists have instituted "hair fairs" to reinforce grooming, dances, and other activities to promote appropriate dating behaviors and social interaction (Blackerby, 1988). Even those with significant cognitive impairment can be included in these "unit parties," complete with music and refreshments. One recreation therapist, a beautician, the nursing staff on the unit, and a few volunteers will ensure that all the patients on the unit can participate. Blackerby (1988) reported one teenager who had such a poor self-concept that he would break mirrors to avoid looking at himself and completely ignore his hygiene needs. After participating in a few hair fairs, he began to cut his hair, he requested a bathroom mirror, and he regularly bathed. Although these types of events are best suited for rehabilitation settings, neuroscience nurses can adapt them to most settings, except possibly the intensive care unit (ICU). When a patient who has experienced a stroke or trauma, such as a head or spinal cord injury, is in the ICU, families and friends often feel helpless. Encouraging the family and friends to take on appropriate hygiene measures of the patient will not only aid in the patient's recovery but also help overcome the families' and friends' anxiety by giving them something to do. After patients are out of the ICU, they may stay on an acute unit for many days or weeks. Families may be willing to arrange and pay for a beautician to come to the unit for hair, nail, and facial care. Early interventions such as these may prevent patients from initially adopting poor hygiene habits after their injury.

Assisting Children to Overcome Sexual Stereotypes About Disabled People

Children with disabilities who are educated about sexuality and taught to accept their own bodies will still experience a great deal of sexual stereotyping from both the general public and health care professionals about their sexuality (Meeropol, 1991). Parents, peers, doctors, and nurses often either downplay sexuality because of ignorance or try to convince disabled children that they will only get hurt if they attempt to establish sexual relationships. To ignore that many able-bodied people see disabled people as sexless will compound the problem. Giving disabled patients recommendations of how to react when confronted with a stereotype and of how to relieve anxiety and inform the ignorant will save them the frustration of figuring this out on their own. Most people with disabilities recommend at least briefly discussing the disability early in any relationship. As children with disabilities mature, they will need to develop a script with which they can quickly describe for others the nature of their impairments in a few minutes in an adult, straightforward manner. Nurses can help them learn to describe themselves in a way that conveys acceptance and humor and emphasizes their abilities. Children learn best by concrete examples, and including some real-life experiences in their script at succeeding developmental ages will help other children and adults understand what to expect in a friendship or romantic relationship with this person. Once these descriptions are conveyed, anxiety about the disability will decrease, allowing everyone to move on to more important things, like having fun and sharing good times with each other. The books *Spinal Network* and *Enabling Romance,* listed in Table 30–1, are excellent resources for nurses, children, and adults with disabilities and for their significant others. In addition to these resources, the reader is also referred to the classic by Bullard and Knight (1981).

SAFER SEX FOR ADOLESCENTS AND ADULTS

Safer-sex practices are recommended for all disabled and able-bodied people regardless of sexual orientation, marital status, and age to ensure protection from sexually transmitted diseases (STDs) and acquired immunodeficiency syndrome (AIDS) (Muma et al., 1997). One study of mortality rates ranked sexual behavior as the sixth most prominent contributor to mortality in the United States in 1990, just ahead of motor vehicle accidents and illicit drug use

(McGinnis & Foege, 1993). As a society, we have a long way to go to ensure that all sexual encounters prevent the spread of disease. Nurses can assist in promoting safer sex in many practice settings—clinics, long-term care institutions, senior centers, hospitals, and homes (Bolus, 1994). The variety of settings allows for unique opportunities for nurses to assess risk and provide protective sex education.

Patients admitted for neurologic trauma or progressive cognitive impairment may discover they are human immunodeficiency virus (HIV) positive during admission to a neuroscience setting. Patients' understanding of routes of HIV transmission needs to be assessed, and, if necessary, patients should be taught the principles of safer-sex practices. The risk of HIV transmission during various sex practices is given in Table 30–2. Protective sex includes sexual activities in which no semen, vaginal secretions, or blood is exchanged between sexual partners. These activities include hugging, kissing, caressing, genital handling in the absence of open lesions, and vaginal or anal intercourse provided a condom and spermicide are used correctly (Flaskerud & Ungvarski, 1994).

Abstinence from penile-vaginal, anal, and oral sex not only prevents the transmission of HIV and other STDs but also prevents pregnancy. Unfortu-

---

TABLE 30–2 • RISK OF SEXUAL TRANSMISSION OF HIV

Absolutely Safe

* Abstinence from penile-vaginal, anal, and oral sex
* Mutually monogamous sex with noninfected partner or any sexual activity between noninfected partners is safe
* Telephone sex, erotic videos or magazines, fantasy, cybersex
* Solo or mutual masturbation

Very Safe (Assuming Intact Skin and No Lesions)

* Noninsertive sexual practices (includes manual stimulation of partner, massage, unshared sex toys, dry kissing)

Probably Safe

* Insertive sexual practices with the use of condoms and spermicide* (includes penile-vaginal and penile-anal intercourse with a barrier as well as cunnilingus, fellatio, and anilingus with a barrier).

Risky

* Everything else

HIV, human immunodeficiency virus.

* Condoms, either the male condom, which fits over the penis, or the female condom, which is inserted into the vagina before intercourse, must be used correctly in conjunction with a spermicide (nonoxynol 9). See Bolus (1994) for complete information on the correct use of both the male and the female condoms.

From Flaskerud, J.H., & Ungvarski, P. (1994). HIV/AIDS: *A guide to nursing care* (3rd ed.). Philadelphia: W.B. Saunders.

nately, learning to "just say no" is not enough for adolescents and adults who want to maintain abstinence. Hatcher et al. (1998) suggested strategies adolescents and young adults can use to ensure that sexual touching stays within the limits they intend. For adolescents to learn these strategies, they will need to practice. Role-playing is an excellent method of practice. For example, some parents practice with a group of boys and girls. The boys come up with statements they have heard from peers to encourage girls to have sex, and then the girls come up with counterstatements. In this manner, everyone learns in a fun, nonthreatening environment how to respect each other when confronted with a high-pressure situation.

FERTILITY CHANGES AND CONTRACEPTION

Closely related to sexual expression are fertility, contraception, pregnancy, and childbirth. Patients may request information about these reproductive issues when asked about sexual concerns. Although most of the content related to these four areas is beyond the scope of this chapter, it is important for neuroscience nurses to recognize that neurologic impairments that affect the spinal cord may have an adverse effect on all four of these areas.

Spinal cord injuries affect the ability of both men and women to have an orgasm. Although this does not interfere with the fertility of women, most men with spinal cord injuries will have some difficulties with fertility because of either absence of ejaculation or retrograde ejaculation. Advances in the treatment of infertility have been made. Even though men with a complete spinal cord injury may not have penile sensation and are not able to feel an orgasm, they may be able to ejaculate through a variety of methods. Most physicians specializing in treatment of fertility problems recommend beginning with a program of penile stimulation, by either hand or vibrator, to see if ejaculation will occur. The amount of time the penis is stimulated needs to be increased slowly to prevent penis swelling or skin breakdown. If these methods are ineffective, electroejaculation may be used. Electroejaculation is conducted by a urologist inserting a electric probe into the man's rectum to stimulate ejaculation. Once semen is obtained, it is inserted into the women's vagina through artificial insemination. For further information, see *Spinal Network* by Corbet et al. (1998) or Seager and Halstead (1993).

Women with spinal cord injuries and other disabilities may encounter obstacles to obtaining routine gynecologic examinations, contraception, and obstetric services. Offices and examination tables may not be accessible so that even going for an examination can be a difficult experience. Nurses can help by identifying clinics that are accessible and providers who have experience working with disabled women. Women with disabilities may have trouble choosing a method of birth control that is both safe for them to use and manageable with some cognitive or physical impairment. Most neurologic disabilities do not adversely affect a woman's ability to conceive, but some disabled women who become pregnant are at high risk of complications from preeclampsia and may be admitted to maternity floors and at times ICUs for extended periods of time. Neuroscience nurses can consult with maternity nurses about the daily care needs of a disabled women, including skin care, bowel and bladder management, and prevention and management of dysreflexia. Sipski and Alexander (1997) and *Spinal Network* (Corbet et al., 1998) provide more information on pregnancy and disability. See Alston and McCowan (1994) for more information on the sexual needs of African-American women with disabilities.

HUMAN RESPONSES TO SEXUAL DYSFUNCTIONS IN ADULTS

Contemporary systems for the classification of sexual dysfunction include five major categories: alterations in sexual desire; alterations in sexual arousal; alterations in orgasm; alterations in sexual self-concept; and alterations in sexual relationships. Each broad category of dysfunction includes several specific types of problems. Moreover, each problem can be described as lifelong or not lifelong and global or situational. Qualifying information can be included in the diagnostic statement. The conventions used by Schover and Jensen (1988) are used in this discussion.

Alterations in Sexual Desire

Alterations in sexual desire include low sexual desire and sexual aversion. Low desire is defined on the basis of frequency of masturbation and partner activity as well as on self-reports of desire for a partner and incidence of fantasy, erotic dreams, or seeking out of erotic stimuli. Aversion to sex is defined as a clearly negative reaction to sex. Low sexual desire and sexual aversion form a continuum.

Alterations in sexual desire, including low sexual desire and aversion, can be attributed to both physiologic and psychosocial factors. Depression, severe stress states, certain pharmacologic agents, low androgen levels, and certain illnesses can interfere with sexual desire. Low sexual desire is a frequent concomitant of depression and may reflect severe stress. Many pharmacologic agents, including narcotics, sedatives, alcohol, centrally acting antihypertensives (such as reserpine and methyldopa), and testosterone antagonists, have been associated with low sexual desire. Illnesses producing discomfort or malaise are also linked to low sexual desire.

Desire phase dysfunctions may occur in response to conscious or unconscious thought processes (Kaplan, 1988). Sexual desire can be turned off by turning on physiologic inhibiting mechanisms associated with anger or fear. Fear and anger can occur as a result of personal conflicts about success and intimacy, complex intrapsychic problems, or severe relationship problems. Anger may be directed at the partner. Anxieties linked to childhood experiences, such as sexual abuse, pressure to have sexual relations, repeated unpleasurable experiences, and guilt, may also interfere with sexual desire.

Diagnosis of alterations in sexual desire is based on the individual's description of frequency of sexual activity and desire for erotic stimuli. Sexual aversion reflects a clearly negative reaction to sex, not just lack of interest. These diagnoses are based on data obtained from a sexual problem history similar to that described in Chapter 29. An important aspect of diagnosis is determining what, if any, qualifying information is pertinent. The diagnosis might be low sexual desire related to malaise from a chronic illness, low sexual desire related to effects of medication, or low sexual desire related to resentment toward a partner. Each of these diagnoses would imply different therapeutic strategies. Several nursing diagnoses related to low sexual desire in clients with nervous system problems are presented, as follows:

Low energy level

Medical regimen

Severe stress

Chronic pain

Partner's poor health

Partner's lack of acceptance of illness

Nursing interventions for low sexual desire and sexual aversion are directed to the underlying causes when they can be identified. When the diagnosis is low sexual desire related to low energy levels in a person with chronic illness, therapeutic strategies might include advising the person to identify times when energy levels are high and attempting sexual activity then. Another strategy might be resting before sexual activity is anticipated. When low sexual desire is related to pharmacologic agents, it is sometimes possible to consult with the client's physician to alter the therapeutic regimen to enhance sexual desire (Table 30–3). When the diagnosis is low sexual desire related to anger directed toward a partner, referral for couples counseling may be the optimum therapeutic alternative. Sexual aversion is most appropriately treated in the context of sex therapy or intensive psychotherapy.

• C A S E   S T U D Y   1

Ms. Thomas, 35 years old, has recently been diagnosed with multiple sclerosis. Her symptoms include transient numbness in her lower extremities, occasional urinary incontinence, and fatigue. She notes a decrease in sexual desire over the past 6 months, which she attributes to her fatigue and her anxiety about being incontinent during sexual activity. Her partner of the last 6 years has been sensitive to her altered sexual desire and attributes it to her illness. Ms. Thomas has been able to give pleasure to her partner by having intercourse but says she just does not feel any motivation to initiate sexual activity with her partner or to stimulate herself sexually. She is "too tired."

A diagnosis of recent low sexual desire related to fatigue and anxiety about potential incontinence suggests the following therapeutic strategies:

1. Enhance sexual desire by planning rest periods before opportunities for sexual activity.
2. Reduce anxiety about incontinence by emptying bladder before sexual activity, discussing the possibility of incontinence with the partner, and using a protective sheet on the bed.

Outcomes of these strategies include improvement in sexual desire and Ms. Thomas's and her partner's understanding of reasons for low sexual desire and concerns about incontinence.

Another example of altered sexual desire is that related to aversion in the partner. Often the sequelae of nervous system dysfunction produce bodily changes in the client and demands on the partner to participate in caretaking situations. Both these situations may alter the partner's sexual desire.

HYPERSEXUALITY OR SEXUAL ACTING OUT

The other end of the spectrum from decreased sexual desire is hypersexual behavior. Often referred to as sexual acting out, hypersexual behaviors in adults have been reported with a number of neurologic impairments, including dementias, head injury, stroke, and Parkinson's disease. These behaviors are thought to occur because of a combination of a loss of inhibitions and memory impairments as sequelae of the injury.

Nurses may experience incidents of patients sexually acting out by masturbating in public areas, requesting sexual favors, making lewd comments, and inappropriately touching breasts and buttocks, primarily by male patients with female nursing staff. Although reported in nursing literature for many years, these incidents are now considered sexual harassment in the work place. One study of nurses working in hospitals found that 70% of nurses had experienced sexual harassment on the job, of which over 50% of the perpetrators were male patients (Libbus & Bowman, 1994). Some nurses in this study also reported that sexual harassment had impaired their ability to work effectively; especially upsetting incidents impaired their ability to problem solve.

Nursing interventions designed to extinguish the inappropriate behavior include immediately telling the patient matter-of-factly that the behavior is inappropriate and what the consequences of the behavior are. An example is, "Your comment asking me to get into bed with you is not appropriate. It is very difficult for me to work with you when you say things like that." Patients who have cognitive impairment may also need to be redirected, as illustrated in the following statement: "When I was helping you transfer just now, you placed your hand on my bottom. I don't like that. Next time, put your hand here on the wheelchair." Nurses may need to let the patient know at the beginning of a shift that they are expected to act appropriately. Patients who are agitated because of neurologic trauma may also need to be approached from their weaker side when providing care. When approaching an agitated patient, a nurse can place a soft object like a washcloth in the patient's hands so

TABLE 30–3 • DRUG EFFECTS ON HUMAN SEXUAL BEHAVIOR

Drug or Drug Category	Effect	Probable Mechanism of Action
Oral contraceptives	Positive	Permits separation of sexual activity from concern about contraception
Antihypertensives Clonidine (Catapres) Guanethidine (Ismelin) Methyldopa (Aldomet) Propranolol (Inderal) Trimethaphan (Arfonad)	Negative	Peripheral blockade of nervous innervation of sex glands
Antidepressants Amitriptyline (Elavil) Desipramine (Norpramin) Imipramine (Tofranil) Nortriptyline (Aventyl) Phenelzine sulfate (Nardil) Protriptyline (Vivactil) Tranylcypromine sulfate (Parnate)	Negative	Central depression; peripheral blockade of nervous innervation of sex glands
Antihistamines Chlorpheniramine (Chlor-Trimeton) Diphenhydramine (Benadryl) Promethazine (Phenergam)	Negative	Blockade of parasympathetic nervous innervation of sex gland Diuresis
Glycopyrrolate (Robinul) Methantheline (Banthine)	Negative	Blockade of parasympathetic nervous innervation of sex gland
Sedatives and tranquilizers Benperidol Chlordiazepoxide (Librium) Chlorpromazine (Thorazine) Diazepam (Valium) Mesoridazine (Serentil)	Negative	Ganglionic blockade of nervous innervation of sex glands
Phenoxybenzamine (Dibenzyline) Prochlorperazine (Compazine) Thioridazine (Mellaril)	Negative and positive	Central sedation, blockade of autonomic innervation of sex glands; suppression of hypothalamic and pituitary function Tranquilization and relaxation
Ethyl alcohol Barbiturates Diuretics Bendroflumethiazide (Naturetin)		Central depression; suppression of motor activity; relaxation
Chlorthiazide (Diuril)	Negative, transiently positive	Release of inhibitions; relaxation
Spironolactone (Aldactone)	Negative	Central depression; suppression of motor activity; hypnosis
	Negative	Diuresis
Sex hormone preparations Cyproterone acetate Nandrolone phenpropionate (Durabolin)	Negative	Antiandrogenic effects on sexual function; loss of libido; decreased potency
Yohimbine	Questionable	Stimulation of lower spinal nerve centers
Strychnine	Questionable	Stimulation of neuraxis; priapism
Amylnitrate	Questionable	Vasodilation of genitourinary tract; smooth muscle relaxation

TABLE 30–3 • DRUG EFFECTS ON HUMAN SEXUAL BEHAVIOR *Continued*

Drug or Drug Category	Effect	Probable Mechanism of Action

Narcotics and psychoactive drugs
   Amphetamines
   Cocaine
	Negative	Central depression; decreased libido and impaired potency

Heroin
   Lysergic acid, diethylamide (LSD)
   Marijuana
   Methadone
	Transiently positive	Release of inhibitions; increased suggestibility; relaxation

Morphine		
Levodopa	Questionable	Improvement of well-being
Caffeine	Questionable	Central nervous system stimulant
Vitamin E	Questionable	Supports fertility in laboratory animals
Selenium	Questionable	Supports fertility in laboratory animals
Lithium carbonate	Questionable	Produces broad endocrine changes; diuresis
Clomiphene citrate (Clomid)	Questionable	Stimulates gonadotropic hormones; enhances expectations of achieving pregnancy
Bromocriptine (Parlodel)	Questionable	Stimulates gonadotropic hormones
Cimetidine (Tagamet)	Negative	Unknown
Clofibrate (Atromid-S)	Questionable	Unknown.
Disulfiram (Antabuse)	None by itself; negative with alcohol	Blocks alcohol metabolism; produces aldehyde syndrome

that the patient is less likely to grab the nurse. A final strategy with cognitively impaired patients is to avoid making statements that can be misinterpreted by the patient. It is better to say, "I'm the nurse who is going to work with you today," rather than "I'm your nurse today," or "I'm going to take care of you."

In the home, the sexual partner may complain of the client's constant requests for sex, spontaneous performance of oral sex, masturbation in the more public rooms of the house, and undressing or spontaneously appearing naked. The impaired adult may initiate sex and then quickly forget what he or she is doing and move onto something else. These behaviors are often quite distressing to the partner, who may seek advice from a nurse or physician on how to handle these situations.

Partners may question whether the impaired adult can give consent to having sex or may express disgust over the thought of sex with someone who is cognitively impaired. These feelings are often accompanied by regret and feelings of having lost a lifelong confidant and lover because of memory impairments and personality changes. Nurses can intervene by informing the partner that behavioral changes are common and occur as a result of the injury; they are not a personality flaw of the caregiver or the impaired adult. Wright (1993) outlined several suggestions nurses can offer partners of people with cognitive impairment.

Alterations in Sexual Arousal

There are several varieties of alteration in sexual arousal (sometimes referred to as excitement phase dysfunctions), including the following:

Decreased subjective arousal

Difficulty attaining an erection

Difficulty maintaining an erection

Difficulty both attaining and maintaining an erection

Decreased subjective arousal coupled with difficulty attaining an erection or difficulty maintaining an erection or both

Decreased physiologic arousal in women (vaginal dryness)

Decreased physiologic and subjective arousal in women

Schover and Jensen (1988) distinguished between feelings of subjective arousal and feelings of physiologic arousal. They stated that some clients report diminished vasocongestion without a loss of erotic sensation. It is possible for both men and women to experience a problem in physiologic aspects of arousal without a problem of subjective feelings of arousal, or vice versa. This diagnostic system offers precision in diagnosis of problems related to erection, because some men have problems attaining an erection, some have problems maintaining an erection, and some have both problems.

Problems related to sexual arousal have their origins in body-mind interaction. It should be noted that transient episodes of difficulty in attaining or maintaining erection are common, with 50% of men experiencing them. Pharmacologic agents, such as those shown in Table 30–3, can interfere with physiologic correlates of sexual arousal in men and women. Disorders that affect vascular function, such as diabetes or Leriche's syndrome, can impair erection in men and vasocongestion in women.

The aging process is associated with less intense vasocongestive response to sexual stimuli. Problems with vaginal lubrication and swelling are associated with menopausal changes in estrogen levels in some women. Performance anxiety and fear of failure are commonly associated with arousal phase dysfunctions. In some instances, anxiety is produced by complex causes.

Diagnosis of arousal phase sexual dysfunction is usually based on defining characteristics obtained from a sexual problem history and a physical examination. The physical examination may or may not provide evidence of arousal phase dysfunction. There may be reflex erection or swelling present with a pelvic or rectal examination, but their absence does not indicate dysfunction. Absence of sensation or alterations of sensation may also be evident in the physical examination (see Chapter 29). As with desire phase dysfunctions, diagnoses can be modified to indicate whether or not the problem is lifelong or situation specific; for example, it is possible to have a lifelong diagnosis of difficulty attaining an erection or decreased subjective arousal that is situational (i.e., linked to an illness).

For people with nervous system problems, it is important to reflect on underlying neurophysiologic mechanisms involved in sexual arousal. The area of the parasympathetic outflow (S2, S3, S4) is important in both reflex erection in men and lubrication and swelling in women. Although sexual function is largely an autonomic function, the neurologic assessment is primarily a somatic examination, and the conclusions about autonomic function are made by inference from somatic findings. The distinction can be made between suprasegmental (upper motor neuron) and segmental (lower motor neuron) types of sexual function by means of data obtained from rectal examination. When reflex tone is present in the external sphincter, suprasegmental (upper motor neuron) disruption to sexual function exists. When reflex tone is not present in the external rectal sphincter, segmental dysfunction exists. The likelihood of experiencing erections is much greater for men with suprasegmental lesions.

Sensation and volitional control are important in assessing sexual function. When all sensation (pinprick, light touch) is absent from the genital area (penile, scrotal, perianal, and vulval skin) *bilaterally* and when volitional control of the external rectal sphincter is absent, it can be inferred that the spinal cord has been functionally transected. The typical consequences are that sexual sensations are not perceived. There are, however, indications that spinal cord–injured women with complete lesions perceive sensations associated with deep vaginal penetration. It is possible that pressure on the cervix causes stimuli to ascend to cortical levels via the autonomic nervous system. When any sensation or volitional control of the rectal sphincter is present, it can be inferred that the spinal cord is only partially transected, and the lesion is termed incomplete. Both the completeness of the lesion and the segmental level have an important effect on prognosis for sexual function. Table 30–4 summarizes the effects of spinal cord injury on sexual functions.

Inhibition of autonomic outflow can interfere with the vasocongestive aspects of sexual arousal, although not with the subjective components of sexual arousal. Although swelling and lubrication may be altered, sensations associated with sexual arousal may be experienced in areas of the body not affected by neurologic description.

Diagnoses of desire phase dysfunctions include the following:

Decreased vasocongestion related to spinal cord injury

Decreased subjective arousal related to fear of failure

Difficulty maintaining an erection related to neuropathy

Nursing interventions for arousal phase dysfunctions are usually directed at reducing anxiety (performance anxiety or fear of failure) and collaborating with the physician in correcting or transcending physiologic problems if possible. Reduction of anxiety is usually accomplished through desensitization exercises in which women and men are instructed to use erotic imagery to approximate the sexual situations that evoke anxiety. Gradually, the erotic images approach the actual situation. Another therapeutic strategy involves structuring sexual encounters so they are not demanding. Exercises in which emphasis is

TABLE 30–4 • SEXUAL RESPONSE OF PEOPLE WITH COMPLETE LESIONS OF THE SPINAL CORD

Location of Cord Lesion	Sexual Function
C1–C3	• Male: Reflex erection from stimulation of genital region or thighs likely. Psychogenic erection from sexual thoughts not possible. Erogenous areas may develop above line of injury. No change in libido. • Female: Little study done. If lubrication analogous to erection, expect reflex lubrication similar to reflexogenic erection. As in male, will not feel sensations or be aware of lubrication unless it is pointed out. No change in libidinal drive. Fertility retained.
C4–C5	• Male: Reflex erection likely. Psychogenic erection impossible. Extragenital erogenous zones above level of injury likely. Nongenital orgasm reported. No ejaculation. Oral sex with partner possible. No change in libido. • Female: Reflex lubrication likely. Psychogenic lubrication unlikely. Extragenital erogenous zones above level of injury likely. Nongenital orgasm reported. Oral sex with partner possible. No change in libido. Fertility retained.
C6	• Male: As for C4–C5 level of injury. Holding and caressing now possible because of ability to use deltoids and biceps. • Female: As for C4–C5, with holding and caressing possible. Fertility retained.
C7–C8	• Male and female: Increased potential for use of hands to give pleasure to self and partner.
T1	• Male and female: As for C7–C8 level of injury, but with increased fine motor hand dexterity.
T2–T5	• Male and female: Commonly reported orgasmic experiences from nipple stimulation. Reflex erection and lubrication not seen.
T6–T12	• Male: Still generally unable to have psychogenic erection. Also unlikely to have reflex erection. • Female: Water-soluble lubricant needed for intercourse because of decreased reflex lubrication. Libidinal drive remains the same. Fertility retained.
L1–L2	• Male: Psychogenic stimulation and erection possible between T12 and L2 level of injury. Reflex erections possible but unlikely below L1 and L2. • Female: Psychogenic erection of clitoris, lubrication, labial swelling, and skin flush possible but unlikely. Fertility retained.
L3–L4	• Male and female: No reflexogenic erection or lubrication. Psychogenic genital sexual reactions unlikely.
L5–S1	• Male and female: Extragenital sexual potential great. Erection and lubrication unlikely through either reflexogenic or psychogenic means.
S2–S4	• Male: Reflex erection possible. Ejaculation possible (may be retrograde). • Female: Reflex lubrication possible.

From Weinberg, J.S. (1982). Human sexuality and spinal cord injury. *Nursing Clinics of North America,* 17(3), 407–419.

placed on pleasure versus performance are suggested. These exercises emphasize sensual aspects of touch; often, genital touching is prohibited. A special form of nondemanding encounter is called *sensate focus* and involves sequential pleasuring by oneself or a partner, gradually approximating the type of sexual activity (masturbation or intercourse) the individual desires. Fantasy or forms of stimulation other than by a partner can be used in conjunction with the sensate focus exercises.

Arousal phase dysfunctions attributable to disrupted neurophysiologic functions are common among people with nervous system problems. Therapeutic strategies can be directed toward altering or transcending the physiologic problem, which sometimes can be altered; for example, medication regimens that interfere with vasocongestion can be modified to restore sexual function. Sometimes, therapeutic agents used to treat underlying medical problems may have positive effects on sexual dysfunction, as is sometimes noted with the use of steroids. For men and women with a total loss of sensation to genital areas, therapeutic strategies directed toward transcending arousal phase problems include techniques that amplify erotic sensations in parts of the body unaffected by pathology. For example, a woman with a sacral and compression injury may learn to amplify the erotic sensations she perceives in her breasts to the point of experiencing orgasm with breast stimulation (Weinberg, 1982). Both men and women report their skin being hypersensitive to erotic touch in the dermatomes between sensation loss and full sensation.

Some neurologic insults leave a survivor with a paraparesis, or partial paralysis accompanied by a partial loss of sensation. These people often have partially impaired genital sensation and function. They may avoid sexual stimulation either because of fear of failure to perform or because of having come to a decision that they will not be able to have sex. These patients often make slow but steady gains in physical and occupational therapy by training the muscles that remain operational, but they need a great deal of strengthening and training to permit gains in activities of daily living or ambulation abilities. More and more of these patients are reporting gains in both genital sensation and genital function with repeated sexual stimulation. One man with an incomplete spinal cord injury following a gunshot wound revealed that it occurred to him that because he had made tremendous gains in learning to walk over the past year as a result of therapy, he ought to regain his ability to achieve an erection through repeated masturbation. He jokingly referred to the masturbation as "physical therapy for my sex life." Others are reporting similar results. Nurses can encourage patients to continue sexual stimulation, either through masturbation or stimulation by a partner, to see if over time both sensation and physiologic excitement improve.

• C A S E   S T U D Y   2

Mr. Williams, 63 years old, had experienced a ruptured cerebral aneurysm 6 months previously during sexual activity with his wife of 40 years. His aneurysm was successfully surgically corrected. He currently desires sexual activity and feels aroused but says he loses his erection too quickly to have intercourse. He is aware that he thinks about the experience of the cerebral hemorrhage and is fearful of its recurrence. Mr. Williams is currently taking propranolol. Mrs. Williams also is concerned about her husband's welfare, worries that her sexual interest may have been responsible for the initial hemorrhage, and fears a recurrence.

A diagnosis of difficulty maintaining an erection, not lifelong, related to fear of a recurrence of cerebral hemorrhage and to medication suggests the following therapeutic strategies:

1. Reduce anxiety about sexual encounters through desensitization exercises using imagery to approximate feeling aroused, feeling an erection, and having intercourse.
2. Monitor response to desensitization exercises, progressing to sensate focus exercises with partner.
3. Monitor response to sensate focus exercises, progressing to intercourse with partner.
4. Monitor medication regimen; if interventions to reduce anxiety are not effective, discuss alteration of medication regimen.

Outcomes of these strategies include improvement in sexual arousal, ability to maintain an erection, and reduction of anxiety about sexual activity for Mr. Williams.

A diagnosis of anxiety related to her husband's well-being and fear of dangerous outcomes of sexual activity for Mrs. Williams suggests the following therapeutic strategies:

1. Advise Mrs. Williams about the slim likelihood of recurrence of cerebral hemorrhage.
2. Involve Mrs. Williams in discussions of desensitization and sensate focus exercises.

Outcomes for Mrs. Williams should include an improved understanding of her husband's low risk of untoward outcomes of sexual activity and reduced anxiety during sexual activity.

The scenario of Mr. and Mrs. Williams needing to overcome fear is included to illustrate how anxiety can interfere with men getting erections after a stroke or chest pain has occurred during sex. However, most times erectile dysfunction is caused by physiologic changes, not fear or anxiety. The inability to experience an erection occurs in most men at some time. The more commonly used term for erectile dysfunction is *impotence.* However, impotence has a negative connotation and implies permanent dysfunction. Erectile dysfunction is a more acceptable term. Older men have a greater likelihood of experiencing erectile dysfunction because of the changes that occur in sexual function with age and the effects of chronic illnesses and medications. Feldman, Goldstein, Hatzichristou, Krane, and McKinlay (1994) estimated that erectile dysfunction affects 18 million American men from 40 to 70 years. In the past, most erectile dysfunction was thought to be psychologic, rather than physiologic, in origin. Estimates are that 90% of impotence is due to chronic illness. The most common cause of erectile dysfunction is atherosclerosis of the vessels in the penis. Other major causes are hormonal alterations because of decreased testosterone and chronic illnesses such as diabetes. Medications, including antihypertensives and antidepressants, and alcohol abuse are also major contributors. Chronic illnesses that cause pain or decrease mobility, such as arthritis, chronic obstructive pulmonary disease, and Parkinson's disease, are also factors. Finally, psychogenic causes such as bereavement, anxiety, and depression can play a role. Often, erectile dysfunction is due to a multitude of factors (Kamel & Mir, 1999a).

Treatment for erectile dysfunction focuses first on the underlying cause. Men with diabetes may find that the better they control their blood sugar, the less erectile dysfunction they experience. Men with vascular disease may benefit from stopping smoking, reducing their cholesterol and fat intake, and adopting an exercise program. These strategies have been shown to actually reduce the amount of coronary artery disease, and it is likely there will be some long-term effect on penile circulation as well.

In addition to treating the underlying factors, medications, penile implants, pharmacologic erection programs, vacuum erection devices, and urethral suppositories are used to treat erectile dysfunction (Kamel & Mir, 1999b). Sildenafil (Viagra) taken 1 hour before intercourse increases blood flow to the penis, leading to an erection. ArginMax, a natural daily nutritional supplement, has been shown to improve men's ability to maintain an erection. For more information, see Table 30–5.

TABLE 30–5 • MEDICAL AND SURGICAL TREATMENTS FOR ERECTILE DYSFUNCTION

Treatment	Method and Outcome
Penile implants	Implants are surgically placed into the penis by a urologist. The two most common types are semirigid rods or inflatable devices. The penile implant affects only the ability to get an erection; ability to reach orgasm and penile sensation are not affected.
Pharmacologic erection programs (PEP)	Pharmacologic erection programs are offered by urologists who specialize in the treatment of erectile dysfunction. As a part of an extensive educational program, men are taught to self-inject the penis with doses of vasoactive drugs to achieve an erection that lasts 30–40 min and is sufficiently hard to permit intercourse. A small syringe and needle are used. Papaverine hydrochloride, used alone or in combination with phentolamine mesylate, has a reported success rate of 65%–100%, with a very low rate of side effects. These agents affect only the ability to get an erection; they do not affect orgasm or ejaculation. PEPs are widely used by men with erectile dysfunction because of diabetes, hypertension, pelvic trauma, and arteriosclerosis who want to continue intercourse and do not wish to have a penile implant.
Vacuum erection device	A vacuum tumescent device with constriction-retention bands is another option for men that does not require surgery or injections. The vacuum device consists of a plastic cylinder that is placed over the penis. Pumping the device creates negative pressure, and blood is drawn into the penis, leading to an erection. The erection is maintained by applying a constriction-retention band to restrict the venous flow of blood out of the penis. Erections may last 15–30 min. A photograph of one brand of vacuum erection device is shown in Figure 30–1.
Medications	Arginmax. A daily nutritional supplement. Order by calling 1-800-STAMINA or at http://www.sexualfitness.com Sildenafil (Viagra). Taken 1 hour before intercourse. Contraindicated in those with cardiovascular disease. Available only by prescription from a physician.
Urethral suppositories (MUSE—Medicated urethral system for erection)	Urethral suppository system of self-administering alprostadil. Rare side effects of burning sensation and minor urethral trauma.

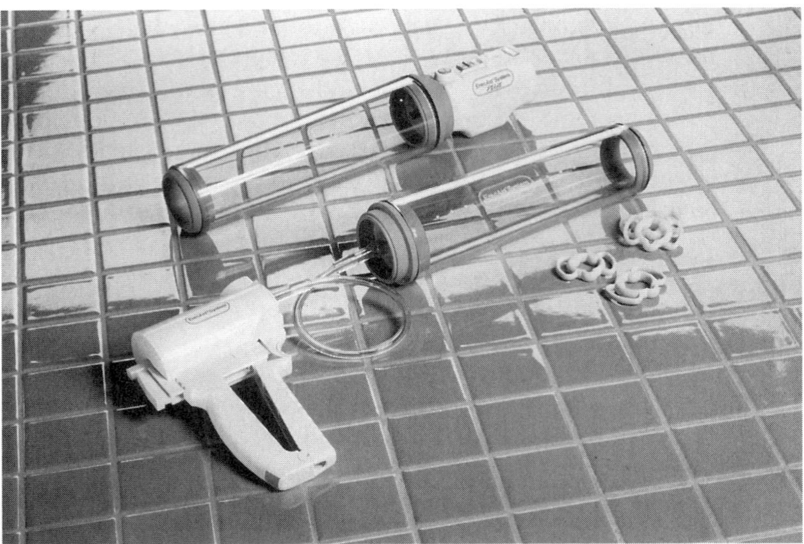

FIGURE 30–1 • Vacuum erection device. (Adapted from Flaskerud, J. H., & Ungvarski, P. [1992]. *HIV/AIDS: A guide to nursing care* [2nd ed.]. Philadelphia: W.B. Saunders.)

Alterations in Orgasm

Orgasm phase dysfunctions include problems with ejaculatory function and orgasm and with perception of pleasure associated with orgasm. Ejaculatory dysfunctions include premature ejaculation and inhibited ejaculation. Premature ejaculation occurs when men ejaculate too rapidly. Usually, the definition is based on the individual's or the couple's definition of what is too rapid rather than on some universally accepted standard. Premature ejaculation may occur before intromission or shortly after intromission. Men who experience premature ejaculation often do not perceive erotic sensations before orgasm and instead progress rapidly from low to very high levels of arousal. Often, an underlying problem is anxiety related to the experience of erotic sensations, and a variety of mechanisms have been suggested, including learned behavior of rapid ejaculation, fear, anger, and anxiety.

Inhibited ejaculation, sometimes termed *retarded ejaculation,* implies an inability to ejaculate at all during sexual activity or the requirement for an extended period of time to ejaculation, even in the presence of adequate stimulation. Some men have never ejaculated, even with masturbation; others have not ejaculated intravaginally. Inhibited ejaculation is often associated with lack of trust or anger in a relationship. Neurophysiologic and other medical conditions, as well as medications, can interfere with ejaculation and stimulation and may be responsible for inhibited ejaculation (see Table 30–3).

Other problems men experience that are related to orgasm include anhedonic orgasm, which occurs when the client ejaculates with normal force but experiences no sensation, or inhibition of ejaculation, in which emission occurs, resulting in seepage of semen rather than forceful ejaculation, and lack of pleasurable sensation is experienced. Ejaculation sometimes occurs with a flaccid penis, and, in other instances, anhedonic orgasms may occur without penile flaccidity. Rapid ejaculation with a flaccid penis may occur, with or without sensation of pleasure.

Orgasmic dysfunctions in women include anorgasmia, a global incapacity to reach orgasm. A woman may be situationally anorgasmic, having orgasms with masturbation or partner manipulation. Anorgasmia with intercourse is common.

Diagnoses include the following:

Inorgasmic except with masturbation

Inorgasmic except with partner manipulation

Inorgasmic except with masturbation and partner manipulation

Infrequent coital orgasms

Inorgasmic except for vibrator or mechanical stimulation

Mechanisms responsible for orgasmic phase dysfunctions include inadequate stimulation or obsessive self-observation. More remote mechanisms include fear or loss of control over sexual or aggressive impulses.

Diagnosis of orgasm phase dysfunctions is based on a sexual history and physical examination. Particular emphasis is placed on differentiating the type of dysfunction and if the problem is lifelong, situationally related, or global in nature. It is important to assume that both physiologic and psychosocial mechanisms may be involved in orgasm phase dysfunctions among people who have nervous system problems. For example, a man who has a spinal cord injury affecting ejaculation may experience retrograde ejaculation— ejaculation of semen into the bladder—or may experience orgasm with a flaccid penis, common outcomes of spinal cord injury. The dysfunction may be premature ejaculation, not simply a consequence of the nervous system damage but also a consequence of the anxiety surrounding sexual activity. In short, a clinician cannot safety assume that because nervous system damage is present, it is the sole explanation for the dysfunction.

Nursing interventions for anorgasmia include structuring the situations for sexual activity to achieve stimulation under the most tranquil conditions possible. Some options include distraction from self-observation through the use of fantasy and the use of imagery or fantasy along with self-pleasuring exercises. In some instances, immobility interferes with pleasuring, and, in others, lack of sensation or altered sensation interferes with orgasmic experience.

Strategies for premature ejaculation include use of the start-stop technique, in which stimulation is withdrawn intermittently to increase awareness of erotic sensations and to increase tolerance of the pleasure associated with sexual arousal. Strategies for retarded ejaculation include the use of manual stimulation, gradually approximating vaginal intercourse. Relaxation and stimulation can be paired, or stimulation, along with distraction by fantasy, can be attempted.

• C A S E   S T U D Y   3

Ms. McCarthy, 28 years old, fell from a horse, sustaining a complete spinal cord transection at L3–L4. Before her accident, she had been orgasmic with intercourse. Since she completed her rehabilitation program, she has had intercourse several times with her husband, has noted vaginal lubrication, has had some sensation with deep penile penetration, but has not experienced orgasms with intercourse.

A diagnosis of anorgasmia related to decreased sensory perception implies, as therapeutic strategies, enhancing erotic sensations through the following:

1. Sensate focus exercises to identify areas of maximum pleasure
2. Use of imagery to enhance sensations of sexual arousal
3. Rehearsal of communication regarding sexual pleasuring with her husband

Outcomes of these strategies include enhancement of erotic sensation, with improved understanding by both Ms. McCarthy and her husband of how to enhance pleasure, and experience of orgasm with intercourse for Ms. McCarthy.

• C A S E   S T U D Y   4

Ms. Fox, a 23-year-old woman with cerebral palsy, has never been orgasmic, although she experiences sexual desire and feels arousal—that is, she perceives vaginal wetness. She does not have a sexual partner. Because of spasticity, she is unable to pleasure herself manually.

A diagnosis of anorgasmia, lifelong, related to limited mobility suggests the following therapeutic strategies:

1. Use of vibrator and hand splint to provide sexual stimulation
2. Use of imagery to enhance sexual pleasure

Outcomes of these strategies include enhanced ability to attain sexual stimulation and orgasm.

Alterations in Sexual Self-Concept

An individual's sexual self-concept can be altered dramatically as a consequence of illness. Sexual self-concept includes the notion we have of ourselves as men or women, masculine or feminine. Sexual self-concept reflects body image and evaluation of one's adequacy as a man or a woman.

Surgery or injuries may cause changes in body image that affect sexual self-concept. Sometimes a person who is ill takes on the identity of the illness, making it difficult to integrate sexuality with the role changes that accompany being sick. Embarrassment and shame associated with changes in one's body because of muscle wasting, spasticity, appliances, and other bodily changes may produce intense anxiety about sexual activity and a pervasive sense of inadequacy.

Nursing diagnoses associated with altered sexual self-concept include the following:

Anxiety about sexual encounters related to altered body image

Altered sexual self-concept related to sick role experiences

Altered sexual self-concept related to partner's response

Diagnoses are based on the sexual history as outlined in Chapter 29. Often, the concerns about sexual self-concept exist independent of experiences of sexual dysfunction.

Nursing interventions for enhancing sexual self-concept include those directed at acceptance and transcendence of altered body image:

1. Transcendence of the sick role

2. Enhanced support from a partner

Particular emphasis is focused on helping the client experience validation of himself or herself in a relationship. Reducing anxiety about sexual encounters because of changed body image involves acceptance and transcendence of a changed body. Often, support from others who have coped with a similar health problem is invaluable. Rehearsing explanations of the health problem with the client may also be helpful. Exchanging information between clients about how to cope in sexual situations contributes to a broader array of coping strategies. Validation of the person's sexual image—that is, comments about the image he or she projects—is helpful.

Transcendence of the sick role is fostered by care environments that encourage client involvement in decision making and emphasize client efficacy. Attributions by others about the illness can either reinforce the client's self-image as sick or encourage the view of self as well and living with a challenge. The client can be encouraged to adopt a self-image consistent with remaining a healthy person in spite of pathology.

Obtaining support from a partner can enhance sexual self-concept. Some clients need assistance in building the social skills necessary to obtain support. These skills include the ability to communicate clearly and comfortably in sexual contexts.

• C A S E   S T U D Y   5

Mr. Anderson, a 22-year-old logger, sustained a crushing cauda equina injury in a logging accident. He has regained some mobility in his lower extremities but does not have bowel control or erections. He has been severely depressed since the injury, referring to the loss of his "manhood" and his occupation as a logger. He refers to himself as "a crip" in front of his male friends and says they pity him.

A diagnosis of altered sexual self-concept related to loss of erections and occupation implies the following therapeutic strategies:

1. Introduce the client to another spinal-cord injured client who has adapted successfully to the injury and has a positive self-concept.
2. Invite the client to rehabilitation unit group meetings that include discussions of sexual adaptation.
3. Rehearse explanations to potential partners about his injury and its effects.
4. Provide anticipatory guidance regarding sexual challenges he may experience.
5. Encourage him to learn to flirt and test out his sexual attractiveness anonymously "online." Levine (1998) is an excellent resource for guidance in learning the "how-to's" of cybersex.
6. Discuss alternative strategies for sexual pleasuring that he may find satisfying for himself or a partner.
7. Refer the client for occupational counseling and retraining.

Outcomes of these strategies should include improved sexual self-concept as evidenced by a decrease in negative references to himself and by an increase in positive self-statements. Long-term goals are a positive sense of his sexuality and his ability to be involved in a sexual relationship.

Nurses may also need to assist some adults who have experienced neurotrauma to protect themselves from being taken advantage of sexually. One of the unfortunate sequelae for some survivors of traumatic head injury is the loss of complex reasoning skills and the loss of social inhibitions, even though basic social skills and physical abilities are maintained. These survivors appear to the casual observer to be able to make competent decisions but are often very trusting and overly friendly, which makes them vulnerable to others who might take advantage of them financially, socially, and sexually (Griffith & Lemberg, 1993). Griffith and Lemberg (1993) presented the case report of a 16-year-old girl who was childish, readily expressed her sexual thoughts verbally, and at times was openly seductive. She casually revealed to her mother her excitement at having befriended a group of male construction workers, for whom she performed various sexual acts. Other authors have described similar incidents where young women and men end up involved in questionable sexual relationships. When head injury survivors exhibit these behaviors, nurses and other health professionals sometimes mistakenly assume the behaviors are due to the survivors' premorbid personality. Nurses can assist both the survivor and the family by anticipating the potential for victimization in those who show these personality traits after head injury. The survivor and his or her significant others need to adopt strategies that will foster independence and yet protect the survivor as well. Role-playing of situations the survivor is likely to encounter and practicing of scripts to use when pressured by others into making a questionable financial, social, or sexual decision are often helpful. Two excellent sources for parents and teachers to assist in dealing with the difficult issues of masturbation, intercourse, HIV/AIDS, homosexuality, and sexual exploitation in those with cognitive deficits are Fegan and Rauch (1997) and Schwier and Hingsburger (2000).

Alterations in Sexual Relationships

Sexual relationships are altered, sometimes profoundly, by illness. Value conflicts about sexual activity, difficulty communicating about sexual issues, dissatisfaction with sexual frequency, partner's inability to provide stimulation, inability to please a partner, and conflicts over the timing of sexual activity are a few of the difficulties couples can experience in their relationships.

In many instances, the partner has no acceptable outlet for sexual activity other than the ill person. When the client is ill, the partner may be forced to inhibit his or her sexual desire. Sometimes, partners who are also caretakers experience fatigue related to caretaking, which lowers sexual desire. In other instances, the partner may experience role confusion when required to care for the client *and* be a lover; for example, performing catheter care or a bowel regimen may be inconsistent with expressing physical love with the same person. In some couples, the partner may feel guilty or abnormal about initiating sexual activity with the person who is ill.

Alterations in sexual relationships as a result of illness are diagnosed through interview, optimally with partners individually and together. Nursing diagnoses related to altered sexual relationships include the following:

Value conflicts related to alternative forms of sexual expression

Dissatisfaction with lowered sexual frequency

Dissatisfaction with partner stimulation

Conflicts over timing of sexual activity

Nursing interventions are directed toward facilitating satisfactory involvement in a sexual relationship and emphasizing sexual desires and dissatisfactions. Primary interventions include helping clients and partners communicate clearly and comfortably about their concerns and problems. Groups of clients and partners dealing with the same concerns are particularly helpful in this regard. Strategies include the following:

1. Modeling effective communication

2. Providing information about the health problem and its effects on sexuality

3. Rehearsing communication about difficulties

• C A S E   S T U D Y   6

Sandra Miller, partner of a 30-year-old man who was involved in an automobile accident with resultant S2–S4 injury, is concerned about lack of vaginal stimulation. Her partner is able to have partial erections, but she has difficulty experiencing orgasm because of resultant decreased vaginal stimulation.

A diagnosis of dissatisfaction with stimulation consequent to partner's erectile dysfunction implies the following therapeutic strategies:

1. Provision of information about the effects of S2–S4 injury and partial erection
2. Provision of information about alternative stimulation—for example, use of the "stuff" technique for insertion of his semi-erect penis, use of vibrator or manual stimulation as a complement; recommendation that her partner obtain a "strap-on erection" into which he inserts his flaccid or semi-erect penis before intercourse (available from the Xandria Collection; see Table 30–5)
3. Rehearsal of communication about sexually satisfying stimuli and providing of feedback

---

One tragic consequence of some neurologic diseases is dementia, as evidenced by memory loss and personality loss. How the sexual partner copes with the sexual losses of dementia varies considerably, as is illustrated in the following paragraphs.

Some spousal caregivers of adults with cognitive impairment will seek out other sexual partners to meet their own needs of intimacy and sexuality, which have been ignored since their spouse became demented. Nurses can help by recognizing that this occurs and by conveying the knowledge that the respite gained from sexual encounters and intimacy outside marriage has helped other caregivers to continue to care for their impaired spouse. Recognizing that even though the spouse is still living, the person the caregiver married and loved for so many years is now gone, will help relieve any guilt the caregiver may be experiencing. Having affairs outside of marriage may be against the values of the nurse, but the nurse should not place blame on caregivers of demented spouses, who often provide care for many years, all alone, with little or no support. Nurses do need to ensure that the caregiving spouse is aware of precautions to use to prevent becoming infected with HIV and other STDs.

Other spousal caregivers are able to maintain the love for their demented spouse until he or she dies. Hepner (1994) wonderfully described the many "goodbyes" she said to her husband as his Alzheimer's disease progressed. Her powerful statements not only reflect her feelings but also are a testament to the willingness of the nursing staff to permit this couple to maintain their relationship to the end. Her memories serve as reminders to nurses that her husband, an end-stage Alzheimer's disease patient, was much, much more than just someone in a coma who died. He was her lifelong love.

ADDITIONAL RESOURCES

In addition to the strategies outlined in this chapter, nurses can help patients with neurologic trauma and diseases find educational resources to assist them to achieve healthy sexual outcomes. Table 30–1 lists written and video resources, as well as catalog companies and organizations, which may be helpful for people who have experienced trauma or diseases, their partners, and the nurses caring for them.

References

Alston, R.J., & McCowan, C.J. (1994). African American women with disabilities: Rehabilitation issues and concerns. *Journal of Rehabilitation 60*(1), 36–40.

Bertosa, H., Cellura, M., Pierce, L., & Rothacker, C. (1993). Women with spinal cord injuries require sensitive reproductive care. *MCN; American Journal of Maternal Child Nursing, 18*(5), 254–257.

Blackerby, W.F. (1988). *Head injury rehabilitation: Sexuality after traumatic brain injury.* Houston, TX: HDI Publishers.

Bolus, J. (1994). Teaching teens about condoms. *RN, 57*(3), 44–47.

Bullard, D.G., & Knight, S.E. (1981). *Perspectives.* St. Louis: C.V. Mosby.

Carrey, N.J., & Adams, L. (1992). How to deal with sexual acting-out on the child psychiatric inpatient ward. *Journal of Psychosocial Nursing, 30*(5), 19–23.

Corbet, B., Dobbs, J., & Bonin, B. (1998). *Spinal network* (3rd ed.). Malibu, CA: Miramar Communications.

Craig, D.I. (1990). The adaptation to pregnancy of spinal cord-injured women. *Rehabilitation Nursing, 15*(1), 6–9.

Feldman, H.A., Goldstein, I., Hatzichristou, D.G., Krane, R.J., & McKinlay, J.B. (1994). Impotence and its medical and psychosocial correlates: Results of the Massachusetts male aging study. *Journal of Urology, 151*(1), 54–61.

Flaming, D., & Morse, J.M. (1991). Minimizing embarrassment: Boys' experiences of pubertal changes. *Issues in Comprehensive Pediatric Nursing, 14*(4), 211–230.

Flaskerud, J.H., & Ungvarski, P.J. (1994). *HIV/AIDS: A guide to nursing care* (3rd ed). Philadelphia: W.B. Saunders.

Griffith, E.R., & Lemberg, S. (1993). *Sexuality and the person with traumatic brain injury: A guide for families.* Philadelphia: F.A. Davis.

Hatcher, R.A., Trussel, J., Stewart, F., Stewart, G.K., Kowal, D., Guest, F., Cates, W. Jr., & Policar, M.F. (1998). *Contraceptive technology* (17th ed.). New York: Irvington Publishers.

Hepner, J.E. (1994). Goodbye, love. *Journal of Neuroscience Nursing, 26*(1), 62.

Kamel, H.K., & Mir, T. (1999a). Impotence and aging. Part I. *Resident & Staff Physician, 45*, 34–46.

Kamel, H.K., & Mir, T. (1999b). Impotence and aging. Part II. *Resident & Staff Physician, 45*, 41–45.

Kaplan, H.S. (1988). *The illustrated manual of sex therapy* (2nd ed.). Philadelphia: Brunner Mazel.

Levine, D. (1998). *The joy of cybersex.* New York: Ballantine Books.

Libbus, M.K., & Bowman, K.G. (1994). Sexual harassment of female registered nurses in hospitals. *Journal of Nursing Administration, 24*(6), 26–31.

Maddox, S. (1993). *Spinal network* (2nd ed.). Boulder, CO: Spinal Network.

McGinnis, J.M., & Foege, W.H. (1993). Actual causes of death in the United States. *JAMA, 270*(18), 2207–2212.

Meeropol, E. (1991). One of the gang: Sexual development of adolescents with physical disabilities. *Journal of Pediatric Nursing, 6*(4), 243–250.

Moglia, R. (1993). Sexual abuse and disability. *National Head Injury Foundations TBI Challenge, 1*(4), 30–31.

Schover, I.R., & Jensen, S.B. (1988). *Sexuality and chronic illness: A comprehensive approach.* New York: Guilford Press.

Schwier, K., & Hingsburger, D. (2000). *Sexuality: Your sons and daughters with intellectual disabilities.* Baltimore: Brookes Publishing.

Seager, S.W.J., & Halstead, L.S. (1993). Fertility options and success after spinal cord injury. *Urology Clinics of North America, 20*(3), 543–548.

Selekman, J., & McIlvain-Simpson, G. (1991). Sex and sexuality for the adolescent with a chronic condition. *Pediatric Nursing, 17*(4), 535–538.

Sipski, M., & Alexander, C. (1977). *Sexual function in people with disability and chronic illness.* Gaithersburg, MD: Aspen.

Weinberg, J.S. (1982). Human sexuality and spinal cord injury. *Nursing Clinics of North America, 17*(3), 407–419.

Wright, L.K. (1993). *Alzheimer's disease and marriage.* Thousand Oaks, CA: Sage.

SELF-CARE PHENOMENA

31 | Self-Care: An Overview

MARGARET AULD BRUYA

The basic role and importance of self-evaluation and self-care in health and during health deviations are of widespread concern to nurses. The concept of self in the maintenance of physical and psychosocial well-being has long been recognized in nursing. This chapter identifies self-care as a range of learned individual behaviors, health maintenance lifestyles, uses of preventive health services, and symptom evaluations. The focus is on developmental aspects of self-care practices, role of the family, and cultural practices. The concept of empowerment (Urbancic, 1992) is intertwined because it facilitates the development of mastery, competence, self-worth, and control, which encompasses nursing strategies and potential studies. Alterations in self-care practices in relation to illness, particularly neurologic illness, are viewed as deviations from the expected or developmental norm. The nurse's collaborative role with patients in identifying and developing strategies that increase patient control over their lives is emphasized.

DEVELOPMENTAL ASPECTS

A growing body of literature is available on self-care and self-care practices. Christiansen, Schwartz, and Barnes (1988) categorized self-care into those daily and routine tasks necessary for living and those that are instrumental, such as food preparation, use of transportation, and housekeeping. Most authors agree that self-care is the basic level of health care in all societies. As such, self-care is considered a deliberate action, the outcome of which is foreseen. It is not considered random or erratic behavior but behavior that is the result of thoughtful and deliberate choices. Common wisdom, the behavior and set of rules and logic, is a pattern many of us learn through acculturation. The patterns of normal self-care practice for each society reflect the extent to which scientific data and knowledge application are developed and available to the public. Some behaviors are enduring and culturally prescribed; others are current fashion and may be more transient (e.g., aerobic exercise). Many self-care actions are known. Middle-aged women in Hartweg's (1993) study identified 8693 diverse self-care actions that promoted well-being.

Achievement of self-care ability in general is an anticipated outcome for humans. Self-care patterns are developed as other skills develop. This presumes the ability to experience sensation (e.g., taste, touch), to move at will (e.g., first crawl, then walk, then run), and to have cognition, consciousness, and affect.

During the course of normal growth and development, the nervous system enables an individual to respond in an integrated fashion to external and internal environments. Integrating the functions of all body systems allows maximal use of the communication network among all body systems and facilitates learning and retention. When the integration function of the human nervous system is impaired, the ability to develop self-care and self-care health practices may be altered. The nurse's essential role in assessing potential for self-care is to evaluate the extent of neurologic dysfunction, including neuroendocrine function or dysfunction; to examine the stages of physical, psychologic, and psychosocial development of the individual; and to consider sociocultural aspects.

The older adult is the focus of many challenges in American health care. Califano (1988), then U.S. Secretary of Health and Human Services, encouraged an investment in time and research to avert conditions that contribute to the decline in older adults' independence and, logically, their ability to perform self-care. The *Healthy People 2000* report is concerned with the rapid increase in the U.S. population older than 65 years (U.S. Department of Health and Human Services, 1993). In 1900, that group composed 4% of the population. The predictions are that persons older than 65 years will compose 13% of the population in 2000 and 22% of the population by 2030. This report emphasizes that quality of life as well as length of life means the years of healthy life. One "indicator of quality of life is an individual's ability to perform activities required for daily living. . . . Difficulty in performing these tasks leads to the need for assistance and often limits opportunity for remaining independent" (U.S. Department of Health and Human Services, 1993, p. 23).

Advanced age is coupled with disabling conditions, including hospitalizations for acute and chronic illnesses, that are encountered by nurses and the aged during convalescence. Modification of self-care activities is often essential after hospitalization (Jopp, Carroll, & Waters, 1993).

ROLE OF THE FAMILY AND SOCIAL GROUP

Cultural variation of self-care practices needs to be examined. Ideologic and cultural incongruities may limit or prohibit the use of self-care practices as many Western nurses view them (Leininger, 1991). The relinquishing to others of self-care in health matters developed early in this country and escalated as technology became institutionalized and industrialized (Northrop, 1993).

Northrop provided a clear analysis of self-care ideology and theory to shape health care policy. She believed that the "adoption of self-care practices and self-care education within the organization of a country's health care system can be used as one instrument for achieving the overall goals of health policy" (Northrop, 1993, p. 65). Families should be viewed as a part of the social group to maximize the nurse's assessment.

The degree of attainment of self-care and self-care health practices is influenced primarily by the family group. In many cultures, it is the wife or mother who assumes the important role of influencing self-care in family members. The practices of self-care espoused by the family are partly determined by the position of the affected individual in that family as well as by the roles assumed in that family. The family primary caregiver's knowledge about health and disease as well as his or her knowledge about health care practices may be limited or erroneous. Some researchers have focused on the various family structures and functions in relation to sociocultural differences, looking for explanations for the findings of poorer health, health practices, and health outcomes among people in lower economic class groups (Jonosik & Green, 1992). One research study reported that 70% of the symptoms documented in a family health calendar were taken care of by the family or through maternal involvement (Pratt, 1976).

Within a family group, people who are expected to produce effective self-care must have essential health care knowledge of themselves as well as knowledge of environmental conditions (Orem, 1991). To effectively care for self or family, the individual making such decisions needs to have the requisite knowledge as well as the ability to be rational and reasonable in judgments. The process of self-care includes ability to perceive symptoms, to weigh options for action, and to initiate self-care behaviors and evaluate their effectiveness (Robinson & Posner, 1992). Disadvantages could occur in family-influenced self-care practices when a considerable lack of knowledge limits the ability to perform home care techniques, even those as simple as body temperature determination.

Other disadvantages of family-influenced self-care health practices could be related to the level of previous life experiences of the members. Orem (1991) claimed without research substantiation that the essential elements to meet specific self-care demands are based on the ability to initiate and persevere in self-care to achieve desired results. She claimed that an ability to achieve these results comes from the following criteria:

1. Having knowledge and skills

2. Being motivated to initiate and continue effects

3. Being committed to meeting particular demands for care

4. Being able to execute the movements required

5. Having energy and a sense of well-being sufficient to initiate and sustain self-care

Cooperative care models, as proposed by Roach and Woods (1993), encourage patient self-care and family involvement. The premise is that active participation by patients and caregivers effects increased and improved self-care practices. This model allows input from patients and care partners and may facilitate meeting Orem's criteria. These authors reported that in the busy medical unit where this model was implemented, patients developed a "sense of responsibility and self-control" and the program fostered "independence and endorse[d] changes in health behavior that result[ed] in more knowledge and self-direction" (Roach & Woods, 1993, p. 29).

CULTURAL FACTORS

In every culture, self-care is learned through human interaction within the context of the sociocultural group. Leininger (1978, 1984, 1991) suggested that culturally variant groups view illness differently. One group perceives illness to be largely a personal body experience. Another group categorizes illness as extrapersonal, or outside the body. For the latter group, illness might be viewed as resulting from angered spirits. Such differences may account for the manner in which self-care practices are learned. The group who believes that illness is a personal and internal body experience tend to use more technical and physical self-care, whereas those who view illness as an extrapersonal experience may not consider self-care as relevant to health.

Birenbaum's (1981) views confirmed this culturally acquired viewpoint. One's group membership and social ties may establish barriers or promote access to seeking professional health care. Working with multiethnic migrants, Byerly (1980) found that there was a great deal of moving in and out of layperson's and traditional health care systems and subsystems as the circumstances dictated.

Early cultural conditioning determines a person's attitudes and reactions to healing beliefs and practices, including self-care practices. When immigration and migration occur, blurring and partial assimilation of one's early and newly acquired health and self-care beliefs may occur. Typically, assimilation into a dominant culture influences an individual, but rather than fully embracing the dominant culture, the individual, and subsequently the family members for whom he or she shares responsibility, develops bicultural values. The family choices reflect this bicultural use of alternative health beliefs and practices (Orque, Block, & Monroy, 1983).

Orque et al. (1983) provided a resource for a full description of cultural variations of health and self-care practices. The emphasis on personal or situational control of self-care practices and health care actions for a number of culturally diverse populations was explored. The belief that culturally prescribed healing remedies may help a person psychologically is subscribed to by many African Americans; however, when such practices fail, a medical person often is sought (Orque et al., 1983). Trust in God and in curanderos (folk healers) characterizes Hispanic culture, whereas Filipino and Chinese people gravitate toward bicultural health practices when assimilated into Western culture (Orque et al., 1983).

Morales-Mann and Jiang (1993) analyzed Orem's conceptual framework of self-care in Chinese nursing. Using the theme of cultural evaluation, these authors chose to examine the applications in Chinese nursing practice. They investigated the central themes surrounding Orem's premise that people require nursing care when their needs for care exceed their own ability to meet these needs (Orem, 1991). Their research demonstrated the utility of this theoretical perspective for Chinese nurses (and therefore Chinese consumers). They proposed that focus on the person with self-care deficits in China as an object of nursing care is "highly practical" for the Chinese nurse. Nurses need knowledge of the variety of cultural influences that have an impact on self-care and health practices. A repertoire of cognitive, perceptual, manipulative, communication, and interpersonal skills is essential to exercising self-care practices, and each person is influenced by cultural values and beliefs. Viewing a client in the context of his or her cultural orientation and heritage should assist the nurse in facilitating the deliberate performance of health behaviors designed to ensure the best outcome. Societal values and influences and individual hierarchies of values in seeking and using the predominant health services of the society all influence health outcomes.

ECONOMIC FACTORS

Economic detriments, such as market supply and demand and distribution of professional health personnel and services, influence one's self-care. Changes and potential changes in health care access and reimbursement will certainly affect nursing and the persons seeking or using nursing services. Abundant layperson's literature is available to the public. The self-treatment component of self-care is thought to represent a growing discomfort and disgruntlement with the perceived dysfunctional aspects and effects of contemporary health service systems. Self-treatment in response to this disgruntlement is not universal but may reflect the historical reliance on one's own emotional and physical resources.

Third-party payment and Medicare and Medicaid programs have made professional care available to more people. Reimbursement patterns are currently being examined and newly regulated. In professional health services, these reimbursement pattern changes have caused drastic cuts in lengths of hospital stay, earlier discharge of more acutely ill persons from acute care agencies, and necessity of greater home nursing skills. The need to learn self-care skills in managing chronic illness is increased by these factors. Nurses' sustained interest in their roles in self-care and self-help movements may prove to be beneficial to their leading other disciplines.

Either as a supplement to or as a substitute for professional services, self-care practices vary among and between individuals. Developmental, social, cultural, economic, religious, and health factors and values have an impact on one's ability to integrate self-care into the living pattern. Nurses must recall that, to exercise self-care, one must have knowledge of one's abilities and limitations. It is said that nursing and the provision of nursing services begin when an individual or groups of individuals do not or cannot meet self-care action requirements for health (Orem, 1991). Jopp et al. (1993) reported that in a sample of persons older than 60 years, 66% of the clients reported self-care deficits after discharge from the hospital. Additionally, 15% reported total inability to care for themselves following discharge. Nurses need to analyze the supportive educational system to promote or enhance self-care at home. Development of nurse specialists, or advanced practitioners in rehabilitation, is supported.

COMPONENTS AND ASSESSMENT OF SELF-CARE

The ability to perform self-care is conceptually automatic after one has learned how to do so. Beginning with childhood, one learns to perfect attainment of a comfortable level of self-care. Empowerment support, as defined by Urbancic (1992), is the deliberate, "collaborative helping relationship [facilitating] the development of feelings of mastery, competency, self-worth and control" (p. 276) useful for persons needing nursing care. Although Urbancic viewed empowerment as largely psychologic support, that view can be broadened to other nursing therapies. Given a broad range of physical, biologic, and social conditions, individuals who have successfully mastered previous learning can adapt their repertoire of abilities and limitations accordingly and are able to estimate their measure of self-care. The power to exercise self-care includes vigilance to the goal; attention to the task; available, usable physical energy; motivation to perform necessary tasks; appropriate technical knowledge; and ability to reason, make reasoned decisions, and conceptualize the self-care plan as an action (Orem, 1991). Support systems, in the form of family, traditions, societal norms, and religious and spiritual values, also affect self-care.

The equilibrium achieved in the prototypical model of an individual able to care for himself or herself can be contrasted with the disequilibrium of one whose skills are no longer operative. Acute or chronic illness, accidents, or extremes in neuroendocrine balance can bring chaos to the individual or to the support systems for that individual. Neurologic or orthopedic damage from an accident may render an individual unable to move, to experience sensations sufficiently to protect vital functions, or to think clearly enough to make decisions. Similarly, a mildly head-injured person whose forte in the past was a strong memory may experience extreme frustrations in coping with the day-to-day short-term memory needed to read the daily newspaper. A person with hypersecretion of a hormone may experience alterations in affect. Habituated self-care practices are severely affected in each of these examples.

The manner in which deviation from usual self-care practices affects an individual relates back to her or his developmental stage. A young child is not expected to perform extensive self-care practices or to exert extensive personal control over health and health actions. Rather, a responsible adult typically does this for the child. The nurse's role is to respect the client's (including the adult's) perceived needs rather than to impose the nurse's perceived need. A parallel exists in the adult whom we anticipate to be developmentally mature but whose role may be altered or deviated from the norm.

Assessment of the impact of a neurologic disorder on self-care is therefore expected to include (1) extent to which the deviation has a impact on mobility, sensation, cognition, coping, consciousness, affect, and support systems; (2) level of development; (3) prior self-care practices; (4) economic and human resources; and (5) cultural beliefs and norms regarding self-care.

When deviations from self-care occur, the effect is not solely on the individual. The nurse must evaluate that person's role in the family, including the patient's age, sex, cultural and social preferences, health care situation (e.g., temporary or chronic), and knowledge, as well as the pathology involved.

The assessment of self-care usually follows a hierarchical model, from being able to perform basic activities of daily living to being able to exercise a degree of perfection in self-care management. When a client appears to have intact neurologic systems necessary for exercising self-care and has the cognitive abilities to do so yet does not exercise self-care options to the extent the nurse thinks optimal, conflict may occur. In such situations, it may be necessary for the nurse to look beyond the physiologic and psychosocial parameters and investigate cultural patterning.

SUMMARY

The concept of self-care is viewed from developmental, sociocultural, and humanistic dimensions. This view serves as the basis for understanding and learning to see the ability for self-care and self-care practices from a broader perspective rather than as simply providing for one's own activities of daily living. Nursing's role in assessing abilities and limitations for self-care is needed when caring for human beings who cannot care for themselves.

References

Birenbaum, A. (Ed.). (1981). *Health care and society.* Lanham, MD: Rowman & Littlefield.

Byerly, E. L. (1980). *Health care alternatives of multiethnic migrants* (Report to the Division of Nursing, Nursing Research Branch, Public Health Service, Grant No. NU00592). Washington, DC: U.S. Department of Health and Human Services.

Califano, J. (1988, March 20). Health care chaos. *The New York Times,* pp. 44, 46, 56–58.

Christiansen, C. H., Schwartz, R. K., & Barnes, K. J. (1988). Self-care evaluation and management. In J. A. DeLisa (Ed.), *Rehabilitation medicine: Principles and practice* (pp. 95–115). Philadelphia: J.B. Lippincott.

Hartweg, D. L. (1993). Self-care actions of healthy middle-aged women to promote well-being. *Nursing Research, 42*(4), 221–227.

Jonosik, E., & Green, E. (1992). *Family life: Process and practice.* Sudbury, MA: Jones & Bartlett.

Jopp, M., Carroll, M. S., & Waters, L. (1993). Using self-care theory as a guide to management of the older adult after hospitalization. *Rehabilitative Nursing, 18*(2), 91–94.

Leininger, M. M. (1978). *Transcultural nursing: Concepts, theories and practices.* New York: John Wiley & Sons.

Leininger, M. M. (Ed.) (1984). *Care: The essence of nursing and health.* Thorofare, NJ: Slack.

Leininger, M. M. (Ed.) (1991). *Culture care diversity and universality: A theory of nursing.* New York: National League for Nursing.

Morales-Mann, E. T., & Jiang, S. L. (1993). Applicability of Orem's conceptual framework: A cross-cultural point of view. *Journal of Advanced Nursing, 18*(5), 737–741.

Northrop, D. T. (1993). Self-care myth reconsidered. *Advances in Nursing Science, 15*(3), 59–66.

Orem, D. E. (1991). *Nursing: Concepts of practice* (4th ed.). New York: McGraw-Hill.

Orque, M. S., Block, B., & Monroy, L. A. (1983). *Ethnic nursing care.* St. Louis: C.V. Mosby.

Pratt, T. (1976). *Family structure and effective health behavior.* New York: Houghton Mifflin.

Roach, K. G., & Woods, H. B. (1993). Implementing cooperative care on an acute care medical unit. *Clinical Nurse Specialist, 7*(1), 26–29.

Robinson, K. D., & Posner, J. D. (1992). Patterns of self-care needs and interventions related to biologic response modifier therapy: Fatigue as a model. *Seminars in Oncology Nursing, 8*(Suppl. 4), 17–22.

Urbancic, J. C. (1992). Empowerment support with adult female survivors of childhood incest: Part 1—Theories and research. *Archives of Psychiatric Nursing, 6*(5), 275–281.

U.S. Department of Health and Human Services. (1993). *Healthy people 2000* (DHHS Publication No. [PHS] 91–502B). Sudbury, MA: Jones & Bartlett.

Bibliography

Aamodt, A. A. (1978). The care component in a health and healing system. In E. E. Bauwens (Ed.), *The anthropology of health* (pp. 37–45). St. Louis: C.V. Mosby.

Antrobus, M. (1981). Self-care in sickness and in health. *Nursing Times, 10*(342), 347.

Brownlee, A. J. (1978). *Community culture and care.* St. Louis: C.V. Mosby.

Cammermeyer, M. (1983). A growth model of self-care for neurologically impaired people. *Journal of Neurosurgical Nursing, 15*(5), 299.

Caporael-Katz, B. (1983). Health, self-care and power: Shifting the balance. *Topics in Clinical Nursing, 5*(3), 31.

Cousins, N. (1976). The anatomy of an illness as perceived by the patient. *New England Journal of Medicine, 295*(26), 1458.

Cousins, N. (1979). *Anatomy of an illness as perceived by the patient.* New York: Bantam Books.

Damant, M. (1981). The meaning of self-care. *Community Outlook, 11,* 373.

Dean, K. (1981). Self-care responses to illness: A selected review. *Social Science Medicine, 15A,* 673.

Decker, S. D., & Kinzel, S. (1985). Learned helplessness and decreased social interaction in elderly disabled persons. *Rehabilitative Nursing, 10*(2), 31.

Dickson, G. L., & Lee-Villasenor, H. (1982). Nursing theory and practice: A self-care approach. *Advances in Nursing Science, 5*(1), 29.

Goodin, B. (1984). Self-care in health. *Lamp, 41*(5), 24.

Harper, D. C. (1984). Application of Orem's theoretical constructs to selfcare medication behaviors in the elderly. *Advances in Nursing Science, 6*(3), 29.

Holzemer, W. L. (1992). Linking primary health care and self-care through case management. *Internal Nursing Review, 393,* 83–89.

Hyde, A. (1975). The phenomenon of caring: Part I. *Nursing Research Report, 10,* 1, 10.

Hyde, A. (1976). The phenomenon of caring: Parts II, III. *Nursing Research Report, 11,* 2, 15.

Hyde, A. (1977). The phenomenon of caring: Part IV. *Nursing Research Report, 12,* 2.

Johns, J. L. (1985). Self-care today in search of an identity. *Nursing Health Care, 6*(3), 153.

Katz, S., Branch, L. G., Branson, M. H., Papsidero, J. A., Beck, J. C., & Greer, D. S. (1983). Active life expectancy. *New England Journal of Medicine, 309*(20), 1218.

Kearney, B. Y., & Fleischer, B. J. (1979). Development of an instrument to measure exercise of self-care agency. *Research in Nursing and Health, 2*(1), 25.

Kerr, J. A. (1985). Adherence and self-care. *Heart and Lung, 14*(1), 24.

Leininger, M. M. (1977). The essence and central focus of nursing: The phenomenon of caring—Part V. *Nursing Research Report, 12*(1), 2, 14.

Leininger, M. M. (1992). Self-care ideology and cultural incongruities: Some critical issues [editorial]. *Journal of Transcultural Nursing, 4*(1), 2–4.

Levin, L. S., Katz, A. H., & Halst, E. (1979). *Self-care: Law initiatives in health.* Canton, MA: Prodist.

Litman, T. (1971). Health care and the family: A three-generation analysis. *Medical Care, 9*(3), 67.

Munkres, A., Oberst, M. T., & Hughes, S. H. (1992). Appraisal of illness, symptom distress, self-care burden, and mood states in patients receiving chemotherapy for initial and recurrent cancer. *Oncology Nursing Forum, 19*(8), 1201–1209.

Nelson, D. (1984). Nurse managed rehabilitation. *Nursing Management, 15*(3), 30.

Orem, D. E., & Nursing Development Conference Group (Eds.) (1979). *Concept formalization in nursing.* Boston: Little, Brown.

Pattulo, A. W., & Barnard, K. E. (1968). Teaching menstrual hygiene to the mentally retarded. *American Journal of Nursing, 68*(12), 2572.

Schlotfeldt, R. M. (1976). Accountability: A critical dimension in health care. In M. M. Leininger (Ed.), *Transcultural health care issues and conditions* (pp. 137–148). Philadelphia: F.A. Davis.

Smits, M. W. (1992). Correlates of self-care among the independent elderly: Self-concept affects well-being. *Journal of Gerontological Nursing, 18*(9), 13–18.

Winegrad, C. H. (1984). Mental status tests and the capacity for self-care. *Journal of the American Geriatrics Society, 32*(1), 49.

Alterations in Self-Care

CHRISTINA MUMMA

When asked about their quality of life, individuals living with multiple sclerosis (MS) emphasized the importance of independence, engaging in desired activities, and being able to care for themselves (Mumma & Gibson, 1997). Study participants' statements included the following:

- Quality of life means functioning well enough to get the things done that you actually have to do, let alone the things you want to do.

- I don't want to be dependent on somebody.

- I used to do all this stuff out in the yard myself; now I have to rely on other people to do a lot of the stuff for me. I have to rely on people to take out my garbage and take the clothes downstairs.

People who acquire neurologic dysfunction as a result of MS, stroke, other diseases, or injuries are likely to experience a variety of alterations in self-care. These self-care deficits vary in both quality, or type of deficit, and quantity, or severity of deficit.

CONTINUUM OF SELF-CARE

The type of self-care discussed most often in the nursing literature can be categorized as performance of activities of daily living (ADLs). Hickey defined ADLs as "activities that must be accomplished independently for patients to assume responsibility for their own needs and to participate actively in society" (1997, p. 239). The self-care activities usually included are self-feeding, bathing, dressing, grooming, toileting, and home care skills (McCourt, 1993; Orem, 1995). Whether a person must be totally independent in the performance of basic self-care tasks to be an active participant in society is debatable. There are many people with disabilities who depend on others for assistance with such personal self-care activities as bathing, dressing, and toileting but maintain full-time jobs and display considerable productivity and creativity. They are certainly active participants in society. The self is considerably more than the body that is fed, bathed, dressed, toileted, and provided with a home. Thus, as discussed in Chapter 31, self-care can be thought of in much broader terms.

Orem (1995) built a model of nursing around the concept of self-care. She described nursing as the assistance of individuals in the provision and management of self-care to sustain life and health, recover from disease or injury, and cope with effects of disease or injury (Fig 32–1). Methods and amounts of nursing care required depend on the type and severity of alterations in self-care. Self-care ability can be considered as a continuum from inability to perform any self-care activities (total self-care deficit) to ability to perform all self-care activities independently. The broadest interpretation of alterations in self-care would allow for growth and expansion of self, not just self-care deficits. Obviously, people are more likely to come to the attention of nurses and the health care system for "too little" self-care rather than for "too much" self-care. Figure 32–1 illustrates the continuum of alterations in self-care, with examples of nursing interventions at various points along the continuum.

The purpose of this chapter is to examine alterations in self-care typically experienced by individuals with nervous system dysfunction. Illustrative case examples are provided in relation to the following areas of the self-care continuum that are depicted in Figure 32–1: protective reflexes, basic hygienic tasks, independent living, and orientation to healthy living. The discussion of each type of self-care alteration includes manifestations and human responses. Manifestations involve the relationship of the alteration in self-care to neuroanatomy and neurophysiology. Each self-care alteration is viewed as a human response to multiple phenomena. The neurologic dysfunction resulting from nervous system injury or disease is usually the most important phenomenon to which the individual responds. Other influencing phenomena include intrapersonal

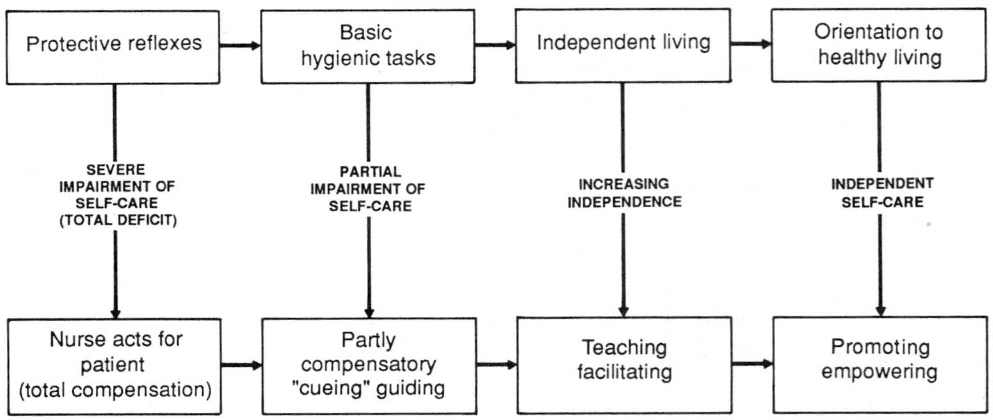

FIGURE 32–1 • Alterations in the self-care continuum.

factors (e.g., beliefs, values, self-esteem), interpersonal factors (e.g., relationships with loved ones and caregivers), and environmental factors (e.g., treatment environment, health care system). Because the phenomena listed are in continuous, dynamic interaction, alterations in self-care are highly complex human responses.

ALTERATIONS IN SELF-CARE

Protective Reflexes

The manifestations, or neuroanatomic evidence, within the nervous system of an individual functioning at the level of protective reflexes have left that person dependent on others to meet all self-care needs. Nervous system dysfunction severe enough to cause coma is the result of cortical damage leading to indirect interruption of the ascending reticular activating system (ARAS) or of a direct lesion of the ARAS—for example, a severe brain stem injury (Copstead, 1995).

• C A S E   S T U D Y   1

Joshua was a 21-year-old man with a medical diagnosis of head injury with coma secondary to a motor vehicle crash. He was being cared for in a neurologic-neurosurgical intensive care unit. One week earlier, on his 21st birthday, he was struck by a speeding car while driving the new car his parents had given him as a birthday present. Paramedics found Joshua unconscious at the scene of the crash. He was transported to a nearby hospital, where an emergency computed tomographic scan indicated bilateral intracerebral hemorrhage and contusion but no bleeding into the subdural or epidural spaces. After admission to the intensive care unit, Joshua remained comatose, with withdrawal response to painful stimuli only. Joshua's parents had been called by the police shortly after the crash and remained with their son almost constantly after his admission to the hospital. They were kept informed of Joshua's condition and treatment and were told that his prognosis for functional recovery was guarded.

ASSESSMENT AND GOALS FOR THE INDIVIDUAL

When an individual has a severely impaired level of consciousness, a detailed assessment of self-care abilities is not appropriate and is not possible. Participation in self-care activities requires an individual to be awake and alert. A comatose person would thus be diagnosed as having a total self-care deficit. The ongoing evaluation of the comatose individual's level of neurologic functioning with regard to protective reflexes would be performed by adding brain stem reflex assessment to a coma scale. Examples of goals that might be established for the individual functioning at the level of protective reflexes are as follows:

- Short-term goal: Basic self-care activities will be done for the patient by nurses and family members.
- Long-term goal: Patient returns to maximum level of independence possible in performance of self-care activities.

NURSING INTERVENTIONS FOR THE INDIVIDUAL

The comatose patient will require what Orem (1995) referred to as a wholly compensatory nursing system. To the extent that an individual cannot independently perform needed self-care functions, others will perform those activities. One important consideration is the environment within which care is provided. During the critical care phase, it would be most appropriate to provide care within a specialty unit (neurologic or neurosurgical intensive care unit) if available. Care should be provided by nurses with knowledge, skill, and experience in providing wholly compensatory care to comatose patients and their families. It would be advantageous to have clinical nurse specialists (critical care, neurology, or neurosurgery) available as resources to the nurses providing direct patient care on a daily basis. The nurse specialists would work in the clinical area with the nurse generalists (staff nurses), participating in the care of the patient to effect facilitating, guiding, teaching, and role modeling. The specialist thus indirectly delivers care to the patient by influencing the care given by the direct caregivers.

ASSESSMENT AND INTERVENTIONS FOR THE FAMILY AND SIGNIFICANT OTHERS

When an individual sustains a brain injury that results in coma, the extent of that person's awareness of the situation is unknown. However, the injured individual's family and significant others are acutely aware of the impact of the profound disability. Their coping capacities are severely tested by having a loved one changed from normally functioning to comatose. Nursing assessment of the family related to the individual's total self-care deficit begins with an evaluation of their understanding of the comatose individual's neurologic conditions, prognosis, and inability to manage any aspect of personal self-care. The assessment also includes the extent to which family members are able and willing to be involved in meeting the patient's self-care needs. The ability and willingness to participate in caregiving activities depend to a considerable extent on family members' own grief experience and coping abilities. Such participation may actually facilitate family coping and resolution of grief. Another area of family assessment is the family members' own self-care activities and the availability and use of support systems. Examples of possible family-focused goals related to self-care—protective reflexes are as follows:

- Family participating in patient's self-care activities (e.g., bathing, grooming)
- Family members effectively meeting their own self-care needs

Nursing interventions provided by nurse generalists and nurse specialists would be based on this assessment and would be specific to the needs of particular families. The staff nurses would assess family understanding of the patient's condition and involve family members in day-to-day care of the patient to the extent that individual family members choose to participate. The neurologic nurse specialist would be consulted as needed to promote family participation and to teach family members particular skills. The specialist's expertise in the area of family adaptation to disability is particularly helpful in the assessment and interventions related to family members' efforts at meeting their own self-care needs. The specialist would also be a teacher and role model to the staff nurses, thereby promoting and facilitating excellent patient and family care.

ASSESSMENT AND INTERVENTIONS FOR THE COMMUNITY

Community assessment related to profound neurologic impairment primarily involves attempts to gauge the knowledge and understanding of people in the community about catastrophic neurologic events, especially those associated with motor vehicle crashes. Other important areas of assessment include availability of motor vehicle crash prevention and safety promotion programs and legislative requirements for safety promotion (e.g., use of child restraints and seatbelts).

Community-focused interventions by both nurse generalists and nurse specialists are based on a systematic community assessment. Nursing interventions toward advocacy, public education, and political action on behalf of persons with profound neurologic impairments and their families should be coordinated with the ongoing efforts of organizations such as the National Head Injury Foundation.

Basic Hygienic Tasks

For many individuals with nervous system dysfunction, alterations in self-care occur in relation to the performance of basic hygienic tasks, such as bathing, dressing, and toileting. The neuroanatomic manifestations of impairment in performance of basic hygienic tasks are primarily in the areas of movement, sensation, and cognitive function. The types of cognitive impairment underlying self-care deficits include memory loss, impaired abstract thinking, easy distractibility, short attention span, impaired judgment, and difficulty transferring learning from one situation to another. Cognitive deficits can often be more impeding to self-care performance and more difficult for family and friends to cope with than other manifestations of neurologic dysfunction—for example, paralysis or communication impairment.

• C A S E   S T U D Y   2

Jack was a 66-year-old man who had experienced a right cortical stroke 5 days earlier. His stroke resulted in left hemiparesis, left hemisensory deficit, left neglect, and impulsiveness. He had a 20-year history of hypertension and was under treatment with antihypertensive medication. He did not take the medication consistently because he "felt fine" without it. Jack and his wife had been married for more than 30 years and had five grown children. He retired last year from his job as a mail carrier for the U.S. Postal Service. His wife was in her mid-fifties and worked part-time as a dental office receptionist. She enjoyed her job and did not want to retire for at least 5 more years. Both Jack and his wife described him as an active, outgoing person who kept busy all the time and could not tolerate sitting around with nothing to do. Jack frequently asked his nurses when his left arm and left leg would return to normal so he could be a "whole man" again.

ASSESSMENT AND GOALS FOR THE INDIVIDUAL

There are a number of possible approaches to the assessment of an individual's ability to perform basic hygienic tasks of self-care. One approach is to evaluate specific aspects of nervous system functioning, such as motor ability, sensation, and perceptual ability, and then make prognostic statements about the individual's basic hygienic task performance. A more direct approach is to evaluate the individual's actual performance of such self-care tasks as bathing, toileting, dressing, and self-feeding. A complete neurologic nursing assessment would include the evaluation of basic hygienic task performance, or ADLs.

One frequently used approach to the assessment of ADLs involves the use of scales that yield functional ability and disability scores. The scales most often referred to in the literature include the PULSES profile and the Barthel Index (Christiansen, Schwartz, & Barnes, 1993; McCourt, 1993).

A scale that is more relevant to the nursing assessment of ADLs is the Enforced Social Dependency Scale (ESDS). The ESDS is a measure of the reliance of the individual on others for the performance of tasks previously accomplished without assistance (Benoliel, McCorkle, & Young, 1980). The ESDS was originally developed within research studies of people with cancer and heart disease. It has also been used to measure enforced social dependency within a sample of individuals after stroke and, more recently, within a sample of persons with MS (Mumma, 1984, 1986; Mumma & Gibson, 1997).

The ESDS is composed of two subscales, Personal Competence and Social Competence (Benoliel et al., 1980). The performance of basic hygienic tasks is measured with the Personal Competence subscale. Assessment of an individual's basic hygienic task performance could lead to the following specific nursing diagnoses (American Nurses Association Council on Medical-Surgical Nursing Practice & American Association of Neuroscience Nurses, 1985, p. 10):

- Self-care deficit: Impaired ability to feed self
- Self-care deficit: Impaired ability to bathe self
- Self-care deficit: Impaired ability to dress self
- Self-care deficit: Impaired ability to use toilet

Examples of possible individual goals related to the performance of basic hygienic tasks are as follows:

- Short-term goal: Participation in self-feeding with setup, cuing, and supervision by nursing staff
- Long-term goal: Demonstration of maximum level of independence possible in performance of basic hygienic tasks (consistent with physical and cognitive limitations)

NURSING INTERVENTIONS FOR THE INDIVIDUAL

The nurse generalist caring for an individual with impaired ability to perform basic hygienic tasks would use a partly compensatory nursing system for the delivery of nursing care (Orem, 1995). A potentially effective approach to the care of people with impaired ability to perform basic self-care tasks is based on rehabilitation nursing principles. Major principles include the following (McCourt, 1993):

- Promotion of health and optimum human potential
- Focus on individual wholeness and uniqueness
- Active partnership with patients and their families
- Provision of supportive environment in which to facilitate independence
- Emphasis on teaching and preparing individuals to return to functional role within family and community
- Continuity of care for patients and families

Facilitating attainment of the goal of independent performance of basic hygienic tasks requires such nursing interventions as teaching, guiding, cuing, and supporting. The nurse collaborates with other members of the health care team to ensure goal attainment. If the patient is transferred to a rehabilitation setting, the involvement of the interdisciplinary rehabilitation team is explicit. In such settings, goal establishment and care planning are usually team endeavors. Nurse specialists would be available as resources for nurse generalists.

ASSESSMENT AND INTERVENTIONS FOR THE FAMILY AND SIGNIFICANT OTHERS

When an individual acquires a neurologic disability that impairs the ability to meet self-care needs, the person's adaptive ability is severely challenged. Adaptive challenges are also faced by the individuals' loved ones. Family assessment related to basic hygienic self-care tasks has a number of components. It is important to assess family members' knowledge and skills related to self-care activities as a basis for involving family members in the patient's care and rehabilitation program. It is also essential to assess how the family is coping with a suddenly disabled loved one. Spouses, in particular, will often describe feeling as if they had lost the person they knew before the disabling event (Bronstein, Popovich, & Stewart-Amidei, 1991; Mumma, 1986). Other aspects of the family assessment include (1) examination of how family members are caring for themselves and (2) assessment of availability and use of support systems.

Family-focused interventions are based on the nurse's sensitivity to the profound stresses experienced by family members coping with the patient's sudden disability. Nursing interventions designed to provide support to family members can be delivered both individually and in a group setting. Support groups provide participants with the opportunity to discuss their experiences with others in a similar situation—as family members of a newly disabled individual. Additional family interventions are similar to those used with the patient, with the added dimension of interaction among family members. Potentially useful interventions include teaching, guiding, modeling, and active listening. These interventions are discussed in Chapter 17. Most interventions could be provided by nurse generalists, with guidance and assistance as needed by nurse specialists.

ASSESSMENT AND INTERVENTIONS FOR THE COMMUNITY

Community assessment related to self-care—basic hygienic tasks can be organized around the following questions: (1) How accessible and receptive is the community to individuals who have impaired self-care ability? (2) Where are the barriers, both architectural and attitudinal, to community involvement of individuals with impaired self-care ability? Attitudinal barriers can often be more of an impediment than architectural barriers. (3) Are educational programs available related to disability? (4) How are individuals with disability portrayed in the media (newspapers, television)? (5) What is occurring in the political and legislative areas related to advocacy for persons with disability?

Nurse generalists and nurse specialists have a responsibility to be involved in community-focus interventions based on systematic community assessment. Interventions include teaching, advocating, and modeling with individuals, groups, and organizations. There are opportunities for nurses to participate in the ongoing work of national and local organizations whose purpose is to provide public education about disabling neurologic conditions.

Independent Living

Cognitive functioning would need to be relatively intact for an individual to have impairment in self-care and yet be capable of independent living. Cortical brain damage to the extent that an individual must rely on others to make decisions and solve problems related to daily living would not be consistent with most definitions of independence. Independence is often a matter of degree and sometimes of definition. No one is totally independent of others, but living independently generally means reliance primarily on oneself to meet the demands of daily living for both personal and social activities (Benoliel et al., 1980; Christiansen et al., 1993).

Neuroanatomic areas in which damage could result in altered performance of self-care with retained ability for independent living include the motor cortex, the primary sensory cortex, the visual system, the subcortical motor system and spinal cord, the autonomic nervous system, and the peripheral nervous system (motor and sensory) (Copstead, 1995).

An example of a nervous system disease that can lead to impaired self-care with retained independent living is MS. The demyelination and plaque formation that occur with MS can result in interruption of nervous system functioning in any of the areas listed above (Copstead, 1995; Hickey, 1992). The interrupted functioning results in impaired ability to perform self-care activities.

• C A S E   S T U D Y   3

Nancy was a 42-year-old woman who was diagnosed with MS at age 30 years. She had had subtle symptoms, including transient blurring of vision in her right eye and numbness and tingling of both legs, for several years before diagnosis. She said she was actually relieved when told that her symptoms were due to MS because she was worried that they were "just in her head" and that she might be "losing touch with reality." She was divorced and lived alone. She had been married at 19 years and thought that she and her husband would have been divorced "with or without the MS" because they had changed and drifted apart over the years. She had two grown children whom she described as close to her and concerned but busy with their own lives.

Nancy's current neurologic deficits were primarily a result of spinal cord damage from MS. She had spastic paraparesis, with more strength in the right leg than in the left leg. She had been unable to walk for the last 5 years but was independent with the use of her wheelchair. Her home was completely accessible by wheelchair. She had continuous numbness and tingling in both legs and for the last year had had intermittent numbness in her left arm, especially when very tired. She was working full-time in a secretarial job but was considering decreasing her work hours because of her problems with fatigue. She was active in her local chapter of the National Multiple Sclerosis Society and was knowledgeable about theories of possible causes of MS and currently available treatments. She considered herself fortunate that she was not more disabled than she was. She was determined to remain as independent as possible for as long as possible.

ASSESSMENT AND GOALS FOR THE INDIVIDUAL

Comprehensive assessment of an individual's capacity for independent living is generally a collaborative effort by various members of the health care team—for example, nurses, physicians, therapists, and psychologists. Nursing assessment of self-care ability may be aided by tools such as the PULSES profile, the Barthel Index, and the ESDS. It is important to assess the individual's ability to perform self-care skills in the broadest sense, beyond basic hygienic tasks. The ESDS includes assessment of such activities as work and recreation (Benoliel et al., 1980). A key aspect of the assessment is an evaluation of the individual's ability to solve problems and make decisions related to daily living. Examples of possible goals for an individual at this level of functioning are as follows:

- To maintain as much independence as possible in performance of self-care activities (activities to be specified)
- To use support systems and community resources as needed to enhance independence in self-care

NURSING INTERVENTIONS FOR THE INDIVIDUAL

As individuals move along the self-care continuum from dependence on others to greater and greater independence, they require less physical nursing assistance. People striving to maintain an independent living situation need less of nurses' doing for them and much more of nurses' teaching, guiding, and facilitating. Not all nurses are comfortable with nursing interventions that empower the patient to make decisions and actively manage self-care. For those who are, it is helpful to have nurse specialists available as resources to guide and promote independence on the part of both staff nurses and patients.

Nursing interventions related to independent living involve collaboration with other members of the health care team to ensure that the chosen living situation is resident friendly—that is, with as few barriers as possible.

ASSESSMENT AND INTERVENTIONS FOR THE FAMILY AND SIGNIFICANT OTHERS

There are several important aspects of family assessment in relation to independent living. It is important to assess family members' knowledge about independent living and about how the patient can maintain as much independence as possible. Family ability and willingness to be supportive of the patient's independent living is a major factor in the success of any independent living situation. It is worthwhile to examine other stresses and problems within the family occurring concurrently. It is rare that a family is faced with one isolated stressor (Butcher, 1994; Williams, 1994).

Family-focused interventions are based on this assessment and on the family's specific goals. Interventions primarily involve teaching, supporting, and facilitating. Nurse generalists and nurse specialists work toward assisting the family to promote the patient's independence.

ASSESSMENT AND INTERVENTIONS FOR THE COMMUNITY

Community assessment related to independent living could be based on the questions suggested in Basic Hygienic Tasks in this chapter. Primary attention should be given to factors within the community that inhibit independent living. Effective community-focused interventions by both nurse generalists and nurse specialists are aimed at strengthening those factors that positively influence independent living and working toward removal of those factors that impede independent living for people with neurologic dysfunction.

Orientation to Healthy Living

Can people who are independent in meeting their own self-care needs benefit from nursing intervention? Is is within the nursing domain to work toward health promotion to help relatively healthy people become healthier? Several authors argue for increased involvement of nurses in health education and self-care promotion for people who are not ill or disabled (Hills & Lindsey, 1994; Pender, Barkauskas, Hayman, Rice, & Anderson, 1992; Spellbring, 1991). A large group of people who might benefit from nurses' guidance and teaching focused on orientation to healthy living are those with stress-related or stress-aggravated headaches (migraine, vascular tension, muscle contraction).

The neuroanatomic manifestations of orientation to healthy living encompass the whole brain and, in fact, the whole person. An individual's approach to life and to maintaining or enhancing health and well-being is an integrated, complex response. Specific areas of the brain that play important parts in orientation to life are the frontal lobe and the association areas of the cortex, the limbic system, and the autonomic nervous system (Copstead, 1995).

• C A S E   S T U D Y   4

Linda was a 34-year-old woman who had had headaches since she was a teenager. She had been recently evaluated by a neurologist, who diagnosed her headaches as mixed vascular tension and muscle contraction headaches and recommended she get counseling in stress management. Linda was married, and her husband was a graduate student in biochemistry. Linda was the primary wage-earner while her husband was in school. They had three healthy, active children, ages 9 years, 7 years, and 18 months. Linda was a registered nurse and worked full-time in a busy family practice clinic. She acknowledged that there were many stressors in her life and that her headaches were much worse during and immediately after particularly stressful times. The major stressors identified by Linda were (1) financial worries, (2) husband too busy with school to have much time for Linda and the children, (3) desire to be at home with her toddler more—to work 3 days per week instead of full-time, and (4) lack of time for herself to do what she wanted to do or to just be alone.

Linda had a headache at least 2 or 3 days each week. The headaches ranged in intensity from mild (3 on a scale of 10) to fairly severe (7 on a scale of 10). When her headache was at its worst, her head throbbed, she felt irritable and nauseated, and she only wanted to get away from everything and go to sleep. She ate a fairly balanced diet, drank too much caffeine (in her opinion), did not smoke, and drank alcohol (wine with dinner) about once a week. She slept about 7 hours per night but did not feel rested in the morning and felt tired by midafternoon. She wanted to exercise regularly but did not know where she would fit it in. She missed work about 1 day per month with a headache; most of the time she kept working even though her head hurt. She occasionally canceled or postponed activities because she had a headache. She expressed high motivation to do something to relieve her headaches and manage stress more effectively.

ASSESSMENT AND GOALS FOR THE INDIVIDUAL

Nursing assessment of an individual who is functioning at the highest level of the self-care continuum (see Fig. 32–1) differs from the assessments previously described in this chapter. A person like Linda has no difficulty meeting her own basic hygienic needs and is living independently. She, in fact, has several people dependent on her to varying degrees. The primary focus of the assessment of someone's orientation to healthy living is an evaluation of lifestyle and health habits, including sleep patterns, diet, exercise, smoking, and consumption of alcohol and caffeine. Special emphasis should be given to exploring identified stressors in the individual's life and current and past coping strategies. On the basis of systematic assessment of an individual's situation, possible goals might be the following:

- Short-term goal: Consistent practice of a relaxation technique three times per day for about 5 minutes, each time resulting in a subjective feeling of calmness and relaxation
- Long-term goal: Decreased frequency and intensity of headaches

NURSING INTERVENTIONS FOR THE INDIVIDUAL

A person with very little difficulty performing personal self-care tasks and living independently may not have much opportunity for interaction with nurses in health care settings. There are nurse specialists in outpatient settings and in the community who provide stress management and health-promotion services. For health-promoting and self-care–enhancing nursing interventions to be used, they must be available and highly visible in the community. It is the responsibility of nurse providers of such interventions to make themselves known.

Appropriate nursing interventions for individuals at the most independent levels of the self-care continuum (see Fig. 32–1) include teaching, facilitating, validating, and role modeling. According to Tomlin, "as nurses engage increasingly in more effective caring for themselves as whole persons, they provide a powerful model for clients to reach ever healthier levels of self-caring" (1983, p. 59). This does not mean that nurses are expected to be perfect in the performance of their own self-care activities but that they are actively moving toward health in their own lives. Nurses have the opportunity and the responsibility to teach the value of healthy living by their own self-care behaviors.

ASSESSMENT AND INTERVENTIONS FOR THE FAMILY AND SIGNIFICANT OTHERS

Human beings are individuals and at the same time members of families and other interacting, reciprocally influencing systems. Thus, a complete assessment of an individual's orientation to healthy living includes evaluating aspects of the individual's key influencing relationships. The assessment focuses on the self-care practices of family members and others identified by the individual as significant. Relationships should be examined in relation to various types of support, emotional and instrumental, received and provided (Dumas & deMontigny, 1993). Another key aspect of relationships is the extent to which they are a source of stress for the people involved.

Family-focused interventions related to healthy living should be similar to those used in the care of the individual. Appropriate interventions with relatively healthy families include teaching, facilitating, supporting, and promoting self-care. In addition to working with family members as individuals, it is important to conduct teaching and support sessions with significant family members and the client as a group. Family sessions provide the opportunity for all involved to hear the same information. The nurses facilitating the sessions should model health-promoting interactions with the client while being observed by family members. These interventions are generally enacted by nurse specialists or by nurse generalists who have developed skills in family assessment and intervention.

ASSESSMENT AND INTERVENTIONS FOR THE COMMUNITY

Community assessment related to orientation to healthy living could be centered on several broad questions. Is the community healthy—environmentally, attitudinally, interactionally? What is the community doing to promote healthy living? Who are the key people in the community who are working toward a healthy community? What are the major barriers or impediments to healthy living within the community? What is the local community doing to promote health in the larger community—the nation, the world?

Interventions toward the goal of community health can be implemented by both nurse generalists and nurse specialists. Nursing as a profession and nurses as individuals have the responsibility to promote an orientation to healthy living within the community (Kulbok & Baldwin, 1992).

SUMMARY

This chapter discusses alterations in self-care that result from nervous system dysfunction. The levels of self-care alteration explored are (1) protective reflexes, (2) basic hygienic tasks, (3) independent living, and (4) orientation to healthy living. Self-care can be thought of as a continuum, from maximum dependence in performance of self-care activities to maximum independence. As such, self-care encompasses more than the frequently referred to ADLs: bathing, feeding, dressing, toileting.

Alterations in self-care are complex human responses to multiple phenomena. Nurse generalists and nurse specialists in various care settings have special opportunities to participate with patients and their loved ones in confronting the effects and challenges of altered self-care performance.

References

American Nurses Association Council on Medical-Surgical Nursing Practice, & American Association of Neuroscience Nurses (1985). *Neuroscience nursing practice: Process and outcome criteria for selected diagnoses.* Washington, DC: American Nurses Association.

Benoliel, J. Q., McCorkle, R., & Young, K. (1980). Development of a social dependency scale. *Research in Nursing and Health, 3,* 3–9.

Bronstein, K. S., Popovich, J. M., & Stewart-Amidei, C. (1991). *Promoting stroke recovery: A research based approach for nurses.* St. Louis: C.V. Mosby.

Butcher, L. A. (1994). A family focused perspective on chronic illness. *Rehabilitation Nursing, 19*(2), 70–74.

Christiansen, C. H., Schwartz, R. K., & Barnes, K. J. (1993). Self-care: Evaluation and management. In J. A. DeLisa & B. M. Gans (Eds.), *Rehabilitation medicine* (2nd ed., pp. 178–200). Philadelphia: J.B. Lippincott.

Copstead, L. C. (1995). *Perspectives on pathophysiology.* Philadelphia: W.B. Saunders.

Dumas, L., & deMontigny, F. (1993). Orem's family evaluation. *Canadian Nurse, 89*(10), 45–48.

Hickey, J. V. (1997). *The clinical practice of neurological and neurosurgical nursing* (4th ed.). J. B. Lippincott.

Hills, M. D., & Lindsey, E. (1994). Health promotion: A viable curriculum framework for nursing education. *Nursing Outlook, 42*(4), 158–162.

Kulbok, P. A., & Baldwin, J. H. (1992). From preventive health behavior to health promotion: Advancing a positive construct of health. *Advances in Nursing Science, 14*(4), 50–64.

McCourt, A. (Ed.) (1993). *The specialty practice of rehabilitation nursing: A core curriculum* (3rd ed.). Glenview, IL: Rehabilitation Nursing Foundation.

Mumma, C. (1984). *The effects of disability following a cerebrovascular accident on older individuals and on their marital relationships.* Unpublished doctoral dissertation, University of Washington, Seattle.

Mumma, C. (1986). Perceived losses following stroke. *Rehabilitation Nursing, 11*(3), 19–23.

Mumma, C., & Gibson, A. (1997). Living in Alaska with multiple sclerosis: A journey. Poster presentation.

Orem, D. E. (1995). *Nursing: Concepts of practice* (5th ed.). New York: McGraw-Hill.

Pender, N. J., Barkauskas, V. H., Hayman, L., Rice, V. H., & Anderson, E. T. (1992). Health promotion and disease prevention: Toward excellence in nursing practice and education. *Nursing Outlook, 40*(3), 106–112, 120.

Spellbring, A. M. (1991). Nursing's role in health promotion. An overview. *Nursing Clinics of North America, 26*(4), 805–814.

Tomlin, E. (1983). Self-care. In J. Lindberg, M. Hunter, & A. Kruszewski (Eds.), *Introduction to person-centered nursing* (p. 51). Philadelphia: J.B. Lippincott.

Williams, A. (1994). What bothers caregivers of stroke victims? *Journal of Neuroscience Nursing, 26*(3), 155–161.

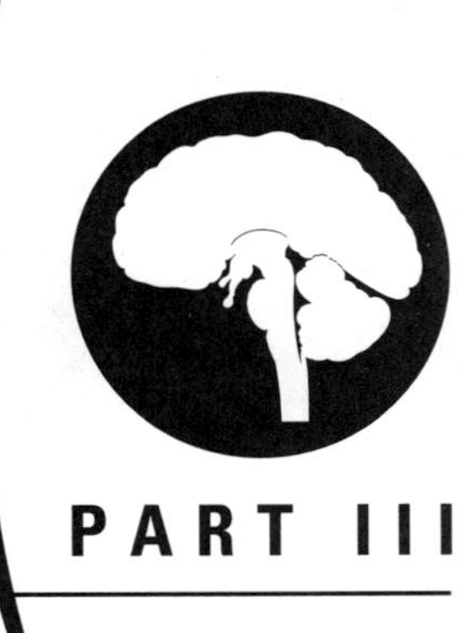

PART III

Integrated Regulation: The Central Nervous System

Integrated Regulation and Altered Integrated Regulation

GERALD A. BANET • CHRIS STEWART-AMIDEI

INTEGRATED REGULATION AND ALTERED INTEGRATED REGULATION

Homeostasis refers to a body's state of equilibrium with respect to its internal environment. The central nervous system (CNS) acts as the primary regulator for homeostasis, although the neuroendocrine system plays an important role. Homeostatic equilibrium is maintained through the balanced influences of the parasympathetic and sympathetic divisions of the autonomic nervous system (ANS), which regulate many of the body's systemic operations and organ systems. This integrated regulation, or control of other organ systems and functions distant to the brain, is critical for the survival of the individual.

Various neurologic dysfunctions may trigger alteration in integrated regulation, with far-reaching implications. Therefore, a clear understanding of the complex physiologic interactions between the brain and the other organs is critical to improved care of neurologic patients (Matuschak, 1994). This chapter reviews ANS function, with an emphasis on neurogenic regulation of cardiovascular, respiratory, and metabolic activities. Such an approach provides a foundation for understanding systemic alterations precipitated by neurologic events and guides nursing interventions.

AUTONOMIC NERVOUS SYSTEM

The ANS primarily regulates the internal environment or the visceral functions of the body not usually under voluntary control (Diamond, Scheibel, & Elson, 1985). The ANS has two major components, the sympathetic and parasympathetic divisions. These two antagonistic divisions delicately counterbalance each other to maintain an optimal functional state (Lefkowitz, Hoffmann, &

Taylor, 1990; Liebman, 1991). Dominance of one division over the other occurs when one division is stimulated or suppressed. For example, iatrogenic sympathetic stimulation may result in a characteristic systemic sympathetic response. Likewise, sympathetic suppression, such as that seen in spinal shock, may result in parasympathetic dominance. Overall, the sympathetic nervous system is more widely distributed than is the parasympathetic system (Lefkowitz et al., 1990; Liebman, 1991).

The ANS exerts its function through nervous tissue, known as ganglia (bunches of nerve fibers), located a distance away from the CNS (Netter, 1983). Preganglionic and postganglionic fibers serve to connect the nervous system with various target organs. Central autonomic fibers originating in the hypothalamus and brain stem synapse in preganglionic fibers in the brain stem and spinal cord gray matter (Netter, 1983). From these areas, preganglionic fibers, usually myelinated, synapse with autonomic ganglia located in a chain adjacent to the vertebral bodies (Fig. 33–1). Postganglionic fibers, usually nonmyelinated, emerge from the ganglia and network in their respective target tissues.

Stimulation of the sympathetic division elicits the generalized "fight or flight" stress response because of its widespread sympathetic innervation (Lefkowitz et al., 1990; Liebman, 1991). This division of the ANS originates in the thoracic and upper three lumbar segments of the spinal cord's intermediolateral cell column (Fig. 33–2). The short, preganglionic sympathetic cholinergic fibers release acetylcholine and terminate in paravertebral ganglionic chains, known as the sympathetic trunk. The postganglionic sympathetic neurons are relatively long and release norepinephrine with stimulation. Norepinephrine binds to adrenergic receptors in various target organs, such as the heart, lungs, blood vessels, and sweat glands; many organs and tissues have sympathetic innervation (Table 33–1). An exception to this pattern is in the adrenal medulla (Fitzgerald, 1992). Here, preganglionic fibers enter directly into the adrenal medulla, which acts as ganglia itself, and postganglionic fibers secrete adrenaline. Adrenaline is then released into the blood stream and contributes to the basic systemic flight or fight response, augmenting local responses of other portions of the system (Katzung, 1994; Keller & Williams, 1993). In summary, norepinephrine provides specific organ response, whereas adrenaline provides a more generalized response (Lefkowitz et al., 1990).

Parasympathetic stimulation, on the other hand, results in vegetative or energy-conserving responses. The bodies of parasympathetic neurons are located in nuclei of the brain stem and sacral spinal cord (see Fig. 33–1). At both levels, preganglionic fibers leave the CNS and synapse at or near the organs they innervate. Preganglionic fibers from the brain stem join the third, seventh, ninth, and 10th cranial nerves and exit via respective ganglia to innervate the eye, face, mouth, heart, lungs, and so on (Table 33–2). Preganglionic fibers from the sacral gray matter emerge as pelvic splanchnic nerves to innervate the rectum, bladder, and genitalia via the pelvic ganglia. Both pre- and postganglionic fibers are cholinergic, releasing acetylcholine (Fitzgerald, 1992; Liebman, 1991; Netter, 1983).

Neuronal impulses are transmitted to target tissues across synaptic junctions by neurotransmitters (Fitzgerald, 1992; Lefkowitz et al., 1990). The two

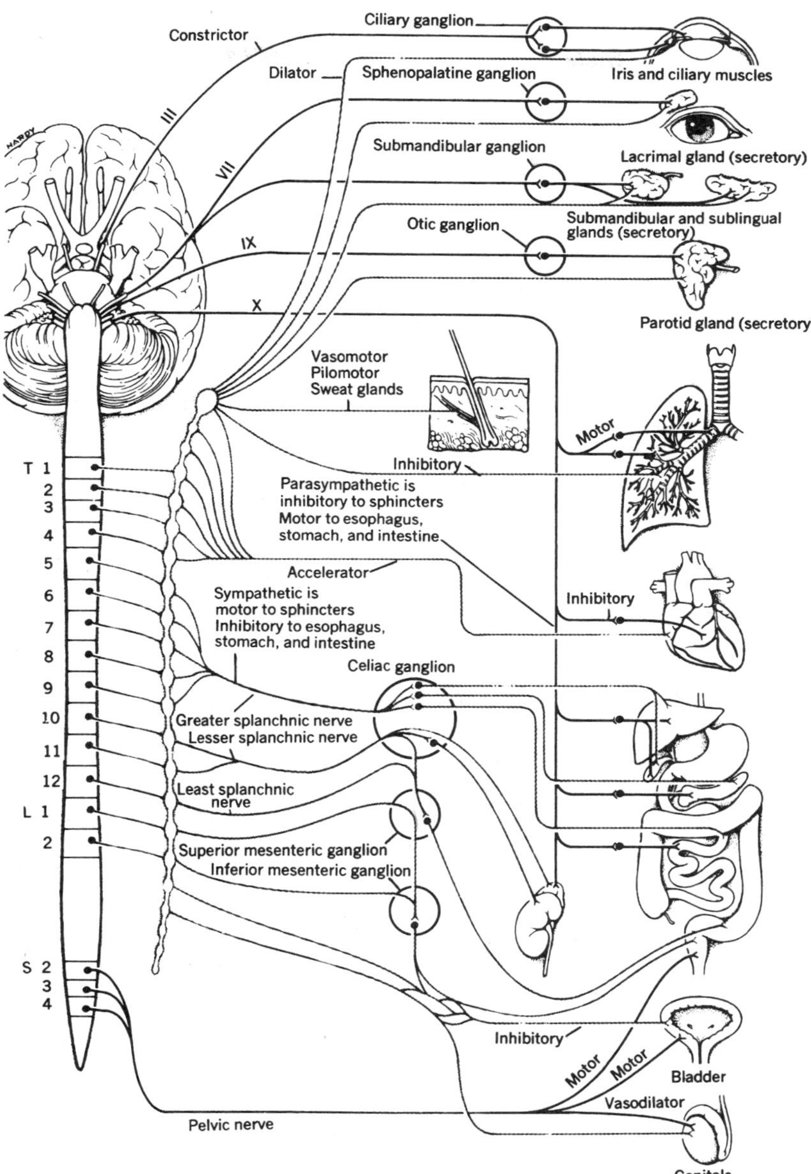

FIGURE 33–1 • Anatomy of the autonomic nervous system, including sympathetic and parasympathetic divisions. Note the dual nerve supply to most organs. (From Chaffee, E.E., & Lytle, I.M. [1980]. *Basic physiology and anatomy*. Philadelphia: J.B. Lippincott.)

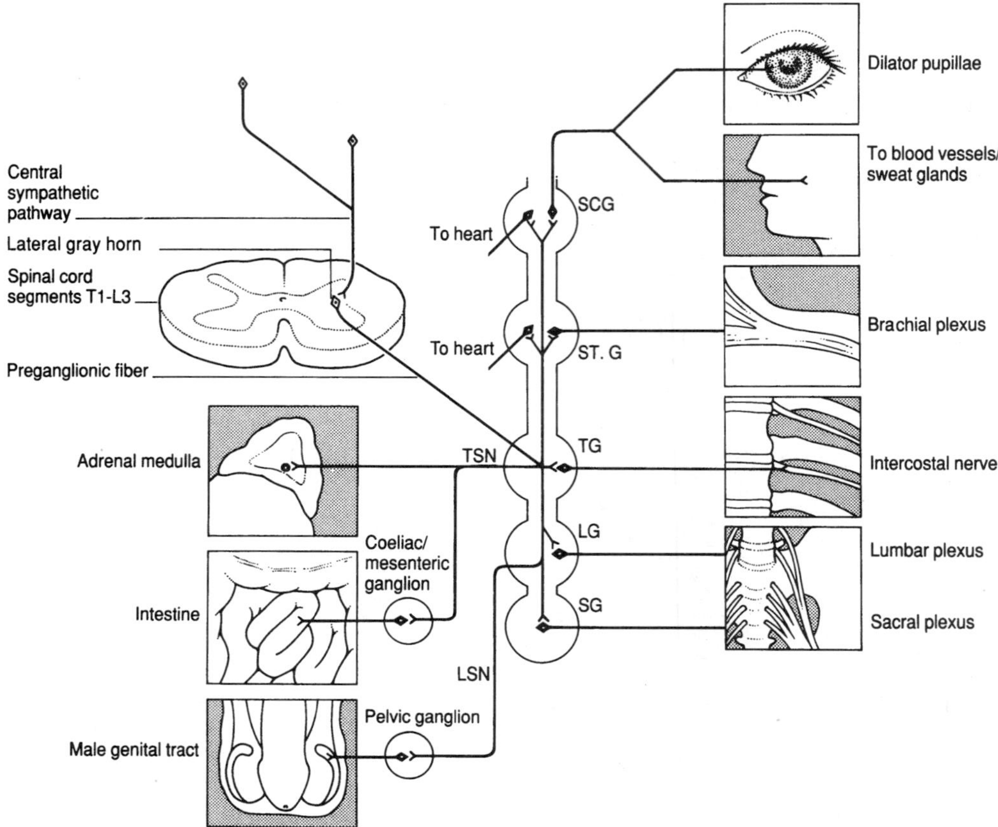

FIGURE 33–2 • Topography of the sympathetic nervous system. LG, lumbar ganglia; LSN, lumbar splanchnic nerve; SCG, superior cervical ganglia; STG, stellate ganglia; TG, thoracic ganglia; TSN, thoracic splanchnic nerve. (From Fitzgerald, M.J. [1992]. *Neuroanatomy: Basic and clinical* [2nd ed.] Philadelphia: Bailliere Tindall.)

main neurotransmitters are acetylcholine and norepinephrine (Table 33–3). Acetylcholine stimulates cholinergic receptors and is the neurotransmitter released by both sympathetic and parasympathetic preganglionic neurons, as well as postganglionic parasympathetic neurons. Cholinergic receptors may be classed as nicotinic or muscarinic. Ganglionic receptors are termed nicotinic because local nicotine may mimic ganglionic excitation (Fitzgerald, 1992). Postganglionic parasympathetic neurons are termed muscarinic because the drug muscarine mimics target receptor excitation (Katzung, 1994; Lefkowitz et al., 1990).

Norepinephrine, the neurotransmitter released by postganglionic sympathetic neurons, stimulates adrenoreceptors (Ruffolo, 1994). There are four known adrenoreceptors, two alpha- and two beta-adrenoreceptors, each with

TABLE 33–1 • AUTONOMIC NERVOUS SYSTEM EFFECTS

Organ	Effect of Sympathetic Stimulation	Effect of Parasympathetic Stimulation
Eye		
Pupil	Dilated	Contracted
Ciliary muscle	None	Excited
Glands	Vasoconstriction	Stimulation of thin, copious secretion containing many enzymes
Nasal		
Lacrimal		
Parotid		
Submaxillary		
Gastric		
Pancreatic		
Sweat glands (eccrine)	Copious sweating (cholinergic)	None
Apocrine glands	Thick, odoriferous secretion	None
Heart		
Muscle	Increased rate	Slowed rate
	Increased force of contraction	Decreased force of atrial contraction
Coronaries	Vasodilated	Constricted
Lungs		
Bronchi	Dilated	Constricted
Blood vessels	Mildly constricted	None
Gut		
Lumen	Decreased peristalsis and tone	Increased peristalsis and tone
Sphincter	Increased tone	Decreased tone
Liver	Glucose released	None
Gallbladder and bile ducts	Inhibited	Excited
Kidney	Decreased output	None
Ureter	Inhibited	Excited
Bladder		
Detrusor	Inhibited	Excited
Trigone	Excited	Inhibited
Penis	Ejaculation	Erection
Systemic blood vessels		
Abdominal	Constricted	None
Muscle	Constricted (adrenergic) Dilated (cholinergic)	None
Skin	Constricted (adrenergic) Dilated (cholinergic)	Dilated
Blood		
Coagulation	Increased	None
Glucose	Increased	None
Basal metabolism	Increased up to 100%	None
Adrenal cortical secretion	Increased	None
Mental activity	Increased	None
Piloerector muscles	Excited	None
Skeletal muscles	Increased glycogenolysis Increased strength	None

From Guyton, A.C. (1995). Textbook of medical physiology (9th ed.). Philadelphia: WB Saunders.

TABLE 33–2 • CRANIAL PARASYMPATHETIC GANGLIA

Ganglia	Innervation	Action
Ciliary	Pupil sphincter	Accommodation reflex
(Oculomotor nerve)	Ciliary muscle	Pupil constriction
Pterygopalatine	Lacrimal glands	Glandular secretion
(Facial nerve)	Nasal glands	
Submandibular	Sublingual glands	Glandular secretion
(Facial nerve)	Submandibular glands	
Otic	Parotid gland	Salivation
(Glossopharyngeal nerve)		
Vagus nerve	Heart, lungs	Slowing of heart rate
		Constriction of bronchioles

a particular function (Table 33–4). The action of endogenous epinephrine from the medulla and of exogenously administered catecholamines is largely mediated through interactions with alpha- and beta-adrenoreceptors (Talman & Kelkar, 1993; Watanabe & Katzung, 1994). Because each receptor has a unique function and many drugs affect individual receptors, an understanding of these receptors is of primary importance for neuroscience nurses.

Both divisions of the ANS include small numbers of nonadrenergic, noncholinergic (NANC) neurons (Fitzgerald, 1992). The exact functions of these neurons are not known, but more than 50 proposed neurotransmitter substances have been found in these neurons. In addition, pain and immune functions are thought to have autonomic interrelationships, possibly through the NANC neurons, but the exact nature is unclear (Liebman, 1991).

The brain stem nuclei involved in ANS activity receive input from other portions of the CNS such as the cortex, hypothalamus, and spinal cord. Such input plays an important role in integrated regulation. For example, fright or excitement may induce an increase in heart and respiratory rates as well as blood pressure. Clinically, a full bladder may produce the same response. Reflex loops include afferent nerves from peripheral receptors that travel to the regulatory nuclei in the CNS, where information is integrated. The efferent component of the reflex consists of descending pathways beginning in the brain

TABLE 33–3 • CHOLINERGIC RECEPTORS

Type	Location	Effects
Nicotinic	Both parasympathetic and sympathetic ganglia	Activates postganglionic nerves
Muscarinic	Parasympathetic junction	Slows heart
		Diminishes force of contraction
		Contracts smooth muscle
		Causes glandular secretion
		Inhibits norepinephrine

TABLE 33–4 • ADRENGERGIC RECEPTORS	
Type	**Effects**
Alpha-1	Contracts smooth muscle in arteries, pupil, sphincters (gastrointestinal and bladder), and vas deferens
Alpha-2	Inhibits neurotransmitter release
Beta-1	Increases heart pacemaker activity, increases force of contraction (causes secretion of renin)
Beta-2	Responds to catecholamines; relaxes smooth muscle; initiates glycogen breakdown

stem nuclei, which recruit input from the parasympathetic and sympathetic divisions of the ANS so that required modifications in the functional state of visceral organs may be made. With a constant interplay between the two divisions, homeostasis is maintained. Direct ANS injury or situations of significant physiologic stress result in autonomic instability. Most often, with a severe neurologic insult, an abnormal hyperactive sympathetic response occurs (Katzung, 1994; Lefkowitz et al., 1990; Richter & Spyer, 1990).

Neurocardiac Integration

NEURAL CONTROL OF THE CARDIOVASCULAR SYSTEM

Although the heart possesses some automaticity, most cardiac function is under neurogenic control (Oppenheimer, 1993; Pinsky, 1993; Richter & Spyer, 1990; Talman & Kelkar, 1993). Some nervous impulses to the heart originate in the limbic cortex and descend by way of the amygdala to the hypothalamus. From the hypothalamus, the parasympathetic and sympathetic divisions of the ANS descend to the brain stem reticular formation where cardiovascular reflexes are mediated.

Both sympathetic and parasympathetic limbs of the ANS innervate the heart. This rich innervation influences heart rhythm, tone of the coronary arteries, and contractile function of the heart's muscles. Sympathetic innervation of the heart is greater than parasympathetic innervation, yet it is the parasympathetic system that provides the overall tone to the myocardium. Efferent parasympathetic fibers descend through the dorsal motor nuclei of the vagus nerve, forming the superior, middle, and inferior cardiac rami of the vagus nerve, contributing to the cardiac plexus. After synapsing in the cardiac ganglia, the short postganglionic fibers terminate in receptors in the heart. Although parasympathetic postganglionic fibers terminate in other organs as well, only the heart is mentioned here. Release of acetylcholine at these receptor sites contributes to slowing of heart rate and decreased force of ventricular contraction, among other responses. Release of norepinephrine is also inhibited.

Axons of the efferent sympathetic fibers that supply the heart exit through the anterior T1–T5 roots of the spinal cord and form portions of the right and left sympathetic chains (Fitzgerald, 1992). In the cervical region, there are three ganglia: upper, middle, and lower. In the thoracic region, the ganglia are generally designated by the segment of origin, such as T1, T2, and so on. The lower cervical and T1 ganglia fuse to form the large stellate ganglia. Postganglionic fibers from the left stellate ganglia terminate in the sinoatrial (SA) and atrioventricular (AV) nodes, as well as in the left ventricle, while right-sided stellate ganglia fibers end in the septum, right ventricle, and atria. Generally, the two stellates function inversely. For example, stimulation of the left stellate ganglia lengthens the QT interval of the electrocardiogram (ECG) and slows heart rate, while excitation of the right stellate ganglia decreases the interval and increases heart rate. Thus, the ECG reflects the complex interaction between sympathetic and parasympathetic influences (Samuels, 1993).

Sympathetic activity also influences coronary vascular tone (Beckwith, 1982; Bishop, 1994; Ruffolo, 1994). The postganglionic sympathetic fibers terminate on alpha- and beta-receptors (Fitzgerald, 1992; Kelly & MacGregor, 1994; Olson, 1994). Alpha-receptors elicit vasoconstriction, while beta-receptors invoke vasodilation (see Table 33–4). Force of ventricular contraction is also increased by beta-adrenergic activity (Ruffolo, 1994).

Neurogenic Cardiac Disorders

Neurogenic cardiac disorders can be caused by various neurologic conditions (Table 33–5), most of which are sympathetically mediated (Barnes, Ferrario, & Conomy, 1979; Barron, Rogovski, & Hemli, 1994; Fincham, Shevapour, Leis, & Martins, 1992; Hachinski, 1993; Hart, Humphrey, & Weiss, 1989; Korpelainen, Sotaniemi, Suominen, Tolonen, & Myllyla, 1994; Matuschak, 1994; Valeriano & Elson, 1993). The mechanism is thought to be stimulation or irritation of the hypothalamus or medulla, which leads to an inappropriate sympathetic stimulation (Hachinski, 1993; Matuschak, 1994). The response is an excessive beta-adrenergic activity, resulting in both a local and a systemic release of catechol-

TABLE 33–5 • RESPIRATORY RHYTHM ABNORMALITIES

Type	Pattern
Cheyne-Stokes	Rhythmic waxing and waning of rate and depth followed by regular periods of apnea; a result of pathology in cerebral hemispheres or diencephalon
Central neurogenic hyperventilation	Increase in rate and depth of respirations; seen with lesions of midbrain or upper pons
Apneustic	Respiratory pause after prolonged inspiration; may be accompanied by an expiratory pause; pathology usually in lower pons
Cluster	Clusters of irregular breaths with irregular periods of apnea; seen with lesions of lower pons or upper medulla
Ataxic	Completely irregular pattern of varying rate and depth, with frequent periods of apnea; seen with lesions in the medulla

amines (Valeriano & Elson, 1993). Parsympathetic activity is also suppressed. The sympathetic hyperactivity ultimately leads to cardiac ischemia, myocardial exhaustion, and cardiovascular collapse (Hachinski, 1993). Manifestations may include dysrhythmias, ECG changes, and elevations in cardiac enzymes (Bronstein, Popovich, & Stewart-Amidei, 1991; Norris, 1983; Oppenheimer & Hachinski, 1992).

Virtually any dysrhythmia may occur with neurologic insult related to abnormalities in impulse formation or repolarization (Cruickshank, Neil-Dwyer, & Brice, 1974; Lane, Wallace, Petrosky, Schwartz, & Gradman, 1992). Life-threatening dysrhythmias associated with acute neurologic disorders, such as ventricular fibrillation, are probably due to repolarization changes within the conduction system (Lane et al., 1992; Marshall, Marshall, Vos, & Chesnut, 1990b). This fatal dysrhythmia results from beta-adrenergic stimulation that increases the length of the vulnerable period when an extrasystole can trigger ventricular tachycardia or fibrillation.

Characteristic ECG changes have been associated with CNS disease (Cruick-shank et al., 1974; Lane et al., 1992; McDermott, Lefevre, Arron, Martin, & Biller, 1994; Oppenheimer, 1994; Valeriano & Elson, 1993). Deeply inverted or peaked ("cerebral") T or P waves can occur, and the ST segment may be depressed. Pro-longed QT intervals and shortened PR intervals can develop. Finally, prominent U waves may be evident. These ECG changes may occur singly or in combination, and they are often intermittent. Additionally, ECG changes indicative of cardiac ischemia may be present in severe cases. Specific changes include inverted T waves and ST segment elevation. Uncommonly, Q waves may be seen. Such changes may be reflective of cellular ischemia produced by sympathetic hyperactivity. Some authors suggest that ECG changes are indicative of poor prognosis (Marshall et al., 1990b; Samuels, 1993; Valeriano & Elson, 1993).

Occasionally, patients with neurogenic ECG abnormalities have elevated CK-MB enymes, an indication of myocardial cell injury (Barnes et al., 1979; Bronstein et al., 1991a; Hachinski, 1993; Norris, 1983). This cellular damage is ischemic in nature and attributed to excessive norepinephrine release that, if sustained, leads to myocardial exhaustion and death.

Studies have shown diffuse myocardial necrosis on autopsy related to myo-fibrillary degeneration (Samuels, 1993; Szabo, Crosby, Hurford, & Strauss, 1993). The myofibrillary necrosis seen with nervous system stimulation is identical to the cellular changes seen with catecholamine infusion, stress, and reperfusion of transiently ischemic cardiac muscle yet distinctly different from the pathology seen in acute myocardial infarction. After myocardial infarction, cardiac muscle cells die in a relaxed state without prominent contraction bands; calcification occurs later. With myofibrillary degeneration, the cells die in a hypercontracted state with prominent contraction bands. In addition, cells demonstrate a mono-nuclear response and may calcify within minutes of the underlying insult. Light microscopy demonstrates myofibrillary degeneration and, in severely injured areas, necrotic debris is infiltrated by mononuclear cells with hemorrhage.

Various models of stress produce myofibrillary degeneration. One model proposes that the hypothalamus, which controls the sympathetic division of the ANS, triggers the release of catecholamines in concentrations toxic to the myocardial cell (Norris, 1983). Catecholamines are released directly into the heart by sympathetic nerve terminals or indirectly into the blood stream from the adrenal medulla. The toxic effect on myocardial cells occurs primarily at the subendocardial layer. Because the cardiac conduction system is located in the subendocardium and catecholamines are dysrhythmogenic, patients with acute neurologic dysfunction that may trigger a sympathetic response are at increased risk for serious dysrhythmias.

Another model expounds on this theory (Samuels, 1993). Through various mechanisms, norepinephrine is released locally into the endocardium from sympathetic nerve terminals. This leads to a failure of the calcium channels with a sudden influx of calcium and a concomitant efflux of potassium, both of which are endotoxic. In addition, free radicals accumulate that contribute to the destruction of cell membranes and subsequent leakage of water and enzymes from myocardial cells. The severity of ECG changes and the degree of cardiac damage are directly related to the extent of catecholamine release. Histologic changes range from complete reversibility to severe myocardial cell necrosis with mononuclear cell infiltration and widespread petechial hemorrhages (Norris, 1983; Oppenheimer, 1994). This mechanism explains the continuum of ECG changes ranging from reversible ECG abnormalities, such as benign ST segment and T wave changes, to permanent repolarization abnormalities reflecting irreversible failure of muscle cells and cardiac necrosis.

To further compound the issue, many patients with neurologic disease have concomitant cardiac disease, making it difficult to clearly understand the brain-heart interaction (Hachinski, 1993; Matuschak, 1994). For example, a stroke may have been caused by emboli from a heart with atrial fibrillation. Often, patients with cerebrovascular atherosclerosis have atherosclerosis in many vessels throughout the body, especially in the heart. Earlier studies even suggested that cardiac dysfunction contributes to neurologic insult, not vice versa. More recently, cardiac dysfunction following neurologic insult has been documented in patients without preexisting history or risk factors, supporting the concept that neurologic insult may instead cause cardiac damage (Marshall et al., 1990b; Norris, 1983). It is important to understand the cause-and-effect relationship and to provide appropriate treatment, because life-threatening dysrhythmias may occur and cardiac alterations may decrease cardiac output, with adverse effects on cerebral perfusion.

In summary, overactivity of the sympathetic limb of the ANS probably underlies major cardiac pathologies associated with neurologic insult. Dysrhythmias, ECG changes, and elevation of cardiac enzymes may be seen. Such changes contribute to the high mortality rates associated with severe neurologic injury (Marshall et al., 1990b; Norris, 1983; Samuels, 1993; Talman & Kelkar, 1993).

Human Responses to Neurocardiac Dysfunction

Nurses need to understand the potential impact of excessive sympathetic stimulation to identify those patients at greatest risk of neurocardiac dysfunction.

Prevention has a limited role; aggressive early intervention is often necessary to improve outcome (Bronstein, Popovich, & Stewart-Amidei, 1991b). Assessment is the initial step.

ASSESSMENT

The nurse must assess the patient with an emphasis on neurologic function (Hickey, 1992a; Smeltzer, 1992; Smeltzer & Bana, 1992). Patients at greatest risk for neurocardiac dysfunctions are those with acute, life-threatening neurologic illness or injury (Marshall et al., 1990b). The frequency of assessment is determined by the patient's acuity and stability. Thus, the nurse uses information from a comprehensive assessment to interpret findings and develop interventions for cardiac dysfunctions associated with severe neurologic insults.

History. The major components of the patient history include chief complaint, details of present illness, medical history, family history, and socioeconomic background (Smeltzer, 1992; Smeltzer & Bana, 1992). Of particular importance is the presence of coexisting heart disease. Particular attention must be paid to a history of coronary artery disease, myocardial infarction, atrial fibrillation, and other dysrhythmias that may confound the clinical picture or contribute to the current cardiac response. Older patients with chronic neurologic problems may have concomitant heart disease, whereas younger, traumatically brain-injured patients often have no cardiac history. Medications should also be reviewed for any cardiac effect or interaction.

Physical Assessment. Initial assessment focuses on ECG configuration and rhythm, noting any abnormalities. Should abnormalities occur, cardiac enzymes may be monitored. If alert, the patient is questioned about cardiac symptoms such as chest pain or palpitations. Nurses should note overall energy level, with attention to intolerance to any activity. Neurologic assessment can be indirectly valuable in determining cardiac status. Severe neurologic deficits signal the need for detailed cardiac assessment because the incidence of cardiac dysfunction increases with severity of neurologic insult. In addition, laterality may play a role in cardiac dysfunction (Oppenheimer, 1994; Oppenheimer & Hachinski, 1992). Patients with right hemispheric involvement often have more severe cardiac effects; the cause of this is yet unknown (Oppenheimer, 1994). Thus, the patient with left hemiplegia should have close attention paid to cardiac status.

Superficial indicators of cardiac function may be helpful in patient assessment. Nurses should observe skin color, moisture, and warmth. Cyanosis, pallor, or cool, clammy skin may indicate cardiac dysfunction. Peripheral pulses and heart sounds should also be evaluated. Weak pulses or abnormal heart sounds may also indicate cardiac dysfunction.

In the critically ill patient, hemodynamic parameters, such as cardiac output, are monitored as well (Roser & Daughton, 1990). Attention must be paid to behavior; subtle changes such as restlessness or confusion may be the first indicators of adverse changes. In the comatose patient, the ECG provides the primary window to the heart. Thus, ECG monitoring in acutely unresponsive patients is of paramount importance (Oppenheimer, 1994).

Vital signs, including temperature, heart rate, and blood pressure, are evaluated (Smeltzer, 1992; Smeltzer & Bana, 1992). Because these parameters relate to neurologic status and cerebral function, they provide clues for possible medical or nursing intervention to help maintain integrity between cerebral and cardiovascular systems. For the first 24 hours after acute neurologic insult, vital signs need to be obtained at least hourly. Subsequently, the patient's condition determines the frequency of assessment. An elevated temperature increases cerebral and cardiac metabolic rates and must be treated early and aggressively to prevent additional insult. Changes in heart rate and blood pressure not only are indicative of neurocardiac dysfunction, but also can contribute to additional neurologic or cardiac injury, mandating close observation. Nurses must also be able to distinguish between anticipated and life-threatening circumstances and be prepared to reverse such events when possible.

Laboratory values may play an important role in assessment. Cardiac enzymes may be monitored for evidence of progression or improvement. Arterial blood gases, hemoglobin, and hematocrit may also be helpful as measures of oxygenation and saturation.

• C A S E   S T U D Y   1

Darlene, a 28-year-old woman, was smoking crack cocaine with friends when she suddenly grabbed her head, screamed, and fell to the floor. On arrival at the scene, paramedics found her drowsy but arousable with stimulation. She complained of the worst headache of her life and of severe neck pain. In the emergency department, her level of consciousness fluctuated and she was irritable on arousal. She had no known past medical or surgical illnesses.

A computed tomography (CT) scan revealed diffuse subarachnoid hemorrhage, likely from a ruptured aneurysm. Angiography confirmed the presence of a right posterior communicating artery aneurysm. Within a few hours, she was taken to surgery and the aneurysm was successfully clipped. On emergence from anesthesia, she was still drowsy but arousable and otherwise neurologically intact. After surgery, neurologic and cardiac status was closely monitored. On the third postoperative day, she developed ECG changes suggestive of cardiac ischemia. She was bradycardic with prolonged QT intervals, inverted T waves, and depressed ST segments and had short episodes of supraventricular tachycardia (SVT). These SVT episodes occurred with any type of stimulation, such as turning, and each episode was associated with a decline in responsiveness. Cardiac enzymes (CK-MB) were elevated, consistent with progressive ischemic changes. On the fourth postoperative day, she had a cardiac arrest following sudden onset of ventricular fibrillation; she was resuscitated. However, her neurologic status deteriorated to a Glasgow Coma Scale (GCS) score of 4. Interestingly, the cardiac changes appeared at the onset of vasospasm.

Her unstable cardiac status made it difficult to treat her with the usual approaches to vasospasm because hypertension and volume expansion are both cardiac stressors. With aggressive life support, she gradually improved. As the vasospasm resolved, her cardiac status stabilized. Three weeks after her hemorrhage, she was discharged to a rehabilitation facility. Permanent ECG changes were noted. She was alert but disoriented at that time and had a mild left hemiparesis with very little activity tolerance. After a 6-week rehabilitation stay, she was discharged home. One year after her hemorrhage, she remained disabled, primarily because of cognitive deficits.

Altered Integrated Regulatory Function

Because of the complex nature of neurogenic cardiac disorders, a collaborative approach, in which neuroscience nurses work with other health care providers, is most effective. Because these patients are critically ill, many cardiac disorders may go unrecognized. By reviewing the associations between cardiac disorders and their neurologic causes, nurses are better able to detect and report such events so that timely interventions may be initiated. Therefore, the balance of this part of the discussion will have a neurocardiac focus.

ALTERATION IN CEREBRAL PERFUSION PRESSURE, DECREASED

The primary nursing diagnosis for patients with neurocardiac involvement is alteration in cerebral perfusion secondary to decreased cardiac output (Bronstein et al., 1991a). Causes for decreased cardiac output include altered electrical factors, such as rate, rhythm, and conduction, or altered mechanical factors, such as preload, afterload, and inotropic state of the heart. Such factors may be present with or without ECG abnormalities or myocardial damage.

Defining characteristics include altered hemodynamic parameters, dysrhythmias, changes in the ECG pattern, fatigue, cyanosis, pallor of skin, and mucous membranes, rales, dyspnea, restlessness, cold and clammy skin, edema, and decreased peripheral pulses along with abnormal heart sounds. In addition, mental status changes, such as confusion or hallucinations, may be noted (Bronstein et al., 1991a).

All patients with acute life-threatening neurologic dysfunction should have cardiac monitoring. Observations indicative of dysfunction include tall or notched T waves, prominent U waves, and shortening and prolongation of the QT intervals. Abnormal T waves are associated with repolarization disorders and along with U waves may be an early warning of intracranial hypertension. As intracranial pressure (ICP) increases, heart rate decreases and the QT interval shortens. In contrast, brain stem involvement and stimulation of the vagus nerve with rostral-caudal deterioration are thought to be related to QT prolongation. Other CNS insults may elicit additional abnormalities including PR interval lengthening, ST segment alteration, and ventricular arrhythmia. The PR interval reflects the time it takes for impulses to travel from the SA node to the ventricles. An increase in this interval may indicate a conduction defect, such as an AV conduction block. Close observation of all these patterns is essential.

Parasympathetic dominance may cause sinus bradycardia or AV blocks. If these rhythms cause hemodynamic compromise, atropine and pacemaker insertion may be indicated. The ST segment reflects the interval between ventricular depolarization and repolarization. Elevation or depression of this segment may indicate cardiac ventricular injury. Significant ventricular arrhythmias, such as premature ventricular contractions (PVCs), may be life-threatening and require immediate intervention. This is especially true if they are frequent (more than six per minute), occur in clusters (two or more together), are multifocal, occur on or near the T wave, or are symptomatic. Lidocaine is administered per advanced cardiac life support (ACLS) protocol until the PVCs are controlled. Additional interventions are dictated by the nature of the problem.

Early intervention is necessary to interrupt the potentially deleterious cycle associated with cardiac events (Keller & Williams, 1993). Therefore, ongoing cardiac assessment is an additional critical component of nursing management. The neuroscience nurse needs a basic understanding of dysrhythmias and appropriate interventions. Patients with cerebral ischemia should be monitored for 2 to 3 days following their event because this is the time period of greatest risk. If they are found to have ECG evidence of ventricular repolarization changes, they should be monitored until these have resolved. If there is insular involvement or a history of preexisting coronary artery disease, risk for sudden death or secondary brain injury as a result of cardiac arrhythmia is increased.

Monitoring of hemodynamic parameters becomes important with greater degrees of cardiac compromise. Adequate cardiac output is essential to cerebral perfusion. When it becomes difficult to balance cardiac and neurologic considerations, hemodynamic monitoring may provide direction for care. However, the risks of the invasive monitoring must be weighed against the benefits of the information provided.

Underlying problems that could contribute to cardiac dysfunction must be prevented when possible or treated early. Electrolyte imbalances must be corrected. For example, mannitol may contribute to changes in serum potassium, which in turn can cause PVCs and tachydysrhythmias. Peaked T waves occur when serum potassium levels reach 5.5 to 6.0 mEq/L. When the level reaches 8.0 mEq/L, interventricular conduction delay occurs, which is reflected by a widening of the QRS complex (Beckwith, 1982).

When controlled mechanical hyperventilation is used, close attention must be paid to the carbon dioxide content. When arterial partial pressure of carbon dioxide (pCO_2) drops below 25 mm Hg, the risk of serious dysrhythmias increases (Beckwith, 1982; Zegeer, 1984). Any medications that compromise cardiac function should be eliminated, if possible, or given cautiously. Hypertension may warrant additional medications. However, blood pressure must be cautiously lowered because higher blood pressure may be necessary for adequate cerebral perfusion. Although it may be impossible to reverse the neurologic dysfunction, every effort must be made to control ICP because increases in ICP are known to contribute to neurocardiac dysfunction. See Chapter 6 for a complete discussion of ICP management.

Airway obstruction or improper suctioning cause hypoxemia, which can contribute to anxiety and decreased cardiac output with resultant cardiac disturbances. Ensuring a patent airway and hyperoxygenating the patient before and after suctioning may minimize the degree of hypoxemia (Rudy, Baun, Stone, & Turner, 1986; Rudy, Turner, Baun, Stone, & Brucia, 1991).

Pain increases ICP and stresses the heart. Unfortunately, pain may be difficult to evaluate in minimally responsive patients, and physicians may be reluctant to medicate patients who are not able to be adequately assessed. Considering the systemic responses to pain and the subsequent cardiac stress of pain, it may be wise to assume that pain is present or, at the very least, to be alert to physiologic changes indicating pain. Morphine is generally the drug of choice for pain because it has a quick onset, provides adequate pain relief, has little effect on ICP, and may be quickly reversed.

Various medications may be administered to protect the myocardium (Katzung, 1994). Oxygen may be used to decrease the overall workload on the heart. Atropine alleviates the effects of the parasympathetic stimulation. Clonidine, an alpha-receptor blocker, or propranolol and other beta-receptor blockers may be used to ameliorate the effects of sympathetic surge (Kelley & MacGregor, 1994). Various medications are used in the ACLS protocols or the critical care guidelines for the treatment of life-threatening dysrhythmias (Lefkowitz et al., 1990). Most of the protocols are directed at increasing the fibrillation threshold by diminishing the alpha- or beta-adrenergic receptor response. Any treatment must be assessed in terms of its risk-benefit ratio in relation to the neurologic problem. Close monitoring for any adverse effects of medications is essential.

Additional nursing interventions focus on minimizing myocardial oxygen consumption (Bronstein et al., 1991a). The patient may be confined to bed while unstable. Once the patient has stabilized, activity may be gradually resumed, with a close eye on the cardiac response to activity. Heart rate and blood pressure must be monitored during activity resumption and activity stopped if adverse responses occur. Cardiac rehabilitation principles may be applied during the recovery period.

Summary

Severe brain insults often elicit autonomic nervous system imbalances that, in turn, may cause cardiovascular dysfunction. These imbalances may be caused by overactivity or depression of either division of the ANS. Diverse brain insults can trigger neurocardiac effects because the ANS is represented at all levels of the brain as well as the heart. Many patients with neurocardiac dysfunction have no history of cardiac disease. Astute nursing care begins with the realization of the brain-heart interaction. Many of these effects may go unrecognized and untreated in their early stages because of lack of awareness or knowledge. Consequently, opportunities for early intervention may be lost, and the brain insults may be compounded. Cardiac effects can contribute to the rapid demise of unstable patients and may compound morbidity. Nursing intervention is guided by an awareness of the life-threatening dysrhythmias and other cardiac changes that may accompany neurologic dysfunction.

NEURORESPIRATORY INTEGRATION

Respiration is the exchange of the gases oxygen and carbon dioxide across the alveolar capillary membrane and at the cellular level (West, 1985). Gas exchange is dependent on several interrelated processes: (1) regulation of ventilation and respiration via feedback from sensors that collect data about concentration of respiratory gases to central control regions that synthesize data and transmit commands; (2) pulmonary ventilation—the process of exchanging air between the atmosphere and alveoli, a mechanical function of the respiratory muscles; (3) diffusion of oxygen and carbon dioxide across the alveolar membrane; and (4) transport of oxygen and carbon dioxide to and from cells. The first three processes are primarily under neural control (West, 1985) This section reviews the respiratory regulation and addresses the pulmonary response to neurologic insult. Knowledge of neuronal control of respiration is critical for assessment and management of the pulmonary responses to neurogenic injury.

Respiratory Regulation

SENSORY RECEPTORS

Respiration is controlled, in part, through a sensory feedback system under neuronal regulation (Fitzgerald, 1992; West, 1985). Sensory afferents are organs that perceive and convey impulses to reflex and higher centers in the brain. In the respiratory system, the primary sensors are chemical and mechanical receptors. Generally, the chemoreceptors determine adequacy of ventilation while the mechanoreceptors regulate how ventilation is to be accomplished.

Chemoreceptors may be peripheral or central. *Peripheral* chemoreceptors are located at the bifurcation of the carotid arteries and in the aortic arch. For their size, these chemoreceptors have a very high blood flow, 200 mL/min/g of tissue, and a very small difference in arterial-venous oxygen content (West, 1985). A decrease in the arterial oxygen pressure (Pa_{O_2}) stimulates these receptors, with feedback into the medulla (Fig. 33–3). Medullary stimulation gives rise to reflex responses that enhance respiration and cause peripheral vasoconstriction in an attempt to bring the gaseous pressures back to normal. If there is a concomitant increase in the arterial carbon dioxide pressure (Pa_{CO_2}), the response is potentiated. Of these two, the receptors in the carotid bodies are more significant because they are additionally stimulated by a decrease in pH (Appenzeller, 1990; Kersten, 1989).

Central chemoreceptors in the brain are located near the ventral surface of the medulla and have more influence on the overall respiratory process than do peripheral receptors (West, 1985). Central receptors respond to chemical changes in the surrounding extracellular fluid—especially to increases in carbon dioxide and shifts in the acid-base balance. Cerebrospinal fluid (CSF) metabolites, regional blood flow, and local metabolism govern the chemical composition of the extracellular fluid. Because CSF has less protein than blood,

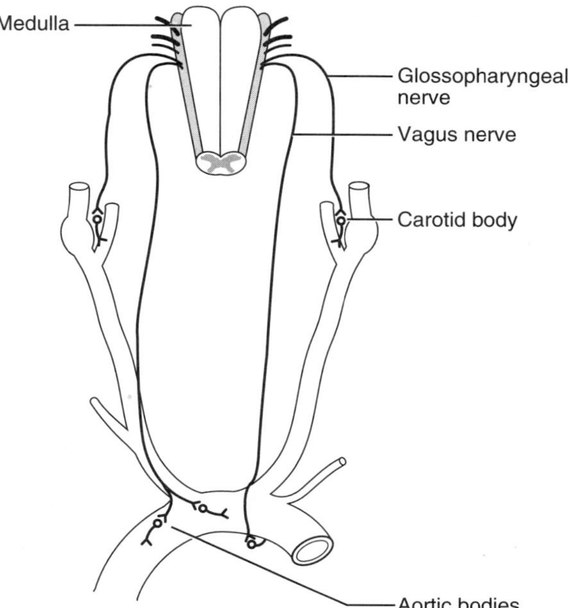

FIGURE 34–3 • Chemoreceptor feedback from the carotid bodies and aortic arch. (From Guyton, A.C. [1995]. *Textbook of medical physiology* [9th ed.] Philadelphia: W.B. Saunders.)

its buffering capacity is much lower than that of blood. Consequently, a change in CSF pH is more significant than a change in blood pH. In response to elevated hydrogen ion concentration—for example, with acidosis or hypoxia— the medulla triggers an increase in respiratory rate (Appenzeller, 1990).

Mechanoreceptors play an important role in regulating ventilation. The three main mechanoreceptors are the pulmonary stretch, irritant, and juxtacapillary receptors. *Pulmonary stretch receptors* lie within the smooth muscles of the airway. Lung distention stimulates these receptors to inhibit further inflation via impulses transmitted through the vagus nerves into the brain stem respiratory center. Referred to as the Hering-Breuer inflation reflex, this prevents overinflation of the lungs (Appenzeller, 1990; Fitzgerald, 1992). In contrast, the Hering-Breuer deflation reflex allows deflation of the lungs so inspiration may begin again. It is thought that stretch receptors cease to be stretched; thus, the inflation reflex ceases, lungs deflate, and inspiration begins (Appenzeller, 1990; Fitzgerald, 1992; West, 1985). The rhythmic inspiration and expiration phases of respiration are regulated through a complex, negative feedback mechanism under central control, which has been characterized as one of reciprocal inhibition. That is, while inspiration is activated, expiration is inhibited.

Irritant receptors are believed to lie between the epithelial cells of the airway. Noxious gases, cigarette smoke, inhaled dusts, and cold air stimulate these rapidly adapting receptors, causing bronchoconstriction and hyperpnea through brain stem mechanisms (Appenzeller, 1990). *Juxtacapillary* or J receptors are located in the alveolar walls near the capillaries. These receptors respond quickly to stretching of the alveolar wall and to chemicals in the pulmonary circulation. Stimulation of these receptors elicits rapid, shallow breathing, again through brain stem mechanisms (George & Chesson, 1990; Kersten, 1989; Malkoff & Borel, 1994).

Other, less important receptors are located in the nose and upper airway, joints, and muscles. Various stimuli, including heat and pain, elicit increases in arterial blood pressure and changes in pressure sensation. They may cause variations in the rate and depth of respiration as well.

BRAIN STEM RESPIRATORY CENTERS

In the brain stem, there are three respiratory centers: medullary, apneustic, and pneumotaxic (George & Chesson, 1990, Kersten, 1989). These specialized centers interact to govern inspiration and expiration. The primary respiratory centers are located in the reticular formation of the medulla (Fig. 33–4).

The *medullary center* neurons appear to have the intrinsic ability to generate a periodic burst of action potentials that ultimately stimulate the diaphragm and other inspiratory muscles. The medullary respiratory center has two distinct areas. The first is the dorsal respiratory group (DRG), which governs inspiration. The other is the ventral respiratory group (VRG), which is associated with both inspiration and expiration. Impulses from the DRG can be inhibited by the pneumotaxic center or modulated by stimuli from the glossopharyngeal and vagus nerves that terminate near the nucleus tractus solitarii (NTS). Because expiration is achieved with the passive relaxation of the inspiratory muscles, the VRG is normally quiet. However, during more forceful breathing, such as with exercise, these neurons elicit active expiration (George & Chesson, 1990).

The *pneumotaxic center*, which is found in the upper pons, shortens the inspiratory phase; as a result, the respiratory rate increases. Overall, it appears to fine-tune the respiratory rhythm by adjusting the depth and rate of breathing. Impulses from this focus excite the DRG and prolong its action potentials. It can also inhibit impulses from the medullary center (Diamond et al., 1985; Malkoff & Borel, 1994; Richter & Spyer, 1990).

The *apneustic center* is located in the lower pons (Diamond et al., 1985). Stimuli from this center tend to excite the VRG. Inspiratory muscle activity is prolonged but can be interrupted by transient expiratory efforts (Malkoff & Borel, 1994; Richter & Spyer, 1990). Spinal cord reflexes and impulses originating in the brain stem regulate involuntary breathing (Malkoff & Borel, 1994). This allows a person to continue breathing while asleep and to not concentrate on breathing when awake. When voluntary control of breathing is desired, impulses from the cortex prevail to some extent. For example, a person can voluntarily hold the breath or take a deep breath on command, such as during speaking and eating. Under certain situations, there is additional input from

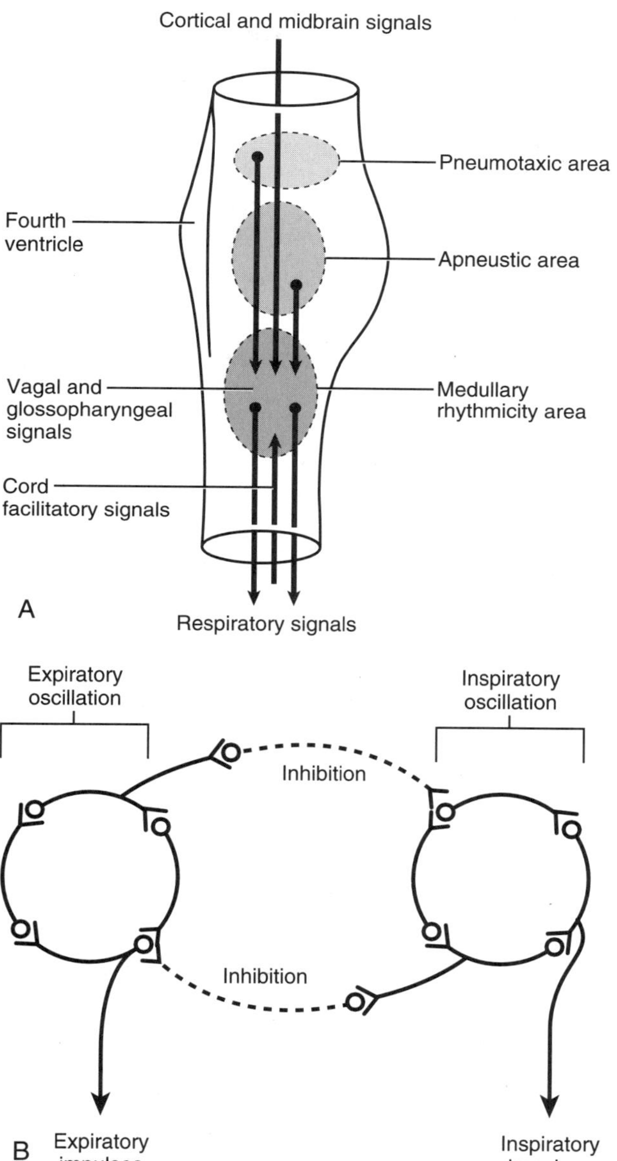

FIGURE 33–4 • *A,* Primary respiratory centers of the brain stem (lower pons and medulla). *B,* Oscillating inspiratory-expiratory feedback mechanism. (From Guyton, A.C. [1995]. *Textbook of medical physiology* [9th ed.]. Philadelphia: W.B. Saunders.)

other parts of the brain. For example, input from areas in the hypothalamus and limbic system cause a person to gasp when frightened.

Within limits, an individual can exert voluntary control over breathing. That is, the cortex can override the automatic respiratory function controlled by the brain stem. By doubling rate or volume with hyperventilation, one is able to decrease the arterial Pa_{CO_2} by half. Because of various factors, deliberate hypoventilation is more difficult to achieve. If a person tries to hold the breath too long, involuntary breathing reflexes take over. Other parts of the brain can also affect the breathing pattern. For example, the limbic system and the hypothalamus can be stimulated by affective states such as rage and sexual excitement, thus increasing respiratory rate (Richter & Spyer, 1990).

RESPIRATORY MUSCLE CONTROL

Via spinal nerves, the respiratory centers of the midbrain regulate the contraction and relaxation of various muscle groups that must work together in a coordinated fashion. Spinal nerves responsible for respiratory control originate in the cervical and thoracic areas. Nerves exiting the cervical spinal cord form the cervical plexus. One of the most important motor branches of this complex is the phrenic nerve, which originates from the C3 to C5 nerve root bilaterally to supply the diaphragm (Fitzgerald, 1992). The phrenic nerve is very important in initiation of respiration. When stimulated by input from the brain stem and spinal cord, the phrenic nerve causes the diaphragm to contract, pulling the chest cage outward and downward, initiating passive flow of air into the lungs. When the phrenic nerve is injured or impaired by disease, such as Guillain-Barré syndrome, the patient loses the ability to initiate respiration. If only one of the phrenic nerves is impaired, the person may appear to have a flail chest, with movement of only one side. If the phrenic nerves are partially impaired, such as with loss of input at C5, the diaphragm may be weak. The intercostal nerves, innervated at the T3–T6 levels, carry impulses to thoracic muscles. These muscles are responsible for elevation of the ribs, which increases the anterior-posterior diameter of the chest, again allowing passive flow of air into the lungs. Relaxation of the diaphragm and intercostal muscles allows passive outflow of air. When these nerves are injured, the patient loses some but not all inspiratory and expiratory function and the ability to cough. The thoracoabdominal nerves, originating at T7–T11, innervate thoracic and abdominal wall muscles. These muscles augment inspiration to a small degree and expiration to a larger degree. When thoracic innervation is compromised, the patient's ability to cough and deep breathe is impaired (Kersten, 1989; Marshall et al., 1990b).

Receptors in the respiratory muscles receive impulses that lead to muscle contraction and the mechanical work of breathing. Any disease that affects the neuromuscular junction can compromise the ventilatory process. For example, in myasthenia gravis, phrenic, intercostal, and thoracoabdominal nerve function is maintained, but a deficit at the muscle receptor site prevents the muscle from receiving the impulse, thus impairing respiration in a potentially life-threatening manner.

AUTONOMIC INPUT

The pulmonary system has both parasympathetic and sympathetic innervation (Diamond et al., 1985; Fitzgerald, 1992). The parasympathetic fibers extend from the trunk of the vagus nerve, and, when stimulated, they elicit vasodilation of the pulmonary vessels and a drop in capillary hydrostatic pressure. The sympathetic impulses are mediated through the thoracic segmental ganglia that innervate the pulmonary vascular bed. As in the heart, stimulation of alpha-receptors in the lung produces vasoconstriction, and stimulation of beta-receptors causes pulmonary vasodilation. Alpha influences also have a more powerful effect on the venous side of the pulmonary circulation. Sympathetic stimulation increases capillary hydrostatic pressure and pulmonary artery pressure without an associated increase in left atrial and systemic blood pressures (Samuels, 1993). Sympathetic stimulation may also cause bronchiolar constriction.

Alpha-receptor sympathetic fibers are widely distributed throughout the body's blood vessels. Thus, a nonspecific "sympathetic storm" could result in systemic hypertension as well as pulmonary venoconstriction, leading to an increase in capillary hydrostatic pressure. If unchecked, pulmonary edema will result. This noncardiac or neurogenic pulmonary edema (NPE) can be caused by at least two different mechanisms: by a potent generalized sympathetic storm stimulating alpha-mediated fibers or from a more specific, localized burst of similar activity affecting only the lungs. In the former case, systemic hypertension and elevated left atrial pressures would be observed, while in the later case, only hypertension would be present (Romand, Donal, & Suter, 1994; Simon, 1993; Taylor & Norwood, 1992; West, 1987).

Respiratory Responses to Neurologic Insult

NEUROGENIC PULMONARY EDEMA

NPE is a potentially fatal complication of a severe CNS insult or injury (Simon, 1993; Taylor & Norwood, 1992). The exact mechanism of this life-threatening complication is unclear. However, a sympathetically mediated pulmonary venoconstriction appears to be the end response (Bleck, 1991). Many of the earlier models of NPE sought a CNS effector site. Yet, most of those models demonstrated centrally induced systemic hypertension with pulmonary edema secondary to heart failure. Early studies suggested that the hypothalamus was the "edemagenic center" of the CNS (Simon, 1993). However, subsequent studies of sympathetic activity observed increases in systemic hypertension, systemic vascular resistance, and ICP, implying that the pulmonary edema may be due to cardiovascular and neurologic factors rather than to pure neurogenic mechanisms (Mayer et al., 1994).

In the medulla, there are two clusters of adrenergic neurons, areas A5 and A1, that may play a role in NPE (Fitzgerald, 1992). The A5 neurons, located in the upper part of the medulla, have projections extending to the preganglionic centers of the spinal cord. In experimental settings, sectioning the cervical cord blocked alpha-adrenergic tone and prevented NPE. Thus, the A5 neurons mediate sympathetic efferent activity, increasing blood pressure and pulse pressure (Nathan & Reis, 1975; Richter & Spyer, 1990).

Area A1 is found in the ventrolateral medulla (Fitzgerald, 1992). Its adrenergic neurons regulate the respiratory process and control sympathetic influences. Autonomic connections from this area extend to the hypothalamus. Studies by Nathan and Reis (1975) noted that NPE was associated with an increase in blood pressure and a decrease in heart rate. Later, Blessing, West, and Chalmers (1981) observed pure NPE after bilateral destruction of the A1 neurons without the associated blood pressure increases.

Two other medullary structures have been associated with NPE, the NTS, and the area postrema (Maire & Patton, 1956). The NTS receives afferent stimulation from the lungs and peripheral chemoreceptors; its efferents terminate in the cord and contribute to respiratory regulation. Bilateral injury to the NTS results in severe hypertension and NPE (Dettbarn & Davidson, 1989; Taylor & Norwood, 1992). Stimulation to the area postrema increases heart rate, cardiac output, peripheral vascular resistance, and blood pressure, as well as causes emesis (Boysen & Modell, 1989; Dettbarn & Davidson, 1989).

Theodore and Robin (1976) proposed the most commonly accepted theory in 1976. In this theory, the initial CNS insult is thought to originate from a massive, hypothalamically mediated sympathetic discharge, causing sudden, severe, transient vasospasm of the systemic and pulmonary systems, resulting in a sharp increase in pulmonary capillary pressure. This sudden pressure change causes dramatic venous congestion, along with platelet sludging. Platelets release substances that, in turn, increase capillary permeability (Dettbarn & Davidson, 1989). Increased capillary permeability allows proteins to leak into the interstitial space and spill over into the alveoli. Fluid follows, with the end result of an extravascular, extracellular edema. The edematous alveoli cannot maintain their normally distended position or an adequate surface for gas exchange, resulting in a decrease in pulmonary compliance. In addition, the pulmonary vasoconstriction decreases pulmonary blood flow, which, if sustained, leads to ischemia. Oxygen is necessary to produce surfactant, the substance required to keep the alveoli open to gas exchange. In an ischemic state, surfactant cannot be produced, further contributing to decreased compliance. Ultimately, atelectasis occurs along with severe respiratory compromise and damage to the pulmonary endothelium (Fig. 33–5). Blood is shunted from the right side of the heart to the left without the needed exchange of carbon dioxide for oxygen. The resultant hypoxemia and hypercarbia further aggravate the initial brain insult as well as other major vital processes (Boysen & Modell, 1989; Theodore & Robin, 1976).

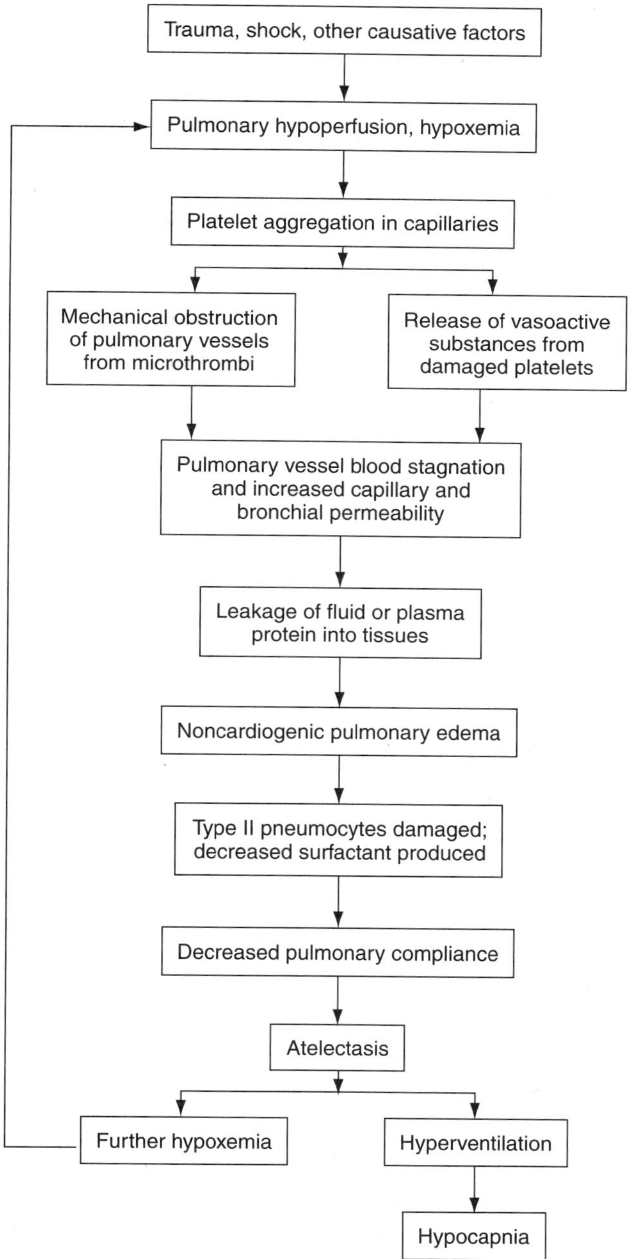

FIGURE 33–5 • Proposed pathophysiology of neurogenic pulmonary edema. (From Stewart, C. [1986]. Multisystem failure associated with neurologic dysfunction. In J. Lundgren, [Ed.], *Acute neuroscience nursing concepts and care.* Sudbury, MA: Jones & Bartlett.)

The hallmarks of NPE are copious, frothy exudate associated with protein-rich, alveolar edema; hypoxemia; and possible carbon dioxide retention. NPE may develop within minutes of the CNS insult or may be delayed in onset by hours or days. Sometimes there is subclinical NPE in which the patient has alveolar edema on chest radiograph with resultant hypoxemia, but carbon dioxide retention is not observed. Although classic NPE is quite rare, subtle subclinical forms of the syndrome are very common. Mild leukocytosis and diffuse, bilateral alveolar filling defects on chest radiography are seen in mild to moderate cases of NPE. Physical examination may reveal tachypnea, cough, and rhonchi without signs of right-sided heart failure. The patient may be lethargic or comatose, have tachycardia, complain of chest pain and shortness of breath, and occasionally have a low-grade fever. Fulminant pulmonary edema with respiratory failure and arterial decompensation may develop within minutes of the CNS event. Consolidation is noted on the chest radiograph. In severe cases, acute respiratory failure can result in death within hours (Misasi & Keyes, 1994).

Because the symptoms of NPE can be subtle, the exact incidence of the syndrome is unknown (Dettbarn & Davidson, 1989; Misasi & Keyes, 1994). Patients at risk for this complication include those with acute open or closed head trauma, intracerebral or subarachnoid hemorrhage, convulsive disorders, other stroke syndromes, brain tumors, hydrocephalus, cervical cord injury, and other pathologic conditions of the CNS (Dettbarn & Davidson, 1989; Pender & Pollack, 1992; Theodore & Robin, 1976).

ASSESSMENT

A comprehensive assessment identifies potential alterations in respiratory status. This assessment consists of history, physical examination, ventilatory measurements, and laboratory evaluation (Hickey, 1992a, 1992c; Smeltzer, 1992). History of respiratory problems should be determined, although patients will often have no contributory respiratory history. Patients with history of asthma, frequent pneumonias or bronchitis, or other chronic respiratory problems may require more frequent or detailed assessment.

The patient's respiratory status is evaluated on admission and as needed. Because neurogenic respiratory alterations are uncommon, initial assessments focus on identifying the more common causes of respiratory dysfunction, such as metabolic imbalance, congestive heart failure, atelectasis, pneumonia, and anxiety. Metabolic, cardiac, and respiratory conditions as well as cervical spine trauma can trigger changes in respiratory function. As the respiratory process becomes compromised, the oxygen supply to the brain is altered and the neurologic status of the patient deteriorates further unless there is timely intervention.

Physical examination focuses on evaluating respiratory parameters such as rate, rhythm, effort, and breath sounds. Although rate will most often be increased with respiratory distress, in patients with neurogenic respiratory alterations, mechanical effort may not be possible, masking respiratory problems. Thus, patients may exhibit a slow, shallow breathing pattern with loss of phrenic nerve function or neuromuscular disease. Fatigue is often evident over time. In addition, in severe respiratory distress, such as late NPE, the patient may not be able to produce the mechanical effort to breathe, thus resulting in bradypnea.

Breath sounds are normally clear. With respiratory problems such as NPE, rales, crackles, and rhonchi may be audible. In patients with poor ventilatory effort, minimal breath sounds may be audible, masking rales or rhonchi until the patient is mechanically ventilated (Boysen & Modell, 1989). When the patient is suctioned or is able to cough productively, attention should be paid to the quantity and quality of secretions.

Respiratory rhythm is usually regular with an even balance between inspiration and expiration. Rhythm abnormalities may be seen with involvement of primary respiratory centers in the brain stem (see Table 33–5). However, true rhythm abnormalities may not be seen because patients are most often intubated and on mechanically controlled ventilation at the onset of problems, overriding the rhythm abnormality.

Comatose patients pose a particular challenge in that they are unable to express concerns about shortness of breath or chest pain, and restlessness may be attributed to the cause of coma and not to respiratory distress (Hickey, 1992c). Often, early respiratory distress goes undiagnosed, and it is not until later signs are evident that diagnosis and intervention take place.

Ventilatory measures are helpful in assessing overall respiratory function. Peak inspiratory pressure, vital capacity and tidal volume, and negative inspiratory force (Table 33–6) are the easiest values to obtain and the most important parameters, particularly when overt signs of respiratory problems are absent. Frequency of measurements is dictated by the patient's condition. Baseline measurements are helpful in all situations where respiratory compromise may occur. Critically ill patients require frequent measurements, whereas more stable patients may be monitored only two or three times a day. A quick bedside measure of ventilatory function when other parameters are not readily available is to ask the patient to sniff. If the patient is unable to sniff, the diaphragm is weak or impaired.

Laboratory studies may reveal different information about ventilatory adequacy. Laboratory data include blood gas measurements, complete blood counts, blood chemistry tests, clotting studies, and sputum cultures. Chest radiographs

TABLE 33–6 • VENTILATORY MEASURES

Measure	Normal Range
Tidal volume	8–10 mL/kg
Vital capacity	15–20 mL/kg
Peak inspiratory pressure	20 cm H_2O
Mean airway pressure	18 cm H_2O
Negative inspiratory force	−2 cm H_2O

are invaluable in documenting infiltrates, atelectasis, and other abnormalities (Dettbarn & Davidson, 1989; Marshall, Marshall, Vos, & Chesnut, 1990a, 1990b).

Human Responses to Respiratory Alterations

• C A S E   S T U D Y   2

AW, a 19-year-old woman, was in good health, was in the sixth month of a normal pregnancy, and had no prior known medical problems. She was brought by a friend to the emergency department with onset of a severe headache following an episode of dizziness. She was not taking any medications on a regular basis. She was vomiting but alert. On arrival, her vital signs were heart rate, 96; respiratory rate, 14; blood pressure, 80/48. She became progressively sleepy with slow, shallow respirations and had coarse breath sounds on auscultation. Her capillary refill was brisk, and her pedal pulses were strong. Within an hour, she was unresponsive to verbal or painful stimuli. Pupils were fixed and dilated; her respiratory rate had dropped to 4 to 5 per minute with very decreased lungs sounds. She was intubated; her lung sounds were very moist, and a moderate amount of frothy, blood-tinged sputum was suctioned from the endotracheal tube (ETT). A portable chest x-ray confirmed ETT placement and presence of pulmonary edema. A catastrophic CNS event was suspected.

After initial stabilization, a CT scan of the head was obtained, which reported an acute intracranial hemorrhage (ICH) into the cerebellar vermis with intraventricular extension. Her ECG showed marked depression of the ST segments with possible anterior subendocardial injury. She was transferred to a tertiary facility via helicopter. Dopamine and intravenous resuscitation were used en route. She remained completely unresponsive. Her GCS was 3 on transfer. Her vital signs were temperature, 35.7°F; heart rate, 122 to 138; blood pressure, 90 to 124/60 to 84. Ventilator settings were tidal volume, 500 mL; assist-control rate, 20 per minute; FIO_2, 40%. Copious amounts of frothy sputum were suctioned from her ETT. Cardiac rhythm strips showed sinus tachycardia with marked ST segment depression and occasional PVCs. Her blood gases revealed pH, 7.56; pco_2, 19; po_2, 334; HCO_3, 17.2. Other laboratory values included serum sodium of 133 mEq/L, potassium of 3.4 mEq/L, carbon dioxide of 19 mEq/L, and hematocrit of 36.8 gm/dL, reflecting respiratory acidosis and hemodilution. A second chest x-ray showed massive pulmonary edema.

In spite of hemodynamic support, including aggressive use of colloids and pressors, AW's heart rate and blood pressure deteriorated, and she was pronounced dead 8 hours after onset of initial symptoms. At autopsy, the ICH was found to be secondary to an arteriovenous malformation. The lungs weighed 540 g on the right and 470 g on the left; left lung weight usually averages 375 g. There was a small amount of pink frothy sputum expressed from both lungs; marked congestion was noted. A number of petechiae were noted anteriorly on the epicardium. However, the cut surface of the myocardium showed no areas of infarction, and the endocardium was unremarkable.

GAS EXCHANGE, IMPAIRED

The etiology of this problem is related to alveolar-capillary membrane changes and altered blood flow. Defining characteristics in mild to moderate impairments include confusion, somnolence, restlessness, irritability, inability to clear secretions, hypercapnia, and hypoxia. Moderate to severe impairments in gas exchange are evidenced by signs and symptoms of respiratory distress. Assessment then focuses on the degree of impaired gas exchange. A detailed respiratory assessment is performed and repeated as necessary. In critical situations, respiratory changes can occur quickly and without warning, as in this case study; thus, interventions need to be quickly instituted.

Nursing interventions begin with prophylaxis. If the critically ill patient is alert and cooperative, he or she should be encouraged to deep breathe and either move around in bed or get out of bed as much as possible because the patient is at risk for respiratory compromise. However, most patients with NPE require intubation and mechanical ventilation and warrant prophylaxis in the form of frequent turning, suctioning, and maintenance of a patent airway.

Early Intervention. Once respiratory compromise occurs, aggressive treatment is warranted. Patients with NPE are likely to be intubated and mechanically ventilated. In these patients, nursing care focuses on promoting optimal respiratory function while minimizing increases in ICP. This is often difficult to balance because medical interventions dictate increasing positive end-expiratory pressure (PEEP) and inspiratory-expiratory ratio to prolong the inspiration phase and raise the mean airway pressure to keep alveoli distended. This may in turn raise the ICP. Thus, use of PEEP must be accompanied by close observation of neurologic status and ICP and aggressive management of increased ICP (Prendergast, 1994; Roser & Daughton, 1990).

Evidence suggests that NPE is more common in patients with significant ICP elevations (Mayer et al., 1994). Further, NPE does not occur as a primary disease but rather as a response to an insult. Thus, treating the underlying disorder may minimize the respiratory response. Nursing measures for preventing secondary brain injury may be found in Chapter 6. Nurses should work with other health care providers in treating the primary CNS disorder and be prepared to intervene quickly if NPE develops (Marshall et al., 1990a, 1990b).

Intubation Considerations. Intubation is considered in a variety of circumstances. Indications for intubation are to prevent or relieve airway obstruction, avoid aspiration, maintain pulmonary toilet, and provide a route for delivery of mechanical ventilation (Bleck, 1991). In the patient with a cerebral insult, intubation is accomplished with sedation when possible, to blunt the usual increase in ICP as a response to intubation. Low-pressure cuff ETTs are advocated because prolonged intubation may be necessary. In patients with greatly prolonged intubation, tracheostomy may be considered. (Hayek & Veremakis, 1993; Marshall et al., 1990b).

Mechanical Ventilation. Early initiation of mechanical ventilation may enhance cerebral perfusion and oxygenation. This intervention is aimed at preventing or relieving obstruction, decreasing the risk for aspiration, decreasing the mechanical work of breathing, reducing ICP, and maintaining pulmonary toilet. Adjustments in ventilatory setting include flow rate, tidal volume, and rate.

With mechanical ventilation, the goal is to maintain optimal ventilation with F_{IO_2} less than 50% and the lowest possible mean and peak airway pressures. PEEP may be considered to distend alveoli and promote adequate ventilation. However, the use of PEEP is controversial in the presence of a cerebral insult, because it can increase intrathoracic pressure, leading to an increase in ICP and a decrease in cardiac output and cerebral perfusion pressure (Moraine, Brimioulle, & Kahn, 1991). Therefore, it should be reserved for those patients who absolutely require additional airway pressure and whose cerebral perfusion pressure and cardiac function can be monitored (Marshall et al., 1990b). Ideally, ventilatory adjustments should be based on neurologic status as well as trends in cerebral perfusion pressure, ICP, and cardiac output (Bleck, 1991; Dettbarn & Davidson, 1989; Marshall et al., 1990b; Pinsky, 1993; Posey & Allen, 1994a, 1994b).

When mechanical ventilation is difficult to accomplish or patient activity adversely influences ventilation, sedation and neuromuscular blockade may be used. Current approaches include use of atracurium and midazolam, although many other agents may be used (Marshall et al., 1990a, 1990b). Pain medication, such as morphine, may also be indicated (Hickey, 1992c).

Suctioning. Endotracheal suctioning stimulates the cough reflex and Valsalva's maneuver, which triggers sharp increases in ICP (Rudy et al., 1986; Rudy et al., 1991; Stone et al., 1991). However, meticulous pulmonary hygiene is required to prevent retention of secretions, airway closure, and accumulation of $Paco_2$. Suctioning may also cause arterial desaturation with resultant increases in ICP. Thus, suctioning should be brief and should be preceded and followed by hyperventilation with 100% oxygen (Rudy et al., 1991; Stone et al., 1991). Topical lidocaine may be applied to the oropharynx to minimize discomfort associated with suctioning (Brucia, Owen, & Rudy, 1992; Kerr, Rudy, Brucia, & Stone, 1993; Rudy et al., 1986).

Positioning. Positioning of the patient has significant implications. Positioning the patient upright, at a 60- to 75-degree angle, decreases the mechanical work of breathing and should be used when possible. However, an upright position may decrease blood pressure and adversely affect cerebral perfusion pressure (CPP). The patient's response to any position change should be noted and the position adjusted according to neurologic status. In addition, the ICP response to position changes should be observed, and CPP should be calculated. Frequent, slow turns, as with a kinetic bed, may be helpful to promote skin integrity and prevent pooling of secretions in the lungs. Postural drainage may help clear secretions as well but must be used cautiously in the patient with increased ICP (Bronstein et al., 1991a; Dettbarn & Davidson, 1989; Hayek & Veremakis, 1993).

Sleep and Rest. Sleep deprivation and lack of rapid-eye-movement (REM) sleep contribute to increased physiologic stress (Zegeer, 1984). Sleep deprivation can lead to restlessness and agitation, which make the work of breathing more difficult and increase the ICP. Measures to promote adequate sleep and rest periods need to be incorporated into the plan of care. Providing total care for the patient in bathing, feeding, and other endeavors may allow the patient to conserve energy for the work of breathing.

Medications. Steroids have been recommended by some to blunt the effects of the sympathetic response on pulmonary tissue, but their use is controversial because of accompanying adverse effects (Bleck, 1991; Boysen & Modell, 1989). Beta blockers such as propranolol have been effective in the treatment of NPE if they are used before massive venous pulmonary hypertension. Even though afterload reduction may be helpful, nitroprusside is contraindicated because it dilates cerebral vessels. Trimethaphan, a ganglionic blocking drug, may be useful; however, it is imperative to monitor the ICP because it can lower the cerebral perfusion pressure (Rossaint et al., 1995). Aminophylline or theophylline may be indicated for severe wheezing and bronchospasm. Some individuals advocate the use of alpha-receptors, blocking agents, or hypothalamic depressants, such as chlorpromazine or meperidine, to block the sympathetic surge, but this remains controversial (Olson, 1994; Wohns, Tamas, Pierce, & Howe, 1985).

Additional Interventions. Nutritional support must be considered because patients are likely to have increased caloric requirements at a time when level of consciousness or intubation prevents oral intake of adequate nutrients (refer to next section). Patients need a great deal of psychologic support during a time when they have very little control over their surroundings. It is important to include patients in decision making and to utilize or develop creative opportunities for patient control. Relaxation techniques may be very useful for these patients. Alternative forms of communication for the intubated patient must be considered and anticipatory care provided.

Summary

The process of respiration is under neuronal control. Severe brain insult or injury can elicit a respiratory response in the form of NPE, which can be fatal. Nursing is critical in the prevention and treatment of NPE. Nursing interventions include intubation and suction guidelines, positioning and sleep considerations, and understanding of various medication effects that may be indicated.

METABOLISM AND THE METABOLIC RESPONSE

Metabolism is the process whereby cells convert nutrients into an energy source useful for cellular function and growth (Ott & Young, 1993). Metabolism is actually a balance between two concomitant processes, anabolism (cellular growth) and catabolism (cellular breakdown), both of which require energy. The rate of metabolism is dependent on cellular demands; the greater the cellular demands, the greater the metabolic rate. Likewise, as cellular function slows, as during sleep, so does metabolic rate. Many factors affect metabolic rate, but actions of the ANS have the greatest impact. Parasympathetic activity slows metabolic rate, whereas sympathetic activity increases metabolic rate. A sympathetically mediated metabolic response to neurologic dysfunction may be seen, in which metabolic rate increases and catabolism dominates, resulting in an inadequate supply of nutrients. Because the metabolic response may adversely affect the patient's outcome, an understanding of normal metabolism, metabolic response, and appropriate intervention is essential. This section reviews normal metabolism and the metabolic response to injury in the context of a case example.

Normal Metabolism

Metabolic requirements are usually met through oral intake of nutrients. Daily nutritional requirements, known as basal energy expenditure (BEE), may be estimated using the Harris-Benedict equations (Ott & Young, 1993).

Male: BEE = 66.0 + (13.7 × W) + (5 × H) − (6.7 × A)
Female: BEE = 66.5 + (9.6 × W) + (1.9 × H) − (4.7 × A)
(W = weight in kg, H = height in cm, A = age in years)

Using this formulation, a 35-year-old man who weighs 70 kg and is 180 cm tall would have a normal daily nutritional requirement of about 1700 kcal.

A simpler formula that may be used to calculate requirements is (Shronts, 1989)

BEE = 25 × weight (in kg)

Using the same example, nutritional requirements would be 1750 kcal. Because nutritional requirements change with illness and activity, correction factors may be applied to accommodate fever, bedrest, and stress (Table 33–7) (Long et al., 1979; Marino, 1998).

TABLE 33–7 • CORRECTION FACTORS FOR NUTRITIONAL NEED ADJUSTMENT IN HYPERMETABOLIC STATES

Minimally active	BEE × 1.2
Febrile	BEE × 1.1 (for each C)
Mild stress	BEE × 1.2
Moderate stress	BEE × 1.4
Severe stress	BEE × 1.6
Multisystem failure	BEE × 2.0

BEE, basal energy expenditure.

Once nutritional requirements are calculated, exact amounts of carbohydrates, proteins, and fats are planned (Long et al., 1979). Approximately 60% to 70% of kcal should be provided in carbohydrate form, while fats should supply 30% to 40% of kcal and proteins 10% to 30% of nutritional supply. Carbohydrates are the most readily used form of kcal, while fats have the highest caloric value. The goal in providing protein is to promote a positive nitrogen balance, delivering more protein than is broken down. In a healthy situation, this is usually not a problem, but when severe catabolism dominates, protein requirements may almost double (Marino, 1998). Additionally, essential vitamins and trace elements are necessary for normal cellular metabolism.

The body has precise daily requirements for each of the nutrients, using what it needs and storing the remainder (Long et al., 1979). The liver and adipose tissue store glycogen and fat, while protein is stored primarily in muscle. These stores, known as endogenous fuel substrates, may be mobilized via the process of glycogenolysis and gluconeogenesis when demand for nutrients exceeds supply.

ASSESSMENT

A detailed nutritional assessment identifies potential alterations in nutritional status. Components of nutritional assessment include history, physical examination, anthropometric measurements, and laboratory evaluation. Nutritional status should be assessed at admission and on an ongoing basis.

History. Preinsult nutritional habits are assessed to identify deficiencies. Recent weight loss or gain of more than 10% of body weight should be noted because this increases risk for nutritional deficits. Concomitant medical diseases that impair nutritional status, such as diabetes, liver and kidney disease, or bowel disease, should be considered as well. Current and previous medication that may affect nutritional status or metabolic rate should also be noted. Cultural and religious food preferences must also be delineated.

Physical Examination. Neurologic examination is helpful in determining any deficits that might impair food intake, such as hypoglossal weakness, incoordination, or hemianopsia. Examination of the skin and mucous membranes may reveal indications of poor nutritional status such as poor skin turgor; dry or edematous skin; easy bruising; bleeding; dry conjunctiva and sunken eyeballs; and tongue swelling. Chronic nutritional deficits are manifested as muscle wasting and atrophy, in addition to ridging in nail beds and hair loss.

Anthropometric Measurements. These measurements provide rough estimations of body composition and state of endogenous fuel stores. Body weights may be taken daily or weekly, depending on the severity of nutritional deficit. Height and weight are compared with standard scales but represent only a rough indication of nutritional state, particularly when edema is present, artificially adding to weight. Subcutaneous fat stores may be estimated through subcutaneous fat measurements, taken at the triceps or subscapular muscle. Low measurements indicate depletion of protein and fat stores.

Laboratory Studies. Laboratory studies provide subjective information on biochemical state, plasma protein, immunocompetence, and protein metabolism. A nutritional screen often includes serum transferrin and albumin and total lymphocyte counts. Other laboratory studies may be ordered, depending on the specific nutritional deficit and treatment given. Table 33–8 lists studies commonly performed to evaluate nutritional status. Should immunosuppression be a concern, the cellular-mediated immune response may be tested

TABLE 33–8 • LABORATORY EVALUATION OF NUTRITIONAL STATUS*

Test	Normal Adult Range of Values	Purpose of Testing
Serum albumin	3.3–4.5 g/dL	Estimates protein stores
Serum total protein	6.6–7.0 g/dL	Estimates protein stores
Serum total iron-binding capacity	Males: 300–400 μg/dL; females: 300–450 μg/dL 0.6–1.2 mg/dL	Estimates protein stores
Serum creatinine		Indicates depletion of muscles mass (protein wasting)
24-hr urine assay for creatinine height index		84–90 mL/min; indicates degree of protein wasting
Blood urea nitrogen	8–20 mg/dL	Indicates rate of protein metabolism
Serum transferrin	250–390 μg/dL	Indicates rate of protein metabolism and iron-binding capacity
24-hr urine assay for urea nitrogen	64–99 mL/min	Measures nitrogen balance
Blood glucose	70–100 mg/dL	Indicates availability of primary energy source
Serum electrolytes		Provides rough measure of fluid and electrolyte balance and overall nutritional status
Sodium	135–150 mEq/L	
Potassium	3.5–5.5 mEq/L	
Chloride	95–115 mEq/L	
Calcium	8.6–10.5 mg/dL	
Phosphorus	3–4.5 mg/dL	
Magnesium	1.5–2.4 mEq/L	
Serum osmolality	286–305 mOsm/L	Estimates fluid balance
Total white blood count	4500–11,000 mm^3	Indicates immune function
Total lymphocyte count	800–4500 mm^3	Indicates immune function
Hemoglobin	Males: 14–17g/dL; females: 12–16 g/dL	Provides rough measure of iron-binding capacity, fluid balance, and absence of anemia
Hematocrit	Males: 40%–54%; females: 34%–51%	Provides rough measure of iron-binding capacity, fluid balance, and absence of anemia

*Additional studies may be ordered as indicated. Examples include serum liver and kidney function studies, free fatty acids, and vitamin and mineral levels.

From Bronstein, K.S., Popovich, J.M., & Stewart-Amidei, C. (1991). Promoting stroke recovery: A research based approach. St. Louis: Mosby–Year Book.

through administration of an energy battery; a delayed response is indicative of immunosuppression.

Human Responses to Metabolic Alterations

The metabolic response and its subsequent consequences may be seen in any patient with neurologic dysfunction. Patients at highest risk for nutritional deficits are those with severe head injury and an inability to take in adequate nutrients because of impaired consciousness or neurologic deficit or those with a premorbid poor nutritional status. Nutritional support is essential in these patients to provide an adequate nutritional intake.

• C A S E   S T U D Y   3

Severe Head Injury

Kevin, a 25-year-old man, lost control while driving a motorcycle and crashed into a tree, sustaining a severe head injury. His admission GCS score was 4. He was intubated in the emergency department and placed on mechanical ventilation. Surprisingly, no other injuries were noted at the time. On the day after admission, mechanical ventilation became increasingly difficult. After frequent ventilator changes and the addition of PEEP, he was determined to have neurogenic pulmonary edema and, although the treatment is controversial, was subsequently placed on high-dose methylprednisolone. His neurologic status remained essentially unchanged; he was unresponsive with decerebrate posturing.

Height on admission was 180 cm, and admission weight was 75 kg. Overall physical condition was adequate; he appeared to be a well-nourished male with good skin turgor. No muscle atrophy was noted. Family members denied any recent weight gain or loss; he was reported to be a healthy eater with an occasional binge of high-fat food. Family members denied alcohol consumption. Admission serum albumin was 4.0 g/dL and, serum transferrin was 300 mg/dL; values were within normal limits (250–390 mg/dL).

Corrected BEE was calculated to be at least 3000 kcal. For the first 3 days, he received only dextrose solution for nutrition for a total kcal amount of 750 kcal. By the third day, his weight had dropped to 71 kg, his serum albumin had dropped to 3.3 g/dL, and his urine was positive for ketones, indicating moderate malnutrition. Feeding via a gastrostomy tube was attempted, but because of high residual gastric volumes, he was unable to be given adequate feedings to meet his estimated metabolic demands. Parenteral nutrition was begun on day 4. By day 8, his weight loss ceased and his weight began to stabilize. Enteral feedings were restarted and gradually increased. Enteral feeding tolerance was initially poor but gradually improved. By day 14, his weight began to increase, and he was tolerating adequate enteral feedings; parenteral feedings were discontinued.

NUTRITION, ALTERED, LESS THAN BODY REQUIREMENTS

Similar to many neurologic patients, Kevin was unable to take in any food orally. Although oral feedings are preferred, neurologic status often precludes this. Even if oral feedings had been possible, it is unlikely Kevin would have been able to take in adequate nutrition to meet his caloric requirements. His metabolic rate was increased not only by the head injury, but also by concomitant respiratory problems, decerebrate posturing, and use of steroids.

Defining characteristics of this diagnosis include inability to feed oneself because of decreased level of consciousness; weight loss and muscle wasting; decline in laboratory values indicative of nutritional status, especially negative nitrogen balance and decreased serum albumin and transferrin; decrease in subcutaneous fat measurements; and immunosuppression. The goal of intervention is to maintain weight and stabilize other indices of nutritional status.

Assessment focuses on the four parameters previously mentioned. Weight should be obtained on admission and at least twice weekly; subcutaneous fat measurements may be taken on admission and weekly. A nutrition screen should be obtained on admission and repeated twice weekly or more often with weight loss. Specific tests may be added on an individual basis (see Table 33–8).

Nursing interventions include early provision of nutritional supplements via the enteral or parenteral route (Hickey, 1992b). Enteral feedings are preferred when short-term nutritional support is anticipated and a gag reflex and bowel sounds are present (Rombean & Caldwell, 1990). Nasopharyngeal to gastric tubes may be used in the absence of orofacial or skull base fractures and gastrointestinal disease (Rombean & Caldwell, 1990). Tubes may cause nasal mucosal erosion; hence, short-term use is preferred. When longer-term feedings are likely, a percutaneous gastrostomy or jejunostomy tube may be inserted (Hickey, 1992b). Tube placement must be verified with an x-ray (Rombean & Caldwell, 1990). Tube-feedings may be given in a continuous pattern if the tube is placed in the small bowel or in a bolus format if placed in the stomach. During gastric feedings, the patient's head should be elevated and the volume of gastric aspirate checked every 4 hours. Feedings may be held or rate changed when the gastric aspirate is greater than 100 mL.

In patients at risk for pulmonary aspiration (those who have limited gag reflex or are otherwise unable to protect their airway), the cuff of a tracheostomy is inflated while feeding and for at least 1 hour after completion to prevent aspiration. The patient should be observed for aspiration, diarrhea, or feeding intolerance. To prevent diarrhea, feedings should be diluted and given slowly, with gradual increases to full strength. Diphenoxylate, fiber formulations, or *Lactobacillus acidophilus* may be used to control diarrhea; metoclopramide may be helpful in stimulating gastric emptying. To prevent aspiration, tube placement should be verified and rechecked before beginning each feeding, and the patient should be placed upright. Suction equipment should be available at the bedside should aspiration occur. Antibiotic treatment may be necessary. Feeding intolerance may be alleviated by changing the formula. Detailed discussion of enteral nutrition complications is found in Table 33–9.

Total parenteral nutrition (TPN) may be the treatment of choice when the patient is unable to eat, is unable to tolerate tube-feedings, or has high metabolic rate that cannot be satisfied by enteral nutrition (Ott & Young, 1993; Wirth & Ratcheson, 1987). Studies have shown that TPN decreases mortality and mor-

TABLE 33–9 • COMPLICATIONS OF ENTERAL NUTRITION

Problem	Possible Causes	Nursing Actions
Diarrhea	Hyperosmolarity of feeding (usually 450 mOsm/L or more)	Begin very slowly, and allow patient to adapt to formula
		Dilute feeding or give free water
		If ordered by physician, a few drops of deodorized tincture of opium may be added
	Rapid rate of infusion	Administer very slowly until gastrointestinal tract adapts to the feeding
		Feeding may have to be discontinued and started again slowly in a diluted form
		If diarrhea is not excessive, paregoric or diphenoxylate (Lomotil) may be given temporarily
	Lactose intolerance	Avoid feeding with lactose unless patient normally drinks milk daily without ill effects
Constipation	Diet high in milk content	Change type of feeding
	Inadequate fluid intake	Give sufficient water in diet
		Record frequency of bowel movements
		Administer stool softeners and mild laxatives if necessary
Vomiting	Feeding too soon after intubation or suctioning	Allow patient a rest period before beginning feeding
	Too-rapid rate of infusion	Run infusion slowly
Dumping syndrome	Too-rapid infusion of hyperosmolar solutions	Run infusion slowly
		Administer free water after intermittent feeding to dilute intake
Dehydration	Rapid infusion of hyperosmolar carbohydrates that cause hyperglycemia, osmotic diuresis, and dehydration	Administer slowly
		Check sugar and acetone periodically (usually every 6 hr)
	Excessive protein and electrolytes (these have an osmotic effect)	May need to administer regular insulin to cover glycosuria
		Adjust formula
		Administer free water

From Hickey, J.V. (1992). *The clinical aspects of neurological and neurosurgical nursing* (3rd ed.). Philadelphia: J.B. Lippincott.

bidity (Ott & Young, 1993; Wirth & Ratcheson, 1987). Nutrients are provided in their simplest, easiest-to-use form via an intravenous (IV) route (Bronstein et al., 1991b). Carbohydrates are provided in the form of glucose, while crystallized amino acids supply protein. Fat emulsions may be administered separately twice a week as necessary; care must be taken to prevent lipemia and a fatty liver. The TPN solution is individualized to patient needs and is a complete source of all essential nutrients, including vitamins and minerals. Solution content and rate may be adjusted on a daily basis to accommodate changing needs. Because the TPN solution is hyperosmolar, a central venous access device is usually necessary for administration; adequate peripheral access may be suitable in some patients (Ott & Young, 1993). Complications of TPN include those related to placement of the venous access device, such as pneumothorax, as well as those related to the solution itself, such as hyperglycemia (Wirth & Ratcheson, 1987). Table 33–10 lists metabolic complications of TPN solution administration. Close observation for adverse effects of TPN is essential.

Once nutritional status is stabilized and the patient is alert enough to swallow or able to swallow without aspirating, oral feedings may be started. Before oral feedings are attempted, an oropharyngeal motility study may be performed to rule out silent aspiration. When beginning oral feedings, the patient must be in an upright position, bent slightly forward. Feedings should not be attempted when the patient is tired. Small amounts of pureed or semi-solid food may be offered with supervision. Liquids are introduced later because they are more difficult to swallow. Thickeners may be added to liquids

TABLE 33–10 • METABOLIC COMPLICATIONS OF TOTAL PARENTERAL NUTRITION

Glucose metabolism

Hyperglycemia, glycosuria, osmotic diuresis, hyperosmolar nonketotic dehydration, and coma
Ketoacidosis in diabetes mellitus
Postinfusion (rebound) hypoglycemia

Amino acid metabolism

Hyperchloremic metabolic acidosis
Serum amino acid imbalance
Hyperammonemia
Prerenal azotemia

Calcium and phosphorus metabolism

Hypophosphatemia, decreased, 2.3-diphosphoglycerate, increased hemoglobin affinity for
  oxygen, erythrocyte metabolic aberrations
Hypocalcemia
Hypercalcemia
Vitamin D deficiency or excess

Essential fatty acid metabolism

Serum deficiencies of phospholipid linoleic acid and arachidonic acid
Serum elevations of 5,8,11 cicosanoic acid

Miscellaneous

Hypokalemia
Hyperkalemia
Hypomagnesemia
Hypermagnesemia
Biochemical liver dysfunction
Bleeding
Anemia
Hypervitaminosis A
Cholestatic hepatitis

From Wirth F.P. & Ratcheson, R.A. (Eds.) (1987). *Neurosurgical critical care*, Baltimore: Williams & Wilkins.

to add substance while allowing adequate oral intake. Suction equipment should be readily available in the event choking or aspiration occur.

As oral feedings become the primary source of nutrition, ongoing attention to nutritional status is required. Daily weights and laboratory values should continue to ensure nutritional stability. Additional attention should be given to other factors influencing oral intake, such as food likes and dislikes, cultural influences, and social environment for eating. Because the metabolic response may continue indefinitely, long-term attention to nutritional status is likely to be necessary.

Summary

Metabolism is a balance between the two antagonistic processes of catabolism and anabolism. Metabolic rate is coupled with cellular demands. A neurogenically mediated sympathetic response may greatly increase metabolic rate, thus making it difficult to maintain adequate nutrition. An understanding of the metabolic response to neurologic insult guides appropriate interventions to enhance optimal nutrition.

References

Appenzeller, O. (1990). Respiration and disorders of ventilation. In *The autonomic nervous system* (4th ed., pp. 339–355). New York: Elsevier.

Barnes, K.L., Ferrario, C.M., & Conomy, J.P. (1979). Comparison of the hemodynamic changes produced by electrical stimulation of the area postrema and nucleus tractus solitarii in the dog. *Circulation Research, 45,* 136–143.

Barron, S.A., Rogovski, Z., & Hemli, J. (1994). Autonomic consequences of cerebral hemisphere infarction. *Stroke, 25,* 113–116.

Beckwith, J.R. (1982). *Basic electrocardiography and vectorcardiography* (pp. 41, 81–82). Lancaster, CA: Raven Press.

Bishop, V.S. (1994). Central nervous system regulation of cardiovascular homeostasis. *New Horizons, 2*(4), 415–418.

Bleck, T.P. (1991). Increased intracranial pressure. In J.E. Parrillo (Ed.), *Current therapy in critical care medicine* (2nd ed., pp. 249–521). Hamilton, ON: B.C. Decker Inc.

Blessing, W.W., West, M.J., & Chalmers, J. (1981). Hypertension, bradycardia, and pulmonary edema in the conscious rabbit after brain stem lesions coinciding with A1 group of catecholamine neurons. *Circulation Research, 49,* 949–958.

Boysen, P.G., & Modell, J.H. (1989). Pulmonary edema. In W.C. Shoemaker, S. Ayres, A. Grenvik, P.R. Halbrook, & W.L. Thompson (Eds.), *Textbook of critical care* (2nd ed., pp. 515–518). Philadelphia: W.B. Saunders.

Bronstein, K., Popovich, J., & Stewart-Amidei, C. (1991a). Alterations in integrated regulation. In *Promoting stroke recovery: A research based approach for nurses* (pp. 69–83). St. Louis: C.V. Mosby.

Bronstein, K., Popovich, J., & Stewart-Amidei, C. (1991b). Alterations in nutrition. In *Promoting stroke recovery: A research based approach for nurses* (pp. 113–131). St. Louis: C.V. Mosby.

Brucia, J.J., Owen, D.C., & Rudy, E.B. (1992). The effects of lidocaine on intracranial hypertension. *Journal of Neuroscience Nursing, 24*(4), 205–214.

Cruickshank, J.M., Neil-Dwyer, B., & Brice, J. (1974). Electrocardiographic changes and their prognostic significance in subarachnoid hermorrhage. *Journal of Neurological and Neurosurgical Nursing, 37,* 755–759.

Dettbarn, C.L., & Davidson, L.J. (1989). Pulmonary complications in the patient with acute head injury: Neurogenic pulmonary edema. *Heart and Lung, 18,* 583–589.

Diamond, M.C., Scheibel, A.B., & Elson, L.M. (1985). *The human brain coloring book* (pp. 1–4). New York: Harper Perennial.

Fincham, R.W., Shevapour, E.T., Leis, A.A., & Martins, J.B. (1992). Ictal bradycardia with syncope: A case report. *Neurology, 42,* 2222–2223.

Fitzgerald, M.J. (1992). *Neuroanatomy: Basic and clinical* (2nd ed.). Philadelphia: Bailliere Tindall.

George, R.B., & Chesson, A.L. (1990). Functional anatomy of the respiratory system. In R.B. George, R.W. Light, M.A. Matthay, & R.A. Matthay (Eds.), *Chest medicine: Essential of pulmonary and critical care medicine* (2nd ed., pp. 3–22). Baltimore: Williams & Wilkins.

Hachinski, V.C. (1993). The clinical problem of brain and heart. *Stroke, 24*(Suppl I), 1–2.

Hart, G.K., Humphrey L., & Weiss, J. (1989). Subarachnoid hemorrhage: Cardiac complications. *Critical Care Report, 1,* 88–92.

Hayek, D.A., & Veremakis, C. (1993). Cerebral resuscitation. In M.R. Pinsky & J.A. Dhainaut (Eds.), *Pathophysiologic foundations of critical care* (pp. 753–777). Baltimore: Williams & Wilkins.

Hickey, J. (1992a). Assessment of neurological signs: Vital signs. In *The clinical practice of neurological and neurosurgical nursing* (3rd ed., pp. 113–143). Philadelphia: J.B. Lippincott.

Hickey, J. (1992b). Nutritional needs of neurological and neurosurgical nursing patients. In *The clinical practice of neurological and neurosurgical nursing* (3rd ed., pp. 147–162). Philadelphia: J.B. Lippincott.

Hickey, J. (1992c). Care of the unconscious patient: Respiratory function. In *The clinical practice of neurological and neurosurgical nursing* (3rd ed., pp. 232–238). Philadelphia: J.B. Lippincott.

Katzung, B.G. (1994). Introduction to autonomic pharmacology. In B.G. Katzung (Ed.), *Basic and clinical pharmacology* (5th ed., pp. 69–80). Stamford, CT: Appleton & Lange.

Keller, C., & Williams, A. (1993). Cardiac dysrhythmias associated with central nervous system dysfunction. *Journal of Neuroscience Nursing, 25*(6), 349–355.

Kelly, J.S., & MacGregor, D.A. (1994). Drugs acting at the cholinergic receptor. In B. Chernow (Ed.), *The pharmacologic approach to the critically ill patient* (3rd ed., pp. 534–547). Baltimore: Williams & Wilkins.

Kerr, M.E., Rudy, E.B., Brucia, J., & Stone, K.A. (1993). Head-injured adults: Recommendations for endotrachea suctioning. *Journal of Neuroscience Nursing, 25*(2), 86–91.

Kersten, L.D. (1989). Mechanics and control of breathing. In *Comprehensive respiratory nursing: A decision making approach* (pp. 71–85). Philadelphia: W.B. Saunders.

Korpelainen, I.T., Sotaniemi, K.A., Suominen, K., Tolonen, U., & Myllyla, V. (1994). Cardiovascular autonomic reflexes in brain infarction. *Stroke, 25,* 787–792.

Lane, R.D., Wallace, J.D., Petrosky, P.P., Schwartz, G.E., & Gradman, A.H. (1992). Supraventricular tachycardia in patients with right hemisphere strokes. *Stroke, 23,* 362–366.

Lefkowitz, R.J., Hoffman, B.B., & Taylor, P. (1990). Neurohumoral transmission: The autonomic and somatic motor nervous systems. In A.G. Gilman, T.W. Rall, A.S. Nies, & P. Taylor (Eds.), *Goodman and Gilman's the pharmacological basis of therapeutics* (8th ed. pp. 84–121). Tarrytown, NY: Pergammon Press.

Liebman, M. (1991). *Neuroanatomy made easy and understandable* (4th ed.). Gaithersburg, MD: Aspen.

Long, C.L., Schaffel, N., Geiger, J.W., Schiller, W.R., & Blakemore, W.S. (1979). Metabolic response to injury and illness: Estimation of energy and protein needs from indirect calorimetry and nitrogen balance. *Journal of Parenteral and Enteral Nutrition, 3,* 452–456.

Maire, R.W., & Patton, H.D. (1956). Neural structures involved in the genesis of preoptic pulmonary edema, gastric erosions, and behavior changes. *American Journal of Physiology, 184,* 345–350.

Malkoff, M.D., & Borel, C.O. (1994). Central nervous system modulation of respiratory function in the critically ill. *New Horizons, 2*(4), 419–425.

Marino, P.I. (1998). Nutrition and metabolism. In *The ICU book* (2nd ed., pp. 721–776). Baltimore: Williams & Wilkins.

Marshall, S.B., Marshall, L.F., Vos, H.R., & Chesnut, R.M. (1990a). Head injury and the treatment of increased intracranial pressure. In *Neuroscience critical care: Pathophysiology and patient management* (pp. 201–203). Philadelphia: W.B. Saunders.

Marshall, S.B., Marshall, L.F., Vos, H.R., & Chesnut, R.M. (1990b). Complications in the critically ill neuro patient. In *Neuroscience critical care: Pathophysiology and patient management* (pp. 400–401). Philadelphia: W.B. Saunders.

Matuschak, G.M. (1994). Organ interactions in critical illness: Paradigms and mechanisms. *New Horizons, 2*(4), 413–414.

Mayer, S.A., Fink, M.E., Homma, S., Sherman, D., LiMandri, G., Lennihan, L., Solomon, R., Klebanoff, L., Beckford, A., Raps, E. (1994). Cardiac injury associated with neurogenic pulmonary edema following subarachnoid hemorrhage. *Neurology, 44,* 815–820.

McDermott, M.M., Lefevre, F., Arron, M., Martin, G.J., & Biller, J. (1994). ST segment depression detected by continuous electrocardiography in patients with acute ischemic stroke or transient ischemic attack. *Stroke, 25,* 1820–1824.

Misasi, R.S., Keyes, J.L. (1994). The pathophysiology of hypoxia. *Critical Care Nurse, 4,* 55–64.

Moraine, J., Brimioulle, S., & Kahn, R.J. (1991). Effects of respiratory therapy on intracranial pressure. *Journal of Critical Care, 6*(4), 197–201.

Nathan, M.A., & Reis, D.J. (1975). Fulminating arterial hypertension with pulmonary edema from release of adrenomedullary catecholamines after lesions of the anterior hypothalamus in the rat. *Circulation Research, 37,* 226–235.

Netter, F.H. (1983). Autonomic nervous system. In *The Ciba collections of medical illustrations: Nervous system* (pp. 69–90). Summit, NJ: CIBA.

Norris, J.W. (1983). Effects of cerebrovascular lesions on the heart. *Neurologic Clinics, 1*(1), 87–101.

Olson, J.M. (1994). *Clinical pharmacology made ridiculously simple.* Tampa, FL: MedMaster.

Oppenheimer, S. (1993). The anatomy and physiology of cortical mechanisms of cardiac control. *Stroke, 24*(Suppl I); 3–5.

Oppenheimer, S.M. (1994). Neurogenic cardiac effects of cerebrovascular disease. *Current Opinion in Neurology 7,* 20–24.

Oppenheimer, S.M., & Hachinski, V.C. (1992). The cardiac consequences of stroke. *Neurologic Clinics, 10*(1), 167–176.

Ott, L., & Young, B. (1993). Metabolic and nutritional management. In B. Andrews (Ed.), *Neurosurgical intensive care* (pp. 163–178). New York: McGraw-Hill.

Pender, E.S., & Pollack, C.V. (1992). Neurogenic pulmonary edema: Case reports and review. *Journal of Emergency Medicine, 10,* 45–51.

Pinsky, M.R. (1993). Heart-lung interactions. In M.R. Pinsky & J.A. Dhainaut (Eds.), *Pathophysiologic foundations of critical care* (pp. 472–490). Baltimore: Williams & Wilkins.

Posey, K., & Allen, S. (1994a). Increased intracranial pressure in stroke patients (part I). *Stroke: Clinical Updates, 4*(6), 29–32.

Posey, K., & Allen, S. (1994b). Increased intracranial pressure in stroke patients (part II). *Stroke: Clinical Updates, 5*(1), 1–4.

Prendergast, V. (1994). Current trends in research and treatment of intracranial hypertension. *Critical Care Nursing Quarterly, 17*(1), 1–8.

Richter, D.W., & Spyer, K.M. (1990). Cardiorespiratory control. In A.D. Loewy (Ed.), *Cerebral regulation of anatomic function* (pp. 189–207). New York: Oxford University Press.

Romand, J.A., Donal, F.A., & Suter, P.M. (1994). Cardiopulmonary interactions in acute lung injury: Clinical and prognostic importance of pulmonary hypertension. *New Horizons, 2*(4), 457–462.

Rombean, J.L., & Caldwell, M.D. (1990). In *Clinical nutrition: Enteral and tube feeding* (pp. 250–262). Philadelphia: W.B. Saunders.

Roser, M., & Daughton, S. (1990). Cerebral perfusion pressure management in head injury. *Journal of Trauma, 30,* 933–939.

Rossaint, R., Falke, K.J., Lopez, F., Slama, K., Pison, U., & Zapol, W.M. (1995). Inhaled nitric oxide for the adult respiratory distress syndrome. *New England Journal of Medicine, 328*(6), 399–432.

Rudy, E.B., Baun, M., Stone, K., & Turner, B. (1986). The relationship between endotracheal suctioning and changes in intracranial pressure: A review of the literature. *Heart and Lung, 15*(5), 488–494.

Rudy, E.B., Turner, B.S., Baun, M., Stone, K.S., & Brucia, J. (1991). Endotracheal suctioning in adults with head injury. *Heart and Lung, 20*(6), 667–674.

Ruffolo, R.R. (1994). Cardiovascular adrenoceptors: Physiology and critical care implications. In B. Chernow (Ed.), *The pharmacologic approach to the critically ill patient* (3rd ed., pp. 167–181). Baltimore: Williams & Wilkins.

Samuels, M.A. (1993). Neurally induced cardiac damage: Definition of the problem. *Neurologic Clinics, 11*(2), 273–292.

Shronts, E.P. (1989). *Nutrition support dietetics.* Gaithersburg, MD: Aspen.

Simon, R.P. (1993). Neurogenic pulmonary edema. *Neurologic Clinics, 11*(2), 309–323.

Smeltzer, S.C. (1992). Nursing management of adults with common neurological problems. In L. Brunner & D. Suddarth (Eds.), *Brunner and Suddarth's textbook of medical surgical nursing* (7th ed., pp. 1062–1096). Philadelphia: J.B. Lippincott.

Smeltzer, S.C. & Bana, B.G. (1992). Nursing assessment of the neurological system. In L. Brunner & D. Suddarth (Eds.), *Brunner and Suddarth's textbook of medical surgical nursing* (7th ed., pp. 1030–1061). Philadelphia: J.B. Lippincott.

Stone, K.S., Preusser, B.A., Groch, K.F., Karl, J.I., & Gonyon, D.S. (1991). The effect of lung hyperinflation and endotracheal suctioning on cardiopulmonary hemodynamics. *Nursing Research, 40*(2), 76–80.

Szabo, M.D., Crosby, G., Hurford, W.E., & Strauss, H.W. (1993). Myocardial perfusion following acute subarachnoid hemorrhage in patients with an abnormal electrocardiogram. *Anesthesia Analgesia, 76*, 253–258.

Talman, W.T., & Kelkar, P. (1993). Neural control of the heart: Central and peripheral. *Neurologic Clinics, 11*(2), 239–256.

Taylor, R.W., & Norwood, S.H. (1992). The adult respiratory distress syndrome: Noncardiogenic pulmonary edema. In J.M. Civetta, R.W. Taylor, & R.R. Kirby (Eds.), *Critical care* (2nd ed., pp. 1240–1241). Philadelphia: J.B. Lippincott.

Theodore, J., & Robin, E.D. (1976). Speculations on neurogenic pulmonary edema (Editorial). *American Review of Respiratory Disease, 113*, 405–411.

Valeriano, J., & Elson, J. (1993). Electrocardiographic changes in central nervous system disease. *Neurologic Clinics, 11*(2), 257–272.

Watanabe A.M., & Katzung, B.G. (1994). Cholinoceptor-activating and cholinesterase-inhibiting drugs. In B.G. Katzung (Ed.), *Basic and clinical pharmacology* (5th ed., pp. 82–96). Stamford, CT: Appleton & Lange.

West, J.B. (1985). Control of ventilation: How gas exchange is regulated. In *Respiratory physiology: The essentials* (3rd ed., pp. 113–129). Baltimore: Williams & Wilkins.

West, J.B. (1987). Vascular diseases. In *Pulmonary pathophysiology: The essentials* (3rd ed., pp. 112–123). Baltimore: Williams & Wilkins.

Wirth, F.P., & Ratcheson, R.A. (Ed.) (1987). *Neurosurgical critical care.* Baltimore: Williams and Wilkins.

Wohns, R.N., Tamas, L., Pierce, K.R., & Howe, J. F. (1985). Chlorpromazine treatment for neurogenic pulmonary edema. *Critical Care Medicine, 13*(3), 210–211.

Zegeer, L.J. (1984). Systemic cardiovascular effects of intracranial disorders: Implications for nursing care. *Journal of Neurosurgical Nursing, 16*(3), 161–167.

On Being Human: Alterations in the Sense of Being

MARLENE REIMER

No part of the body is more closely associated with being human than the nervous system. Without the nervous system there would be no thought, no movement, no awareness of that which is beautiful or horrible, no hope or despair, no sense of time, no sexual pleasure, no enjoyment of music, no joy, and no pain. The impact of neurologic illness on the person as a whole is the focus of this chapter. Concepts such as body image, self-perception, self-concept, coping, and grieving are addressed elsewhere in this book. Discussion in this chapter is limited to reflections on what neurologic dysfunction may mean to the integrated whole, the sense of being.

The meaning of being human touches the essence of philosophical inquiry (Harrison, 1993). It is also a very personal, individual quest. Reflection on human responses to actual or potential threats to humanness is a matter of practical importance. Neuroscience nurses are there when patients struggle with threats to their being, to the self as they have known and experienced it, to personhood, and to their taken-for-granted body.

The knowledge of human responses to these threats is embedded in practice. The topic has received scant attention in the health literature. Sacks' (1987) observation, "Constantly my patients drive me to question, and constantly my questions drive me to patients," echoes the belief that knowledge is extended and developed in practice (Benner & Wrubel, 1989). In this section, the reader is invited to reflect on what has been learned through patient encounters when humanness is threatened.

Philosophically, humanness and personhood have included consciousness, self-awareness, ability to communicate, and rational thought (Harrison, 1993). The concept of personhood is also assumed to include some degree of psychologic and social continuity (Cassell, 1991). However, the effects of trauma, amnesia, or dementia are such that the continuity of the person often seems broken, to himself or herself and to others. Families are heard to comment that their brain-injured son is "not the same person." In early stages of dementia, individuals themselves may express the sense that they are losing their very self.

Yet clinical experience suggests that personhood remains in spite of profound deficits. Harrison (1993) suggested that viewing an individual's life as a narrative can give a sense of unity even though personality and behavior may seem radically changed or almost nonexistent. By considering the narrative of a life, the neuroscience nurse has a context in which to establish relationship. Such simple measures as putting up photographs of the patient and the family taken before the neurologic insult are commonly used. However, Harrison (1993) challenged the status quo, recommending development of much more person-oriented assessments that facilitate exploration of an individual's life story even when that person is unable to tell it directly. Part of the person-oriented approach is identification of positive behaviors, abilities, values, and experiences. For example, Harrison described the behavior of an elderly woman with Alzheimer's disease who became particularly distressed whenever a homemaker came to help. Finding out that this woman had always considered the kitchen "her territory" and therefore might resent the homemaker as an "intruder" opened space to consider other alternatives.

The social construction of humanness in relationships between nondisabled and severely disabled people has been the subject of a series of qualitative studies (Bogdan & Taylor, 1989). Rather than focus on patterns of stigmatization and dehumanization, the studies specifically examined the perspectives of nondisabled people who were in caring and accepting relationships with profoundly disabled children and adults. More than 20 sites were visited, primarily small community settings and natural, foster, and adoptive homes. Unfortunately, the methods used were insufficiently described to permit replication in other contexts. Nevertheless, the four dimensions identified as characterizing the perspectives of people who continue to see humanness even in disabled individuals merit reflection:

- Attributing thinking to the other
- Seeing individuality in the other
- Viewing the other as reciprocating
- Defining a social place for the other (Bogdan & Taylor, 1989, p. 135f)

These dimensions have remarkable similarity to those that Sheehan (1992) presented as a basis for ethical decision making regarding persons with advanced Alzheimer's disease and health care rationing. He made three points with respect to those who have lost cognitive continuity with their past: they remain persons who have a history even if they cannot recall it; they continue to be in relationship with others, albeit a very dependent relationship; and they are part of a community, a community of family and caregivers.

CONSCIOUSNESS

Consciousness has two components: awakeness and awareness (Boss, 1994). For the human being to be aware, there must be some minimum level of awakeness. However, as neuroscience nurses recognize, awakeness does not ensure awareness. States of awakeness follow a continuum from deep coma to hypervigilance, as discussed in Chapter 5. States of awareness are more complex and variable. Two types of awareness are particularly relevant to discussion of humanness: awareness of environment and awareness of self.

Awareness of Environment

The essential evidence for determining brain death is absence of responsiveness to the external and internal environments. Research has confirmed clinical accounts of persons who can recall the presence of certain people and other sensations experienced during a period of deep coma. Tosch (1988) explored the recollections of 15 survivors of posttraumatic coma (Glasgow Coma Score [GCS] 3 to 8 for more than 6 hours). The eight survivors with recall had GCSs and types of injuries similar to those of the seven survivors without recall; the only difference was a tendency for recall to be associated with a shorter period of coma. Patients remembered being pinched (probably as part of assessment), being comforted by touch or voice tone, and hearing bits of conversation. Themes were related to being held against their will; having intensified visual, olfactory, or auditory perception; and having deathlike experiences. One patient's coma recollections were vividly described in a journal article (Paul & Littlejohns, 1994).

The assumption, even without research validation, that comatose patients may be aware of some external stimuli has been integral to the practice of neuroscience nursing. To talk to the unconscious patient is normal practice to the experienced clinician but is often perceived as strange behavior in the eyes of beginning nursing students. Likewise, the almost intuitive sense that accompanies the first flickers of response is one of the ways of knowing of the expert neuroscience nurse.

Awareness of Self

Loss of self has been identified as a fundamental form of suffering in chronic illness (Charmaz, 1983). The chapter on coping with neurologic illness in *The Primacy of Caring* opens with the statement, "People with neurological illnesses sustain damage to their 'selves' in a way that people with no other illness do. . . . Even if the personality and linguistic abilities are spared, there can be motor or sensory damage, damage of the sort that makes people feel that they are trapped in someone else's body" (Benner & Wrubel, 1989).

Sacks (1987) also spoke specifically about how neurologic disease affects the self. In *The Man Who Mistook His Wife for a Hat and Other Clinical Tales*, he stated, "It must be said from the outset that a disease is never a mere loss or excess—that there is always a reaction, on the part of the affected organism or individual, to restore, to replace, to compensate for and to preserve its identity, however strange the means may be" (p. 6). Earlier, he made the comment that "the patient's essential being is very relevant in the higher reaches of neurology, and in psychology; for here the patient's personhood is essentially involved and the study of disease and of identity cannot be disjoined" (p. viii).

Illnesses that result in loss of control are especially damaging to the sense of self, given the high value that society places on controlling the body and its functions in socially accepted ways (Charmaz, 1983). Unpredictability, loss of function, and dependence may further reduce the sense of self and connectedness with others. Some neurologic deficits with these characteristics, such as tics, seizures, or ataxia, have evoked responses of avoidance and stigmatization from others (Hartshorn & Byers, 1994). Increasing social isolation further weakens the sense of self in relation to others and becomes a source of further suffering (Cassell, 1991).

Thus far the discussion has focused on ways in which neurologic illness may damage the self. As Charmaz (1983) found in interviewing 57 chronically ill adults with varied diagnoses, the loss of the previous self is a major source of suffering for most people, even those with no evidence of cognitive impairment. Suffering associated with conscious awareness of change is also seen in patients with many neurologic conditions including spinal cord injury, peripheral syndromes, and left-hemisphere insults. However, neuroscience nurses also work with individuals who seem to lack awareness of how they have changed. Cassell (1991) made the point that suffering associated with loss of the former self does not occur at just a cognitive level. He argued that the meaning of the experience is also perceived emotionally, bodily, and spiritually and, furthermore, that these different meanings may be contradictory and jumbled. This author argued that even when the cognitive ability to assign meaning is lost, we do not know what other levels of personal meaning and selfhood are still being perceived. Thus the elderly lady with Alzheimer's disease who was upset about a homemaker "intruding" into her kitchen can be seen as expressing awareness of her self in the felt role of cook and homemaker even though the cognitive continuity of selfhood seemed broken.

Impaired self-awareness has been a major focus in Prigatano's work with brain-injured adults. He described self-awareness as "the highest of all integrated activities of the brain" and as "perhaps the single most salient factor deterring reintegration" of brain-injured individuals (Prigatano, 1992, 1994). Self-awareness is conceptualized as the capacity to perceive oneself in a relatively objective manner and yet also to subjectively interpret that experience.

From clinical experience, many neuroscience nurses can relate to the "self-centeredness" commonly seen among patients recovering from traumatic brain injury. The dynamics of facilitating increased insight into the nature and severity of disability are complex and individualized. First, the patient and family need time to mourn losses, to put them into perspective, and to begin to construct a new view of the self. However, the nature of brain injury in itself interferes with normal grieving. Memory impairments may distort recall, reduced attention span may interfere with working through grief processes, and the sheltered environment of a rehabilitation center or home may limit reality testing (Sachs, 1984). The term *mobile mourning* has been applied to the particular pattern of grieving seen in brain-injured individuals and their families (Muir & Haffey, 1984). It is organized around the "partial death" of the patient and is characterized by prolonged uncertainty of outcomes, wide fluctuations between euphoria and despair, tension within support systems, feelings of rage, and learned helplessness (Muir & Haffey, 1984).

ACKNOWLEDGMENT OF HUMANNESS

As stated in the American Association of Neuroscience Nurses (AANN) Scope of Practice Statement, neuroscience nursing encompasses care at "all levels of human existence, from basic bodily functions to advanced processes of the human mind" (AANN, 1994, p. 47). Central to our practice in neuroscience nursing are the ways in which we relate to persons who are comatose, grossly deformed with contractures, or unable to communicate, affording them respect and dignity. Even after death, respect for the body is a basic expectation.

Respect

Respect is defined as "to feel or show honor or esteem for; hold in high regard . . . to concern; relate to" (*Webster's New World Dictionary*, 1979). It includes the ethical sense of special obligations that we have to others simply because they are persons (Harrison, 1993). Respect is fundamental to caring. Respect gives the benefit of the doubt even when all cognitive functions normally associated with personhood are destroyed by disease or trauma. As Harrison (1993) stated, "their moral worth and equality persist, grounding our duty to care for them" (p. 431).

Dignity

The introduction to the Canadian Neuroscience Nursing Certification Examination includes the statement, "An important goal of neuroscience nursing practice is to ensure that the dignity of all clients is respected even in the absence of cortical functioning. This goal is based on the belief that a physically and/or cognitively incapacitated client with a body that . . . no longer functions or a brain that cannot reason or remember requires special protection and care" (Canadian Nurses Association, 1990).

SPIRITUALITY AND DEATH

Fundamental to acknowledgment of humanness are concepts of spirituality and death. Spirituality means personal views and behaviors that express a sense of relatedness to something greater than oneself, to something that transcends what can be perceived in space and time (Hastings, 1992). The content of beliefs can vary widely, but respect and dignity are closely related to the sense that to be human is to be more than a body. Spiritual well-being has been described as a harmonious interconnectedness among self, others, nature, and the Ultimate Other that gives an inner state of peace, freedom from abnormal anxiety and guilt, and a sense of security and direction in life (Hastings, 1992).

It has been argued that belief in the finality of death has constrained modern society either to try to master death or to ignore its presence (Hastings, 1992; Hungelmann, Kenkel-Rossi, Klassen, & Stollenwerk, 1989). An alternative, openness in the face of death, is proposed as part of a spiritual humanism. Reaching out in caring for another can transcend the self and give meaning to life and to being human (Frank, 1991; Reinsmith, 1989). Out of openness to death can come comfort, dignity, and awareness of a transcendence that goes beyond the boundaries of brain functioning. An exploration of the mind-brain issue is beyond the scope of this chapter. However, the interested reader is referred to the references listed at the end of this chapter for further reading on the subject.

QUALITY OF LIFE

The concept and measurement of quality of life can also be considered in the context of "being human." Some ethicists argue that there are two essential preconditions to quality of life: biologic life and capacity for self-awareness (Faden & LePlege, 1992). However, those who have worked closely with severely disabled children and adults challenge the taken-for-granted position that health care professionals can determine whether or not these individuals have capacity for self-awareness. Bogdan and Taylor (1989) make the point that "clinical perspectives are based on different ways of knowing and seeing than the perspectives of people involved in intimate relationships with those who have disabilities" (p. 141).

Quality of life can be conceptualized as the overall state of well-being that individuals experience as assessed by subjective and objective measures of functioning, health, and satisfaction with the important dimensions of their lives (Brown, Bayer, & MacFarlane, 1989; Hunt & McKenna, 1993; Schipper, Clinch, & Powell, 1990). It is common in health care research and practice to limit the concept to health-related quality of life, that which is affected by disease, trauma, or treatment thereof (Romney, Jenkins, & Bynner, 1992). Essential dimensions of health-related quality of life are physical function, social function, emotional or mental state, burden of symptoms, and sense of well-being (Spitzer, 1987; Stewart, 1992; Ware, 1986, 1987).

However, the sequelae of diseases and trauma affecting the nervous system can be so intrusive as to permeate all dimensions of human life: individual (e.g., enjoyment of leisure activities, economic status), family (e.g., marital relationship), and community (e.g., service demands).

Measurement of quality-of-life outcomes in persons who have experienced neurologic dysfunction is important but difficult. The importance of research and social policy planning arises because of the large proportion of patients in critical care, acute care, rehabilitation, long-term care, and community support programs who have been affected by different neurologic dysfunctions; the spiraling costs of health care; and the increasing emphasis on quality-of-life outcomes as a basis for planning and evaluation of services. The importance of clinical decision making lies in the very difficult choices faced by patients, families, and health care providers in the face of devastating threats to life, humanness, and quality of life from neurologic disease and trauma. The difficulty arises from the impact many neurologic dysfunctions have on the ability of affected individuals to cognitively process or communicate judgments about what is important to their quality of life. There is also an ethical basis for involving individuals with neurologic dysfunction in determining what is important to their quality of life. The concept of respect for persons includes the idea that all persons should have the opportunity to express their views about what affects them and protection when they cannot express these views (Council for International Organizations of Medical Sciences, 1991).

Cognitive impairment affects both quality of life and ability to respond to its measures (Bergner, Bobbitt, Carter, & Gilson, 1981; Cohen & Mount, 1992; Kinsella, Moran, Ford, & Ponsford, 1988; Ron & Feinstein, 1992; Shindler, Brown, Welburn, & Parkes, 1993; Tempkin, Dikmen, Machamer, & McLean, 1989). To be useful as a measure in the condition of cognitive impairment, a quality-of-life instrument should have four qualities:

First, it should tap indicators that are responsive to the kinds of impact that cognitive impairment has on quality of life. For example, safety has been identified as an important indicator of quality of life in this population, yet it is not included in most quality-of-life measures (Brown et al., 1989; Lehman, Possidente, & Hawker, 1986; Massion, Warshaw, & Keller, 1993).

Second, the measure should be responsive to programs and interventions targeted at the condition or its underlying cause (e.g., cognitive rehabilitation).

Third, the quality-of-life measure should be understandable in the presence of mild to moderate cognitive impairment (Tompkins, Jackson, & Schulz, 1990). To be understandable to individuals with mild to moderate impairment, the measure may need to be briefer, simpler, and more concrete in its wording than measures for cognitively normal adults (Wyness, 1987).

Fourth, the measure should be usable by proxies, especially when impairment is severe. A proxy is someone who knows the affected subject well and undertakes to answer questions from the subject's perspective. To be usable by proxies, a measure must not ask for information that they cannot know. Proxies can observe behavior, including what individuals may communicate verbally and nonverbally about feelings, but they cannot "know" the individuals' feelings. Therefore, the General Health Questionnaire, which has items such as "Have you recently felt you couldn't overcome your difficulties?" (McDowell & Newell, 1996) is less suitable for proxies than is the Sickness Impact Profile, which asks about behaviors such as "talk[ing] about the future in a hopeless way" (Bergner et al., 1981; McDowell & Newell, 1996).

A common assumption in outcome studies with cognitively impaired persons is that self-report data are of little value because of the patients' limited self-awareness, lack of insight, limited comprehension, or impulsivity in responding (Hunt & McKenna, 1993; Kinsella et al., 1988). It has been argued, however, that it is those distortions that represent reality for these individuals (Massion et al., 1993; Tyerman & Humphrey, 1984). It has also been argued that there are degrees and types of cognitive impairment that do not automatically preclude reliability of self-report (Awad, 1993; Lehman, 1983).

HOPE

Hastings (1992) made the point that "to inspire hope is an acknowledged part of nursing care. . . . Hope nurtures a person's transition from being weak and vulnerable to that of functioning or living as fully as possible." Miller (1992b) went so far as to say that "everything human beings do in life is based upon some level of hope" (p. 414). One of the profound challenges of neuroscience nursing is to help patients and families grapple with multiple and devastating challenges to hope—hope for recovery; hope for the future for oneself or one's child, partner, or friend; hope for continued meaning in life. Two spheres of hope can be distinguished: particularized hope and generalized hope. Particularized hope is anticipation of achieving a specific desired goal (e.g., walking unaided), whereas generalized hope refers to a sense that life is worthwhile. This latter form of hope is closely related to the concept of quality of life.

SELF-CONCEPT

Self-concept has to do with the self, being human, the whole person. Self-concept is affected by developmental and situational stressors, as discussed in Chapter 19. As neuroscience nurses, we are usually acutely aware of the situational stressors that sudden or chronic neurologic dysfunction precipitates. However, the patient population with whom we work usually represents a broader mix of ages than is the case for other specialties. It is, therefore, important that we continually consider how the impact of neurologic dysfunction may be interacting with developmental evolution and modifications to self-concept. Probably the most frequent example is that of the brain-injured adolescent. As Worthington (1989) pointed out, "Nurses are in a unique position to observe the conflicts of adolescent development as the patient progresses through recovery." The abrupt disruption of brain injury, set against the often-turbulent adolescent struggle for increasing independence, may be one of the major stressors for families as well as for patients. But are we as sensitive to the premature aging in appearance associated with Parkinson's disease? What meaning does that have for individuals?

Acute stressors on self-concept are more easily recognized than are chronic ones, particularly to the individuals most involved—patients and their families. Charmaz (1983) identified four threats to self-perception through the experience of chronic illness: living a restricted lifestyle, existing in social isolation, experiencing discredited definitions of self, and becoming a burden. As Miller (1992a) pointed out, "Personal worth is needed for all individuals, sick or well" (p. 410). Integration of an altered self does not have to mean integration of a devalued self. However, the challenge of helping patients through this process is one of the major challenges of neuroscience nursing.

"Neversameness"

Rice (1992) captured the sense of irrevocable change in the powerful description of his own experience with "neversameness." The sequela of mild head injury has been acknowledged for the major disruption it can cause in human functioning. With that recognition has come increasing awareness of how sequelae such as slower information processing, decreased concentration, and reduced ability to attend to two things at once demand more attention and effort on the part of the individual. Benner and Wrubel (1989) referred to a "state of chronic effort" (p. 319). To the individual, the injury may be minor, something that should take no more than a few days to get over. Social and work contacts may not even be aware of the injury and thus reinforce the expectation that nothing has really changed. However, the individual may be noticing that it seems to take more effort to perform at preinjury levels and that the taken-for-granted body is no longer responding with the usual ease. Teaching injured persons and family members that normal responses to the physiologic damage of concussion may include decreased concentration, some loss of memory, sleep disturbances, distractability, and irritability has been shown to improve family coping and to facilitate earlier return to social and work activities (Hinkle, Alves, Rimell, & Jane, 1986; Mahon & Elger, 1989; Sanguinetti & Catanzaro, 1987).

Reintegration and Social Interaction

Social interaction is a major forum for the reintegration of the new self. Most neurologic dysfunctions potentially affect the frequency and nature of social interaction. Some of these differences may seem minor, except to the persons involved. For example, what does loss of customary height mean to the wheelchair-bound individual as he or she interacts with someone who is standing up or sings as part of a choir?

The ability to communicate is a major factor in social interaction. The difficulties associated with dysphasia after stroke are relatively well recognized. However, there are other, more subtle, forms of altered communication associated with most types of neurologic dysfunction (for impact of altered mobility, see Chapter 20). From speech therapy and psychiatry come increasing recognition of the effects of more subtle deficits on linguistic processing and comprehension (Butler-Hinz, Caplan, & Waters, 1990; Gouvier, Coon, Fuller, & Arnoldi,

1992; Liles, Coelho, Duffy, & Zalagens, 1989; Penn et al., 1993; Sarno, Buonaguro, & Levita, 1986). For further discussion, see Chapters 14 and 15.

An interest in impaired nonverbal communication was stimulated by a 5-year-old's comment, "Grandpa doesn't smile anymore" (Reimer, 1993). To the family, this 74-year-old grandfather with advanced Parkinson's disease had always been seen as a man who loved to laugh and joke. It took a 5-year-old to point out the change—to the family who was taking him for granted as he had been and to the home care nurse who was taking him for granted as he now appeared, not recognizing the personality now trapped within the rigidity and masklike face of parkinsonism.

The symbolic interactionist perspective has framed numerous investigations into the effect of illness on self-concept (Bogdan & Taylor, 1989; Charmaz, 1983). From that perspective, the sense of self is developed, maintained, and modified through social relations. Thus, from that perspective, reintegration of a new, equally valued self is largely dependent on a supportive, normalizing environment. Unfortunately, our focus as professional caregivers on helping patients to cope with disease and disability reinforces a tendency for the disease or disability to become a major component of the new identity. Creating a different identifier for the person can be a helpful intervention. For example, a previously brain-injured young man was chosen to be known as the "fellow with the funny cap" rather than be recognized by friends for his slightly ataxic gait.

The Taken-for-Granted Body

The concept of the "taken-for-granted body" has particular relevance to neuroscience nursing (Benner & Wrubel, 1989). It is the taken-for-granted body that is an integrated, smoothly functioning unit. With disruption, the taken-for-granted body begins to demand attention. The presenting symptom may be the pain of trigeminal neuralgia. But for the person experiencing the pain, the previously integrated functions of chewing, talking, concentration, and so on are disrupted. It is the integrated whole that is disrupted; it is not just the symptom of pain nor the impairment of one specific function (e.g., chewing). The whole person responds to this disruption. As Frank (1991), a sociologist, said in describing his own illness experiences, "What happens when my body breaks down happens not just to that body but also to my life, which is lived in that body" (p. 8).

Risk Taking and Injury Prevention

The concept of the taken-for-granted body can also be useful in considering prevention of neurologic trauma. Developmentally, the taken-for-grantedness of life and health, of being invincible to injury, often lasts into the middle years of adulthood. Likewise, individuals vary widely in their attitudes to risk taking (Mawson, Jacobs, Winchester, & Biundo, 1988; Zucherman, 1990).

A psychologic model representing the concept of danger in human activity is useful to consider in this context (Apter, 1992). The model, based on reversal theory, depicts three parallel zones of variable width: the safety zone, the danger zone, and the trauma zone (Fig. 34–1). The boundaries of these zones are entirely subjective and may apply to anything from a conversation with one's partner to mountain climbing. *Safety zone* means the state in which there is little awareness or concern about danger. The *danger zone* involves awareness that the situation could escalate into what would be traumatic for the individual. The *dangerous edge* is the boundary between the danger zone and the *trauma zone*. Foundational to the model is the understanding that it can be applied in almost any context. For example, some conversations can approach the dangerous edge of physical assault or emotional trauma just as a false step can lead to a major fall.

Physiologic variations in preferred level of arousal have been described by numerous investigators (Lipowski, 1975; Zucherman, 1990). Apter (1992) took these observations one step further by proposing that these differences are not only biochemical but also states of mind. The relevance of these differences can be seen in such daily activities as preferred sound level in listening to music, degree of darkness preferred for sleeping, and so on. Risk-taking behavior involves the seeking of an increased level of arousal—excitement. In activities that are perceived as exciting (in contrast to those that arouse feelings of anxiety and avoidance), Apter (1992) hypothesized the existence of a protective frame just inside the dangerous edge (i.e., the boundary between the danger zone and the trauma zone). In situations that are perceived as anxiety inducing rather than exciting, there is no sense of a protective frame; even approaching the dangerous edge is feared. However, when the individual is in the excitement-seeking state of mind, the assumptions ''Nothing can happen to

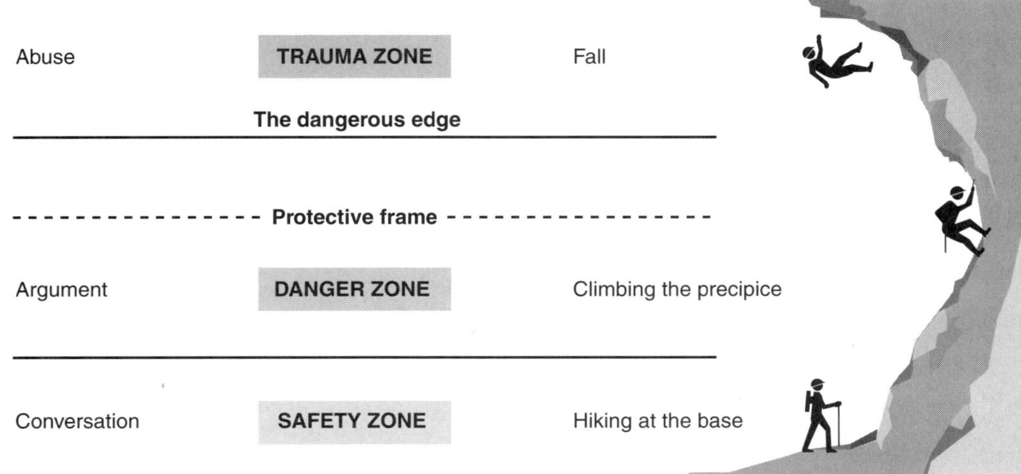

FIGURE 34–1 • Flirting with danger: excitement or anxiety?

me" and "I can handle it" are predominant. Indeed, the closer to the dangerous edge, the higher and more satisfying the arousal, the state of excitement.

Excitement seeking varies among people and within the same person, over time and in different contexts. A detailed discussion of the biologic and environmental factors influencing excitement seeking is beyond the scope of this chapter. However, the implications have become an important area of research for neuroscience nurses involved in trauma-risk–reduction programs.

SUMMARY

The sense of being is intricately linked with the functioning of the nervous system. Neuroscience nursing is intricately linked with helping patients and families cope with threats to their sense of self. Throughout this chapter, the reader has been encouraged to reflect on patient encounters in which humanness has been threatened. As neuroscience nurses, we have learned to be sensitive to the subtle cues of awareness of environment and self. Our interventions are directed to preserving quantity and quality of life. We experience the struggle of supporting hope. Perhaps we have given less thought to the part we play in integration of the changed self. We must ask ourselves whether our interaction with patients is supportive of reintegration of a new, equally valued, self or whether it reinforces a new identity as a damaged, diseased self.

References

American Association of Neuroscience Nurses. (1994). Scope of practice statement. *Journal of Neuroscience Nursing, 26*(1), 47.

Apter, M. J. (1992). *The dangerous edge: The psychology of excitement.* New York: The Free Press.

Awad, A. G. (1993). Methodological and design issues in clinical trials of new neuroleptics: An overview. *British Journal of Psychiatry, 163*(S22), 51–57.

Benner, P., & Wrubel, J. (1989). *The primacy of caring: Stress and coping in health and illness.* Reading, MA: Addison-Wesley.

Bergner, M. (1989). Quality of life, health status and clinical research. *Medical Care, 27*(3), S148–S156.

Bergner, M., Bobbitt, R. A., Carter, W. B., & Gilson, B. S. (1981). The sickness impact profile: Development and final revision of a health status measure. *Medical Care, 19,* 787–805.

Bogdan, R., & Taylor, S. J. (1989). Relationships with severely disabled people: The social construction of humanness. *Social Problems, 36*(20), 135–148.

Boss, B. (1994). Coma and cognitive deficits. In E. Barber (Ed.), *Neuroscience nursing* (pp. 175–202). St. Louis: Mosby–Year Book.

Brown, R. I., Bayer, M. B., & MacFarlane, C. (1989). *Rehabilitation programmes: Performance and quality of life of adults with developmental handicaps.* Toronto, ON: Lugus Publications.

Butler-Hinz, S., Caplan, D., & Waters, G. (1990). Characteristics of syntactic comprehension deficits following closed head injury versus left cerebrovascular accident. *Journal of Speech and Hearing Research, 33,* 269–280.

Cassell, E. J. (1991). *The nature of suffering and the goals of medicine.* Don Mills, ON: Oxford University Press.

Charmaz, K. (1983). Loss of self: A fundamental form of suffering in the chronically ill. *Sociology of Health and Illness, 5*(2), 168–195.

Council for International Organizations of Medical Sciences. (1991). *International guidelines for ethical review of epidemiological studies.* Geneva, Switzerland: Author.

Canadian Nurses Association. (1990). *Neuroscience nursing certification examination blueprint*. Ottawa, ON: Author.

Cohen, S. R., & Mount, B. M. (1992). Quality of life in terminal illness: Defining and measuring subjective well-being of the dying. *Journal of Palliative Care, 8*(3), 40–45.

Faden, R., & LePlege, A. (1992). Assessing quality of life: Moral implications for clinical practice. *Medical Care, 30*(5S), MS166–MS175.

Frank, A. (1991). *At the will of the body*. New York: Houghton Mifflin.

Gouvier, W. D., Coon, R. C., Fuller, K. H., & Arnoldi, K. R. (1992). Evaluation of linguistic variations by college students with and without head injuries. *Rehabilitation Psychology, 37*(3), 165–174.

Harrison, C. (1993). Personhood, dementia and the integrity of life. *Canadian Journal of Aging, 12*(4), 428–440.

Hartshorn, J. C., & Byers, V. L. (1994). Importance of health and family variables related to quality of life in individuals with uncontrolled seizures. *Journal of Neuroscience Nursing, 26*(5), 288–297.

Hastings, D. (1992). Adjustment, coping resources and care of the patient with multiple sclerosis. In J. F. Miller (Ed.), *Coping with chronic illness: Overcoming powerlessness* (2nd ed., pp. 222–254). Philadelphia: F. A. Davis.

Hinkle, J. L., Alves, W. M., Rimell, R. W., & Jane, J. A. (1986). Restoring social competence in minor head-injury patients. *Journal of Neuroscience Nursing 18*(5), 268–271.

Hungelmann, J., Kenkel-Rossi, E., Klassen, L., & Stollenwerk, R. (1989). Development of the *JAREL Spiritual Well-Being Scale*. In R. M. Carroll-Johnson (Ed.), *Classification of nursing diagnoses. Proceedings of the eighth conference* (pp. 393–398). Philadelphia: J. B. Lippincott.

Hunt, S. M., & McKenna, S. P. (1993). Measuring quality of life in psychiatry. In S. R. Walker & R. M. Rosser (Eds.), *Quality of life assessment: Key issues in the 1990s* (pp. 343–354). Norwell, GBR: Kluwer Academic Publishers.

Kinsella, G., Moran, C., Ford, B., & Ponsford, J. (1988). Emotional disorder and its assessment within the severe head injured population. *Psychological Medicine, 18*, 57–63.

Lehman, A. F. (1983). The well-being of chronic mental patients: Assessing their quality of life. *Archives of General Psychiatry, 40*, 369–373.

Lehman, A. F., Possidente, S., & Hawker, F. (1986). The quality of life of chronic patients in a state hospital and community residences. *Hospital and Community Psychiatry, 37*(9), 901–907.

Liles, B. Z., Coelho, C. A., Duffy, R. J., & Zalagens, M. R. (1989). Effects of elicitation procedures on the narratives of normal and closed head-injured adults. *Journal of Speech and Hearing Disorders, 54*, 356–366.

Lipowski, Z. (1975). Sensory and information inputs overload: Behavioral effects. *Comprehensive Psychiatry, 16ff*(3), 199–219.

Mahon, D., & Elger, C. (1989). Analysis of posttraumatic syndrome following mild head injury. *Journal of Neuroscience Nursing, 21*(6), 382–384.

Massion, A. O., Warshaw, M. G., & Keller, M. B. (1993). Quality of life and psychiatric morbidity in panic disorder and generalized anxiety disorder. *American Journal of Psychiatry, 150*(4), 600–607.

Mawson, A. R., Jacobs, K. W., Winchester, Y., & Biundo, J. J., Jr. (1988). Sensation-seeking and traumatic spinal cord injury: Case-control study. *Archives of Physical Medicine and Rehabilitation, 69*, 1039–1043.

McDowell, I., & Newell, G. (1996). *Measuring health: A guide to rating scales and questionnaires* (2nd ed.). Wolfe City, TX: University Press.

Miller, J. F. (1992a). Enhancing self-esteem. In J. F. Miller (Ed.), *Coping with chronic illness: Overcoming powerlessness* (2nd ed., 397–412). Philadelphia: F. A. Davis.

Miller, J. F. (1992b). Inspiring hope. In J. F. Miller (Ed.), *Coping with chronic illness: Overcoming powerlessness* (2nd ed., 413–433). Philadelphia: F. A. Davis.

Morse, J. M., & Johnson, J. L. (1991). *The illness experience*. Thousand Oaks, CA: Sage Publications.

Muir, C. A., & Haffey, W. J. (1984). Psychological and neuropsychological interventions in the mobile mourning process. In B. A. Edelstein & E. T. Couture (Eds.), *Behavioral assessment and rehabilitation of the traumatically brain damaged* (pp. 247–271). New York: Plenum Press.

Paul, M., & Littlejohns, L. R. (1994). Coma recollections. *Journal of Neuroscience Nursing, 26*(5), 319–322.

Penn, D. L., Van Der Does, A. J., Spaulding, W. D., Garbin, C. P., Linszen, D., & Dingemans, P. (1993). Information processing and social cognitive problem solving in schizophrenia: Assessment of interrelationships and changes over time. *Journal of Nervous and Mental Disease, 181*(1), 13–20.

Prigatano, G. P. (1992). Neuropsychological rehabilitation and the problem of altered self-awareness. In N. von Steinbuchel, D. Y. von Cramon, & E. Poppel (Eds.), *Neuropsychological rehabilitation* (pp. 55–65). New York: Springer-Verlag.

Prigatano, G. P. (1994, June 10). *A neuropsychologically oriented rehabilitation program following traumatic brain injury: Philosophy, treatment procedures and outcome data.* Paper presented at the Brain Injury Symposium, Alberta Hospital, Ponoka, Canada.

Prigatano, G. P., & Schacter, D. L. (1991). Introduction. In G. P. Prigatano & D. L. Schacter (Eds.), *Awareness of deficit after brain injury: Clinical and theoretical issues* (pp. 3–16). Don Mills, ON: Oxford University Press.

Reimer, M. (1993). Impaired non-verbal communication: A photo investigation. In R. Carroll-Johnson (Ed.), *Nursing diagnosis: Proceedings of the tenth conference.* Philadelphia: J. B. Lippincott.

Reinsmith, W. A. (1989). Finality of death: The underlying issue. *Humane Medicine, 5,* 31–36.

Rice, M. J. (1992). Minor head injury: Is anybody listening? *Journal of Neuroscience Nursing, 24*(3), 173–175.

Romney, D. M., Jenkins, C. D., & Bynner, J. M. (1992). A structural analysis of health-related quality of life dimensions. *Human Relations, 45*(2), 165–176.

Ron, M. A., & Feinstein, A. (1992). Multiple sclerosis and the mind. *Journal of Neurology, Neurosurgery and Psychiatry, 55,* 1–3.

Sachs, P. R. (1984). Grief and the traumatically head-injured adult. *Rehabilitative Nursing, 9*(1), 23–27.

Sacks, O. (1987). *The man who mistook his wife for a hat and other clinical tales.* New York: Harper Collins.

Sanguinetti, M., & Catanzaro, M. (1987). Comparison of discharge teaching on the consequences of brain injury. *Journal of Neuroscience Nursing, 19*(5), 271–275.

Sarno, M. T., Buonaguro, A., & Levita E. (1986). Characteristics of verbal impairment in closed head injured patients. *Archives of Physical Medicine and Rehabilitation, 67,* 400–405.

Schipper, H., Clinch, J., & Powell, V. (1990). Definitions and conceptual issues. In B. Spilker (Ed.), *Quality of life assessments in clinical trials* (pp. 11–14). Fort Collins, CO: Raven Press.

Sheehan, M. N. (1992). Persons with Alzheimer's disease and health care rationing. *Journal of Geriatric Psychiatry, 25*(2), 195–210.

Shindler, J. S., Brown, R., Welburn, P., & Parkes, J. D. (1993). Measuring quality of life of patients with Parkinson's disease. In S. R. Walker & R. M. Rosser (Eds.), *Quality of life assessment: Key issues in the 1990s* (pp. 289–300). Norwell, GBR: Kluwer Academic Publishers.

Spitzer, W. O. (1987). State of science 1986: Quality of life and functional status as target variables for research. *Journal of Chronic Disease, 40*(16), 465–471.

Stewart, A. L. (1992). Conceptual and methodological issues in defining quality of life: State of the art. *Progressive Cardiovascular Nursing, 7*(1), 3–11.

Tempkin, N. R., Dikmen, S., Machamer, J., & McLean, A. (1989). General versus disease-specific measures: Further work on the Sickness Impact Profile for head injury. *Medical Care, 27*(3S), S44–SJ53.

Tompkins, C. A., Jackson, S. T., & Schulz, R. (1990). On prognostic research in adult neurologic disorders. *Journal of Speech, Language, and Hearing Research, 33,* 398–401.

Tosch, P. (1988). Patient's recollections of their posttraumatic coma. *Journal of Neuroscience Nursing, 20*(4), 223–228.

Tyerman, A., & Humphrey, M. (1984). Changes in self-concept following severe head injury. *International Journal of Rehabilitation Research, 7*(1), 11–23.

Ware, J. E. (1986). The assessment of health status. In L. H. Aiken & D. Mechanic (Eds.), *Application of social science medicine and health policy* (pp. 204–227). Piscataway, NJ: Rutgers University Press.

Ware, J. E. (1987). Standards for validating health measures: Definition and content. *Journal of Chronic Disease, 40*(6), 473–480.

Webster's new world dictionary (2nd college ed.) (1979). Cleveland, Ohio: William Collins.

Worthington, J. (1989). The impact of adolescent development on recovery from traumatic brain injury. *Rehabilitation Nursing, 14*(13), 118–122.

Wyness, A. (1987, June). Patient and family education: A key component of neuroscience nursing. *Axon:* 95–98.

Zucherman, M. (1990). The psychobiology of sensation seeking. *Journal of Personality, 58*(1), 313–345.

Index

Note: Page numbers in *italics* refer to illustrations; page numbers followed by t refer to tables.

ISBN 0-7216-2288-7